Consumer-Driven Health Care

Consumer-Driven Health Care

Implications for Providers, Payers, and Policymakers

Regina E. Herzlinger

Editor

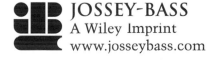

JOSSEY-BASS
A Wiley Imprint
www.josseybass.com

Published by Jossey-Bass
A Wiley Imprint
989 Market Street, San Francisco, CA 94103-1741   www.josseybass.com

Jossey-Bass books and products are available through most bookstores. To
contact Jossey-Bass directly call our Customer Care Department within the U.S.
at 800-956-7739, outside the U.S. at 317-572-399386 or fax 317-572-4002.

Jossey-Bass also publishes its books in a variety of electronic formats. Some
content that appears in print may not be available in electronic books.

Library of Congress Cataloging-in-Publication Data
Consumer-driven health care: implications for providers, payers, and
policymakers / [edited by] Regina E. Herzlinger.
p. ; cm. Includes bibliographical references and index
ISBN 0-7879-5258-3 (alk. paper)
1. Health planning—Citizen participation. 2. Patient satisfaction—Evaluation
3. Consumer Satisfaction 4. Medical Care—Evaluation.
5. Medical economics. 6. Consumer protection
[DNLM: 1. Consumer Participation. 2. Delivery of Health Care—economics
3. Delivery of Health Care—organization & administration. 4. Health Care Costs.
5. Insurance, Health.   W 84.1 C7584 2004] Herzlinger, Regina E.
RA394.C685 2004
362.1'068-dc22
2003026854

Printed in the United States of America
FIRST EDITION
HB Printing 10 9 8 7 6 5 4 3

To George Herzlinger, my husband—
My life partner and best friend
and
Ella and Alexander Elbinger, my parents—
Whose iconoclasm and optimism, in the face of
overwhelming opposition, inspired me

CONTENTS

Preface   xvii

Introduction   xix

PART ONE: WHY WE NEED CONSUMER-DRIVEN HEALTH CARE   1

1 Fear and Loathing of Defined Benefit Health Insurance   3

2 The Frayed Safety Net   28

3 The Solution   57

4 Consumer-Driven Health Insurance: What Works   74

5 Health Care Productivity   102

6 The Silent Revolution   127

7 Scare Stories, Opponents, and the Role of Government   153

8 How to Make Consumer-Driven Health Care Happen   195

PART TWO: VISION AND MODELS 199

9 The Future of Twenty-First Century Health 203
William W. George

10 How Employers Can Make Consumer-Driven Health Care a Reality 213
Brian J. Marcotte

11 Designing Health Insurance for the Information Age 224
John C. Goodman

12 Risk Adjustment: An Overview and Three Case Studies 242
Lisa I. Iezzoni

13 Consumer-Driven Health Care: Dialogues with Socrates 262
Stephen S. Hyde

14 Employee Tax Payments and Consumer-Driven Health Care 270
Jeanne A. Brown

15 The Implications of Tax Rulings on "Savings Accounts" 279
Charles H. Klippel

16 You Just Can't Pay Tom, Juan, and Ashley the Old Way Anymore 284
Bonnie B. Whyte

17 The Federal Employees Health Benefits Program 291
James W. Morrison Jr.

18 Health-Based Premium Payments and Consumer
Assessment Information 298
*Vicki M. Wilson, Jenny M. Hamilton, Mary K. Uyeda,
Cynthia A. Smith, with Graydon M. Clouse*

19 The Buyers Health Care Action Group:
Creating Incentives to Seek the Sick 309
Ann L. Robinow

20 An Insurance CEO's Perspective on Consumer-Driven Health Care 317
Leonard D. Schaeffer

21 An Alternative to Managed Care: A European
Perspective on Informed Choice 322
Bruno L. Holthof

22 Medical Savings Accounts and Health Care
Financing in South Africa 330
Shaun Matisonn

23 European Health Care: The Cost of Solidarity and the Promise of
    Risk-Adjusted Consumer-Driven Health Care   338
    Paul Belien

24 Consumer-Driven Health Care: An International View   362
    Alvaro Salas-Chaves

25 Challenges of Consumer-Driven Health Care   368
    Eugene D. Hill III

26 Making the Transition to Consumer-Driven Health Care   371
    Jesse S. Hixson

27 The New Consumer-Driven Health Care System   373
    Daniel H. Johnson

28 The Patient's Right to Decide   376
    Warner V. Slack

29 Comments on Consumer-Driven Health Care   380
    Corbette S. Doyle

30 The Evolution of Consumer-Driven Health Care   384
    Robert W. Coburn

31 Will Consumer-Driven Health Care Work for Employers?   391
    John C. Erb

32 The Perspective of an Advocate for the Elderly   394
    John Rother

PART THREE: THE NEW INTERMEDIARIES   399

33 Where Will Consumer-Driven Health Care Take
    the Health Care System?   403
    Bernard T. Ferrari

34 The Role of Information: J. D. Power's Paradigm Lessons
    from the Automotive Industry   410
    J. D. Power III

35 Providing Information to Consumers   419
    David Lansky

36 Consumer-Driven Health Care and the Internet   428
    Mark A. Pearl

37 The Present and Future Roles of Information in a
   Consumer-Driven Health System   440
   Russell Ricci

38 Who Has Star Quality?   443
   Jon A. Chilingerian

39 Grounding Consumer-Driven Health Care
   in Social Science Research   454
   Arnold Milstein, Nancy E. Adler

40 Providing the Most-Wanted Information When Most Needed:
   Best Doctors   458
   Steven W. Naifeh, Gregory White Smith

41 The Half-Billion Dollar Impact of Information About Quality   467
   Becky J. Cherney

42 Buyers Health Care Action Group: Consumer Perceptions
   of Quality Differences   475
   Katherine M. Harris, Roger Feldman, Jennifer S. Schultz, Jon Christianson

43 Helping Consumers Choose Among Complex Insurance Plans   487
   Colleen M. Murphy

44 CareCounsel: Consumer-Driven Health Care Advocacy   490
   Lawrence N. Gelb

45 Access Health Group: A Medical Management Perspective   501
   Joseph P. Tallman

46 Consumer's Medical Resource: Helping Consumers Evaluate Medical
   Treatment Options   510
   David J. Hines

47 The Cost Effectiveness of Consumer-Driven Lifestyle Changes in the
   Treatment of Cardiac Disease   516
   Dean Ornish

48 Healthtrac: Proven Reduction of the Need and Demand
   for Medical Services   523
   James F. Fries

49 The Healthwise® Approach: Reinventing the Patient   532
   Donald W. Kemper, Molly Mettler

PART FOUR: INNOVATIVE CONSUMER-DRIVEN SOLUTIONS TO CHRONIC PROBLEMS 543

50 The Role of Providers   549
Michael L. Millenson

51 A Disease Management Approach to Chronic Illness   561
Jessie C. Gruman, Cynthia M. Gibson

52 Consumer-Driven Health Care: Management Matters   570
Richard M. J. Bohmer, Amy C. Edmondson, Gary P. Pisano

53 Consumer-Driven Health Care for the Chronically Ill   589
Al Lewis

54 A Cost-Effective Model for High-Quality Catastrophic Care   595
Bernard Salick, Seth M. Yellin

55 Collaborating with Consumers to Advance Health Knowledge and Improve Practice   602
S. Robert Levine, Laura L. Adams

56 Package Pricing at the Texas Heart Institute   612
Denton A. Cooley, John W. Adams Jr.

57 Helping Patients Manage Their Asthma: The National Jewish Approach   619
Lynn M. Taussig, David Tinkelman

58 A Model of Focused Health Care Delivery: Shouldice Hospital   627
Daryl J. B. Urquhart, Alan O'Dell

59 Chronic Problems, Innovative Solutions: Paving the Way to the Focused Factory   635
Stuart Lovett

60 Improving Health and Reducing the Costs of Chronic Diseases   643
Robert E. Stone

61 The Impact of Horizontal Integration in Hospitals: HCA Healthcare Corporation   651
Thomas F. Frist Jr.

62 An Innovative Approach to Population Health: Kaiser Permanente Southern California   661
Les Zendle

63 The Right Care: Vanderbilt Medical Center 669
Harry R. Jacobson

64 Achieving Focus in Hospital Care: The Role
of Relational Coordination 683
Jody Hoffer Gittell

65 Consumer-Driven Health Care Is a Message of Hope 696
James F. Rodgers

66 An Academic Health Center Perspective 699
Roger J. Bulger

67 Consumer Choice in Consumer-Driven Health Care 703
François Maisonrouge

68 Individual Genetic Profiles: The Empowerment of
the Health Care Consumer 707
Tony L. White

69 Delivering the Right Drug to the Right Patient 716
Mark Levin

PART FIVE: THE ROLE OF GOVERNMENT 727

70 The Uninsured: Understanding and Resolving
an American Dilemma 731
Jon R. Gabel

71 A Health Insurance Tax Credit: The Key to More
Coverage and Choice for Consumers 749
David B. Kendall

72 The Politics of Consumer-Driven Health Care 764
Eric S. Berger, Carrie Gavora, Daniel H. Johnson

73 Health Care: What Role for Regulation? 774
Karen Ignagni

74 Adult Health Insurance 779
Ken Abramowitz

75 AmeriChoice Corporation: The Personal Care Model 781
Anthony Welters

76 The Uninsured and Access 789
Constance G. Jackson

77 Consumer-Driven Health Care for the Uninsured   794
    Kevin Vigilante

78 A Health Care SEC: The Truth, The Whole Truth,
    and Nothing But the Truth   797
    Regina E. Herzlinger

79 Keep 'Em Honest: The Health Care SEC   811
    Robert N. Shamansky

80 The U.S. Needs a Consumer-Driven Medical Care System   816
    Rita Ricardo-Campbell

81 Government's New Roles in the Era of
    Consumer-Driven Health Care   820
    Richard A. D'Amaro

The Editor   829

The Participants   831

The Contributors   833

Name Index   841

Subject Index   857

PREFACE

Consumer-driven health care is fundamentally about empowering health care consumers—all of us—with control, choice, and information. Consumer control will reward innovative insurers and providers for creating the higher-quality, lower-cost services we want and deserve. In this consumer-driven system, government will protect us with financial assistance and oversight, not micromanagement.

In these ways consumer-driven health care is a revolution—a radical turn away from the technocratic, top-down policies that just say no to providers and consumers both in the United States and abroad.

This book explains how consumer-driven health care works.

The eight chapters in Part One of this book, which I wrote, explain the theory and workings of consumer-driven health care. Parts Two through Five amplify these themes in chapters written by some of the leaders who will make this vast transformation work. Throughout this book the chapters describe the shortcomings of our present third-party health insurance system, delineate the desired characteristics of a consumer-driven health care insurance system, and assess the impact of the consumer-driven system in some early adopter organizations. They also explain how consumer-driven health insurance will increase the productivity of the health care system, and describe the innovations created by the insurance, provider, technology, and government entrepreneurs who have already begun to craft the essential ingredients of this insurance.

In the last chapters of Part One, I rebut those critics of consumer-driven health care who aver that it will fail to control costs, injure the sick, increase disparities in access, confuse the consumer, and focus on the role of government in overseeing and enabling a consumer-driven health care system.

To your health!

February 2004

Regina E. Herzlinger
Boston, Massachusetts

INTRODUCTION

This book is about consumer-driven health care—the why and the how of enabling people to obtain the health care they want at a price they are willing to pay. The American public supports the idea of consumer-driven health care. When people ask me the title of my latest book, the almost invariable reaction to its name, *Consumer-Driven Health Care,* is, "Well, it's about time!" whether the person is the barista at the local Starbucks, a business executive, a cabdriver, or a doctor.

Like them, I favor the notion of consumer-driven health care.

ABOUT CONSUMER CONTROL

Indeed, I like the idea for all spheres of human endeavor. You see, I owe my academic career to consumer control.

Back in 1972, when I joined the Harvard Business School faculty, student evaluations of courses and instructors were coming into their own, one aspect of the revolution in higher education fashioned by the self-absorbed, self-actualizing baby boomers. Student evaluations are one form of consumer control, through which the customer holds providers accountable for the quality of their services. I viewed them as my savior.

Before the 1970s, prior to the counterculture revolution that asserted the students' pivotal role, higher education was controlled primarily by the faculty and staff. The students' role was to listen adoringly to the wisdom of their elders. An archival photograph, circa 1950, of a Radcliffe program for women interested in business administration exemplifies this role. It shows a lecturer, nattily attired in a bow tie and horn-rim glasses, standing on a pedestal surrounded by a sea of upturned, smiling, beatific women's faces.

In those days students had no evaluative voice. Peer review was the norm. I recall the baffling, lobotomizing lectures I endured at MIT and Harvard, my alma maters, that were mysteriously hailed as pedagogical miracles by the instructors' peer group. Irrelevant, pedantic harangues on Bayesian statistics, feathers falling in elevators, and the miracles that accompanied government "investments" were lauded as the equals of Warren Buffet's thoughts on finance or Crick and Watson's views on the future of genetics. Of course the instructors' peers loved the stuff—many of their lectures were dull and abstract too.

Yes, student evaluations existed even back then, but they were ignored. A standing joke at MIT was that the winner of the Best Teacher prize would never receive tenure. Like most comedy the joke was a callus that protected against the painful kernel of truth within. Students were bright, empty vessels to be filled by the teacher's erudition. Faculty who valued students' feedback were seriously flawed—clowns who catered to the masses. (Even today, student evaluations continue to be scorned. In 2002, the dean of faculty of Williams College said of a student-run faculty-rating Web site, "It is incredibly humiliating," denouncing it as part of the "troubling trends of consumerism" in higher education.[1])

I had no chance of success in a peer-reviewed academic institution. I was so different from my peers.

I believed in Jefferson: I sought feedback from all sources.

They believed in Hamilton: they sought feedback only from the elite.

And to top it all off, I was a woman in male-dominated academia. A professor who had consulted for me in the job I held prior to joining the Harvard Business School faculty spoke for others when he asked of my appointment, "Surely, they are not asking a woman to teach business?"

But the advent of serious student evaluations, driven by the relentlessly self-seeking 1970s' counterculture, changed my view of my career prospects. A consumer-centered system of accountability would give an out-of-the-mold person like me the chance to succeed—or to fail. A peer-led educational system would have consigned me to the trash heap.

Mind you, I did not know whether I would succeed as a teacher. Indeed, the thought of leading the one hundred–person, primarily male, Harvard Business School MBA sections, composed of people roughly my own age, filled me with dread. The school's famous case method is a very challenging teaching technique. A case is like real life. It is an open script. The learning process comes from the students' participation in analyzing and solving the issue it poses. Orchestrating the discussion is like herding cats. A case cannot be taught by dusting off last year's lecture notes. The case method demands deep preparation, immense concentration, quick response, and broad competence from all its participants. I worried that I was not up to the job.

But I loved my subjects, loved research, loved people, loved to write, loved to talk, loved to listen. Rightly or wrongly, an academic career seemed appropriate for me.

Then, too, I had benefited from accountability before. The New York State Regents examinations, administered to all the high school students in the state, and the national SAT exams, had convinced MIT that I was the equal of their other admits, although they had never before had an applicant from the small, women's parochial high school in which I was enrolled.

Gambling on my future, with a consumer-led accountability system as my sole support, I left a position in which I had the title of vice president, a large staff, and an even larger salary, and took a two-thirds cut in pay to become an assistant professor at the Harvard Business School, with a staff of one-third of one secretary.

My first student evaluations, from the participants in an executive health care program, were disastrous. But I learned from the feedback. To my own surprise, and that of my peers who believed that women could not teach business, the students' ratings of my teaching typically topped the charts in my area. In 1980, I became the first woman to earn tenure at the Harvard Business School (HBS).

Nearly thirty years after teaching my first class, I continue to learn from my students' feedback. Although I was elected one of HBS's two best instructors in an inaugural vote by first-year MBAs, I found some of my other students less enthusiastic about my efforts. My peers benefited from student feedback as well, even in an institution as dedicated to teaching as the Harvard Business School. Published evaluations of business schools in *U.S. News & World Report* helped all of us too.

Accountability has had similar effects on public schools in states that publish school performance ratings. Alabama's 750,000 public school students, for example, performed better on the Stanford Achievement Test in 1997 than in 1990, with fourth and eighth graders scoring higher than the national average in many subjects. The reason? "The only variable that changed statewide . . . was the implementation of a (public) ranking system," noted one official.[2]

When the consumer's voice was finally heard, it improved education.

Consumer control has improved other sectors as well. For example, a newly found focus on consumers' notions of quality has enabled U.S. manufacturers to succeed in the international businesses where they had once failed. Pressured by competition and the loss of the vast camera, watch, and color TV markets to high-quality, foreign competitors, manufacturers tossed out their old notion of quality—conformance to internal requirements—and supplanted it with quality measures that internalized their customers' preferences.[3]

Better quality reduced failures.

Reduced failures lowered costs.

But only when quality was defined from the consumers' perspective.

THE NEED FOR CONSUMER-DRIVEN HEALTH CARE

All of this is to clarify why I compiled this massive tome, *Consumer-Driven Health Care*. When consumers drive health care, it too will become better and cheaper.

Presently, health care systems are controlled by third parties who are neither consumers nor providers. In the United States, it is the employers and their human resource agents who select, price, and purchase health insurance policies and their insurance intermediaries. Many employees have a "choice" of only one policy. Even those who have a choice of more than one find all the policies depressingly similar, with features that are largely standardized. And most of the public sector payers, both here and abroad, offer no choice at all. They are monopolies.

The absence of health care information that can help consumers choose also hobbles their role. The little information that exists comes primarily from health policy experts residing in academia and think tanks; captive, industry-dominated accreditors; foundations; and lobbying groups, who advise the third-party payers and insurers. This information only rarely responds to consumer needs. To see their mind-set more clearly, review this bit of prose from a member of a self-styled health care "policy elite": "There is one foe confronting a policy elite that seeks universal entitlement—Americans. . . . National health insurance can be attained in America [only] if the policy elite imposes a solution that (the) . . . electorate has not attained." As for those who advocate consumer-driven health care, they are "an ideological fox in sheep's clothing."[4] (Apparently the policy elite's mastery does not extend to simple English.)

Thus, when I purchase a pair of eyeglasses in a consumer-controlled market, I can readily find many evaluations of the quality of different stores and price comparisons to inform my selection. But when I chose a physician to oversee the birth of my children, I had no information at all about the quality of his care or his price. Because the information that exists is only the little that is voluntarily disclosed, bad news can be hidden. For example, in 2002, low-quality health insurers were found to be much more likely to suppress quality disclosures about their performance than were higher-quality ones.[5]

The health care system is much like the old higher-education system—controlled by insiders, closed to consumers.

Do not get me wrong. Most of these people—bureaucrats, insurers, and technocrats—are like most of us: they do the best they can. They want to do good.

They do not want to do bad. But their perspective is upside-down. Rather than supporting consumer choice and control, they choose to supplant it. Their view is top-down, not bottom-up.

Thus it should come as no surprise that many of them oppose consumer-driven health care. In the fall of 2002, Blue Shield of California launched a first strike when it threatened the brokers who sell such products with termination: "There are some companies that are using high-deductible plans in the 2–50 (employee) market. . . . The employer, [sic] through the help of the company, purchases a high-deductible plan and then uses the savings to self-fund the actual benefits they want. Blue Shield of California does not endorse or encourage any type of these programs. . . . Any deviation from the broker responsibilities outlined . . . may result in termination of the Producer Agreement with Blue Shield."[6]

But in the absence of consumer-input, costs can run rampant, while consumers cannot obtain the health care they want. No wonder the productivity of health services has declined over the past two decades.[7]

Health care will not improve until consumers drive it.

This book, *Consumer-Driven Health Care,* describes how to make that happen. The new consumer-driven health insurance system will enable consumers to choose from a large array of differentiated health insurance options with the support of employers or other groups who will help to provide the pretax money to buy them. New intermediaries will supply enrollees with information and assistance so they can select intelligently among these options. Consumer-driven innovators will create newly productive, high-quality health care services and technology that respond to consumers' needs. And a newly consumer-driven government will oversee the suppliers and protect the consumers.

THE HISTORY OF CONSUMER-DRIVEN HEALTH CARE

I believe so strongly in consumer-driven health care, that I have been writing various versions of this book for more than twenty years. My first public advocacy for consumer-driven health care came in a 1979 *Harvard Business Review* article, "Can We Control Health Care Costs?"[8] I echoed the theme in a 1983 *Wall Street Journal* editorial,[9] which was followed by a series of mid-1980s' *Harvard Business Review* articles.[10] Although my work won research awards, it had the practical impact of a feather. To the contrary, by the late 1980s, the managed care plans then coming into vogue had turned away from consumer-driven health care. To me, they were a wrong turn—right into an abyss. Although they were marketed as "market-driven," in truth most of them were controlled by third-party technocrats rather than innovative providers intent on re-creating health care in a way responsive to consumers' needs for efficient, personalized services.

Virtually the sole exception was Kaiser Permanente, a well-established, California-based managed care organization with a deep-rooted, provider-driven culture. But most of the managed care plans were no Kaisers. They lacked its organizational structure, leadership, and culture. Then too, the Kaiser model was hardly a universal favorite. Busy, assertive Americans have so disliked its stringent requirements that limit care to Kaiser-affiliated physicians and hospitals that the market share of this type of HMO plummeted from 40 percent of enrollees in 1993 to 18 percent in 1998,[11] and some, including its own nurses and government officials, grew concerned about the quality of its care.[12] The model was also ferociously expensive to set up, requiring massive up-front outlays for financing the physician groups and hospitals exclusively devoted to the insurance plan.

In lieu of following Kaiser's costly model, most managed care plans cobbled together a network of independent providers who reluctantly accepted low payments and "gatekeeper" oversight in exchange for the custom of the patients enrolled with the plan. As a gatekeeper, a provider had to obtain approval for many patient referrals from an insurance executive.

Managed care as market driven?

What an odd idea.

Market-driven solutions rely on interaction between supply and demand, customers and providers. But with managed care, a third party, a technocrat, controlled all the action. To most Americans, this version of managed care had the cold, hard heart of an underripe cheese.

A technocrat's notion of managing care is to reduce payments to hospitals and doctors and to wean consumers away from wasteful, expensive specialists. Most managed care organizations did not seek to re-create the way health care is delivered through competition among different services for the consumers' custom. Noted an expert 2002 analysis, "Most (but not all) HMOs have not accomplished what their proponents had promised: changing clinical practice processes and improving quality of care relative to the existing system."[13]

To the contrary, the founders of the managed care movement wanted to standardize insurance products.[14] Their version of managed care inhibited innovation. Instead of fostering change, it controlled costs with "just-say-no" policies—no to enrollee requests for referrals to specialists and hospitals and no to providers' price schedules.[15] In 1999, for example, 72 percent of physicians with managed care contracts were financially rewarded for productivity by the insurers and only 24 percent were rewarded for patient satisfaction.[16] Of course, many of the no's were justified, to redirect inappropriate, extravagantly priced care, but they were not consumer driven. (Chapter Two analyzes managed care's impact on costs.)

It did not take long for this version of managed care to unravel.

Following the principles of Economics 101, fragmented providers who felt bullied by large buyers combined into groups whose united front could effectively counter managed care's demands for discounts. In Boston, for example, the 1993 "partnership" of the world-famous Massachusetts General Hospital with the Brigham and Women's Hospital created a Goliath that employed more than 4,000 of the area's doctors and 2,500 of its registered nurses.[17] When a health care plan demanded discounts from this renowned institution, guess who blinked first?[18] Meanwhile, consumers, frustrated with gatekeeper hurdles, placed massive pressure on their employers to loosen access to the health care providers they wanted.

Today, these managed care policies are so widely deplored that they have become the stuff of political humor. For example, one Web site posted a satirical article that began:

New HMO Strategy: Pay Health Claims
Analysts Skeptical; Doubt Insurers Equipped to Handle Job
Minneapolis, Minn. (SatireWire.com)—Moving into what insurance executives concede is "uncharted territory," five of the nation's leading HMOs announced yesterday they will begin paying health insurance claims for sick and injured people.[19]

Plans that provide easier access to specialists and hospitals now dominate.[20] Yet even when their just-say-no strategy was coming apart at the seams, some managed care executives retained much of the expensive gatekeeper infrastructure—and their organizations' administrative costs significantly exceeded those of loosely managed plans.[21] This time around, the executives promise to control costs by actually managing care, especially for the victims of chronic diseases and disabilities, rather than just saying no.

Yet this new version of managed care is unlikely to reverse upward cost trends. Sure, it is the right idea, because most health care costs are incurred by people who suffer from chronic diseases and whose care is mismanaged.[22] But insurers are unlikely agents of change. Ostrichlike executives moan and groan about providers' "low compliance" with insurers' care management advice, mysteriously baffled by the reluctance of independent professionals who are legally liable for the quality of care to "comply" with the strictures of health insurance officials who not so long ago made these professionals' lives a misery.[23]

Indeed, the fundamental premise of a top-down strategy that asks an insurer to re-create how hundreds of thousands of independent physicians, multibillion-dollar medical technology firms, and thousands of hospitals deliver medical care to millions of people is dubious. It is as questionable as a premise that automobile insurers could rescue the automobile industry by telling manufacturers how to make better, cheaper cars.

Productivity gains arise primarily from innovations in production, not from saying no. Entrepreneurs, not technocrats, create the innovations that increase productivity. We celebrate Thomas Edison, Henry Ford, and Sam Walton because they transformed how energy was used, cars were manufactured, and goods were sold. We do not celebrate them because they muscled down their suppliers' prices and barred consumers from needed goods.

Nevertheless, the health care policy world was delirious about the happy prospects of managed care. After all, it put policymakers' technocratic skills of evaluating people and things front and center. A 1984 article in the prestigious *New England Journal of Medicine* presented the Twin Cities in Minnesota, whose insurance markets were heavily penetrated by HMOs, as a national model. "The Twin Cities system is as good an example of health-care reform—American style—as one can find."[24] Even politicians as astute as former U.S. president William Clinton and his wife, Hillary Rodham Clinton, swallowed the bait. It was a costly mistake. They failed to achieve their laudable aim of universal insurance, in large part because they chose managed care as the centerpiece of their health care reform plans.[25]

Bucking the tide, I predicted the downfall of managed care in a 1989 *Harvard Business Review* article, "The Failed Revolution in Health Care," and a 1991 *Atlantic Monthly* article, "Healthy Competition." This time around, my predictions elicited a response: they were greeted with almost universal loathing.[26] No more research awards for me. To the contrary, the *Harvard Business Review*'s mailbag bulged with negative responses and the *Atlantic*'s editors even tried to rewrite my article into a more politically acceptable, pro–managed care formulation. Fittingly, one of the earliest negative voices came from the CEO of Oxford Health, a major U.S. managed care organization that heralded the failure of the movement with its collapse in 1998.[27]

Despite this response or, more accurately, because of it, I felt my message was getting warmer. After all, where there is smoke, there is usually a fire.

In 1997, I tried once again, with the book *Market-Driven Health Care.* It was about markets—suppliers and demanders, health care providers and consumers.[28] *Market-Driven Health Care* told the tales of industries entirely reshaped by paying attention to their customers—retailing, finance, manufacturing—and of the entrepreneurs who were beginning to do the same in health care. The book argued that the assertive, smart consumers who had already reformed much of the U.S. economy could, and would, do the same for health care, acting in concert with providers. As a result the reconstructed U.S. health care system would become better and cheaper, like the rest of the U.S. economy. Once again, I stressed that technocratic, third-party fixes—managed care organizations and hospitals vertically integrated with salaried physicians and owned insurers—were doomed to failure because they could not respond to the consumers' needs. Their just-say-no and big-is-beautiful philosophies ran counter to the decentralized, personalized responses Americans wanted and deserved.

Stung by their omission from this calculus, the policy types struck back. Their journals roundly panned the book. For example, *Health Affairs* titled its scathing review with what was apparently the most negative headline the editorial staff could imagine—"The Apotheosis of the Health Care Consumer."[29] Horrors!

But *Market-Driven Health Care* received positive reviews in the provider and business press, such as the *Journal of the American Medical Association, Fortune,* the *Wall Street Journal,* and *The Economist.*[30] Ultimately, the book became a current events bestseller for a number of years, won the Health Care Executives' book of the year award, was translated into foreign languages, and remains available today in paperback. It had obviously hit a responsive chord. I continue to receive letters from new readers six years after the book's initial publication.

WHY THE TIME IS RIGHT FOR CONSUMER-DRIVEN HEALTH CARE

Buoyed by the success of this message, I felt the time for a consumer-choice health care system was finally nearing. Many factors were pushing it along, but fundamentally, a consumer-driven health care system was inevitable because activist U.S. consumers and other powerful groups in our society wanted it.

Consumers wanted it because the type of managed care so ardently advocated by the health care policy experts had failed them so badly. The promises that managed care would lead to better quality and cost control had not been kept; employers were once again facing large increases in health care expenses—13 percent for Fortune 100 firms in 2002 alone,[31] and employees both disliked it—even top HMOs earn only 55 percent approval ratings[32]—and questioned its impact on their health.

Providers were also dejected. Everywhere I went on my lecture tour for *Market-Driven Health Care,* I met physicians who told me they were leaving the field because they could no longer practice medicine as it should be practiced. The persistent decline in medical school applications has been widely attributed to managed care's hobbling of the profession.[33] A nurse who is no longer caring for patients speaks for many others with the statement, "I love nursing. I just can't do it anymore."[34] Many providers thought that consumer-driven health care would free them of the shackles of managed care.

Even the sorts of politicians who view government as the solution, not as the problem, got the message. Thus, the activist former U.S. senator Bill Bradley advocated a consumer-driven health care system during his bid for the Democratic nomination for U.S. president.[35]

Other powerful forces wanted it too. One was the employers who in the early 2000s were facing double-digit health insurance premium increases while their profit growth was languishing. Many knew that when it came to costs, the worst was yet to come. For one thing, the patient protection legislation pending in various legislatures seemed likely to unleash a squadron of skilled lawyers, armed with costly pain-and-suffering lawsuits, on vulnerable managed care insurance plans.[36] If they won, one way or another, it would be the business community that would fund the resulting massive judgments. The magnitude of the anticipated haul was indicated by the caliber of the lawyers showing an interest in this legislation. Among them were David Boies, who pled Al Gore's presidential election case before the Supreme Court, and "Dicky" Scruggs, an architect of the successful multibillion dollar tobacco lawsuit settlements.[37] Adding to employers' concerns about future costs was the surge in the baby boomer population; now in their fifties baby boomers are used to getting their way. Although the boomers will experience less disability than prior elderly cohorts, these empowered, manipulative elders will insist on treatment with the drugs that will be developed through the marvelous new genomic cartography of our bodies.[38] The cost of such drugs is staggering—for example, Genzyme's designer drug for the victims of Gaucher's disease, a rare, deadly genetic disorder, costs approximately $170,000 a year per user.[39]

Concerned CEOs correctly feared that corporations' bottom lines would bear the brunt of all this.

Because health care is such a large expense—accounting for 10.5 percent of total gross payroll in 2000—and so highly valued by employees—outranking even compensation in importance by a 2 to 1 margin in a 2002 survey—employers are desperately seeking a silver bullet.[40] Short of a government-run health care system, there are no more arrows in the quiver. After all, managed care had not only annoyed their employees but also failed to control costs.

From this perspective, why not switch to consumer-driven health care?

In 2000, the tide began to turn.

A number of powerful, well-regarded firms offered innovative consumer-driven health care products to their employees. These firms included such titans of U.S. industry as Medtronic and Johnson & Johnson.[41] Simultaneously, a bevy of entrepreneurial firms sprang up to deliver consumer-driven health care products—innovative health insurance plans, information, support, and health care services.

In late 1999, I felt that consumer-driven health care was so imminent that I hosted a large conference at the Harvard Business School to discuss the subject. The Consumer-Driven Health Care Conference was a major stylistic departure for me. I rarely attend academic health care conferences because I am repelled by their elitist, micromanaging content. But to advance awareness of consumer-driven health care, I broke my mold. I invited major health care figures, most of whom were unaware of each other's views on the subject, to discuss the topics that inform the four sections of this book: the theory and models of consumer-driven health care, the new intermediaries who will support consumer-driven health insurance, the providers of services and technology who will create the new consumer-driven health care system, and the government that will oversee it.

The conference created visibility for the topic, as illustrated by the front-page story written by a *Wall Street Journal* reporter who attended it.[42] Its participants represented virtually all the many aspects of the health care system: doctors, insurers, CEOs of technology and hospital firms, health care financiers, advocates for health promotion and the uninsured, Internet propeller-heads, lobbyists, consultants—you name the sector, a representative of it was likely in attendance. Participants came from as far away as Costa Rica, Germany, and South Africa. Some of them told the story of their own contributions to consumer-driven health care. Others assessed it. Not all were advocates. Not all were opponents. Instead, they presented a balanced assessment of consumer-driven health care from their many vantage points. And the chapters in Parts Two through Five of this book are updated versions of a selection of the excellent papers written by the conference attendees, supplemented with other, equally excellent chapters that describe the most recent developments in the rapidly evolving consumer-driven health care sector.

ACKNOWLEDGMENTS

Thank you to the consumer-driven health care entrepreneurs who graciously reviewed my warts-and-all portraits of them and their works in Chapter Six: William George, retired CEO of Medtronic; Ray Herschman, senior health care consultant at Mercer Human Resource Consulting; Gregory White Smith and Steven Naifeh, founders of Best Doctors; Denton Cooley, surgeon-in-chief and president of the Texas Heart Institute; Andy Slavitt, CEO of HealthAllies; Mark Levin, chair and CEO of Millennium Pharmaceuticals; David Kendall of the Progressive Policy Institute; and Anthony Welter, president and CEO of AmeriChoice Corp.

And my gratitude to those who reviewed various other parts of this manuscript: John C. Bogle, founder and former chairman of The Vanguard Group; Mark Chassin, professor and chairman of the Department of Health Policy at Mount Sinai School of Medicine; David Cutler, professor of economics at Harvard University; Roger Feldman, professor at University of Minnesota; James Fries, professor at Stanford Medical School; Lawrence Gelb, president and CEO of CareCounsel; Leo Henikoff, CEO, Rush-Presbyterian-St. Luke's Medical Center; Ray Herschman, senior health care consultant of Mercer Human Resource Consulting; Stephen Hyde, managing partner of Clear Creek Resources; Arthur L. Kelly, managing partner of KEL Enterprises, LP; Dana E. McMurty, vice president for health policy and analysis, WellPoint Health Network; Peter Madras, former chairman of the Massachusetts Board of Medicine; Robert F. Monoson, adjunct associate professor at the University of Colorado Institute of Bioenergetics; Robert Pozen, former vice chairman of Fidelity Investments; Ann Robinow, president and COO of Patient Choice Healthcare, Inc.; Andrew Samwick, professor at Dartmouth University; Ralph Snyderman, executive dean of the School of Medicine, Duke University; and Mark Tierney, chairman of eBenX. Thanks too to Howard Wizig, founder of the Consumer-Driven Health Care Association, for contributing the section of Chapter Four entitled "Consumer-Driven Health Care: Early Innovators."

All remaining errors and lapses in logic, clarity, and good taste are mine.

Kudos too to my former MBA students who traveled from all over the United States, at their own expense, to help facilitate the conference—Sarah Bua, Amy Burroughs, Judith Toran Cousin, Matthew Eyring, Todd Farha, Jefferson Greyling, Michael Kaswan, Stacey Lauren, Alfred Martin, Thomas Nagle, Joanne Nardone, Steve Nelson, Thomas Policelli, Sharon Reich, Jenny Ulin, and Scott Walton. I also appreciate the work of Leon White and Meryl Comer, who helped me to organize the massive Consumer-Driven Health Care Conference.

Many thanks to the Harvard Business School for its generosity in sponsoring the conference and to its marvelously able staff: Jeffrey Cronin of the Baker Library, the maestro of research, and Aimée Hamel at the Case Services Center, who personifies professionalism. Jackie Baugher orchestrated the reading, living, dining, and conference arrangements.

My admiration to the two formal speakers for the conference: William George, then CEO of Medtronic, and Robert Waller, CEO of the Mayo Clinic. My gratitude too to Richard D'Amaro, who with assistance from KPMG conducted a consumer-driven health care survey expressly for the conference.[43]

And my thanks to my able, supportive editor, Andy Pasternack, for his patience as I repeatedly updated this book while waiting for the "right time" for its publication.

SO, WHERE IS THE CONSUMER?

You may have noticed somebody's absence amid all these names and titles.

Of course. There are no consumers present—because in the health care system, both here and abroad, consumers are missing in action.

I have long wanted consumers to drive health care.

I waited to publish this book until the time for the consumer-driven health care revolution to occur was right.

The time is now.

Notes

1. Healy, P. "Student Web Site for Rating Faculty Drives a Rift at Williams." *Boston Globe,* June 3, 2002, p. A1.

2. Steinberg, J. "Public Shaming: Rating System for Schools." *New York Times,* Jan. 7, 1998, p. A19.

3. Cole, R. E. "Learning from the Quality Movement: What Did and Didn't Happen and Why." *California Management Review,* Fall 1998, *41*(1), 43–73.

4. Melhado, E. M. Review of T. Rice, *The Economics of Health Care Reconsidered* (Chicago: Health Administration Press, 1998). *Journal of Health Politics, Policy and Law,* Feb. 2000, *25,* 252, 248.

5. McCormick, D., and others. "Relationship Between Low Quality-of-Care Scores and HMOs' Subsequent Public Disclosure of Quality-of-Care Scores." *Journal of the American Medical Association,* 2002, *288,* 12, 1484.

6. Blue Shield of California. "Important Announcement." Nov. 2002.

7. Corrado, C., and Stifman, L. "Decomposition of Productivity and Unit Costs." *American Economic Association Papers and Proceedings,* May 1995, *89*(2), 320.

8. Herzlinger, R. E. "Can We Control Health Care Costs?" *Harvard Business Review,* Mar.–Apr. 1978, *56,* 102.

9. Herzlinger, R. E. "Limit Employee Health Plans to the Big Bills." *Wall Street Journal,* June 6, 1983, p. 30.

10. Herzlinger, R. E., and Schwartz, J. "How Companies Tackle Health Care Costs: Part I." *Harvard Business Review,* July–Aug. 1985, *63,* 68–82; Herzlinger, R. E. "How Companies Tackle Health Care Costs: Part II." *Harvard Business Review,* Sept.–Oct. 1985, *63,* 108–112; Herzlinger, R. E., and Calkins, D. "How Companies Tackle Health Care Costs: Part III." *Harvard Business Review,* Jan.–Feb. 1986, *64,* 70–81.

11. Healy, P. "Student Web Site for Rating Faculty Drives a Rift at Williams." *Boston Globe,* June 3, 2002, p. A1.

12. See, for example, Ornstein, C. "Kaiser Clerks Paid More for Helping Less." *Los Angeles Times,* May 17, 2001, pt. 2, p. 1; Ornstein, C. "Cases Reveal Lapses in Kaiser Emergency Care." *Los Angeles Times,* Jan. 2, 2002, p. 1; Olmos, D. R. "Kaiser Is Facing Threat of a Shutdown in Texas." *Los Angeles Times,* Apr. 3, 1997, p. D1; Auge, K. "Hospital Workers See Appeal of Unions: Walkout Against Kaiser Watched Across Nation." *Denver Post,* Mar. 26, 2000, p. B1.

13. Miller, R. H., and Luft, H. S. "HMO Plan Performance Update." *Health Affairs,* July–Aug. 2002, *21,* 80–81.

14. See Enthoven, A., and Kronick, R. "Universal Health Insurance Through Incentives Reform." *Journal of the American Medical Association,* 2001, *265,* 2532–2536.

15. Stone, T. T., and Mantese, A. "Conflicting Values and the Patient-Provider Relationship in Managed Care." *Journal of Health Care Finance,* Fall 1999, *26*(1), 48–62; Schauffler, H. H., McMenamin, S., Cubanski, J., and Hanley, H. S. "Differences in the Kinds of Problems Consumers Report in Staff-Group Health Maintenance Organizations, Independent Practice Association–Network Health Maintenance Organizations, and Preferred Provider Organizations in California." *Medical Care,* Jan. 2001, *39,* 15–25.

16. "Findings from the Center for Studying Health System Change (HSC)." Issue Brief No. 48. Washington, D.C.: Center for Studying Health System Change, Jan. 2002.

17. Pham, A. "HM—Oh Yes We Can." *Boston Globe,* June 15, 1997, p. G1; Golden, D., and Stein, C. "MGH, Brigham Plan to Merge." *Boston Globe,* Dec. 8, 1993, p. 1.

18. Kowalczyk, L. "Partners, HMO Reach Deal on Care." *Boston Globe,* June 20, 2001, p. A1.

19. SATIRE.COM. [www.satirewire.com/news/022800/satire/hmo.shtml], Jan. 2002.

20. Draper, D. A., Hurley, R. E., Lesser, C. S., and Strunk, B. C. "The Changing Face of Managed Care." *Health Affairs,* Jan.–Feb. 2002, *21,* 11–23.

21. Douglas Sherlock, personal communication to the author, 2002.

22. Hoffman, C., Lice, D., and Sung, H.-Y. "Persons with Chronic Conditions." *Journal of the American Medical Association,* 1996, *226,* 1473–1479.

23. Wojcik, J. "HMOs Still Using Gatekeeper Model." *Business Insurance,* Dec. 11, 2000, *34,* 3, 13.

24. Iglehart, J. K. "The Twin Cities' Medical Marketplace." *New England Journal of Medicine,* 1984, *311,* 348; But the chorus was not universal. As early as 1986, Roger Feldman and his colleagues at the University of Minnesota warned that HMOs did not lower hospital costs or diminish hospital profits. They presciently concluded that "public policy created to induce competition must go beyond the simple stimulus of HMO growth." See Feldman, R., Dowd, B., McCann, D., and Johnson, A. "The Competitive Impact of Health Maintenance Organizations on Hospital Finances: An Exploratory Study." *Journal of Health Politics, Policy and Law,* Winter 1986, *10*(4), 675–697. And a 1994 report by the U.S. government's Office of Technology Assessment questioned the wisdom of a national model based on the Twin Cities experience. The report concluded: "It is difficult to accurately assess whether expenditures for health care in the Twin Cities are higher or lower than in other metropolitan areas." See "A Model in Dispute." *Minneapolis Star Tribune,* July 27, 1994, p. 1A.

25. "Health Care in Minnesota: Model for U.S. or Novelty?" *New York Times,* Oct. 9, 1993, p. A1.

26. Herzlinger, R. E. "The Failed Revolution in Health Care: The Role of Management." *Harvard Business Review,* Mar.–Apr. 1989, *67,* 95–104; Herzlinger, R. E. "Healthy Competition." *Atlantic Monthly,* Aug. 1991, pp. 69–82.

27. Winslow, R., and Lipin, S. "Health Care: Oxford's Chief to Resign in Expected Shake-Up." *Wall Street Journal*, Feb. 23, 1998, p. B1.

28. Herzlinger, R. E. *Market-Driven Health Care: Who Wins, Who Loses in the Transformation of America's Largest Service Industry.* Cambridge, Mass.: Perseus Books, 1999.

29. Robinson, J. C. "The Apotheosis of the Health Care Consumer." *Health Affairs,* Nov.–Dec. 1997, *16,* 254–255. See also Herzlinger, R. E. letter in "Letters to the Editor." *Health Affairs,* May 1, 1998, *17,* p. 277.

30. Henkoff, R. "Why HMOs Aren't the Future of Health Care." *Fortune,* June 9, 1997, pp. 38–39; Anders, G. "The Impatient Patient." *Wall Street Journal,* Jan. 7, 1997, p. A14; Hixson, J. S. Review of "Market-Driven Health Care: Who Wins, Who Loses in the Transformation of America's Largest Service Industry" (New York: Addison-Wesley, 1997). *Journal of the American Medical Association,* 1997, *278,* 686; "Hamburgers and Hernias." *The Economist,* Aug. 9, 1997, p. 55.

31. "Premium Rates: The Trend Is Up." *On Managed Care,* Jan. 2002, *7*(1), 2.

32. Appleby, J. "Top 25 HMOs with High Satisfaction Ratings." *Managed Health Care Executive,* Jan. 2002, p. 52.

33. Romero, M. "Lost Luster." *Modern Healthcare,* Oct. 30, 2000, p. 16.

34. Benko, L. B. "Loosening Their Grip." *Modern Healthcare,* Apr. 15, 2002, p. 30.

35. Dan Balz, D., and Amy Goldstein, A. "Bradley Unveils Health Care Plan." *Washington Post,* Sept. 29, 1999, p. A1.

36. "Suits Have Managed Care Facing 'Very Perilous Times.'" *Business Insurance,* Apr. 1, 2002, *36*(13), 4; Albert, T. "Doctors Win Latest Round in Court Battle Against HMOs." *American Medical News,* Apr. 8, 2002, *45*(14), 1, 4.

37. "Big Cases Nothing New to These Lawyers: Supreme Court Veterans to Make Arguments for Bush and Gore Today." *San Francisco Chronicle,* Dec. 11, 2000, p. A9; Meier, B. "The Spoils of Tobacco Wars: Big Settlement Puts Many Lawyers in the Path of a Windfall." *New York Times,* Dec. 22, 1998, p. C1.

38. Barrett, M. J., and others. *Personalized Medicine.* Cambridge, Mass.: Forrester Research, Aug. 2000.

39. Aoki, N. "The Price of Success: Orphan Drug Act Has Spurred Advances and Disputes." *Boston Globe,* July 25, 2001, p. F1; Olendorf, D., Jeryan, C., and Boyden, K. (eds.). *The Gale Encyclopedia of Medicine.* Farmington, Mich.: Gale Research, 1999, p. 1262.

40. For the costs, see U.S. Chamber of Commerce. *The 2001 Employee Benefits Study.* Washington, D.C.: U.S. Chamber of Commerce, 2002; for the importance, see "Rank Health Care as No. 1 Benefit." [www.Hewitt.com/Hewitt-resource/ newsroom/pressrel/s00s/02-25-02.htm], Feb. 25, 2002.

41. Herzlinger, R. E. *Consumer-Driven Health Care: Medtronic's Health Insurance Options.* HBS Case No. 302-006, Rev. Sept. 2002. Boston: Harvard Business School, 2001.

42. Winslow, R., and Gentry, C. "Medical Vouchers—Health Benefits Trend: Give Workers Money, Let Them Buy a Plan—Advocates Say Pluses Include More Choice for Patient, Less Hassle for Employer—A Reaction to Managed Care." *Wall Street Journal,* Feb. 8, 2000, p. A1.

43. KPMG. "A New Direction for Employer-Based Health Benefits." Publication No. 99-12-05. KPMG, LLP, Nov. 1999.

Upon this gifted age, in its dark hour,
Rains from the sky a meteoric shower
Of facts . . . they lie unquestioned, uncombined.
Wisdom enough to leech us of our ill
Is daily spun; but there exists no loom
To weave it into fabric[.]
—Edna St. Vincent Millay, "Upon This Age"

PART ONE

WHY WE NEED CONSUMER-DRIVEN HEALTH CARE

The eight chapters in Part One of *Consumer-Driven Health Care* present both an overview of the main themes and much essential background. Chapter One delineates how consumer control improved our financial and automobile markets and how the absence of consumer control adversely affects the health insurance sector. It explains the mystery of how individual consumers improve quality and cost, despite their lack of clout or expertise.

Chapter Two describes how current, standardized health insurance policies injure the sick, the self-employed, the poor, employers, providers, and even insurers themselves, and explains why managed care policies have failed to ameliorate these problems.

An extended analogy to Breakfast Insurance is used in Chapter Three to explain health insurance, a topic many find mysterious, and how consumer-driven health care insurance policies can resolve the problems of the sick, the uninsured, employers, providers, and insurers that are discussed in Chapter Two and can improve pricing.

Chapter Four outlines the essential characteristics of consumer-driven health insurance policies, describes early examples of such policies and their impact, and illustrates how these policies could have helped the victims of the frayed safety net described in Chapter Two.

Some believe that consumer-driven health care will lower costs only by causing people to skimp on needed health care. Chapter Five illustrates how consumer-driven health care will simultaneously improve quality and control costs not by rationing but by motivating productivity-enhancing changes in health care: integrated record systems, focused factories, and personalized medicine.

Today, some visionary entrepreneurs are creating the elements of a consumer-driven health care system. Chapter Six discusses these new insurance policies, new intermediaries, new consumer-driven services and technologies, and new consumer-oriented government programs.

Chapter Seven debunks the scare stories about consumer-driven health care, mostly promulgated by those who fear loss of stature or market position as this new model is put into practice. This chapter also explains the oversight role that government must play in a consumer-driven health care system.

A wise book editor once told me that the reason for the commercial failure of most books on health care is the overuse of the word *must*—as in "the government must," "the doctors must," "the consumers must." This shower of Mosaic commandments neutralizes the intrinsic humanity of the subject and lobotomizes the reader. I have tried my best to heed his advice throughout this book, but I cannot avoid the dreaded word *must* in a chapter entitled "How to Make Consumer-Driven Health Care Happen." I hope that Chapter Eight's brevity provides some compensation for its hectoring tone.

 CHAPTER ONE CHAPTER ONE

Fear and Loathing of Defined Benefit Health Insurance

My heart sank when I spied the familiar large envelope, emblazoned with Harvard's classic maroon and white colors, on my mail table. The words "Benefit Selection" were gaily festooned on the face of the envelope, as if it were an invitation to a party. But selecting benefits was no party.

Inside the envelope an ominously fat booklet listed the many benefits offered by my employer, Harvard University: investment options for the money the University and I were setting aside for my retirement and insurance choices for my life, disability, teeth, and health.

Do not get me wrong: I do not dislike most of the benefit selection process. For one thing, the process is easy, requiring only a phone call on my part to log in my choices. A booming baritone male voice or a silkily seductive female one then guides me. And the selection of disability, life, and dental benefits is relatively straightforward, one of those many chores we mindlessly perform to get through life, like brushing our teeth.

I even enjoy one part of the process—that of picking investment vehicles for my retirement benefits. Like many other Americans, I have benefited from my freedom to choose the mutual funds that best meets my needs. Sure, I took a hit when the overheated U.S. stock markets cooled down, but even with that hit, many still have substantial unrealized gains in their retirement assets. Most

---

I deeply appreciate John Bogle's review of the section "My Heart Belongs to Vanguard."

3

Americans recognize this as a temporary lull. They are in the market for the long run. No wonder the number of households invested in the stock markets rose from 1999 to 2001.[1]

So what was my problem?

My fear and loathing of health insurance benefits overwhelmed my feelings about the rest of the process.

The lack of real choice among the policies made me feel powerless.

The lack of information about my health care insurers and providers made me feel dumb.

And the lack of coverage for the benefits and providers I wanted and the high prices of the insurance made me worry about my future were I ever to become sick or change my job.

Why do I feel so good about the selection of retirement benefits? Why do I feel so bad about my health insurance options?

MY HEART BELONGS TO VANGUARD

I found the process of selecting investment options for my retirement kind of fun because it made me feel smart and powerful. This process goes by the moniker of *defined contribution,* an unappealing name for a very appealing concept—my direct management of the investments in my retirement funds, using a pretax "contribution" by my employer and me and a vast array of choices vetted by my employer.

With good reason, I do not normally feel smart and powerful. But the plethora of good information about each of my choices made me feel smart. And to me, as to most other people, choice equals power. A quirky study underscores the correlation between these qualities and consumer satisfaction—it found that people who were donating blood felt less pain when they controlled the choice of the arm from which the blood was drawn.[2] (Who thinks up these studies?)

Talk about choice. I could pick from many different types of investments: mutual funds for money markets, bonds, and equities were all readily available. More than 90 percent of employers with these plans offer seven or more distinctly different investment options to their employees, ranging from index funds to microcap equity funds, and 58 percent offer more than eleven.[3] In some firms, employees can even specify their retirement desires and a "lifestyle fund," tailored to their needs, is dispatched to them. And I could allocate my money largely as I chose. If I felt ill at ease about the future of the stock market, I could invest my funds in other types of securities, including money markets. But if I felt exuberant about the future of stocks, I could readily invest a large chunk of my money in them.[4] Indeed, investors can now design their own investment portfolios—baskets of stocks whose future they manage.[5]

I even had a personal favorite among the choices. For its sheer smarts, my heart belonged to Vanguard. The Vanguard Group was created by John Bogle, a crusty, brilliant man, whose 1951 college thesis proposed the formation of mutual funds that followed stock market indices. Bogle asserted that these passively managed index funds (funds with a broad portfolio linked to a stock index such as the Standard & Poor's 500 Index) would outearn actively managed ones, over the long run, and require much lower administrative costs. He also proposed that these funds be sold directly to consumers.[6]

Like many other consumer-driven advocates, Bogle was derided as a kook by the members of the establishment.[7] After all, he espoused two heretical ideas that deeply threatened them: indexing and consumer focus. At the time, most retirement funds were managed by professionals who picked the securities in which your retirement funds were invested, absent any guidance from you. *Defined benefit* (DB) is the title for retirement funds like these, run by smart-money investors and promising retirees a "defined" level of retirement "benefits."

In the heyday of defined benefits, consumer-focused index funds were hard to find. The clubby money managers pooh-poohed the notion that the stock market as a whole was smarter, or at least a better performer, than they. Notes one historical account, "The indexing concept went against the best interests of the professional fraternity—securities analysts, Wall Street firms, pension consultants."[8] And this fraternity considered the idea that consumers would buy mutual funds to be ludicrous. What did consumers know about the mysteries of finance? Because we are so stupid, ordinary people like you and me are appropriately timid about buying mutual funds. Only the smart-money managers of the pension and endowment funds of institutions would buy such funds with intelligence and confidence. Or so they said.

When Bogle introduced his first indexed mutual fund, in 1976, he noted that it "went nowhere." It drew only $11.4 million—less than 10 percent of the amount he had hoped to raise. But the advent of the consumer-controlled, defined contribution concept in pension funds accelerated the growth of index funds. Employers found that employees liked them.[9]

Ultimately, Bogle triumphed over the naysayers. In 2000, The Vanguard Group accounted for about 20 percent of the $1.5 trillion in U.S. index assets. Thirty-plus years after the first index fund was sold, indexing is so well accepted that benefit consultants find the likelihood that "active management will outperform [it] over the long term a dubious prospect at best."[10] By March 2001, Vanguard's index fund had outperformed "large blend" stock funds and diversified funds by 2 percent a year over a twenty-year period.[11] Vanguard's fund family, which now includes more than a hundred investment choices, ranging from bonds to foreign securities, manages $550 billion in assets and generally achieves among the top rankings in performance, administrative expense, and customer satisfaction.[12]

Unfortunately, like all of us, Bogle has not been totally immune from life's cruel twists. Although he lived long enough to savor the triumph of becoming a lionized, wealthy man, he also experienced an Oedipal fate. He was ousted from the board of the company he created by his hand-picked successor. Enough about that.

THE STARS TOLD ME

How did I know that the Vanguard funds were so good?

Simple.

The stars told me.

The Morningstar stars, that is, that indicate evaluations of mutual funds. With a five-star rating system, Morningstar evaluates the following dimensions of each fund it analyzes: performance, risk, ownership, management, and cost. As you can guess I am a Morningstar fan. I like the clarity and expertise of its presentations. Like a bantamweight boxer, those little stars pack a big wallop.

Morningstar's history is similar to Vanguard's. It too was formed by an eccentric, competent visionary. In this case the founder, Joe Manseuto, was no MBA. Instead, he had earned a degree in American literature from the University of Chicago. His literary leanings are apparent in Morningstar's name, borrowed from Thoreau's *Walden*—"The sun is but a morning star"[13]—and its clarity of exposition. His University of Chicago background also brought an expertise gained from the university's brilliant business school—packed with Nobel economics prize laureates—to the rating process.

One of the university faculty's major contributions was to demystify the measurement of risk. In theory a mutual fund manager who invests in risky ventures can earn a better return than more risk-averse managers. More risk, more reward. But suppose you do not like risk. Suppose you want your investments to be the risk equivalent of a Raisin Bran-eating, Volvo-driving, suburb-living, golf-playing kind of life. How can you separate the go-go players from their conservative siblings? Considerable hand-wringing accompanied the pre-risk measurement days.[14] Once again, the smart-money, leave-the-investments-to-us crowd worried that ordinary investors would be raped and pillaged if they could not identify the risk-return relationship. (Left unexplained was the question of how the smart money could evaluate risk in the absence of good measures.)

Enter Harry Markowitz, one of the University of Chicago's stellar products.[15] He popularized *beta,* a measure of the riskiness of an investment. The risk of a stock with a beta of 1 is equal to the risk of the market as a whole; a stock with a beta much greater than 1 is for an investor on steroids; and one with a beta much lower than 1 hints that the investor is your grandfather. The first measure of beta, limited to one variable, was suggested in Markowitz's 1952 University of Chicago doctoral thesis in economics. Although Milton Friedman, later to be a Nobel laureate in economic science, voted against accepting the thesis, Markowitz too ultimately won the Nobel prize. The model was then refined by yet another Nobel laureate and used as the basis of the capital asset pricing model that serves as the theoretical foundation for index funds. Since then, the measure of beta has been sharpened to incorporate more than one variable and in other ways.[16] As the refinement of this measure of financial risk continued, investors had access to ever-better data with which to evaluate the performance of their mutual funds and stocks.

Sure, there are shortcomings to the beta measure. For one thing, like all statistical measures, it is a historian rather than a futurist. And there was endless nitpicking about and improvement in the measurement process.[17] But on the whole it does the job. It enables people to compare risk-adjusted measures of investment performance.

These measures of investment performance are vitally important to the success of consumer-driven retirement funds. They enable people who cannot differentiate a debit from a credit to choose investments competently.

Many credit Morningstar with enabling "democratized investing."[18] Morningstar's accessible rating system changed information from an institutional business to a consumer one.[19]

The current pervasiveness of measures of investment performance underscores their importance. If I were not a believer in reading the stars, I could turn to many other sources of information. I could tune into the many talking financial heads—fat, thin; plain, attractive; old, young; bald, hirsute—who are televised round-the-clock, worldwide. Or I could read the fund evaluations in the *Wall Street Journal, Consumer Reports, Forbes,* or *USA Today.* Or I could target Vanguard with evaluations written by a self-styled Bogle's Bogle, who bird-dogs the funds.[20] Or, if I were an Internet propeller-head, I could query the hundreds of certified financial planners and accountants or the message board staffed by pros at various Internet sites.[21] Or, being the old accounting hot dog that I am, I could read the annual reports of the mutual funds.[22]

IMPACT OF CONSUMERISM ON THE U.S. FINANCIAL SYSTEM

Consumer-driven information and control created enormous wealth for investors. The Dow-Jones index zoomed from 777 in 1982 to more than 10,000 a decade later.[23] From 1980 to 1998, the total annual return on stocks exceeded

17 percent, whereas the treasury bill return averaged a meager 5 percent from 1990 to 1998.[24]

These benefits accrued to average consumers, not only to Big Bops. By 2002, millions of Americans, nearly 50 percent of all households and 84 percent of adults, were invested in the stock markets, as compared to 19 percent of households and individuals in 1983.[25] In 1980, Americans saved most of their money, $160 billion, in low-interest-earning bank accounts and money market funds and placed only $2 billion in mutual funds, but by 1996, they had reversed these strategies: investments in the low-earning funds increased by only $40 billion, and mutual fund investments grew by $195 billion.[26] In 1998, the median family with the head of the household aged fifty-five to sixty-four held $58,000 in mutual funds and $21,000 in stocks.[27]

The benefits were widely spread. All income classes invested. In 1998, middle-class households, earning less than $100,000 a year, accounted for half of all the households owning mutual funds. Low-income households, earning less than $25,000, accounted for 10 percent, and lower-middle-income ones, earning more than $25,000 but less than $50,000, accounted for another 14 percent.[28]

Investors also benefited from the increasing efficiency of the market. As the volume of transactions rose, fueled by broader participation, the cost of executing these transactions declined. In 1980, the commission earned per share traded was roughly $.44; by 1997, these charges had decreased to $.02 per share.[29] Put another way, the commissions earned by the securities industry declined from 1.4 percent of the value of the stocks exchanged in 1980 to .05 percent in 1997.[30]

As a result of this broad participation and efficiency, the capital markets in the United States became the envy of other developed countries. A reporter noted of his meeting with Jiang Zemin, the president of China, "[He] spoke wistfully of the Nasdaq . . . being the crown jewel of all that is great about America."[31] The U.S. securities industry grew increasingly efficient. For example, in 2000, New York Stock Exchange fees and commissions for an average trade were 38 percent of the average figure for forty-two countries.[32]

Those who had predicted that consumers would be raped and pillaged in the investment field were disproved in a landmark study that compared the returns earned by consumers in defined contribution plans and by smart-money investors in defined benefit plans.[33] Study coauthor Andrew Samwick summarized the results this way: "When control was devolved from the central fund to the individuals, they organized their compensation, contributions, and . . . choice in such a way as to increase their own retirement security relative to the DB regime."[34] Watson Wyatt Worldwide determined that the returns of 401(k) plans outperformed the smart-money DBs not only in the boom period from 1995 to 1998 but also in the down market years of 1990 and 1993 to 1994.[35] These results are all the more remarkable because they were achieved by employees who were operating with one hand tied behind their back as their employers stuffed their 401(k)s with company stock, a matching employer contribution that participants often could not readily sell. In 1999, 19 percent of their assets were allocated to company stock.[36]

Why did the returns earned by consumer-led retirement plans outperform those supervised by their employers? Simply put, agents whom you do not directly supervise may not necessarily work in your best interests. For one thing, they cannot know your individual preferences. Further, the interests of some agents may differ from yours, and in the absence of your direct input, you cannot steer them right.

Consider this hypothetical example, drawn from my experiences while serving on the boards of directors of twelve publicly traded companies. An old-line, New York City firm invested its defined benefit retirement funds through an old-line, New York City money management firm. The two institutions enjoyed historical ties, a tradition maintained by the firm's CFO and the money manager, who regularly played squash together. Unfortunately, the money manager's results were abysmal. Yet the CFO was reluctant to dismiss him. He worried that his squash partner would lose his job and was concerned about disrupting the historical relationships between the firms. Such conflicts are rife in public pension management.[37] One public pension official notes, "In places where politicians are up to their eyeballs in handling investment operations, there's always the potential for a conflict of interest."[38] For example, the California state treasurer's decision, made on social grounds, to sell some $800 million of tobacco stocks owned by public retirement funds may have cost retirees nearly half a billion dollars in lost appreciation. A *Business Week* editorial noted that "state pension funds are steered into treacherous waters when political grandstanding forces them to mix controversial social goals with their clear financial mandate."[39]

Last, the absence of direct oversight by investors may also tempt managers to commit out-and-out fraud. Pension scandals abound, including the kickbacks paid a Connecticut treasurer by private equity firms for his outsize investments in them and the free patio furniture given to an Ohio public pension fund manager who bought 8,258 imported lightbulbs and fifty-gallon drums of floor wax for his largely carpeted office space in return.[40]

This is not to say that agents are unnecessary; to the contrary they can be invaluable. One analysis pegged the savings achieved by the customers of the automobile information aggregator Autobytel at $20 million, for example.[41] Similarly, *Consumer Reports* found substantial savings, up to $54 a night, between the rates hotels quote to on-line brokers and those quoted to individual consumers. Two of the brokers achieved better rates 60 percent or more of the time.[42] In pension investing too, most investors rely on mutual funds as agents that select stocks on their behalf. Reliance on them can be well rewarded: for example, a dollar invested in large company stock funds in 1980 was worth $14 in 2000.[43]

The critical question is who controls the agent? In consumer-controlled retirement plans it is the investor. In defined benefit plans, in contrast, the mutual funds are selected by an agent who is acting on your behalf but who is not directly controlled by you.

To observe the same agent effect in health insurance, consider the following vignette:

In the first year of performance measurement of hospital outcomes in the Cleveland, Ohio, area, the only hospital to achieve better-than-expected ratings was the Mount Sinai Medical Center. Though little known, it expected major shifts as a result. "We thought for sure that if we were on top of the heap that, by golly, it should direct some business to us," noted its then CEO.

Guess what? The shifts did not happen.

To understand the reason, consider the response of Lubrizol Corp., a 3,000-person local employer. Although it included Mount Sinai among the five hospitals its employees could use under their insurance, it also included some that achieved "worse-than-expected" mortality ratings. "We were not all that aggressive" on the quality issue, noted Lubrizol's global quality manager.[44]

This manager is not alone. Although employers aver that quality of care is very important in selecting health plans, only one-third obtain quality information, and health plans say that employers are much more concerned with cost than with quality.[45] Although the range of employers that formed the Leapfrog Group are working valiantly to improve this situation by paying the providers who meet their selected quality criteria more than those who do not, would employees choosing for themselves be more "aggressive" on the quality issue?[46] The success of high-quality foreign car firms in decimating low-quality U.S. manufacturers' domestic market share testifies to the American public's interest in that characteristic.

WHY 401(K)S ARE A GOOD MODEL FOR CONSUMER-DRIVEN HEALTH CARE

During a recent briefing on the subject of consumer-driven health care, the members of the *Boston Globe*'s editorial board listened to me with interest, courtesy, and some sympathy. But they cringed when I used 401(k)s as an example of a consumer-driven product. "These plans are a disaster, workers have lost their shirts, how will their retirements be funded?" they correctly noted. When we left the meeting, James Aisner, the brilliant communication director for the Harvard Business School, advised me to drop the analogy. I typically treasure his advice. But this time I decided not to follow it.

Sure, 401(k) assets dropped as the stock market declined in the early 2000s; but in the long run, they have performed well. And the "expertly" managed assets of the defined benefit plans declined as well. Real life is never a straight uphill climb. Neither 401(k)s nor DBs are foolproof. In down stock markets, both lose value. Many DB plans were underfunded: by as much as $4.5 billion at General Motors, $1.2 billion at Ford, and $1.4 billion at United Technologies.[47] Between 1999 and September 2001, the liabilities of DB plans outstripped their assets by 45 percent.[48] A 2002 study indicated a staggering $243 billion short-fall among 360 firms in the Standard & Poor's 500 Index.[49] The assets of consumer-controlled plans also dropped.[50] But of the $1.1 trillion increase in the value of 401(k) plans between 1995 and 2000, $846 billion was earned through the market appreciation of the assets that consumers selected.[51]

Of course, 401(k) plans must be reformed to ensure that participants receive adequate retirement income. Who can ignore the plight of employees in stumbling companies like Lucent, whose 401(k)s shriveled as the stock plummeted from a price of $63 in December of 2000 to $1 in August of 2002? But concerns about the adequacy of 401(k)s to fund retirement income do not negate the fundamental point of my analogy. These are important concerns, to be sure; but my interest is to demonstrate that when consumers invest for themselves, they do a good job of it: *to my mind, 401(k)s demonstrate the ability of consumers to manage their financial affairs.*

HOW CONSUMERISM IMPROVES THE ECONOMY

The explosion of U.S. productivity from 1995 to 1999 also illustrates the impact of consumerism. A 2002 McKinsey report revealed that six sectors accounted for virtually all the growth. When I ask my lecture audiences to identify them, most correctly cite the high-tech manufacturers—companies that produce computers, semiconductors, and telecommunications equipment. But the primary contributors to productivity were three low-tech sectors that virtually nobody names: wholesale trade, retail trade, and securities and commodity brokerages.[52] Two of these three sectors that jump-started U.S. productivity are consumer driven, and all are service providers.

The ferociously competitive retailing sector illustrates how consumers drive productivity. Challenged by customers who demanded more, better, and cheaper services, smart companies, like Wal-Mart, responded with numerous innovations such as everyday low pricing and cross-training of employees that enabled the company to simultaneously control prices, increase profits, and grow sales volume. Savvy competitors emulated Wal-Mart.[53] An explosion of choice in consumer products helped consumers get their way: in 1997, there were 77,000 book titles, 790 magazines, and 1,742 community colleges. The choice in each of these categories has increased by at least 150 percent from 1970.[54]

How can these essential productivity-creating characteristics be replicated in health care?

Consumer-driven health care requires that employees have two "C"s and an "I": substantially greater *choice* of highly differentiated health plans, *control* over how much they spend for various health care needs, and *information* to aid their choices. The expansion in choice and control responds to the employees angered by managed care's just-say-no constraints. Competition among newly differentiated products helps to control health care costs, and direct selection by informed employees ensures that costs are moderated by improving quality and not by jettisoning appropriate standards of care.

HOW MARKETS WORK

How does all this happen? After all, the average person is not an expert about most of his or her purchases.

One reason that average people can reshape whole industries is that markets are guided not by the average consumer but by the marginal one. In English, this economic jargon means that producers respond to their *last* customers, not to their *average* customers. Typically the last ones to buy drive the toughest bargain; they are the show-me crowd. These hard-nosed buyers are heavy consumers of information and are adept in interpreting and using that information.

To understand how this market mechanism works, consider my purchase of a car. I confess: I have only the dimmest notion of how a car functions. After all, a car is a high-tech device, studded with microchips. My notions of the mechanical compression and ignition of gasoline that lead to an explosion whose energy ultimately rotates the wheels of a car are as dated as my first car, the 1957 Dodge that I purchased in 1966. It got seven miles to the gallon, rivaled a stretch limo in length, and belched pollutants.

I do not think that I am alone in my ignorance. When I see someone in an automobile showroom peering under the hood of a car, I think to myself, "What the heck are you looking at?" Nevertheless, like all Americans, I can now readily find the kind of car I want at a price I am willing to pay. My quality choices have increased substantially since 1966, at the same time as the cost of a car has decreased as a proportion of income.

How is it that an ignoramus like me can easily find cars that are better and cheaper?

And as only one person in a vast sea, why am I not pillaged in the automobile market?

The answer to these questions illuminates how markets work so that even ignorant solo participants, like me, are offered better and cheaper products.

Two ingredients are crucial to an effective market.

One of these ingredients is information.

Information enables me to be an intelligent car shopper, despite my ignorance.

How does it work? It's simple. I review the rating literature to look for a car that embodies the attributes I seek: safety, reliability, and price. Thus, when I studied *Consumer Reports* for cars with these attributes, two brands caught my eye: Volvo and Buick. I confess. I skipped the earnest reviews of how the engines work, the fuel efficiency, the comfort, the handling, the styling, and so forth. These attributes of an automobile are important to many people, but I am not among them. Safety, reliability, and price—that is what interests me. And objective information about the attributes in which I am interested is easily available to me.

I opted for the Buick. Although it was not as reliable as the Volvo, it was cheaper and had more of the heft that I associate with safety.

But many of those who shared my views of a car's desired characteristics opted for the Volvo. The car grew from an obscure Swedish brand to a substantial one with sales of 100,000 cars in 2001.[55] During this period of growth, Volvo's rivals came to understand that a meaningful number of their customers were interested in safety and reliability and introduced these qualities into their cars. In the quest for safety, some of them acquired rival brands. Thus, *Business Week* labeled Ford's 1999 acquisition of Volvo as an attempt to obtain "cars for safety-minded yuppies."[56] Other automobile manufacturers improved their reliability. By 2000, U.S. cars equaled European ones in reliability, and the Japanese cars had only a small edge. Quite a change from 1980 when U.S. cars were three times as unreliable as Japanese ones and twice as unreliable as European vehicles.[57]

So that is how cars became better even when the consumer is a doofus like me.

Information makes dumb people like me smart.

But what stops the car manufacturers from refusing to cut their prices?

After all, I am only one person.

I buy only one car.

Why should they reduce their prices for me?

The answer is that in the competition for my business, they will continue to cut their price up to the point where the revenue from the extra volume they bring in is equal to the extra cost of making and selling that additional car.

Do you smell something in the air? It is the stale aroma of your freshman college economics course. Price equilibrium is achieved at the point where marginal revenue equals marginal cost.

Yes, the second key ingredient in a competitive market is a downward-sloping demand curve, the old standby of Economics 101. The psychology behind a downward-sloping demand curve demonstrates the importance of the last few buyers in determining the price.

At a high price, there are only a few buyers and they are more or less indifferent to price. The good news is that they are willing to pay a very high price. The bad news is that there are only a few of them. As providers reduce their prices, they attract more and more customers. The increased volume of customers more than compensates for the cut in price. Providers continue to reduce their price until they hit a brick wall: the last picky, tough-minded customers who set the price. At this price, the extra revenue the providers generate from sales to the hard-bargain drivers is roughly equal to the extra cost of manufacturing their purchases. All the rest of us benefit from the assertiveness of the last-to-buy crowd.

This relatively small group of demanding consumers seek out the suppliers who will reduce price and improve quality. For example, a fascinating McKinsey study showed that a small group, only one hundred investors, "significantly affect the share prices of most large companies."[58]

The car market also illustrates their prowess. Currently, automobile prices are the lowest they have been in two decades. In 1991, for example, the average family had to spend thirty weeks of income to purchase a new vehicle, but by 1999, a new vehicle required only twenty-four weeks of their income—a 20 percent decline.[59] Simultaneously, automobile quality is at an all-time high. The range of choices is better too, as the quality differences between the best and worst manufacturers have declined.

How did automobiles become both better and cheaper?

Ford Motor's ex-CEO knows the answer:

> Automobile prices are at all-time relative lows as customer affordability and values are at best-ever levels. This situation is primarily driven by excess worldwide production capacity, more open global competition, and much better informed customers. In this environment, prices are relatively stable while quality, technology, safety, and upgraded features improve customer value. Additionally, although the power of the brand remains a strong customer differentiator, it is important that the promise of the brand is absolutely delivered.
>
> The customer is the clear winner.[60]

In the auto market and most other markets, these two characteristics—information and a group of picky consumers—enable the rest of us to obtain a good product at a good price.

ARE AVERAGE JANES AND JOES SMART ENOUGH TO BUY CONSUMER-DRIVEN HEALTH INSURANCE POLICIES?

Some policy analysts argue that a consumer-driven health care system cannot work because average consumers will be stymied by the process of selecting among differentiated health insurance products. Instead, they say, the process must be increasingly centralized into the analysts' able hands. As one notes, "The approach of trying to give people the purchasing power to operate in the current insurance market assumes too much about individual purchasing abilities."[61]

Like some others who denigrate the astuteness of consumers, the author of this statement, Lawrence Lewin, is hardly a disinterested observer. As the leading industry journal *Modern Healthcare* has noted, his firm, The Lewin Group, is known for its "very very expensive" studies, often used by the health care organizations that commission them "to advance the client's political positions."[62] A consumer-driven health care system, in contrast, depoliticizes the environment because it relies on consumers, not politicians, to allocate resources. It also threatens the interests of those who rely on the status quo.

Although it is hard to understand why we should continue to entrust the selection of health insurance to those who have made such a hash of 15 percent of our GNP to date, critics like Lewin raise an interesting question: how do average consumers fare when they buy other complicated products, such as computers, cars, and mutual funds? After all, most of us have little idea of how high-tech computers and cars work, and as an old accounting teacher, I can personally attest to the fact that most people lack the expertise needed to evaluate the performance of mutual funds. Yet average consumers do surprisingly well in buying complex products. The price of cars and computers, as a percentage of income, has steadily decreased while their power, safety, quality, and reliability has increased. And when it comes to mutual funds, even after the downturn in the U.S. stock market, the American public was sitting on billions of dollars in unrealized stock market gains in their defined contribution funds.

How do consumers who are baffled by the functioning of a microcircuit, an internal combustion engine, and an investment portfolio, nevertheless obtain better and cheaper products over time?

Information and a group of assertive consumers, as I have discussed, are key. Another critical element is the changing face of the American consumer. Current generations of Americans are much better educated than prior ones. In 2000, 25.6 percent of the population had attained a college education or more and 84.1 percent were high school graduates. In 1960, in contrast, fewer than half the people were high school graduates and only 7 percent had a college education.[63] These higher levels of educational attainment have increased individuals' ability to obtain and interpret information as well as their self-confidence. One example of this change is manifested by the Christians who increasingly stand rather than kneel at church, likely to express their notion that the service provides an opportunity for a personal encounter with God rather than an opportunity only to reverentially worship him. About 80 percent of the pews ordered from the country's largest manufacturer now come without kneelers.[64]

Affluent Web surfers also typify the characteristics of this better-educated group—they spend much more time than others searching for information on the net before making a purchase and are much more likely to buy, once they have found a good value for the money.[65] Policy analysts who focus on their affluence miss the point. Affluent or not, they eat the same bread, buy the same appliances, wear the same t-shirts, and use the same gasoline and oil as we. Their activism improves these products for the rest of us.

Do not get me wrong. If I were queen, I would push hard to ensure universal literacy. But markets function well even when consumers have very mixed abilities, as long as they contain information and a small group of smart, picky, I-want-what-I-want-when-I-want-it-at-a-rock-bottom-price consumers who force providers of goods and services to offer many choices from which they can select.

Health care consumers who typify these characteristics abound. Some express their activism directly by mastering medical skills, such as CPR and the use of external defibrillators.[66] Others search for information, such as the 1.8 million people who spent an average of twenty minutes each at the government's National Institutes of Health Web site, studded with highly technical medical journal articles, in September of 2000.[67] A 2002 report found that seventy-three million people in the United States had used the Internet for health information, six million of them daily.[68]

The assertiveness and self-confidence that typify American consumers are even more strongly evident among health care Internet users. They agree more than average U.S. adults with the following statements: "I like to investigate all options, rather than just ask for a doctor's advice," and, "people should take primary responsibility and not rely so much on doctors."[69] Their pragmatism is apparent too. They do not search idly. More than 70 percent want on-line evaluations of physicians,[70] and when they obtain the information, they use it.[71] Nor is consumer assertiveness limited to the United States. For example, 70 percent of Canadian doctors say that their patients are briefed by Internet information.[72]

Although the characteristics of these Internet health care users mirror those of general users—they are primarily affluent and college educated—interest in health care information crosses all demographic categories; thus the percentage of non-college-educated users who searched for health care information, 40 percent, almost equaled the percentage of college-educated users, 50 percent.[73]

In response, some nascent sources of helpful information about heath care and insurance have already emerged. For example, the Massachusetts firm Consumer's Medical Resource provides information on forty-three medical conditions, derived from sources such as the Harvard Medical School and the *New England Journal of Medicine.* This information "helps you know everything about a disease," notes the company's founder. The service has helped individuals locate additional medical advice that aided one to avoid a heart transplant for her child and another to disprove a diagnosis of Parkinson's disease.[74] Similarly, CareCounsel, of San Rafael, California, helps mediate and expedite HMO or insurance-related questions and problems. For example, it gave one employee guidelines for writing an appeal of Kaiser's denial of coverage. Kaiser officials agreed with his appeal arguments and paid the bills. "The only thing I had to pay were some charges on my deductible," he reported.[75]

Nevertheless, as the old blues song noted about men, good sources for health care information "are hard to find. You always get the other kind."[76] Sure, plenty of data are available, but the information about the quality of health care providers, which is what people want and need to make intelligent decisions, is notable for its absence. (For a fuller discussion, see Part Five and the section of Chapter Six entitled "Health Care Policy Revolutionaries: The Role of Government," which discusses how government can ensure data availability, relevance, and integrity.)

LESSONS FROM CONSUMER-DRIVEN RETIREMENT PLANS

The very scale of the shift to consumer-driven health care is worrisome. Its monumental size creates opportunities for more and bigger mistakes than a smaller, more modest shift would offer. Those who have already been badly burned by the large-scale shift to managed care are rightly concerned about yet another mistake.

Fortunately, we can learn from the similar change that took place in the retirement benefits area more than two decades ago, when many employers expanded their pension plans from defined benefits (DB) options to include defined contribution (DC) as a choice. This shift was propelled by forces similar to those prompting a shift in health care benefits. For one thing, employers became ensnarled in spiraling mountains of red tape as the U.S. Congress increased regulations on the pension field, causing potentially embarrassing full disclosure of underfunding of DB plans. The 1974 Employee Retirement Income Security Act gave employers a way out of these administrative and financial nightmares by increasing the tax advantages of DC plans. Then too, the changing face of U.S. business was evident even back then, and newer, smaller firms naturally gravitated toward the administrative simplicity of DC plans. And last, mobile U.S. employees welcomed the portability of DC plans and, likely, the personal control they enabled.[77]

Although not precisely analogous, the characteristics of DC plans are similar to those of consumer-driven health care in the following ways:

1. *Both have similar roles for employers.* The employer's role is to enable a contribution to the employee's retirement plan, provide a menu of pretax investment options, and support the employee's decision-making process about these

options. Similarly, under consumer-driven health care, the employer's role is that of enabling contribution of pretax money and providing a rich menu of choices and support to the employee. (The employer's role in health insurance is fostered by our tax laws. Under 2002 U.S. income tax laws, the employer's payments for health insurance are tax deductible, and the employee does not pay income taxes for them. Conversely, individuals who purchase health insurance must pay for it with after-tax funds and, in most cases, cannot deduct these expenses from their taxes. The 2003 Medicare Drug Reform Act also changed the status of health-savings accounts, as discussed in Chapter Fifteen.)

2. *Both have similar roles for employees.* The employee has primary responsibility for selecting specific investment vehicles in DC plans. Similarly, under consumer-driven health care, employees choose the health options that best meet their needs.

3. *Both enable pretax employer contributions.* As in DC plans, in consumer-driven health care, contributions for the purchase of health insurance are made with pretax funds. And in the judgment of most experts, employer contributions to health savings accounts that fund discretionary purchases of health care are not taxable.

4. *Both support choices that are more portable.* Balances in DC retirement accounts belong to the employees and can be moved by them if and when they change their employment situation. Similarly, because the insurance policy in a consumer-driven health care system is tailored to the needs of individual employees, it can be more readily transferred if they change their employers, and deposits to the health savings accounts are portable.

Lessons About Investors and Employers

Many of those who worried about the shift from DB to DC plans were concerned about the investment acumen of employees and the integrity of employers. They feared that Americans would not participate or, conversely, that firms would seize the opportunity to abandon their support of employees' retirement needs. Others focused on the equity of the arrangement; they wondered if low-income employees or those in smaller firms would get locked out of the market. Last, some fretted that employees would misuse their ability, in some DC plans, to borrow against their savings or would fail to diversify their holdings.[78]

A Fidelity Investments study of its DC plans, which the firm claims are representative of the national average, disproved many of these concerns. The study showed that 75 percent of eligible employees participated. Participation rates varied inversely with plan size. Contrary to prior expectations, Fidelity found higher participation rates, 84 percent, in smaller plans. Highly compensated participants and less-well-paid participants defer approximately equal percentages of their income for retirement, regardless of the employer size.[79] A 2002 survey by another firm pegged the average percentage of income deferred at 9.[80] In the

Fidelity study, 62 percent of lower-income earners, with incomes between $20,000 and $29,999, saved for the future. Overall, plan participants had healthy savings, with average balances of $60,000. Nonparticipants in DC plans cited their financial situation as their main reason for not enrolling, but they were more likely than plan participants to hold financial assets other than DC plans. For example, 24 percent of nonparticipants owned CDs as contrasted with 2 percent of DC participants.[81]

All in all, Fidelity concluded that "[p]articipants appear to approach retirement saving sensibly." They do not churn their investments: "only a small fraction make more than one exchange a year, and 80 percent do not borrow against their balances." Those who borrow likely do so for financing other investments for the future, such as the purchase of a home or education. They also diversify their holdings: "In plans with more than ten investment options . . . over half of the participants hold at least three funds and one-quarter hold five or more."[82]

As for the concern that employers would opt out of funding retirement plans, in the period between 1989 and 1998 employers increased their annual contributions to pensions by more than $20 billion.[83] Seventy-six percent of Fidelity's plans had some form of employer matching. A majority offered a 26 percent to 50 percent match of the participant's contribution, and a quarter offered a match of 75 percent or more. The effective match averaged between 2.1 percent and 3 percent of the participant's income. Matching was independent of the size of the firm.[84]

Many defined contribution plans offer their participants convenient, fair access to their services with withdrawal, conversion, and vesting features. Fidelity's analysis indicated that 83 percent of plans permit some form of in-service withdrawal (although partial withdrawal is generally forbidden by federal regulations), 90 percent allow participants loans against their balances, and 98 percent permit daily exchanges among funds.[85]

Lessons About Suppliers

Some critics also questioned the vaunted administrative simplicity of the switch. Who would provide employees with the choice, information, and support they required? After all, at that time, few investment vehicles were targeted to consumers. Most were aimed at institutional investors. Information was virtually nonexistent. And would small firms lock their employees out of the pension market because of the prohibitive cost of administering DC plans?

Most of these concerns proved unfounded.

To begin with, entrepreneurial, consumer-oriented mutual funds entered the market. Their number increased from 600 in 1980 to 5,800 in 1995.[86] "By making the capital markets easily accessible to ordinary citizens, mutual funds have made an important contribution to both the democratization and the strengthening of the U.S. economy," notes one expert.[87]

The history of the entrepreneurial, DC mutual fund providers is instructive to the consumer-driven health care movement. In the early 1980s, a few mutual fund companies—Fidelity, Vanguard, and T. Rowe Price—targeted the new 401(k) market. Their decision to compete on the basis of their returns, services, and costs proved successful. For example, as Vanguard shaved its operating costs to become the low-cost producer and focused on its service, its assets boomed. Noted one Vanguard official, "The big thing we did differently . . . was to treat the participants in the 401(k) plan the same way as the other (institutional) investors in our funds. This meant valuing their accounts every night, giving them an 800 phone number, and allowing them to switch from one fund to another."[88]

These entrepreneurial providers took substantial market share away from the banks that in 1988 held 32 percent of all 401(k) assets while mutual funds accounted for only 14 percent. A decade later mutual funds commanded a 37 percent market share while the banks' share plummeted to 22 percent. Entrepreneurial mutual fund firms provided employers with a full spectrum of services that the banks struggled to match. Fidelity, for example, offered a number of different types of funds, a brand name, and record-keeping and administrative services. When banks tried to compete, they "started to blow up," noted one retirement services specialist. "They experienced substantial service problems and loss of personnel."[89]

A relentless focus on the consumer was critical to the success of the mutual fund firms. "[B]anks had no culture of dealing with the individual," said a Vanguard spokesperson. "What separated us . . . was putting emphasis on participants' needs, in addition to the corporate clients."[90] This focus is implemented through detailed management techniques. Vanguard's CEO checks daily on how fast the firm's telephone representatives respond to callers and sustains a corporate culture in which employees are called "crew members."[91]

A focus on costs has been key too. Fund expenses declined steadily from 1993 to 1999. The reason? Investors rewarded low-cost firms. They understood that seemingly minor differences in costs can cumulate to substantial differences in returns. For example, $10,000 invested in a sample Vanguard fund in 1982 would have been worth $163,000 in 2002, with an expense ratio of .22 percent, and $110,000 in a general equity fund, with a ratio of 1.29 percent.[92] Last, most funds offered educational assistance to investors. Some even tailored their educational messages to the specific attributes of the audience. American Express, for example, segments its educational messages to forty-four classifications of investors. Its "East Coast" immigrant group, for instance, is targeted with video-based education because of the group's high rate of video rentals.[93]

These entrepreneurial firms turned to the small employer market. In 1999, Fidelity's entrance into that market reduced the costs of a 401(k) to a small company by an estimated 50 percent.[94] At that time only 32 percent of firms with fewer than one hundred employees had DC retirement plans;[95] but the rate was expected to grow at 15 percent a year.[96] The number of attractive vendors was one reason for the expected growth. For example, a plan jointly marketed by Fidelity and the U.S. Chamber of Commerce contained features equal to those offered to large employers: 24/7 access, daily valuation, ample information, and eight fund options. Similar plans were offered by the payroll processing firm ADP,[97] Travelers Insurance, Smith Barney, Metropolitan Life Insurance, and others.[98]

Once again, entrepreneurs gave the status quo providers a run for the money. The insurance companies and banks that once dominated the small-employer markets were forced to change their ways. For example, Aetna, then one of the largest providers of small plans, lowered its fees by as much as 33 percent and added many new investment options in response to Fidelity's planned entrance. Yet even with these decreases Aetna's expense ratio of 1.3 percent to 1.55 percent remained higher than Vanguard's.[99]

But the DC movement was not entirely successful.

For one thing, some of the employers who were permitted to match employees' contributions with stock did so with a vengeance. The 401(k) assets of a few large firms, such as Abbott Laboratories, Coca-Cola, and Procter & Gamble, were more than 80 percent invested in company stock and some firms locked their employees into long-term prohibitions against selling these stocks.[100] In 1999, 19 percent of the assets of all 401(k) participants were in company stock, but in plans that offered company stock, the percentage jumped to 36.[101] As the market value of firms such as Lucent collapsed, the value of the employees' underdiversified 401(k) assets took a commensurate nose-dive.

Then, too, the quality of the disclosure and oversight of corporate financial performance proved less than optimal. For example, when the energy trading firm Enron filed for the largest bankruptcy in U.S. history in 2001, a number of shenanigans were uncovered. For starters, major debts had been kept off the balance sheet, and self-dealing partnerships between the firm and purportedly independent corporations led by Enron's top management had been only murkily revealed.[102] In addition, the auditors and lawyers hired to protect Enron's shareholders with professional, expert oversight, appeared to be paper tigers.[103] Government oversight of corporate disclosure has already become much more aggressive as a result. In the first two months of 2002, the SEC more than doubled its financial accounting inquiries, for example.[104]

Applying These Lessons to Consumer-Driven Retirement Plans

What conclusions can we draw from all this?

On the plus side the DC retirement plans democratized investment. More than one hundred million Americans were able to participate in the booming equity markets through entrepreneurial, low-cost, high-performance mutual funds that tailored their services to these individuals' needs. Many participants benefited substantially from the process.

Employees demonstrated that they were sensible investors: they participated substantially in DC plans, made prudent investment choices, and employed their saved capital in useful ways. Employers too continued to contribute to DC plans, negating concerns that they would opt out of the retirement benefits area.

Competent entrepreneurial mutual funds firms, including well-regarded financial giants such as Fidelity and Vanguard, responded to this new market by providing excellent, low-cost services. These firms offered their services to small customers as well as large ones. Intense competition among them led to continuing cost decreases and quality improvements. In addition, raters, such as Morningstar, that provided authoritative, objective, easily comprehended evaluations made it possible for those who were not financial wizards to participate intelligently.

On the negative side the remaining corporate restrictions on the ability of employees to invest freely, in the form of company stock matches locked in for the long term, subjected these employees to great risk. And government must act more aggressively to ensure transparency and integrity in the market.

When these lessons are applied to consumer-driven health care, they imply that employers, employees, and entrepreneurial firms will behave rationally and responsibly. Specifically:

- Employers will continue to offer health insurance benefits and pay a share of the costs, in line with their economic circumstances. As the U.S. economy boomed from 1987 to 2000, U.S. employers increased their share of the payment of health insurance premiums from 69 percent to 76.4 percent.[105]

- Employees will purchase insurance and act to protect their health status. In a 2002 survey a majority considered the choice of health plans to be the most critical benefit decision they make.[106]

- Entrepreneurial firms will supply the innovative insurance and information products that consumer-driven health care requires. They will force status quo providers to shape up or ship out. The competition among them will continually improve products and reduce costs.

- Consumer-driven health care may well *expand* the number of small employers that offer insurance, just as many small employers are now offering 401(k) plans, and also expand the market for individuals. For example, by 2002, 800,000 Californians had already purchased the innovative consumer-driven insurance plans first offered by Blue Cross in the individual market in 2001.[107] One likely reason for their popularity is their low cost. For example, a mother in her early forties who lived in

Los Angeles could purchase a plan for her children and herself for as little as $1,400 a year.[108]

At the same time, consumer-driven retirement plans underscore the importance of the government's role in creating the performance disclosure and oversight that is the key to any consumer-driven activity. As *Business Week's* Michael J. Mandel notes, "while voluntary risk-taking in the pursuit of innovation and growth is both desirable and commendable . . . transparency is an essential [characteristic]."[109]

Notes

1. Norris, F. "Outside 401(k) Plans." *New York Times,* Sept. 28, 2002, p. B1.

2. Mills, R. T., and Krantz, D. S. "Information, Choice, and Reactions to Stress: A Field Experiment in a Blood Bank with Laboratory Analogue." *Journal of Personality & Social Psychology,* Apr. 1979, *37,* 608–620.

3. "Option Overload?" *Institutional Investor,* Dec. 24, 2001, p. 121.

4. Brenner, B. "A Wealth of Choices." *Business Week,* July 10, 2000, p. F36.

5. McGeehan, P., and Hakim, D. "2 Fund Giants to Introduce Self-Directed Portfolios for Investors." *New York Times,* Feb. 14, 2001, p. C1.

6. Slater, R. *John Bogle and the Vanguard Experiment.* Chicago: Irwin, 1997, pp. 8–9.

7. Goldberg, S. T. "John Bogle Retire? Are You Kidding?" *Kiplinger's Personal Finance Magazine,* Dec. 1999, *53,* p. 38.

8. Damato, K. "Index Funds: 25 Years in Pursuit of the Average." *Wall Street Journal,* Apr. 9, 2001, pp. R4, R9.

9. Damato, "Index Funds."

10. Williams, F. "Special Report: Indexing and ETFs." *Pensions & Investments,* Mar. 5, 2001, p. 28.

11. Damato, "Index Funds."

12. Waggoner, J. "Vanguard Refuses to Be Shaken: Firm Famous for Low Costs Stays the Course Even as Index Funds Have Cooled." *USA Today,* Aug. 21, 2000, p. 3B.

13. Whitford, D. "My Favorite Job." *Inc.,* Oct. 1994, pp. 70–77.

14. Schwenditman, C. J., and Pinches, G. E. "An Analysis of Alternative Measures of Investment Risk." *Journal of Finance,* Mar. 1975, *30,* 193–211.

15. Miller, M. H. "The History of Finance." *Journal of Portfolio Management,* Summer 1999, *25,* 95–101.

16. Miller, "The History of Finance."

17. Black, F. "Beta and Return." *Journal of Portfolio Management,* Fall 1993, *20,* 8–18.

18. McCormick, J. "Morningstar's New Shine." *Newsweek,* June 22, 1998, pp. 53–54.

19. Block, S. "Morningstar Strives to Stay Bright: Fund Tracker Rises and Shines." *USA Today,* June 12, 1997, p. 1B.

20. See Wiener, D. (ed.). *The Independent Adviser for Vanguard Investors.* Monthly Newsletter. Potomac, Md.: Phillips Investment Resources.

21. "Free Advice from Knowledgeable Folks." *Business Week,* May 15, 2000, p. 186.

22. Caggiano, C. "Some Annual Reports Are Worth Reading." *Inc.,* July 1999, p. 88.

23. Norris, F. "With Bull Market Under Siege, Some Wary About Its Legacy." *New York Times,* Mar. 18, 2001, p. A1.

24. U.S. Census Bureau. *Statistical Abstract of the United States, 1999.* Washington, D.C.: U.S. Government Printing Office, 2000, p. 532, table 835; see also Norris, "With Bull Market Under Siege."

25. "Small Investors Now a Big Bloc." *Wall Street Journal,* Sept. 27, 2002, p. A4.

26. U.S. Census Bureau, *Statistical Abstract of the United States, 1999,* p. 470, table 736.

27. U.S. Census Bureau, *Statistical Abstract of the United States, 2001.* Washington, D.C.: U.S. Government Printing Office, 2002, p. 796, table 1167.

28. U.S. Census Bureau, *Statistical Abstract of the United States, 2001.*

29. Computed by dividing total commissions by total number of shares sold, for all exchanges in 1980 and 1997; see *Statistical Abstract of the United States, 1999,* pp. 535, 539, tables 842, 854.

30. Computed by dividing the value of stocks traded into commissions earned by the securities industry in 1980 and 1997; see *Statistical Abstract of the United States, 1999,* pp. 535, 539, tables 842, 854.

31. Cox, J. "U.S. Success Draws Envy." *USA Today,* Aug. 3, 2000, p. 1B.

32. Computed as the ratio of fees and commissions/average price of stock for the NYSE and in forty-two countries; see "Double Whammy." *Institutional Investor,* Nov. 2001, p. 98.

33. Samwick, A. A., and Skinner, J. "How Will Defined Contribution Pension Plans Affect Retirement Income?" Working Paper, National Bureau of Economic Research, Oct. 2001.

34. Andrew Samwick, personal communication to the author, Apr. 2002.

35. "Do Amateurs Do Better than DB Professionals in Bull Market?" *Pensions & Investments,* Jan. 21, 2002, pp. 3, 77.

36. Employee Benefit Research Institute (EBRI). "401(k) Plan Asset Allocation, Account Balances and Loan Activity in 1999." Issue Brief No. 230. Washington, D.C.: EBRI, Feb. 2001, p. 10.

37. Walters, J. "Pension Fund Follies." *Governing,* Aug. 2000, pp. 54–58. See also Willoughby, J. "Out of Options." *Institutional Investor,* Apr. 1999, pp. 36–43; Walsh, J. "Police Fund Risked Millions, Audit Says." *Star Tribune,* Aug. 15, 1998, p. 1B; Ramsey, R. "Questionable Real Estate Loans Shrink Teachers' Pension Fund." *Houston Chronicle,* May 15, 1994, p. 1A; Patge, M. "U.S. Probes Pension Trustees." *The Plain Dealer,* Mar. 7, 1994, p. 1A; Gladstone, M. "Public Pension

Systems Looking at Inner City." *Los Angeles Times,* Feb. 25, 1993, p. J6; Vise, D. A. "A Billion-Dollar Battle over Pension Plans' Purpose." *Washington Post,* Dec. 6, 1992, p. H1.

38. "Politicians Should Butt Out of Pension Funds." *Business Week,* June 11, 2001, p. 150.

39. "Politicians Should Butt Out of Pension Funds," p. 150.

40. Rehfeld, B. "The Toughest Job in Pensions." *Institutional Investor,* Feb. 2000, *34,* 56–65; "Mission Impossible?" *Institutional Investor,* July 1999, *33,* 45–48.

41. Zettelmeyer, F., Morton, F.M.S., and Silva-Risso, J. "Cowboys or Cowards: Why Are Internet Car Prices Lower?" Working Paper E6-16, Yale School of Management, Oct. 2001.

42. "Hotels vs. Brokers: Comparing Rates." *Consumer Reports,* July 2001, p. 13.

43. "Mutual Fund Performance, 1980–2000." *Pensions & Investments,* Dec. 24, 2001, p. 24.

44. Jaklevic, M. C. "Hospital Report-Card Model in Peril." *Modern Healthcare,* Jan. 18, 1999, p. 14; "The Clinic Takes a Walk." *The Plain Dealer,* Jan. 13, 1999, p. 8B.

45. Watson Wyatt Worldwide, Washington Business Group on Health, and Healthcare Financial Management Association. *Changing Role of Health Care Benefits 2001.* Washington, D.C.: Watson Wyatt Worldwide, 2001, p. 8.

46. Ulin, J., and Herzlinger, R. E. *Health Care–Focused Factories.* Boton: Harvard Business School Publishing, Oct. 2003.

47. "The New Pinch from Pensions." *Business Week,* Aug. 5, 2002, pp. 44–45.

48. "Funds' Liabilities Outpace Assets by Record 45%." *Pensions & Investments,* Jan. 21, 2002, pp. 1, 73.

49. "The Pension Plan Pit." *Wall Street Journal,* Oct. 11, 2002, p. C1.

50. "Top 200 DC Plans Sustain Back-to-Back Losses for the First Time in History." *Pensions & Investments,* Jan. 21, 2002, pp. 11, 62.

51. "Good Times May Be Over for 401(k)s." *Pensions & Investments,* Apr. 30, 2001, p. 1.

52. Lewis, W. W., Palmade, V., Regout, B., and Webb, A. B. "What's Right with the U.S. Economy." *McKinsey Quarterly,* 2002, 1, 31–40.

53. Johnson, B. C. "Retail: The Wal-Mart Effect." *McKinsey Quarterly,* 2002, *1,* pp. 40–43.

54. "The Economics of Panty Hose." *Forbes,* Aug. 23, 1999, p. 70.

55. Ward's Reports. *Ward's Automotive Yearbook.* Detroit, Mich.: Ward's Reports, 2002, p. 202.

56. Kerwin, K. "At Ford, the More Brands, the Merrier." *Business Week,* Apr. 3, 2000, p. 58.

57. "Twenty Years of *Consumer Reports* Surveys Show Astounding Gains." *Consumer Reports,* Apr. 2000, p. 12.

58. Auto Affordability Index. [http://www.comerica.com/cma/cda/main/0,00,1 A 1299.00.html], Aug. 21, 2003.

59. Coyne, K. P., and Witter, J. W. "What Makes Your Stock Prices Go Up and Down." *McKinsey Quarterly,* 2002, *2,* 29–39.

60. Jacques Nasser, former CEO, Ford Motor Company, personal communication to the author, Feb. 2003.

61. New York Business Group on Health (NYBGH). *Conference Proceedings: The Nation's Health Insurance System.* New York: NYBGH, 1992, p. 61.

62. "Defense! Defense!" *Modern Healthcare,* Apr. 25, 2002, p. 20.

63. U.S. Census Bureau, *Statistical Abstract of the United States, 2001,* p. 139, table 215.

64. "An Uprising in the Pew." *USA Today,* Apr. 16, 2001, p. 1.

65. Forrester Research. "The Millionaire Online." Cambridge, Mass.: Forrester Research, May 2000, p. 11.

66. "Just Another Day at the Office." *USA Today,* Apr. 16, 2001, pp. 1B–2B.

67. PricewaterhouseCoopers. *HealthCast 2010.* New York: PricewaterhouseCoopers, Nov. 2000, p. 22; Reents, S. *Impact of the Internet on the Doctor-Patient Relationship: The Rise of the Internet Health Consumer.* New York: Cyber Dialogue. [www.cyberdialogue.com/pdfs/wp/wp-cch-1999-doctors.pdf], 1999, p. 4.

68. Fox, S., and Rainie, L. *How Internet Users Decide What Information to Trust.* [www.perInternet.org/reports/pdfs], May 2002.

69. Reents, *Impact of the Internet on the Doctor-Patient Relationship,* p. 4.

70. Reents, *Impact of the Internet on the Doctor-Patient Relationship,* p. 2.

71. Miller, T. E., and Reents, S. *The Health Care Industry in Transition: The Online Mandate to Change.* New York: Cyber Dialogue. [www.cyberdialogue.com], 1998.

72. "Internet Not Saviour of Health Care," *Medical Post,* Nov. 28, 2000, p. 1. [www.ephams.com/news_article.asp?_FINP_0034200044].

73. Brodie, M., and others. "Health Information, the Internet, and the Digital Divide." *Health Affairs,* Nov.–Dec. 2000, *19,* p. 258, exhibit 2.

74. Appleby, J. "Firms Offer Medical Data Services." *USA Today,* Jan. 22, 2002, p. 3B.

75. "Helping Navigate Health Insurance." *Marin Independent Journal,* Mar. 11, 2002, p. 4.

76. Scalise, D. "Who's Rating You?" *Hospitals & Health Networks,* Dec. 2001, pp. 36–40.

77. Samwick and Skinner, "How Will Defined Contribution Pension Plans Affect Retirement Income?"

78. Lucas, L. "Under the Microscope: A Closer Look at the Diversification and Risk Taking Behavior of 401(k) Participants and How Plan Sponsors Can Address Key Investing Issues." *Benefits Quarterly,* 2000, *16*(4), 24–30.

79. Fidelity Investments. *Building Futures.* Boston: Fidelity Investments, 1999, pp. 12, 17, 21.

80. *2002 Radford Benefits Survey.* Chicago: Aon Consulting Inc., 2002, p. E8.

81. Fidelity Investments, *Building Futures,* pp. 18, 27, 56–57.

82. Fidelity Investments, *Building Futures,* p. 23.

83. "Pension Changes Have Put the Burden on the Worker." *New York Times,* Apr. 5, 2002, p. C2.

84. Fidelity Investments, *Building Futures,* pp. 44, 45.

85. Fidelity Investments, *Building Futures,* pp. 58, 60, 63.

86. Slater, *John Bogle and the Vanguard Experiment,* p. 142.

87. "Where Main Street Meets Wall Street." *Harvard Business School Bulletin,* June 1999, p. 38.

88. Slater, *John Bogle and the Vanguard Experiment,* pp. 144, 146.

89. Slater, *John Bogle and the Vanguard Experiment,* p. 146.

90. "What Banks Can Learn from Mutual Funds." *U.S. Banker,* Mar. 1998, pp. 45–55.

91. "Mutual Funds Report." *New York Times,* July 5, 1998, sec. 3, p. 27.

92. Oppel, R. A. "Fund Expenses: They're Going Down, Down, Down." *New York Times,* July 4, 1999, sec. 3, pp. 11, 28; John Bogle, personal communication to the author, Apr. 4, 2002.

93. Pozen, R., with Crane, S. D. *The Mutual Fund Business.* Boston: MIT Press, 1998, p. 416.

94. "A Newfangled 401(k)." *Institutional Investor,* Aug. 1999, p. 163.

95. "Small Employers Adopt 401(k) Plans." *Employee Benefit Plan Review,* Mar. 1998, *52,* 40–44.

96. "401(k)s Catch On at Small Companies." *National Underwriter,* June 9, 1997, pp. 7, 22.

97. "Small Employers Adopt 401(k) Plans," p. 44.

98. "401(k)s Catch On at Small Companies."

99. Brenner, B. "A Wealth of Choices," p. F36.

100. "Too Much of a Good Thing?" *Institutional Investor,* Feb. 2000, p. 121.

101. Employee Benefit Research Institute. "401(k) Plan Asset Allocation . . ."

102. Mclean, B. "Why Enron Went Bust." *Fortune,* Dec. 24, 2001, pp. 58–68.

103. Grimaldi, J. V. "As Enron Irregularities Mount, Outside Law Firm Subtly Tries to Deflect, and Reassign, Blame." *Washington Post,* Mar. 25, 2002, p. E11; Eichenwald, K. "Enron's Many Strands: The Accountants." *New York Times,* May 8, 2002, p. C1.

104. "Revenge of the Bean Counters." *Fortune,* Apr. 29, 2002, pp. 22, 110.

105. Cowan, C. A., McDonnell, P. A., Levit, K. R., and Zezza, M. A. "Burden of Health Care Costs." *Health Care Financing Review,* Spring 2002, *23,* 131–159.

106. CIGNA. "Survey Shows 92% Want to be More Informed Health Consumers." *PR Newswire,* Oct. 7, 2002.

107. Blue Cross of California. *Monthly Rates for Individual and Family Medical Plans, Effective 1/1/01.* Newbury Park, Calif.: Blue Cross of California, n.d., pp. 2–5.

108. Dana E. McMurty, vice president for health policy and analysis, WellPoint, personal communication to the author, May 3, 2002.

109. Mandel, M. J. "A New Economy Needs a New Morality." *Business Week,* Feb. 25, 2002, p. 115.

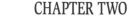

CHAPTER TWO

The Frayed Safety Net

A ll of this is to explain why I am whining about Harvard's benefit selection process.

When it came to health insurance, I felt weak and dumb.

Because I had no real choices, I was weak.

Because I had no real information, I was dumb.

Sure, I had a few health insurance options. But although they differed somewhat in ease of access to health care providers, they all offered more or less the same benefits.

Since 1996, many employers have steadily narrowed health care choice. In 2001, 40 percent of all employers and 92 percent of small ones were offering only one plan. Compared to the number of choices in defined contribution retirement plans—twenty-five choices in most large firms, seven in small ones[1]—the choice in defined benefit health insurance was ludicrously narrow: nearly 90 percent of firms offered three or fewer health insurance policies.[2] One reason, notes an Employee Benefit Research Institute official, is that "there aren't all that many health plans out there to choose from."[3] From 1990 to 2002, for example, the number of Blue Cross Blue Shield plans declined from seventy-two to forty-four.[4]

And even the employees who are offered more than one plan may find that choice illusory.[5] The managed care products currently offered by large employers are remarkably standardized—most feature the same benefits, insure virtually identical levels of expenses, reimburse providers for a limited array of traditional services, generally pay all local providers at similar rates, and last for only one year. They are like Henry Ford's notion of the acceptable color for a car, in a comment widely attributed to him, "You can paint it any color, so long as it's black."[6] Product differentiation in these policies consists largely in the ease with which enrollees can access providers—tight plans force them to jump through hoops, for a lower price, while looser ones offer readier access to the provider of choice, at a higher price.[7] Notes one frustrated Massachusetts buyer, "Three managed care plans have most of the market and their plans have less than 10% variation."[8]

Many people are not happy with this constricted choice. In a poll conducted by a Democratic party think tank, 64 percent of the respondents agreed with the statement, "individuals are best able to choose the health care coverage they want so they should have that option and not have to take just what coverage their employer provides."[9]

In terms of choice, my few, standardized defined benefit health insurance options were a mere shadow of the many, clearly differentiated retirement investment options available to me.

But that is not all that worried me. I was also concerned about my ability to pay for the health care I needed if I got sick. Like me, only 24 percent of privately insured respondents to a 2000 survey were confident that they "will be able to afford health care without financial hardship," and the percentage dropped to 14 for Medicare enrollees.[10] I was also concerned about whether I could choose the best providers for my needs. Where was the information to help me find them?

What an irony—when it came to investing retirement money, defined contribution plans gave me excellent choices and information. I felt smart and powerful. But when it came to my health, something much more important to me, the defined benefit approach laid out in my university's benefits enrollment guide gave me virtually no choice, no information, and all-too-little assurance about my future. I felt weak and dumb. If I wanted to be covered for nursing home care in my old age, and were willing to exchange a higher deductible for long-term care insurance coverage, there was no way to express that choice. And, if I preferred Dr. A to Dr. B, good luck to me. I might be able to visit Dr. A, and then again, I might not, as the following vignette illustrates:

My friend, I'll call her "Molly," showed me a small growth near her neck. Round, solid, with the gleam of a pink pearl. It had the seductive beauty of evil. We recognized it immediately—a cancerous growth, insidiously hidden within a glowing shell.

Her primary care provider (PCP) was not nearly so sure of the diagnosis, but he approved a diagnostic visit to the dermatologist Molly had been seeing for many years. As soon as she saw it, the dermatologist's nurse diagnosed the growth. After all, unlike Molly's PCP, she had seen many of them. It was a cancer. The dermatologist recommended immediate removal.

Unfortunately, Molly's PCP would not allow her dermatologist to remove the growth. Molly's dermatologist was not a member of her PCP's "network." Instead, the PCP referred Molly to the dermatologist who was part of his network group—Dr. Scar as she called him.

Molly was told to visit Dr. Scar, for yet another diagnosis. (And you wonder why health care costs are so high.) Instead, Molly, a feisty, busy woman, called Dr. Scar to discuss the surgical techniques he would consider using to remove her visible growth. Understandably, she preferred a surgical technique that would minimize scarring.

The Mohs surgical technique, which requires precise calibration of the excision, sounded like the right way to achieve her goals, but Dr. Scar hemmed and hawed, attempting to convince Molly that the old dig out, cut, and stitch would do the trick. Finally, Dr. Scar confessed that he could not perform the Mohs technique because he was not trained in it.

Back Molly went to her PCP. He reluctantly approved a visit to her usual dermatologist. Had the PCP not approved, Molly would have been forced to pay for the removal of the cancer out of her own pocket.

The PCP was hesitant because this referral would result in his citation on a "leakage report"—physicians in his network who "leaked" referrals outside their system. The PCP's leakage would likely affect his compensation.

Did Molly know about these constraints on her freedom of choice before she selected her health insurance?

Did she know that Dr. Scar was not a master of all dermatological surgical techniques before she spoke to him?

Did she know the risk-adjusted results of a surgical procedure performed by Dr. Scar and the same procedure performed by her own provider?

Did she know the financial incentives and disincentives faced by her PCP?

Molly knew as much about these issues as I do about quantum physics. Not a whole lot, I assure you.

Most Americans sympathize with people who have experiences like Molly's. In a large survey they registered major dissatisfaction with their current ability to choose a doctor and obtain referrals to and appointments with specialists. The largest source of dissatisfaction was with "health costs not covered by insurance."[11] Yet the problems faced by fundamentally healthy people like Molly and me are dwarfed by those endured by the sick, the uninsured who are self-employed or poor, the employers, and even the dedicated health care providers and their insurers.

The health insurance safety net is frayed. Like the retirees who were once stuck with a smart-money, defined benefit system, health care insurance enrollees too are at the mercy of a third party who will not or cannot readily respond to their needs. Standardized, one-size-fits-all insurance plans leave many important needs uncovered: they fail to provide the sick with the integrated, supportive health care they require; they impose substantial productivity losses on the U.S. economy; and they offer insufficient insurance coverage. They injure providers as well.

In a consumer-driven health insurance system, insurers will respond to these unmet needs with differentiated products that offer far greater choice in benefits, levels of insurance coverage, bundling and payment of providers, and policy duration.

Consider the following examples of differentiated, consumer-driven insurance policies that could help to fill currently unmet needs:

• People with debilitating, chronic diseases, such as AIDS, diabetes, or asthma, frequently find that the integrated care they need is unavailable, in part because providers are paid only for episodes of care, or because integrated care is uninsured, or because they are unable to identify the providers who excel in treatment of their disease. Chronic disease patients are now forced to wend their way from one provider to the next to obtain full treatment of their complex disease. Some of the services they need are uninsured. The sickest 10 percent of the population spent $1,736 for their care in 1996, even though they were insured.[12] Those who were in poor health spent $3,600 out of their own pockets in 2001.[13]

In a consumer-driven health insurance system sick people will be offered fully insured access to integrated teams of the many different kinds of providers they need. Performance ratings will enable consumers to separate the wheat from the chaff.

• Middle-class Americans are hard pressed to pay for expensive medical events that are presently often uninsured, such as prescription drugs and long-term care. In 1996, the out-of-pocket medical expenses of about 5.4 million fully insured households exceeded 5 percent of their income.[14] Small wonder that the overwhelming response when people are asked, "What do you think is the most important reason to have health care coverage?" is, "To cover the costs associated with major, life-threatening illness or accidents."[15] Most insurance policies for long-term care are sold to individuals or group associations, not through employers.[16]

In a consumer-driven health care system, enrollees will be able to trade in insurance coverage they do not want for the benefits they do want, such as coverage for catastrophically expensive care, including long-term care.

• People who require extensive, presently uninsured support to maintain their health do not find the assistance they require. These include people with diabetes who struggle to comply with their daunting, painful, minutely detailed quotidian regimens of care and individuals morbidly addicted to tobacco, food, or drugs. The economic rewards of promoting health are well known, but these payoffs are thought to be generally long term. As Stanford Medical School professor James Fries says: "The most effective health promotion programs improve health and reduce costs even in the first year. . . . But other benefits, such as prevention of chronic lung and heart disease or lung cancer, accrue only after a number of years."[17] Because many insurers lose about 20 percent of their enrollees every year to other insurers, why should they invest now in health-promoting activities that will benefit their competitor some time in the future?[18]

In a consumer-driven health insurance system, multiyear insurance policies will motivate the insurer to provide enrollees with this support and motivate those who need this support to comply with prevention regimens.

• Employees are losing wages and their employers are losing work time because of the perverse economic incentives in the present insurance system. From 1997 to 2001, the length of a wait for a needed appointment increased substantially. For example, 28 percent of sick and injured patients waited more than seven days for an appointment in 2001. Nearly a third of patients in 2001 cited their inability to get a timely appointment as the reason they did not obtain care, up from 23 percent in 1997.[19] The cost of unscheduled absences for medical reasons, many caused by the fragmentation and lack of consumer focus in the present system, accounted for $810 per employee in 1999 and 4.4 percent of payroll in 2000.[20] Ironically, the conditions on which the most money is spent are typically not those that account for the most bed-days, work loss, or impairment. For example, ischemic heart disease ranks number one in costs but number nine in work-loss days. Conversely, back problems rank number one in work loss and number six in expenditures.[21]

Insurers and providers are at times rewarded for acting in ways that may increase this work loss. For example, because the cost of an open gall bladder repair is substantially lower than the cost of a minimally invasive one, the insurer may prefer it. Hospitals may prefer it too, because of the shorter surgical time for an open procedure. But the average return to work time is nine days for the minimally invasive procedure versus seventeen for the open one. So what is good for the employer and employee, a procedure that minimizes recovery time, is not necessarily good from the insurer's and hospital's perspective.[22]

In a consumer-driven health care insurance system, differentiated policies will permit enrollees to trade off the cost of the more convenient care against the value of their time. These policies will highlight convenience from the consumers' perspective.

• Providers too are shortchanged by today's insurance system, in which the insurer dictates the precise episodes of health care for which it is willing to pay and the price. Entrepreneurial providers who bundle medical care in innovative ways may not receive any reimbursement because their activities do not fit the insurers' codes. Dedicated caregivers struggle to adjust insurers' reimbursement schedules so their patients can obtain needed care.[23] And efficient or slothful, master or tyro, compassionate or indifferent, providers are paid the same (although insurers are now beginning to use tiered systems that require higher out-of-pocket payments for higher-cost hospitals).[24]

In a consumer-driven health care system, providers will be free to bundle care in the ways they feel are appropriate and to name their own prices. As in other consumer-driven markets, excellent information will enable users to evaluate the quality of the providers.

The remainder of this chapter examines in more detail the failure of defined benefit health insurance to provide the safety net that health insurance should put in place. Moreover, it is not adequate for the sick, not for the self-employed, not for the poor, not for the employers, not for the doctors, not for the chronically ill, not for the insurers.

NOT FOR THE SICK

"When your eyes meet mine, call out the name of a loved one who is sick or in pain. The congregation will then pray for them." Slowly, the clergyman panned his eyes around the congregation.

My husband, George, and I were in the front row, a penalty for our late arrival. The clergyman's eyes met George's first.

George's resonant voice rang out. "Bea Herzlinger," he said, naming his brilliant mother, robbed of her speech by the massive electrical short circuits in her brain, a sneaky, cruel series of ischemic attacks.

I was next. "Jacqui,"[25] I said, naming a valiant, charming friend who woke up one morning to find she had lost her sense of taste. The diagnosis? The worst. Stage IV breast cancer.

George and I were not alone. Virtually half the congregants named a loved one. The cloud of sorrow that rose from their breath filled the room. Even our ebullient rock-and-roller, once a drummer in a famous band, was subdued. So much pain. So much suffering.

Both Bea and Jacqui died, despite our prayers. Sadly, the U.S. health insurance system abetted their suffering.

One of my memories of Bea is of a small-boned woman, wearing a pink sweater, her back a "U," hunched by osteoporosis. Her soft, fluffy hair frames her face. She is wearing old-fashioned, little-old-lady glasses with thickish, two-toned plastic frames.

Bea is playing cards. Her surprisingly large hands shuffle the cards adroitly. She is a skilled, but not Las Vegas–level, shuffler.

Bea is playing bridge with three other old ladies. I smile inwardly. I can predict how this game will end. Bea will clean their clocks. Because underneath all that pink, old-lady fluff lies a computer-like brain, an atavistic, sharklike will to succeed, and an encyclopedic memory.

I picture Bea as she is now, an eighty-pound bird, seated in her wheelchair in the nursing home. "Where are your glasses?" I ask, knowing she cannot see without them. I find them buried in her bedstand drawer, the lenses filmed with grease. Yes, her attendants are kindly, but she lacks humanity in their eyes.

The wipeout of Bea's speech was foreshadowed by a year filled with sudden falls. Why was she falling? Nobody knew for sure. But the falls coincided with transient ischemic attacks on those brilliant brain cells. And now here she was, sitting in a wheelchair.

Like her Depression-era peers, all her life Bea scrimped and saved, applying her intelligence equally to the purchase of tuna fish in advance of a price increase and to puts and calls on stocks. And now that modest amount of capital, so painfully accumulated, was flowing out to support her stay in the nursing home.

Sure, she had long-term insurance, but its coverage was laughable. And Medicare, our health insurance for the elderly, offers limited coverage of the major financial catastrophe of nursing home care. Only Medicaid, our health insurance for the poor, pays for ongoing long-term nursing home care. In 2000, it paid for 45 percent of nursing home expenses, whereas Medicare covered only 14 percent;[26] but because Bea was not poor, she was not enrolled in Medicaid.

How many children illegally secrete elderly parents' assets so that they can qualify for Medicaid? Why do we have tax-financed health insurance that causes people to commit fraud? Why do we have health insurance that does not insure? Because until the provisions of the 2003 Medicare Prescription Drug Act came into effect, Medicare did not cover most prescription drugs and long-term care services, whether in institutions or the home, the financial consequences can be devastating. Retirees' 1999 health care expenditures nearly equaled what they spent for food.[27] The cost of health insurance to supplement Medicare was their single largest item of expenditure. Low-income Medicare beneficiaries are especially hard hit, spending an average of 40 percent of their income on health care.[28] It is no wonder that 50 percent of nonelderly respondents to a survey about the future of Medicare doubted that they would be able to afford health care "without financial hardship."[29]

Bea was well aware of the problem. She knew that the long-term costs for women were high—they average $124,370.[30]

"What can I do?" she said, shrugging her thin shoulders. "I would like to change my Medicare coverage and trade in insured visits to my internist for long-term care insurance. But how can I communicate my wish to those people in Washington? They are out of touch. They do not know how worried I am about the hundreds of thousands of dollars I may need to pay for long-term care.

"Why do I need insurance for an $80 doctor visit? I need insurance for big items."

As I said, Bea was smart.

Underinsurance is not limited to long-term care. In 2000, U.S. consumers spent $419 billion out of their own pockets for health care:[31] in addition to paying for long-term[32] and complementary health care, they spent $194.5 billion for professional services that insurers do not cover,[33] including expenditures for items labeled as cosmetic, such as orthodontics and vision-correcting surgery; lifestyle enhancing, such as drugs and devices for impotence; and experimental, such as new, potentially life-saving drugs and devices.[34]

Victims of chronic diseases are also especially hard hit: 12 percent of them spent more than 10 percent of their income for uninsured care.[35] Those with asthma, diabetes, and hypertension paid approximately 40 percent of the direct costs of their care out of their own pockets.[36] And in 1996, the small fraction of prescription drug users who accounted for 70 percent of all drug spending were forced to pay for 35 percent of their massive expenditures.[37]

Ironically, present-day health insurance policies all too often fail to provide insurance when it is needed most, for catastrophically expensive medical bills. In addition, a growing percentage of the uninsured are people who have access to group health insurance through an employer but who turn it down, most likely because they consider it a bad value for the money.[38]

I remember Jacqui too—a woman filled with love. She had love to spare—for her children, husband, family, friends, life. She even loved the secretive, unresponsive Siamese cats that snaked around her household. Jacqui loved her country too. She was a civil rights lawyer and a darn good one. Jacqui needed all these assets—the goodwill she engendered, her considerable legal prowess, and her sassiness—to manage her breast cancer. Her insurer simply refused to pay for the therapy she wanted—a stem cell bone marrow transplant.

In retrospect, her request was misplaced. More recent evidence indicates that bone marrow transplantation does not improve the survival rate of breast cancer patients.[39] But at the time the jury was out. Jacqui's insurers understood the ambiguity. They were not bad guys. They were prepared to pay for the transplant, but only if it were performed in a local Boston hospital. Jacqui wanted it done elsewhere; she had researched the matter and selected an out-of-state hospital that specialized in the procedure. "Those Boston guys are amateurs. I do not want them practicing on me," she said.

Although the breast cancer specialty hospital charged lower fees, the insurer refused her request. Like many HMOs, they covered a narrow range of providers, with the idea that they could thus squeeze down the costs of those lucky few—a practice known as *selective contracting.*

Jacqui fumed, "The operation will cost a quarter of a million dollars. We cannot afford to pay for it ourselves. How dare they turn me down!" She furiously lobbied her friends to intervene with the insurer. The combination of her fire-hose energy and a vast and powerful Rolodex ultimately caused the insurer to cover the procedure. It acceded not only to Jacqui's request but changed its policy for all its insureds.

Yet her life force seeped out. A few weeks after we prayed for her health, Jacqui died of liver failure.

Some of her rage transferred to me with her death. She died at the prime of her life. She could not enjoy the success of her brilliant, beautiful children and husband. But my anger brought me small relief because it was largely inappropriate.

After all, her doctors and she did their best to stave off the attacks of the rav-enous cancer cells that ultimately disabled her liver. But a small flicker of my anger was deserved. It was aimed at an insurance system that denied sick peo-ple the care they need.

Sure, Jacqui ultimately got what she wanted. But she was a turbo-charged lawyer with a powerful network of allies. What happens to us more ordinary mortals when we get sick? Must we blindly accede to the insurer's notions of where we receive our care and what kind of care we get? After all, my home-owners' insurance does not specify the carpenter I should use to repair damage to my house.

One physician uses the term *selective chaos* to sum up his personal experi-ences with this process. He says: "[let's imagine]) a medical care system in which patients are not allowed to go to a good-quality laboratory two floors above their doctor's office but have to drag themselves four miles across town to get their blood drawn. Everyone would say, 'That's a ridiculous idea.' Yet across this country the architects of managed care have turned this ridiculous idea into reality."[40]

The problem sick people encounter with their third-party controlled health insurance systems are not limited to the United States.

Paul Belien writes in Chapter Twenty-Three of this book of his Belgian grand-father, a great believer in "solidarity," who for years paid taxes to Belgium's national health care system. When his grandfather fell ill, for the first time in his life, he was treated with an antibiotic. The drug was low cost and effective: its only drawback was the small incidence of an unhappy side effect—deafness. Yes, an antibiotic without that side effect was available, but it cost more. To the state's health care planners, the choice of drug was obvious, especially for an elderly person.

Bad luck. Paul's grandfather suffered the side effect. He lost his hearing. Trapped in the isolating shell of deafness, he fell into a dark depression and died a lonely, premature death. After a lifetime of "solidarity," of paying for other people's health insurance, he was prematurely robbed of his life the one time he used that insurance.

"Oh well," I thought, "this is the price of our survival to middle age. We get sick." But the next day, when I asked my twenty-something MBA students about their experiences with illnesses, I was stunned by the problems they had encountered.

Eleanore's story was typical. A doctor herself, she is a brilliant researcher and entrepreneur to boot. Eleanore spoke of the inhumanity of the treatment of her parents, both stricken with cancer. Delays, long waits, and "lost" pieces of medical records were but some of the problems they encountered. "One day after a three-hour wait for a scheduled appointment, my father and mother went home," Eleanore recounted. "An official called my father. 'Where were you?' he demanded angrily. 'Why did you leave? Why did you not wait? After all, you do not have anything important to do with your time.'"

Would this problem have occurred had her parents been paying directly for their care? Perhaps because the care is paid for by a health insurer, Medicare, and because Medicare generally pays the same amount for every provider— prompt or tardy, compassionate or cruel—the official felt little compunction about his rudeness or the length of the wait.

Like Eleanore and her parents, for the past fifteen years patients have grown increasingly dissatisfied with waiting times. In a California survey nearly three out of four rated the length of the time they spent in the waiting room as less than excellent, and 61 percent were hardly satisfied with the promptness of phone responses to their phone queries.[41]

NOT FOR THE SELF-EMPLOYED

Even healthy, wealthy people encounter considerable health insurance problems. Take my friend Sam, a self-employed, high-level businessman: smart, articulate, successful.

While Sam and I were being driven to a joint business destination, he made the mistake of asking me what I was doing. Politely listening to my lengthy, enthusiastic description of this book, Sam finally broke in:

"Consumer-driven health care would solve my problems," he said.

"What health problems can you possibly have?" I asked, dubiously studying his robustly healthy face.

"Since I went into business for myself, about fifteen years ago, my wife and I have had great difficulty obtaining major medical insurance," he said. "Although neither one of us has ever had a claim or has a preexisting condition, the best package currently available to us costs more than $12,000 per year and has a $10,000 deductible. We live in fear that the carrier will cancel the policy if either of us gets sick.

"It is not right," he continued. "The price of my policy is much higher than a fair actuarial calculation of my likely costs would yield. The health insurer can stick it to me because I am self-employed and not a member of a group. What kind of bargaining power can I have in a market dominated by buyers composed of large groups?"

Sam's story explains why many people who are not poor remain uninsured.[42]

The individual insurance market limits access—with strict individual medical underwriting—and frequently provides limited coverage.[43] In other words, many find health insurance a bad buy. For example, 43 percent of the nonpoor uninsured surveyed in California agreed that "health insurance is not a very good value for the money."[44]

It costs too much. It delivers too little.

Those enrolled in group insurance paid $1.07 in 1996 to receive $1 worth of health care benefits. In contrast, those enrolled in individual insurance policies paid $1.40 in 1996 to receive $1 of health care benefits.[45]

Health insurance is intrinsically expensive, even in group settings.

Just how expensive is health insurance?

In 2000, the cost for a family paying a group rate for enrollment in an HMO—typically among the lower-priced health insurance options—averages around $5,000 a year.[46] In the individual market, that family would likely pay more for the same policy. For example, applying the cost-per-benefit-dollar statistics given earlier, individual insurance would cost 1.40 ÷ 1.07 more than group insurance, or approximately $6,500. A family earning $50,000 would thus consume 13 percent of its income to buy that $6,500 health insurance policy, a percentage equal to the average family's expenditures on shelter and larger than its food expenditures.[47]

As further evidence of the "bad value for the money" perception of individual health insurance policies among the nonpoor, consider the following:

- *Lack of access to insurance is not the sole impediment.* Twelve percent of those offered group health insurance coverage rejected it. Most of them do not insure themselves at all—few of those offered group coverage took individual coverage instead.[48]

- *Lack of income is not the sole impediment.* Although higher-income people are more likely to have individual health insurance coverage than lower-income ones, both groups have low rates of individual insurance. Over 27 percent of California's and 18 percent of the nation's uninsured earned more than $50,000 a year.[49] (To calibrate these earnings, note that the 1999 median income of households was $35,232.[50])

- *Lack of confidence in the ability to purchase health insurance is not their major concern.* Three-quarters of California's uninsured disagreed with the statement, "getting health care through a health insurance plan is too complicated for me."[51]

NOT FOR THE POOR

The year 1999 marked a banner event—the percentage of uninsured in the United States declined for the first time since 1987.[52] By 2001, the percentage shrank even further. But the benefits of this decline were not evenly shared.[53] The poor or near-poor continue to dominate the ranks of the uninsured.[54] In 1999, 46 percent of the uninsured earned below $20,000 a year and an additional 25 percent earned less than $35,000. By 2002, 52 percent of those who had lost health insurance were casualties of the rising unemployment rates in the United States.[55]

The absence of health insurance inhibits the appropriate utilization of health care resources. Fewer than half of the uninsured have a usual source of care, compared to 73 percent of those with insurance. They are two or three times as likely as the insured not to visit a doctor; to defer other needed medical or dental care; and to omit filling a prescription, having a test, or scheduling a follow-up visit because of the expense. Nearly a third have been dunned by a collection agency for medical bills.[56]

The impact of these dry statistics on the productivity of our economy is likely substantial. Sick people account for significant time off and treatment costs. In one firm, for example, depressed employees incurred, on average, ten sick days and $2 million in costs a year; people with diabetes, seven sick days and $1 million; and those with heart disease, 7.5 sick days and $4 million.[57] These effects could be modified with early intervention and integrated care, but currently there are pronounced deficits in the care of the long-term uninsured who suffer from chronic illnesses such as high cholesterol, diabetes, and AIDs.[58]

How do the poor uninsured obtain needed services?

Their options are far from wonderful.

Some practice self-care. For example, an ethnographic study of eighteen uninsured families in Arizona revealed self-care strategies such as stockpiling and swapping unused medicines, obtaining free medication samples from doctors, and buying low-cost prescription drugs in neighboring Mexico. The results can be less than optimal. One mother's self-treatment of her "cold" with Mexican-purchased ampicillin, for example, deferred for three months a doctor's diagnosis of bronchitis and prescription of amoxicillin, the appropriate drug for the problem. And the absence of health insurance creates continual stress in these families' lives.[59]

Other poor, uninsured individuals receive care from the federally funded clinics whose use has grown substantially. Victims of chronic diseases may receive symptomatic relief, but are unlikely to receive integrated follow-up care. Notes one emergency room physician of his largely uninsured patients: "When they look at us and ask 'Where do I go after you take care of me tonight?' I often do not have a good answer."[60]

What accounts for this situation?

The conventional view is that the government and employers have failed to discharge their obligations to their citizens and employees, respectively. Following this logic, the government or the employers, or both, should extend health insurance coverage to all.[61] (However, those who favor such proposals overwhelmingly want them funded by someone other than themselves. Raising income taxes is the least-favored funding option.[62])

But the plain fact is that despite decades of "shoulds," Medicaid, our health insurance for the poor, provides increasingly less coverage for them. And private sector employers have left 15 percent of their full-time workers without health insurance.[63]

Why? Are they heartless? Callous?

Perhaps. But a more likely reason is that they simply cannot afford to provide more health insurance. Like my friend Sam, they may well judge it a bad value for the money. And many simply find it unaffordable.

While Medicaid's expenses grew sixfold from 1980 to 1997 and the federal government's share of Medicaid funding nearly sevenfold,[64] the number of recipients increased by only about 50 percent.[65] To calibrate these expenditure growths, consider that the total expenditures of federal, state, and local governments grew threefold during this period.[66] Medicaid spending grew roughly twice as fast as those substantial growth rates.

As for private sector employers, they celebrated their recent prosperity by reducing their number of uninsured by 9.4 million.[67] Nevertheless, significant pockets of uninsured remain among small employers and those in the retail, finance, and service sectors. The low profit margins of these employers cannot support the expansion of health insurance benefits, and, as the economy declines, the number of uninsured grows.[68]

Medicaid Coverage

How is this for a statement that "should" be true? *Medicaid, our country's health insurance for the poor, covers all poor people.*

Unfortunately, it is not true. Medicaid's eligibility criteria are so stringent and vary so considerably across the United States that many poor people are left without health insurance. In Orlando, Florida, for example, only 4 percent of residents were covered by Medicaid in 1997, whereas in Knoxville, Tennessee, 21 percent were covered. As a result, only 8 percent of low- and moderate-income people in Orlando received Medicaid benefits, but 42 percent of low- and moderate-income people in Knoxville were covered.[69]

Nationwide, Medicaid *decreased* the share of the uninsured it covered by 3.5 percent annually between 1994 and 1998. A careful analysis concluded that "this reduction in Medicaid enrollment of 3.1 million seems to be more attributable to the drop in the likelihood of coverage than to the decline in the number of low-income persons."[70]

Employer Coverage

Fortunately, employers took up some of Medicaid's slack. As just mentioned, from 1994 to 1998 they added 9.4 million people to the insured rolls. Yet despite their efforts, the number of uninsured grew by 8.9 million people, driven by cutbacks in Medicaid and a reduction in the numbers of the self-insured.

So how about this for another statement that "should" be true? *Employers provide health insurance for all their employees.*

Again, it is not so. Although virtually all firms with more than two hundred workers offer insurance, a number of smaller employers do not provide any health insurance. Only 67 percent of firms with fewer than two hundred workers do so. The firms in the retailing, service, and finance industries are least likely to provide coverage.[71] These exceptions account for a considerable number of the uninsured. After all, small firms and those in the finance, retailing, and service sectors constitute a major proportion of U.S. employees. In 1996, about 80 percent of the country's employees worked in firms with fewer than five hundred employees, and 55 percent worked in firms with fewer than one hundred employees. The finance, retailing, and service sectors accounted for 60 percent of employees.[72]

OK, one last try. *The employers who offer health insurance do so for all their employees.*

Once again, not so. Employers can exempt employees from health insurance coverage for many reasons—because they work part time; are classified as temporary; suffer from preexisting, severe health problems; have not completed the waiting period for enrollment; or cannot afford either their share of health insurance premiums or the out-of-pocket maximums of the policy. As a result, in 2000, only 10 percent of part-time and temporary workers were offered health insurance. In small firms, especially those in the retail and service sectors, only 31 percent of part-time workers were offered health insurance. Small firms also caused their employees to wait for two months before their coverage began, and retailers for nearly three months. The modal wait was one year.[73] Last, only 13 percent of larger employers and 19 percent of smaller employers paid for the entire cost of a family plan. In 2000, employees paid on average 27 percent of a family plan premium, and those in the retail and service sectors paid 32 percent.[74] Not surprisingly, only three-quarters of the employees in low-wage firms, those in which 35 percent or more of the employees earned less than $20,000 a year, enrolled in their employers' health plan.[75]

These exemptions cast a wide shadow. There are many part-timers and newly employed people in the workforce. In 2000, for example, 25 percent of employees spent fewer than thirty-four hours a week at work, and 27 percent had worked for fewer than twelve months.[76] Some of the industries with the highest requirements for workers' contributions to health insurance were those with the lowest wages and salaries. The average hourly 2000 earnings of $13.88 for service industry workers and of $11.72 for the finance industry's large number of depository institution employees was lower than or roughly equal to the U.S. private sector average of $13.74.[77]

All these details compound to one grim statistic: 68 percent of the uninsured work.[78] Like Sam, the wealthier ones consider health insurance a bad value for the money. And the poor among them simply cannot afford it.

NOT FOR THE EMPLOYERS

So, why do employers not pay up for all of their employees' health insurance?

Typically they simply cannot afford the expense.

It is not that employers are Scrooges. Most of them want to provide health insurance. They may want to do it because it is the right thing to do. But they surely want to offer health insurance because it is the smart thing to do. Even small businesses know that health benefits have been ranked as the top incentive by nearly 40 percent of job applicants surveyed, topping other benefits, such as paid vacations, by nearly 30 percent.[79] Employers also understand the positive impact of health insurance on employee retention, performance, and health.[80]

But they simply cannot afford to provide all the health insurance for all employees.

Private, employer-based health care costs are staggeringly high. In 2000, at $335 billion, they dwarfed all other employment-based benefits.[81] The average midsize employer paid $5,144 for health benefits per employee in 2000. Larger employers' costs were even higher, $5,459.[82] Across the United States, the average cost for a family was $6,351.[83] And large as they are, health care costs are inflating rapidly. For 2003, the increase in premium costs was 14.3 percent. It ranged from 20 percent in Denver to 14 percent in Dallas/Fort Worth.[84]

Numbers of this magnitude dramatically affect employers' profits. They accounted for nearly 60 percent of after-tax profits in 2002.[85]

For example, consider the service sector, whose uninsured record stands at 38 percent.[86] With profits of 3 percent, average wages of $31,184, and family insurance costs of $6,403, it can hardly afford widespread health insurance payments for its workers.[87] The service sector also currently suffers from high bankruptcy rates. In 1998, services and retailing accounted for nearly 60 percent of all U.S. business failures.[88]

But cost is not the employer's only health insurance concern. The very act of offering health insurance may place employers at risk for employee lawsuits. Although the current professional liability status of health insurance plans is ambiguous, if the enrollees' right to sue them is affirmed, employers will wind up footing the bill. And there is support for this right. U.S. Representative Charles Norwood (R-GA), for example, has argued that "[s]ince 1974, managed care plans have enjoyed a near-total immunity from any legal accountability for injuring and killing the citizens of this country for monetary gain. No thinking, feeling American can let that stand."[89] One expert articulates the argument that supports the right to sue this way: "Only in limited circumstances has a health plan been held legally accountable for the actual quality of care delivered to a patient. . . . But there is a certain inconsistency to allowing corporate health plans to assume responsibility for the cost of care while making it easy for them to exempt themselves from more than nominal responsibility for quality."[90] The U.S. Supreme Court advanced this movement when it upheld the rights of states to protect patients in disputes with managed care firms.[91] The right of enrollees to sue self-funded plans, that are exempted from state regulation, remains a major open question in this arena.

If liability suits against health plans swell, employers will pay for them in the form of increased premiums.

Will this occur?

I would not bet on attempts to limit the American public's right to sue.

The awesome array of legal talent lined up to press the cause of the right to sue health plans buttresses the notion that it is not only a just cause but also a lucrative one. The lawyers include David Boies, who argued the U.S. government's successful case against Microsoft and Vice President Gore's case in the contested 2000 presidential election, and Richard "Dickie" Scruggs, whose folksy nickname belies his pivotal role in the hugely successful class action suits against the tobacco industry.[92] Currently, their suits argue that health plans violate the federal laws that require "fiduciary duty," under the Employee Retirement Income Security Act, through undisclosed financial incentives to physicians to limit care, and that they crossed the Racketeer Influenced and Corrupt Organizations Act, commonly known as RICO and carrying heavy penalties, by defrauding consumers.[93] Although these theories of the case may not prevail, the stakes are sufficiently large that other, more successful complaints may well emerge.

Employers' fears of these risks are so pervasive that a new insurance product, marketed since the mid-1990s, covers the liability of such lawsuits. The costs of the insurance are hardly insignificant, ranging from 15 percent to a hefty 20 percent of the policy premium.[94] Notes one trenchant analysis, "Although the direct costs of liability are uncertain . . . the prospect of litigation may effect employers' involvement in health coverage."[95] A 2001 report by Hewitt Associates found that 46 percent of employers would likely cut their provision of health care coverage if they were subject to expanded liabilities.[96]

Last, and perhaps most important, employers receive little credit for their purchase of health insurance. Although employers expend considerable effort in choosing these plans and their benefits,[97] employees are considerably more satisfied with the quality of their health care than with their employers' choice of health insurance plans. In a 2000 survey, for example, 65 percent of respondents were somewhat or not satisfied with their HMO-type plans, nearly 20 percent more than those who registered such feelings about the quality of their health care.[98]

NOT FOR THE DOCTORS

Consumers and employers are not the only ones who suffer from the present health coverage system.

Doctors suffer too. In a recent survey, over half believed their ability to provide quality health care has deteriorated over the past five years. Topping their list of concerns were insurers' efforts to control costs by external reviews of physician decisions and limitations on the drugs they can prescribe, specialist referrals, and hospital care. And 43 percent of generalists bemoaned "not having enough time with patients" because of insurance payment constraints.[99]

Dedicated providers who want to empower their patients are especially hard hit. The health insurance system pays physicians for seeing patients and treating their illness. It typically either does not pay, or pays low prices, for services that help patients to help themselves. With 20 percent of the client base consisting of new enrollees every year, it hardly makes financial sense for an insurer to cover health-promoting services.[100] After all, years later, when the benefits of the health promoting approaches become evident, the person will likely no longer be enrolled in the health insurance plan. Why should insurers invest if they cannot reap the reward?

One study found that physicians who are rewarded for productivity, as many are, tend to skimp on time-consuming health-promoting activities. The authors speculated that productivity incentives induce more volume and less time per patient.[101] One result, for example, is that physicians promote healthy practices among those coping with diabetes largely through giving them written information. Not surprisingly, according to another study, many diabetic patients are not well-versed in managing their disease. For example, more than 30 percent of literate diabetics studied did not know that exercise, a key health-promoting activity for them, lowers blood pressure.[102]

Robert F. Monoson, M.D., gave me a vivid example of the consequences of this lack of knowledge when he told me the history of one of his diabetic patients.

Vivian was diagnosed with Type 1 diabetes at the age of seven. By the age of twenty, she had significant eye and kidney disease. She was headed for kidney dialysis, blindness, and premature death.

After Vivian's twenty-third birthday, she married. I was quite concerned when Vivian appeared in my office, pregnant. I found her diabetes treatment regimen depressingly similar to what I had observed in most patients. She had received no more than a little education when first diagnosed sixteen years earlier. Tight glucose control had never even been mentioned. Instead, her doctor recommended strongly against pregnancy and even suggested a tubal ligation.

Poor glucose control at the beginning of her pregnancy dramatically increased its risk. My worst fears were realized when a later ultrasound examination revealed that the baby suffered from a fatal condition often associated with poorly controlled diabetes. Vivian and her husband were devastated. I expected never to see her again.

But a year later, there she was. Since I had last seen her, Vivian had rejected her physician's disregard for tight glycemic control. Based on what I had taught her, she had adjusted her own treatment regimen. Her blood glucose results improved dramatically.

I recommended that we aim for even tighter control. I felt she was now as ready as ever to attempt pregnancy. She agreed. We spoke daily throughout the pregnancy to fine-tune her treatment.

Today, Vivian has two healthy children. As a new believer in tight, self-directed glucose control, she even arrested the progression of her kidney and eye disease.

I recently received a letter from Vivian in which she thanked me for saving her kidneys, her eyes, and her life, as well as making possible her wonderful family. But she complained bitterly about the health care system that for many years had failed to help her to help herself.

No one had told her about the possibility of a better outcome in a different health care setting, such as mine, that enabled consumers to control their own health care.[103]

Many providers share this physician's view. As a recent *American Medical News* headline put it: "Everyone talks about quality, few pay for it."[104]

But lack of payment for health promotion is hardly providers' only problem. Dedicated caregivers are generally hard pressed to adjust reimbursement schedules so they can obtain needed care for their patients. Providers are shortchanged by an insurance system in which the insurer dictates the precise episodes of health care for which it is willing to pay and the price it will pay. In a 2000 *Journal of the American Medical Association* report, a majority of the responding doctors said that they "exaggerate the severity of a patient's condition to help them avoid an early discharge from the hospital" and even "change a patient's official billing diagnosis to help them secure coverage for a needed treatment or service." These physicians were aware of the dangers. They worried about the consequences of their behavior—nearly 60 percent of those who did not manipulate the rules were concerned about prosecution for fraud— but those who did so overwhelmingly felt that "today, it is necessary to game the system to provide high-quality care."[105]

Small wonder that the American Medical Association's plan for national health insurance is entitled "Putting Power into Patient Choice."[106]

NOT FOR THE CHRONICALLY ILL

Vivian is not alone. Others with debilitating, chronic diseases, such as AIDS or asthma, are now forced to wend their way from one provider to the next to obtain full, supportive treatment of their complex disease. All too frequently they find that the integrated care they need is unavailable, in part because providers are paid only for episodes of care and in part because some of the services they need are uninsured: the sickest 10 percent of the population spent $1,736 on average for their care in 1996, even though they were insured. Further, because patients do not influence the prices paid to providers, they cannot financially reward excellence.

Presently, providers generally cannot name their price for a bundle of services. They usually are forced to accept the insurers' prices for episodes of care. The resulting fragmentation imposes devastating consequences on the health status of those with chronic diseases and, ultimately, on the costs of the health care system. For example, when Duke University's hospital system integrated the component parts of care for congestive heart disease through a self-funded disease management program, this improved patient oversight saved more than $8,000 per patient in hospital costs in only one year through decreased admission rates and lengths of stay. But the current hospital-based payment system penalized Duke for the innovations. It pays Duke for hospital care. The healthier its patients, the more money it lost. Ironically, it was penalized for improving health status.[107] Further, when Duke is paid the same price per procedure as Joe's drive-in heart center, the incentive to innovate is diminished.

NOT FOR INSURERS

Ironically, health insurers are none too pleased with their current situation either.

For one thing, the HMO sector is unstable. Some eighteen HMOs failed in 2000, following the twenty-four that failed in 1999. Only 39 percent of HMOs were profitable in 1999[108] because many found increases in their medical expenses outstripping their ability to raise their rates.[109] Although in 2002 most large managed care plans were profitable,[110] buoyed by sky-high premium increases,[111] the sustainability of these profits can be questioned.

The managed care movement has hit a brick wall of consumer, employer, and political resistance that has undermined its cost-control potential. Urged by consumers, legislators have raised barriers that handcuff the ability of managed care firms to manage the medical care for which they pay. These barriers include mandates to provide certain forms of care and patients' bills of rights that enable consumers to sue for the absence of appropriate care.[112] A 2003 U.S. Supreme Court Decision that bars HMOs from excluding "any willing providers" who follow their terms cripples their ability to form restricted provider networks.[113] To compound the managed care cost-control problems, providers have smartened up too. To avoid being pushed around by just-say-no prices, fragmented small providers have bulked up to counter the market power of large managed care firms. For example, when the Boston-based insurer then known as the Harvard Community Health Plan decided to play off its traditional hospital provider,

Brigham and Women's Hospital, against another Boston hospital, Massachusetts General Hospital, it received an unpleasant surprise: the two hospitals did not engage in price-cutting warfare. Instead, they "merged." Partners Healthcare System, the name of the new entity, indicates their strategy. It suggests an affiliation to pursue joint interests much more than a cost-cutting, efficiency-creating merger—a relationship, rather than a marriage.[114] The merger created a giant, accounting for 20 percent of the hospitals in the market and 25 percent of the physicians in Massachusetts. In 2000, Partners Healthcare System successfully faced down an insurer who balked at the price increases it wanted. It simply canceled its contract with the HMO. When the insurer considered the prospect of excluding Partners' many doctors and world-famous hospitals from its roster, it blinked first.[115]

Hospitals around the country are employing a similar strategy. Notes the Center for Studying Health System Change, "One of the most extreme examples . . . is Cleveland where two local hospital systems now control 70 percent of the . . . capacity. In Indianapolis and Phoenix, hospitals [are] at times creating virtual monopolies in . . . submarkets.[116]

Although Wall Street analysts lauded managed care firms' return to profitability in 2000, from a long-run perspective the plaudits are misplaced. The profits were earned only with double-digit hikes in prices. These sorts of increases are simply not sustainable.[117] In 2001, HMO profits dipped. Noted one analyst, in 2002 "their profits are probably going to stay flatter and start declining again."[118]

Double-digit health insurance premiums are what drove American corporations into managed care.

Double-digit premium increases are what will drive them away from it.

Further, in addition to these financial strains, it cannot be rewarding to be part of an industry whose service is consistently rated as poor by consumers. HMOs are ranked even lower by consumers than tobacco companies.[119] One can only imagine the low morale of the many good people working in the sector.

So what should managed-care insurers do?

The choice is clear. They must exit the business of managing care and enter the business of offering the health insurance that gives Americans what they want. As *Business Week*'s Ellen Licking puts it, "It seems that managed care companies have little choice but to invest in more consumer-friendly solutions. Their continued survival depends on it."[120]

THE STORY OF AETNA

What went wrong with managed care?

The sad saga of Aetna,[121] the venerable 148-year-old insurance company that insures the health care of one of every ten Americans, illustrates two aspects of the problem.

First, for too long a time Aetna was a company in denial. Its forceful just-say-no tactics enraged providers and customers alike. Moreover, these hard-ball tactics failed to produce commensurate profits. To the contrary, Aetna's operating margin was half that of its competitors. After spending $10 billion on acquisitions, its market value plummeted to $5 billion. This is not the kind of news that gladdens the hearts of a company's board of directors.

In late 1999, the CEO who was the architect of Aetna's strategy and acquisitions was forced to resign. His resignation and his successor's rapid actions to reverse his policies illustrate the second aspect of the problem. Although the CEO's resignation was widely anticipated by Wall Street, the health policy experts who were wedded to a view that the technocratic micromanaging of health care costs was effective appeared unaware of Aetna's difficulties. Indeed, *Health Affairs,* a prominent health policy journal, published "James C. Robinson Interviews Aetna CEO: At the Helm of An Insurance Giant" as its cover story on nearly the same date as that CEO's forced resignation.[122] Robinson earnestly solicits the views of Aetna's CEO on the future of health insurance. The contrast between his reporting and the *Wall Street Journal's* trenchant critique of these self-same policies after the CEO's departure highlights the managed care problem: when an industry is not consumer driven, its managers and the experts who advise them can all too easily deny the consumers' point of view.

Consider the following examples of the differences in perspective between these two reports on Aetna.

Choice

Health Affairs

"Human resource departments clamor for efficiency in dealing with the huge number of differing types of health carriers. . . . We've seen a shift to using fewer carriers."[123]

The Wall Street Journal

"'There's no business model in the world that succeeds by making customers angry,' noted the CEO's successor."[124]

Physician Relationships

Health Affairs

"If (physicians) wish to do business with us . . . they must be willing to handle all of our members"—a statement made in reference to Aetna's all-products policy, which compelled physicians to participate in all of the company's products.[125]

The Wall Street Journal

> "Aetna became . . . the only major company to force doctors to participate in low-paying HMO plans if they wanted to (participate) in higher-paying ones."

> "Aetna acts like we're liars"—a statement from a physician.[126]

The Future

Health Affairs

> *Question:* "Do you see the system evolving [to] increase the level of satisfaction . . . of the U.S. population?"

> *Answer:* "I'm not sure I'm going to live long enough to see that era."[127]

The Wall Street Journal

> "In retrospect, Aetna concedes that . . . its . . . public posturing simply made no sense."

> The company now notes that its prior CEO seemed insensitive to the growing criticism of managed care.[128]

As the Aetna saga illustrates, the problems of managed care were caused by an addiction to a failed set of just-say-no policies and a denial of this failure. And those experts who supported these anticonsumer, antiprovider policies served as the industry's enablers.

I take no personal pleasure in the failures of Aetna or its CEO. Far from it. But failures they were.

JUST SAY NO TO JUST-SAY-NO HEALTH INSURANCE

Managed care's just-say-no strategy is generally conceded to be a failure. Health care costs are once again rising at double-digit rates.

Nevertheless, some advocates point to past reductions in the annual increases of the insurance premiums paid by employers as evidence of managed care's efficacy;[129] for example, they might attribute the reduction from the 8.5 percent increase in premiums in 1993 to the mere 0.8 percent increase in 1996 to managed care. But this causal chain is difficult to swallow: after all, many other cost-reducing events occurred during this period too. For one, general inflation dropped dramatically—the consumer price index declined from a 3 percent increase in 1993 to a 1.6 percent increase in 1998.[130] And from 1997 to 1999, Medicare's harsh new payment rules caused substantial cost decreases among providers. For example, Medicare's rate per beneficiary declined by a staggering 27 percent for home health costs, 5 percent for outpatient hospital costs, and 0.5 percent for hospital costs, for an overall decline of 0.7 percent per beneficiary.[131] (And these cost decreases were not caused by shifting health care costs to others. To the contrary, during this period, Medicare paid 100 percent or more of its costs.[132]) Last, some insurers suffered significant losses during this period, effectively creating price decreases by absorbing cost increases. For example, the underwriting gains of the Blue Cross and Blue Shield plans of 1.3 percent in 1994 reversed to losses of 1.2 percent in 1997.[133]

In other words, reductions in the inflation of health insurance prices paid by employers were also affected by the general low level of inflation in the economy, the cost-reducing pressure from Medicare, and the price competition among insurers in an attempt to gain market share.

Indeed, the intrinsic cost effectiveness of the gatekeeper concept in managed care has been thrown into question by the results achieved by plans that enable enrollees to choose their own providers. A 2001 *Journal of the American Medical Association* article concluded that more than 93 percent of enrollees in point-of-service plans did not self-refer to specialists.[134] Similarly, after a tightly managed Boston group practice eliminated its gatekeeping requirement, analysts could not find changes in the enrollees' relative use of primary care providers and specialists.[135] As for claims that managed care has profoundly improved quality of care, Robert H. Miller and Harold Luft, the latter a long-time, expert analyst of HMOs, concluded in a 2002 report that "HMOs have not accomplished what their proponents had promised: changing clinical practice processes and improving quality of care relative to the existing system."[136]

All in all, the cost-controlling efficacy of managed care remains unclear.

At any rate, reductions in health insurance premiums are a relic of the past. The underwriting losses incurred in 1998, 1 percent in the case of the Blues, were the last straw. Health insurers raised their rates by 8.3 percent in 2000, in successful efforts to restore their underwriting profitability.[137] Meanwhile, underlying health care costs have shot up once again. And patients are so annoyed by what they perceive as the sneaky ways in which managed care organizations inappropriately limit their use of the health care resources, that they have urged patient protection bills—legislative barriers that handcuff the ability of managed care organizations to manage care. By 2001, forty-five states had granted patients the right to sue or to appeal medical decisions by HMOs.[138]

Say good-bye to the cost-control efficacy of managed care, such as it was.

Notes

1. Fidelity Investments. *Building Futures.* Boston: Fidelity Investments, 1999, p. 67.
2. McLaughlin, C. G. "Health Care Consumers: Choices and Constraints." *Medical Care Research and Review,* 1999, *56* (supplement: "The Power of Choice in the Health Care Marketplace and Its Consequences"), 40–42.
3. Gillette, B. "Take the Bull by the Horns." *Managed Healthcare,* Dec. 2000, p. 24.

4. Benko, L. "Numbers Game." *Modern Healthcare*, May 6, 2002, p. 18.

5. Rice, T., Gabel, J., Levitt, L., and Hawkins, S. "Workers and Their Health Plans: Free to Choose?" *Health Affairs*, 2002, *21*, 185, exhibits 1, 2.

6. Although according to the Henry Ford Museum, there is no proof that Ford ever said this; see [www.hfmgv.org/exhibits/showroom/1908/model.t.html].

7. With deep thanks to Ray Herschman and Mark Tierney for their review of these differences in Feb. 2002.

8. Dutton, G. "The Shrinking Pool of Plans." *Business & Health*, 2001, p. 14.

9. Penn, M. J. "Health Care Is Back." *Blueprint*, Spring 2000, p. 70.

10. Employee Benefit Research Institute (EBRI). *2000 Health Confidence Survey.* Washington, D.C.: EBRI, June 2000, p. 8.

11. Employee Benefits Research Institute (EBRI). *Health Confidence Survey: 2000 Results.* Washington, D.C.: EBRI, Nov. 2000, p. 3.

12. Consumers Union. *Hidden from View: The Hidden Burden of Health Care Costs.* Washington, D.C.: Consumers Union, Jan. 22, 1998, p. 32.

13. Achman, L., and Gold, M. *Out-of-Pocket Health Care Expenses for Medicare, HMO Beneficiaries.* New York: Mathematica Policy Research, Feb. 2002, p. 4.

14. Consumers Union, *Hidden from View,* table 5a.

15. Penn, "Health Care Is Back," p. 69.

16. Coronel, S. A. "Long-Term Care Insurance in 1998–1999." [www.hiaa.org/research/usefulfacts.Cfmhlongtermcare], Sept. 8, 2001.

17. James Fries, personal communication to the author, Jan. 2002.

18. Reed, M. C., and Trude, S. *Who Do You Trust? Americans' Perspectives on Health Care, 1997–2001.* Tracking Report No. 3. Washington, D.C.: Center for Studying Health System Change, Aug. 2002.

19. "Lack of Insurance Not the Only Obstacle to Health Care." *American Medical News*, Apr. 8, 2002, pp. 12–13.

20. Andrea Joyeaux, Medstat, personal communication to the author, 2002; Mercer Human Resource Consulting. *Employers' Time-Off and Disability Programs.* New York: Mercer Human Resource Consulting, June 2002.

21. Druss, B. G., Marcus, S. C., Olsfson, M., Tanielian, T., and others. "Comparing the National Economic Burden of Five Chronic Conditions." *Health Affairs*, Nov.–Dec. 2001, *20*, 233–241.

22. Sinclair, J. L. "Total System Costs and the Case of the Executive's Hernia." *Benefits Quarterly*, 1998, *1*, 1, 14, 45–54.

23. Werner, R. M., Alexander, G. C., Fagerlin, A., and Ubel, P. A. "The 'Hassle Factor': What Motivates Physicians to Manipulate Reimbursement Rules?" *Archives of Internal Medicine*, May 27, 2002, *162*, 1134–1139.

24. Greenwalk, J. "Taking Cost Control to Another Level." *Business Insurance*, Feb. 11, 2002, p. T3.

25. "Jacqui" is a pseudonym.

26. Wagner, L. "Saving the Seeds." *Provider*, July 2002, p. 23.

27. U.S. Census Bureau. *Statistical Abstract of the United States, 2001*. Washington, D.C.: U.S. Government Printing Office, p. 431, table 59.

28. Medicare Payment Advisory Committee. *Report to the Congress: Medicare Payment Policy*. Washington, D.C.: Medicare Payment Advisory Committee, Mar. 2000, pp. 36–45.

29. Employee Benefit Research Institute. *2000 Health Confidence Survey*, p. 8.

30. Moffitt, R. E., Teske, R., and Moses, S. "How to Cope with the Coming Crisis in Long-Term Care." *Heritage Lectures* No. 659. Washington, D.C.: Heritage Foundation, Apr. 27, 2000.

31. Cowan, C. A., McDonnell, P. A., Levit, K. R., and Zezza, M. A. "Burden of Health Care Costs." *Health Care Financing Review*, Spring 2002, *23*, 131–159.

32. Levit, K., and others. "Inflation Spurs Health Spending in 2000." *Health Affairs*, Jan.–Feb. 2002, *21*, 172–181.

33. Cowan and others, "Burden of Health Care Costs."

34. Levit and others, "Inflation Spurs Health Spending in 2000," pp. 172–181.

35. Hwang, W., Weller, W., Ireys, H., and Anderson, G. "Out-of-Pocket Medical Spending for Care of Chronic Conditions." *Health Affairs*, Nov.–Dec. 2001, *20*, 267–278.

36. Druss and others, "Comparing the National Economic Burden of Five Chronic Conditions."

37. Danzon, P. M., and Pauly, M. V. "Insurance and New Technology." *Health Affairs*, Sept.–Oct. 2001, *20*, 86–100.

38. Blumberg, L. J., and Nichols, L. M. "The Health Status of Workers Who Decline Employer-Sponsored Insurance." *Health Affairs*, Nov.–Dec. 2001, *20*, 180–187.

39. Stephenson, J. "Bone Marrow with Stem Cells: No Edge in Breast Cancer." *Journal of the American Medical Association*, May 5, 1999, pp. 1576–1578.

40. Bodenheimer, T. "Selective Chaos." *Health Affairs*, July–Aug. 2000, *19*, 200–205.

41. Jacob, J. A. "Patients Like Their Physicians, But Hate All the Waiting." *American Medical News*, Nov. 6, 2000, p. 29.

42. Duchon, L., and others. "Listening to Workers." [www.cmwf.org], Jan. 2000, p. 3.

43. Pollitz, K. "The Health Care Crisis of the Uninsured: What Are the Solutions?" Hearing before the U.S. Senate Committee on Health, Education, Labor and Pensions, Mar. 12, 2002. Washington, D.C.: U.S. Government Printing Office, 2002.

44. Yegian, J. M., Pockell, D. G,. Smith, M. D., and Murray, E. K. "The Nonpoor: Uninsured in California, 1998." *Health Affairs*, July–Aug. 2000, *19*, p. 173.

45. U.S. Census Bureau. *Statistical Abstract of the United States, 1999*. Washington, D.C.: U.S. Government Printing Office, 2000, p. 539, table 855. Some believe that this pricing reflects the outsize charges billed to the sick in individual markets. But when individual premiums are adjusted for age and location, they are not significantly higher than those for high-risk enrollees in groups; see Pauly, M. V., and Herring, B. *Pooling Health Insurance Risks*. Washington, D.C.: AEI Press, 1999.

46. Harrington, C. " Health Care Costs on the Rise." *Journal of Accountancy,* May 2003, *195,* 59–63.

47. U.S. Bureau of the Census, *Statistical Abstract of the United States, 1999,* p. 471, table 738.

48. Pauly, M., and Percy, A. "Cost and Performance." *Journal of Health Politics, Policy and Law,* Feb. 2000, *25,* 15.

49. Yegian and others, "The Nonpoor," p. 172; U.S. Bureau of the Census, *Statistical Abstract of the United States, 1999,* p. 127, table 185.

50. U.S. Bureau of the Census, *Statistical Abstract of the United States, 2001,* p. 478, table 661.

51. Yegian and others, "The Nonpoor," p. 174.

52. Mills, R. J. *Current Population Reports: Health Insurance Coverage 1999.* P60–P211. [www.census.gov/prod/2000pubs/p60-211.pdf], Sept. 2000.

53. Centers for Disease Control and Prevention. *Early Release: Estimates Based on 2001 National Health Interview Survey.* [www.cdc.gov/nchs/about-/mgor/ nhis/ released_200207.html], July 15, 2002.

54. Mills, R. J. *Health Insurance Coverage 1999.*

55. Commonwealth Fund. *Listening to Workers: Findings from the National Survey of Workers' Health Insurance.* New York: Commonwealth Fund, 2000, p. 41; Commonwealth Fund. *The Erosion of Employer-Based Health Coverage.* New York: Commonwealth Fund, Aug. 2002.

56. Commonwealth Fund. *The Erosion of Employer-Based Health Coverage,* p. 46.

57. Druss, B. G., Rosenheck, R. A., and Sledge, W. H. "Health and Disability Costs of Depressive Illness in a Major U.S. Corporation." *American Journal of Psychiatry,* Aug. 2000, *157,* 1274–1278.

58. Ayanian, J. Z., and others. "Unmet Health Needs of Uninsured Adults in the United States." *Journal of the American Medical Association,* Oct. 25, 2000, *284,* 2061–2069.

59. Vuekovic, N. "Self-Care Among the Uninsured: 'You Do What You Can Do.'" *Health Affairs,* July–Aug. 2000, *19,* 197–199.

60. Landers, S. J. "Uninsured Often Get Second Class Care." *American Medical News,* Aug. 20, 2000, p. 8.

61. Commonwealth Fund, *Listening to Workers,* p. 51.

62. Commonwealth Fund, *Listening to Workers,* p. 52.

63. Commonwealth Fund, *Listening to Workers,* p. 20.

64. Commonwealth Fund, *Listening to Workers,* pp. 314, 316, tables 508, 511.

65. U.S. Bureau of the Census, *Statistical Abstract of the United States, 1999,* p. 124, table 179.

66. U.S. Bureau of the Census, *Statistical Abstract of the United States, 1999,* pp. 316, 348, tables 511, 542.

67. Holahan, J., and Kim, J. "Why Does the Number of Uninsured Americans Continue to Grow?" *Health Affairs,* July–Aug. 2000, *19,* 190.

68. Freudenheim, M. "Small Employers Severely Reduce Health Benefits." *New York Times,* Sept. 6, 2002, p. C1.

69. Brown, E. R., Wyn, R., and Teleki, S. *Disparities in Health Insurance and Access to Care.* New York: Commonwealth Fund, Aug. 2000, p. 13.

70. Holahan and Kim, "Why Does the Number of Uninsured Americans Continue to Grow?" p. 191.

71. Kaiser Family Foundation and Health Research Educational Trust (HRET). *Employer Health Benefits 2000.* Menlo Park, Calif., and Chicago: Kaiser Family Foundation and HRET, 2000, pp. 33, 35.

72. U.S. Census Bureau, *Statistical Abstract of the United States, 1999,* p. 384, table 596.

73. Kaiser Family Foundation and HRET, *Employer Health Benefits 2000,* pp. 4, 46, 134, 135–138.

74. Kaiser Family Foundation and HRET, *Employer Health Benefits 2000,* pp. 74, 81, 83.

75. Kaiser Family Foundation and HRET, *Employer Health Benefits 2000,* p. 48.

76. U.S. Census Bureau, *Statistical Abstract of the United States: 2001,* p. 378, tables 588, 589.

77. U.S. Census Bureau, *Statistical Abstract of the United States: 2001,* pp. 378, 395, table 602.

78. Commonwealth Fund, *Listening to Workers,* p. 53.

79. "Prospective Employees Have Edge in Recruitment." *Journal of Accountancy,* Sept. 2000, p. 28.

80. Fronstin, P., and Helman, R. *Small Employers and Health Benefits: Findings from the 2000 Small Employer Health Benefits Survey.* Issue Brief 226 and Special Report SR-35. Washington, D.C.: Employee Benefit Research Institute, Oct. 2000.

81. Cowan and others, "Burden of Health Care Costs," p. 136.

82. Mercer Human Resource Consulting. *Mid-Sized Employer Health Plans, 2001.* New York: Mercer Human Resource Consulting, 2002.

83. Kaiser Family Foundation and HRET, *Employer Health Benefits 2000,* p. 26.

84. Hewitt Associates. "Health Care Costs 2004." (www4.hewittcom/hewitt/resources/ newsroom/pressrel/2003/HC_costs_2004.pdf), Oct. 13, 2003.

85. Cowan and others, "Burden of Health Care Costs," p. 140.

86. Kaiser Family Foundation and HRET, *Employer Health Benefits 2000,* p. 29.

87. U.S. Census Bureau, *Statistical Abstract of the United States: 1999,* pp. 443, 551, tables 697, 871; Kaiser Family Foundation and HRET, *Employer Health Benefits 2000,* p. 29.

88. U.S. Census Bureau, *Statistical Abstract of the United States: 1999,* p. 561, table 886.

89. Pear, R. "House Passes Bill to Expand Rights on Medical Care." *New York Times,* Oct. 8, 1999, p. A1.

90. Havighurst, C. C. "American Health Care and the Law . . . We Need to Talk." *Health Affairs,* July–Aug. 2000, *19,* 98.

91. Greenhouse, L. "Court 5–4, Upholds Authority of States to Protect Patients." *New York Times,* June 21, 2002, p. A1.

92. "Big Cases Nothing New to These Lawyers: Supreme Court Veterans to Make Arguments for Bush and Gore Today." *San Francisco Chronicle,* Dec. 11, 2000, p. A9; Meier, B. "The Spoils of Tobacco Wars: Big Settlement Puts Many Lawyers in the Path of a Windfall." *New York Times,* Dec. 22, 1998, p. C1; McGinley, L. "Humana Faces Suits on Matters of Coverage." *Wall Street Journal,* Oct. 5, 1999, p. A3.

93. Hagland, M. "Blood In the Water." *Healthcare Business,* Mar.–Apr. 2000, p. 42.

94. Toran, M. W. "The Emerging Managed Care Risk." *Risk and Insurance,* Sept. 1, 2000, *11,* 19–22.

95. Studdert, D. M., Sage, W. M., Grensburg, C. R., and Hensler, D. R. "Suing Health Plans." *Health Affairs,* Nov.–Dec. 1999, *18,* 24.

96. Hewitt Associates. "U.S. Employers Are Frustrated with Health Care Delivery." Lincolnshire, Ill.: Hewitt Associates, Feb. 12, 2001.

97. Kaiser Family Foundation and HRET, *Employer Health Benefits 2000,* p. 174.

98. Employee Benefits Research Institute, *Health Confidence Survey: 2000 Results.*

99. Commonwealth Fund. "Doctors in Five Countries See Decline in Quality of Care." News release. [www.cmwf.org/media/releases/hsph_physicians_release_10122000.dsp], Oct. 2, 2000.

100. Kaiser Family Foundation and HRET, *Employer Health Benefits 2000.*

101. Wee, C. C., and others. "Influence of Financial Productivity Incentives on the Use of Preventive Care." *American Journal of Medicine,* Feb. 15, 2001, *110,* 181–187.

102. Williams, M. V., Baker, D. W., Parker, R. M., and Nurss, J. R. "Relationship of Functional Health Literacy to Patients' Knowledge of Their Chronic Disease: A Study of Patients with Hypertension and Diabetes." *Archives of Internal Medicine,* Jan. 26, 1998, *158,* 166–176.

103. Robert Monoson, M.D., personal communication to the author, 2002.

104. Croasdale, M. "Everyone Talks About Quality, Few Pay for It." *American Medical News,* Feb. 18, 2002, p. 1.

105. Wynia, M. K., Cummins, D. S., Van Geest, J. B., and Wilson, I. B. "Physician Manipulation of Reimbursement Rules for Patients: Between a Rock and a Hard Place." *Journal of the American Medical Association,* Apr. 12, 2000, *283,* 1858–1865.

106. Dickey, N. W., and McManamin, P. "Putting Power into Patient Choice." *New England Journal of Medicine,* Oct. 21, 1999, *341,* 1305–1308.

107. Ralph Snyderman, M.D., personal communication to the author, 2002.

108. "The Competitive Edge: HMO Industry Report 10.2." *Medical Benefits,* Dec. 15, 2000, pp. 4–5.

109. J.P. Morgan, *Managed Care Outlook.* New York: J.P. Morgan, Jan. 6, 2003, p. 51.

110. J.P. Morgan, *Managed Care Outlook,* p. 12.

111. J.P. Morgan, *Managed Care Outlook,* p. 12.

112. Pear, R. "White House and Senate Hit Impasse on Patients' Rights." *New York Times,* Aug. 2, 2002, p. 17; Lankford, K. "Patients Flex Their Muscle." *Kiplinger's Personal Finance Magazine,* Jan. 2002, *56,* 90–92; Flanigan, J. "Patients' Rights and Health Care Costs Are Expanding Together." *Los Angeles Times,* Aug. 5, 2001, p. 1.

113. Strauss, P. "Providers, HMOs Could Benefit from Supreme Court's AWP Ruling. *Managed Care Week,* Apr. 14, 2003, pp. 5, 6.

114. Knox, R. A. "New Name, New Slant on Hospital 'Merger.'" *Boston Globe,* Mar. 22, 1994, p. 21.

115. Kowalczyk, L. "Hospitals Raising Rates for HMOs." *Boston Sunday Globe,* Mar. 18, 2000, pp. A1, A22.

116. Lesser, C. S., and Ginsberg, P. B. *New Cost and Access Challenges Emerge.* Washington, D.C.: Center for Studying Health System Change, Feb. 2001, p. 2.

117. Licking, E. "Health Care." *Business Week,* Jan. 8, 2001, p. 116.

118. "Blues Plans Drive Increase in Health Insurance Profits." *Reuters Medical News,* Sept. 3, 2002.

119. "How Business Rates." *Business Week,* Sept. 11, 2000, p. 148.

120. Licking, "Health Care."

121. See Martinez, B. "Aetna Tries to Improve Bedside Manner in Bid to Help Bottom Line." *Wall Street Journal,* Feb. 23, 2001, pp. A1, A9.

122. Robinson, J. C. "At the Helm of an Insurance Giant." *Health Affairs,* Nov.–Dec. 1999, *18,* 89–99.

123. Robinson, "At the Helm of an Insurance Giant," p. 89.

124. Martinez, "Aetna Tries to Improve Bedside Manner," p. A9.

125. Robinson, "At the Helm of an Insurance Giant," p. 96.

126. Martinez, "Aetna Tries to Improve Bedside Manner," pp. A1, A9.

127. Robinson, "At the Helm of an Insurance Giant," p. 99.

128. Martinez, "Aetna Tries to Improve Bedside Manner," p. A1.

129. Hogan, C., Ginsberg, P. R., and Gabel, J. R. "Tracking Health Care Costs: Inflation Returns." *Health Affairs,* Nov.–Dec. 2000, *19,* pp. 217–223.

130. U.S. Census Bureau, *Statistical Abstract of the United States: 1999,* p. 495, table 776.

131. Medicare Payment Advisory Commission. *Report to the Congress,* p. 14.

132. Jaklevic, M. C. "What Hospitals 'See' They Get." *Modern Healthcare,* Mar. 6, 2000, p. 61.

133. Sherlock, D. *Blues.* Gwynedd, Penn.: Sherlock Co., 2000.

134. Vogeli, C., and others. "Self-Referral in Point-of-Service Health Plans." *Journal of the American Medical Association,* May 2, 2001, *285,* 2223–2231.

135. Ferris, T. G., Chang, Y., Blumenthal, D., and Pearson, S. D. "Leaving Gatekeeping Behind." *New England Journal of Medicine,* Nov. 1, 2001, *345,* 1312–1316.

136. Miller, R. H., and Luft, H. "HMO Plan Performance Update." *Health Affairs,* May–June 2002, *21,* 80–81.

137. Hogan and others, "Tracking Health Care Costs."

138. Pear, R. "Kennedy and Bush Negotiate on Patients' Rights, Alarming Their Allies." *New York Times,* Jan. 23, 2002, p. 12.

CHAPTER THREE

The Solution

The problems of our health insurance system appear overwhelming. Many people cannot obtain reasonably priced health insurance, even though our governments and employers break the bank to pay for it. And despite these high prices the health insurance sector is struggling to stay afloat.

Nor do the high prices yield services that satisfy those who do have health insurance. In their eyes, our standardized, managed care health insurance policies all too often fail to provide the health care they need. Americans worry that payment practices needlessly fragment and limit care. They also worry about the influence of health insurance rules on their doctors' medical care decisions. These concerns are pervasive: in one survey 44 percent of those with regular physician relationships voiced them.[1]

All too often, sick people and their loved ones also despair of the inhumanity of their treatment. Yes, the doctor was great—only 7 percent of Americans think that doctors fail to put their needs first[2]—but they are frustrated by the waits, the rudeness, the abuse, the lack of information and support, the pain thoughtlessly and needlessly foisted on the sick. Most blame the growth of

In this chapter I use the metaphor of "breakfast insurance." A similar metaphor is used by Gerald L. Musgrave, Leigh Tripoli, and Fu Ling You in "Lunch Insurance," *Regulation*, Fall 1992, *15*(4), 16–24. I was not aware of it when I wrote this essay; but an early reader, Steve Hyde, kindly called it to my attention. Gerry Musgrave has graciously allowed me to use my essay if I acknowledge his, which I do most gratefully and happily.

managed care for these problems. Although the satisfaction levels with a doctor's visit have remained at 85 percent, or more, since 1978, the majority of Americans have come to believe that managed care will harm the quality of care and is generally "a bad thing."[3] And the health care system's lack of attention to self-care fails those who want to help themselves and fails their dedicated doctors, who are increasingly depressed by the loss of professional autonomy they perceive. Although insurers have recently relaxed access to providers, in itself, easier access will not correct these other problems.

Former U.S. vice president Al Gore's intervention to secure Aetna's continued support for a brain-damaged child exemplifies some of these concerns. It is wonderful that Gore persuaded the insurer to revise its decision to abandon this child; but if we all need a U.S. vice president's intervention to manage our health insurance benefits, we are in deep trouble.[4]

How did we get here?

This question is all the more puzzling in view of the massive expenditures on health care, a seventh of our gross domestic product in the United States and nearly 10 percent in other developed countries.

To me, the reason is obvious: health care systems worldwide are guided by someone other than the consumer.

In the United States, health insurers and employers hold sway. In most of Europe, Asia, South America, and the Middle East, government officials are firmly in control. No consumer is in sight.

Do not get me wrong. Most of these people—bureaucrats, insurers, and technocrats—are like most of us: they do the best they can. They want to do good. They do not want to do bad. But their perspective is elitist. Rather than supporting consumer choice and control, they want to supplant it. Their kind of thinking views the consumer as muted, muddled, malleable; a pawn in someone's grand health care design; a statistic in a health care benefit-cost analysis.

The results? Bea, an elderly woman stripped of her assets; Jacqui, a middle-aged woman who spent her dying years fighting her health insurer; Paul's grandfather, an old man killed by a wayward social calculus; Eleanore's parents, humiliated in the search for care; Sam, a healthy man who struggles to find reasonably priced health insurance only because he is self-employed; Vivian, a diabetic woman nearly robbed of her life by the lack of supportive information that would help her to help herself; and doctors like Rob Monoson, valiantly fighting to deliver the best care for their patients.

The cure is as obvious as the diagnosis: we need a new health care system, one guided by consumers.

After all, who can better right these wrongs than the people who endure them? Armed with money, choice, and information, consumers can reward those who cherish their humanity and punish those who treat them as ciphers and statistics.

Bea, Jacqui, and Paul's grandfather would reward insurers whose policies featured the benefits they wanted: coverage of long-term care for Bea; of focused, experienced breast cancer providers for Jacqui; and of drugs with minimal side effects for Paul's grandfather. Eleanore's parents would reward the providers who treated them with the courtesy they deserved. Vivian's custom would be sought by the physicians who wanted to help her to help herself. People like her would in turn reward physicians like Dr. Monoson.

And in a consumer-driven system, health insurers would act like automobile and life insurers who sell directly to the consumer. They would court all consumers, including self-employed people like Sam, and not only those employed in large organizations.

As delineated in Chapter Five, these results can be accompanied by improved cost control that would help employers to broaden their safety net. After all, who can better weigh the costs versus the benefits of health insurance and health care—the user or an agent miles removed from the user's concerns? When manufacturers adopted consumer-driven quality control, products became both better and cheaper. Similarly, health care organizations that are clearly focused on consumers' needs for integrated, supportive care raise quality and thereby control costs.

Controlled health care costs will enable more of the uninsured and their employers to afford the health insurance they need and may increase the willingness of the U.S. Congress to expand coverage.

To appreciate the impact of consumer-based competition on the service sector, recall the productivity gains of the U.S. economy from 1995 to 1999. A 2002 McKinsey report revealed that three sectors accounted for much of the growth: wholesale and retail trade and securities and commodity brokerages.[5] Two of these sectors are consumer driven and all provide services. In contrast, from 1978 to 2001, the defined benefit, third-party-driven health care sector demonstrated productivity *losses* of 24 percent compared to the nonfarm productivity gain of 42 percent. Physicians' output per employee decreased by a hefty 29 percent, in part because of the massive administrative demands of coping with managed care's just-say-no policies.[6]

AETNA *REDUX*

Happily, Aetna points the way to the future. In 2001, Aetna joined the consumer-driven health care movement. It introduced Aetna HealthFund:

> [A]n innovative health product that gives employers additional flexibility in customized product design and gives consumers greater choice and control in directing the health benefits provided by their employers. Aetna HealthFund combines a preferred provider plan with [an] . . . employer-funded health savings account

that can be rolled over at the end of the year with any remaining funds going toward covered services in subsequent years. [It] also includes Aetna Navigator, [an] . . . online resource that [enables] members to manage their health and track health expenditures on a personalized website and to obtain pertinent information about health issues.

Noted an Aetna official, "We believe this new product may be of particular interest to employers who are looking for new ways to give employees more flexibility to choose a plan that meets their own unique health care needs. Aetna HealthFund is the first plan of its type to be offered by a national, full-service health benefits company."

The first employer to select Aetna HealthFund as an option for its employees was Aetna itself. "We believe Aetna HealthFund will give Aetna employees an attractive alternative to the other Aetna (managed care) plans they can select currently," said Aetna's senior vice president of human resources.

Aetna HealthFund is the first product introduction resulting from Aetna's new strategic focus on customer segments. "Aetna has a history of working closely with our customers to evaluate next generation products and determine what makes the most sense for them," said an Aetna official, without a trace of irony. "We will be working with a number of employers in the middle market segment, specifically those with 300 to 3,000 employees, to help them evaluate consumer-directed product offerings which are just now coming to market and offer guidance on matching plan design to individual employer needs."[7]

By 2003, over one hundred thousand people were enrolled. Aetna's new CEO, Dr. John Rowe, was lauded for these and other steps that resulted in a near doubling of the firm's stock price.[8]

IN HEALTH INSURANCE IT'S THE DETAILS THAT MATTER

Aetna's plan is a harbinger of what is to come.

But it is merely a harbinger—one small marker on a map. If consumer-driven health insurance follows the model of other consumer-driven sectors, the market will be flooded with choice. These newly differentiated products will correct the flaws of what we have available today.

The fault lines lie deep, buried in the limited choice, lack of consumer control, distorted pricing, and nonexistent information that characterize the present system. It is the details of our present third-party-driven health insurance system that caused these problems. And it is the details of the new consumer-driven products that will correct them.

Some ideologues assert that the mere act of consumer control will fix the problems. I wish I could agree with them. But as the tragedies that unfolded during the transformation of the former Communist USSR to a market-driven economy vividly demonstrated, mere consumer control does not do the trick.

The transformation must attend to the details; the characteristics that foster the problems must be identified and corrected.

As a society, we Americans love to believe in quick fixes. That is why we are bombarded with miracle diets, seven-minute managers, and thirty days to firmer thighs. But in our bones, we know that detail, detail, detail is the key to success. "Life is 5 percent inspiration, 95 percent perspiration"; "God [the Devil; someone powerful] is in the details"—the ubiquity of these sentiments about the importance of detail underscores the widespread acceptance of the message. Details account for Oprah's success and Roseanne's failure as a talk-show hostess, for Red Auerbach's winning streak and Rick Pitino's failure with the Boston Celtics, and for the delicious flavor of home-baked bread and the cotton texture of its commercial counterpart.

When it comes to our health care system too, success is going to depend on getting the details right. This chapter identifies the detailed characteristics that are essential to a consumer-driven health insurance system and assesses their impact in some early-adopter organizations.

BREAKFAST INSURANCE: A METAPHOR FOR HEALTH INSURANCE

To understand the functioning of health insurance, consider a hypothetical insurance product—insurance for breakfast.

I hope you will find this metaphor as amusing as I intend it to be. Health insurance is no laughing matter, of course. It is vitally important and deadly serious. Indeed, from my teaching experience I know that the "deadly" serious aspect of health insurance causes a problem when I begin describing the details that plague the market. Intelligent people go into a stupor when the health insurance industry is discussed. Its complexity boggles their minds. Breakfast insurance, however, is a humorous, approachable insurance product, yet the origins and cures of its problems largely echo those of the health insurance sector.

Of course it is only a metaphor. Unlike breakfasts, health care services have long-term consequences and their costs are highly concentrated: 80 percent of the costs are attributable to roughly 20 percent of the users. And eating breakfast does not mirror the life or death consequences of health care. But its very ordinariness makes the subject more accessible. And the salient dimensions of the breakfast insurance product I describe are identical to those of health insurance.

It's the Nooks: No, It's the Crannies

I hope that you will agree with my assessment of the power of metaphor when you finish reading it. (As an old teacher, I know that a more realistic statement would conclude with the phrase "*if*" you finish reading it.)

Do you remember that ridiculous Thomas' English Muffins ad?

In the ad, a Casper Milquetoast and a great big guy are sitting next to each other at a food counter, blissfully munching on some toasted Thomas' English Muffins, slathered with butter.

"It's the nooks," ventures the little guy.

"No. It's the crannies," thunders the big one.

A battle royal ensues over the inherent message: Thomas' English Muffins have extra deep nooks and crannies that trap whatever you spread on them.

Stupid, huh?

Well, the ad worked for me. I love those English muffins. Sure they cost a little more. But to me they taste much better than the limp, bland supermarket brands. I find them so much better that I will not eat an English muffin other than Thomas'.

Each of the millions of people like me across the United States has his or her own little breakfast preferences. Some prefer Post's Raisin Bran to Kellogg's, Bigelow's tea to Lipton's, white eggs to brown ones, skim milk to whole milk.

Some like to eat breakfast at home, some swear by their local diner, and still others get their jollies eating a power breakfast while seated conspicuously in a plush booth in a fancy restaurant.

I may not approve of all their food preferences or restaurant venues. But their choices are none of my business. They can do what they like. After all, their money pays for their preferences. As for me, I will stick with my Thomas' English Muffins.

As a consumer-driven industry, the breakfast sector works pretty well. You can get a darn good breakfast for very little money. You have access to many choices and continued innovations in both products and services. You can obtain mountains of readily accessible information about your choices: *Consumer Reports* and other publications evaluate various brands of breakfast foods, and Zagat's *America's Top Restaurants* and local reviewers in individual cities evaluate restaurants. And the government protects you too. It oversees the cleanliness and safety of your food and its preparers. The U.S. government's Food and Drug Administration monitors food processors, and local public health officials oversee the cleanliness of restaurants and publish their findings in local media.

In the consumer-driven restaurant sector, chefs hold an honored professional status. Charlie Trotter exemplifies this breed. A sampling of his thoughts on the subject of dessert illustrates the intelligence and expertise that chefs devote to their craft. For example, writing in the "The Chef," a regular *New York Times* column, Trotter notes: "The kind of planning that goes into . . . the meal, the careful thinking of how to balance every dish against every other . . . breaks down when it comes to [dessert]. What comes last is usually just sweetness and heft. [But] I want something that takes time to appreciate, a last course you don't spoon up mindlessly but one that you can linger over and contemplate."[9] OK. It is only dessert. But who can deny Trotter's intellect, passion, and skill? Following his essay is a recipe that exemplifies these qualities and explains Trotter's elevated status.

Defined Benefit Breakfast Insurance: Phase One

Now, imagine that your employer has provided you with breakfast insurance.

Her motives were pure.

She knew that you need to eat breakfast and that many people were skipping breakfast. They were too busy to cook at home and did not want to spend the money to eat in restaurants. The "skipped breakfast" problems of those with special needs—such as eating disorders and illnesses linked to nutrition, such as diabetes and metabolic diseases—were of special concern to her.

Your employer was deluged with information about her role in solving this major national problem. All urged her to offer breakfast insurance to her employees. Breakfastologists demonstrated that skipping breakfast caused dire effects: lower productivity, reduced life-span, and increased illness, depression, and bad breath. And U.S. breakfast economists bemoaned the absence of insurance for breakfasts eaten in restaurants in the United States. They pointed to the European economies that had universal breakfast insurance, controlled by the government. We Americans would be as productive, long-lived, healthy, jovial, and sweet-smelling as the Europeans if we only provided breakfast insurance, they averred.

Your employer sympathized with these pleas.

And anyway, a quirk in the income tax code favored her paying for breakfast insurance: a corporation like hers could deduct the expenses of breakfast insurance in computing the income taxes it owed to the U.S. government. And you, you lucky person, would not owe income taxes on the value of the breakfast insurance she paid on your behalf, but if you purchased breakfast insurance for yourself or ate breakfast at home, your costs could not be deducted from your individual income for tax computation purposes. In most cases only corporations could take this deduction.

Your employer was a sweetheart. She decided to offer breakfast insurance. To simplify things, she decided to choose one insurance company and to pay it the same price for each enrollee. She thought it was only fair to have the lettuce nibblers subsidize the expense of those with special nutritional needs. But to protect herself from the possibility of rampant breakfast expenditures that might accompany insurance, she listed the "covered items" you could eat for breakfast—eggs, milk, coffee, sugar, bread, cereal, and so on. She even threw in steak for the former football players on her payroll and vegetables for the lettuce nibblers. These were your breakfast insurance "benefits."

She signed up with the venerable Baetena as the insurer.

Heaven, huh?

Initially, it seemed that way.

But it's a funny thing about human nature: we take advantage of the things we perceive as "free."

Pretty soon, people stopped eating breakfast at home. Instead, they scarfed down three-course breakfasts in restaurants. And they ate large quantities of very expensive meals—steak, five eggs, and a side order of out-of-season tomato salad. To the eaters the prices for these meals presented no problem. After all, they were not paying. Some anonymous insurer was paying.

Prices began inflating wildly. To obtain payment for the covered items, restaurateurs disaggregated their menu offerings.

Oh, you want sugar with your coffee? That will be another $.50. And cream? Hand over another dollar.

An order of toast? Five bucks.

A cup of coffee? Three bucks.

No more $3.99 breakfast specials—eggs, juice, toast, and coffee. Say goodbye to the heart-healthy delight—$4.99 for yogurt, whole-wheat cereal, skim milk, fresh fruit, and tea.

The chefs who once took pride in their ability to present wholesome, inexpensive meals grew increasingly unhappy. The days of creating such meals were gone.

Managed Breakfasts: Phase Two

Now, your employer was starting to worry. Her breakfast insurance expenses were going through the roof.

She considered rescinding the benefit, but the tax-code advantages virtually dictated that she should pay for it. And restaurant breakfasts had become so expensive that employees rated breakfast insurance as their number one benefit.

In despair, she turned to a new kind of insurer: a managed breakfast plan. These managed breakfast guys had some nifty stratagems to control her costs. They planned to

- *Limit the restaurants that were eligible for insurance.* In exchange for the volume of business they would send to these lucky few restaurants, the managed breakfast guys planned to muscle down the prices those restaurants charged.

- *Restrict access to expensive food items.* So, if you wanted to eat steak, you needed a referral from the breakfast gatekeeper. After all, for most people a couple of strips of soy-based protein would do the job.

- *When possible, require the use of cheaper, generic items.* No more Thomas' English Muffins for people like me.

The managed breakfast crew assured your employer that they would provide better breakfasts at a lower price. They even tossed in some extra "covered benefits" that were important for health, such as soy products and vitamin pills.

Bruce: The Human Resource Managed Breakfast Movie Star

To encourage competition your employer wanted to offer plans from several different managed breakfast insurers. But the breakfast insurance thing was getting out of hand. She had a business to run. She was not a breakfast insurance specialist. So she turned the whole thing over to Bruce, newly designated as the human resource (HR) department's breakfast benefits maven.

Bruce was a red-blooded American. He believed in competition as much as the next guy. But in his eyes there were too many breakfast insurers. He could not possibly offer all of their plans to the employees. Instead, he decided to limit the choice of insurers to a few—two or at most three. And to make it easy to compare the value for the money of these different breakfast insurers, he standardized their covered items so all the insurers offered identical benefits: eggs, yes, but employees had to pay for fresh fruit out of their own pockets.

Unwittingly, Bruce was enforcing a defined benefit approach to breakfast.

Like many human resource people, Bruce was not a finance guy. Far from it, he had a master's degree in organizational behavior. So when he evaluated the financial aspects of breakfast insurance, he couldn't follow the numbers exactly. Nevertheless, Bruce believed that U.S. Breakfast's people were the sharpest of the breakfast manager tacks. They sure looked the part—they were all lean and talked fast and confidently. And all the breakfastologists assured him that U.S. Breakfast was among the best of the managed breakfast crowd.

To induce employees to sign up for U.S. Breakfast's insurance plan, he offered it for free; at the same time, he charged the employees who wanted to sign up with their old-fashioned breakfast insurer, Baetena, a very high price. Although both U.S. Breakfast and Baetena charged the company roughly equal prices, Bruce believed that in the long run, those skinny guys at U.S. Breakfast would lower costs much more effectively than the old-fashioned, unmanaged breakfast Baetena folks. The breakfastologists and breakfast economists applauded Bruce's wisdom.

They featured him as the keynote speaker at the National Managed Breakfast Convention and the meetings of the National Academy on Breakfast Insurance Policy and Administration, a self-selected group of experts.

After all, Bruce was their agent of change. He was finally realizing their vision of how breakfast should be prepared. The breakfastologists had long documented that those farmers, food processors, chefs, and restaurateurs were out of control. Their studies showed that there was simply too much variability among these people in the breakfast food chain, but their important messages had been ignored. As for breakfast eaters, well, they too needed managing.

Consider the important issue of scrambled eggs, for example. The breakfastologists were worried about inconsistencies in the way chefs scrambled eggs. Different chefs used different ingredients and cooking techniques—some added milk, some favored brown eggs, some fried in butter, and some cooked the eggs over low heat in a copper pan on a gas range. The scrambled egg guidelines derived by the expert breakfastologists, on the basis of many laboratory studies, specified brown or white eggs, quickly fried in a bit of margarine in an iron skillet on an electric range. The eggs were to be cooked to a firm consistency, with curds less than one-half inch but more than one-eighth inch in size.

But those pesky chefs failed to follow the guidelines. The chefs felt that cooking was an art more than a science. They thought that their responsibility was to respond to their customers' needs. These needs differed by region of the country, ethnicity, race, and gender and even by education. The chefs found the breakfastologists' rigid guidelines ludicrous, a fantasy created by those who had little contact with the customer.

The criticisms stung. Although some of the breakfastologists were former chefs, they no longer practiced the art. In reality most of the breakfastologists could not actually scramble eggs, but they had learned the sociology and economics of the breakfast industry in the course of their lengthy Ph.D. studies. Many had devoted their careers to the development of expert guidelines about important breakfast items, such as preparing oatmeal and baking bread, derived from extensive econometric studies and the advice of the experts in the National Academy on Breakfasts, but the breakfast industry continued to ignore them.

Managed breakfast insurers would change all that.

Like the breakfastologists, the breakfast economists also favored the idea of managed breakfasts. If the United States were going to pass up the wonderful European example of breakfasts provided by the government, then managed breakfasts were the next best thing.

But despite the support of the experts, one thing worried Bruce. He had no way of judging the quality of the breakfasts and the consumers' satisfaction with the restaurants and their products.

The restaurant reviewers had pretty much died out when the breakfast industry was transformed to a managed breakfast payment system. After all, if consumers have little choice, what is the point of reviews? And the limited restaurants and standard benefits of managed breakfast insurance obviated the feedback that could have been obtained from consumer selection.

Bruce's only information was about the costs.

Yet he was ambivalent about hiring experts to rate quality and employee satisfaction. What if the raters revealed that the employees were dissatisfied with the choices he had made on their behalf?

And his boss, the CEO, was primarily interested in controlling costs.

The heck with measuring quality.

Bruce began to mousse his hair and wear black turtlenecks, Armani suits, and sunglasses. He became a star—the managed breakfast movement's poster child.

All Hell Breaks Loose: The Yolk's on You

Pretty soon, your employer was longing for the good old days.

Her breakfast insurance prices were zooming out of sight.

The few restaurants selected for coverage by the managed breakfast insurers became so powerful that they could enforce substantial price increases. Oligopolistic "partners"—loose mergers of the few remaining restaurant establishments—negotiated on behalf of their members. The insurer had no choice but to meet their price demands.

Simultaneously, the restaurants tried to reduce their costs, primarily by substituting cheap, high-profit covered items for more expensive, low-profit ones. The salsa that once sparkled with fresh tomatoes and parsley was now goopy with canned tomatoes and stuffed with inexpensive chopped onions.

And the vitamin pill providers, newly covered by the managed breakfast insurers, were increasing their prices, inventing new vitamin formulations, and advertising directly to consumers to increase vitamin pill utilization.

The expenses of the breakfastologists, many of whom now consulted for the managed breakfast insurers, were only adding to these costs.

Ironically, the insurers were unhappy too. All those cost increases were cutting their profits.

But the CEO's biggest concern was that her employees were mad—really, really mad. Bruce's price subsidies for U.S. Breakfast's managed breakfast plans had caused most of them to switch away from Baetena. But they disliked the limited restaurant choice of the managed breakfast insurers. And they resented the fact that their favorite restaurants were not included in the managed breakfast list. They were also dissatisfied with the interaction with U.S. Breakfast's gatekeepers. Some disliked the hassles needed to obtain payment for the foods they wanted. After all, many wanted fresh fruit, not soy milk. And the seriously ill among them claimed that the managed breakfast insurers had worsened their health status by making it difficult for them to obtain the expensive food they required.

As for people like me, they disliked the denial of their old favorite, Thomas' English Muffins.

This anger did not go unnoticed. A flotilla of sharks—plaintiff's lawyers—swam in, smelling the prospect of juicy class-action settlements.

The food industry was angry too—especially those companies whose products were not included among the covered benefits.

Finally, the talented, artistic chefs who made it all happen were leaving the industry in droves. They did not like all the second-guessing by the breakfastologists and breakfast economists, and they did not want to spend their time negotiating with them for payments.

A few brave chefs continued to follow their vision and offer creative meals tailored to the needs of their clients—"value" meals, heart-healthy meals, gourmet meals, and so on. But few paid them for meals anymore. Instead, the restaurateurs were constantly urging chefs to whip up recipes that used high volumes of low-cost ingredients. The chefs felt that good taste and nutrition was being sacrificed for cost.

Worst of all, the problem your CEO had tried to solve by offering breakfast insurance in the first place, skipped breakfasts, was at an all-time peak.

People skipped breakfast because restaurant service and food quality were deteriorating. The restaurateurs seemed more interested in glad-handing Bruce than in serving their patrons. After all, Bruce paid the bill, not the patrons. And the chefs felt handcuffed and depressed.

The employees with serious eating problems were not receiving the help they needed. The insurers received the same payment for each enrollee, and these folks had very expensive eating needs. To make their earnings, the managed breakfast insurers could not become excessively interested in serving the employees with eating disorders—morbidly obese or anorexic—or those with illnesses linked to nutrition, such as diabetes and heart disease.

Especially hard hit were the uninsured self-employed and the poor. Breakfast prices were now so high that they simply could not afford to eat a regular breakfast any more.

Consumer-Driven Breakfast Insurance: Back to the Future

In response the CEO switched to a consumer-driven breakfast insurance.

Although she continued to pay for her employees' breakfast insurance, to maintain the favorable tax treatment and the market power that group purchasing enabled, she made the following changes:

- She switched to consumer-driven breakfast insurance. She gave her employees a fixed sum of money and a large array of breakfast insurance policies to choose from. She thus provided the enrollees with incentives to treat the money she spent as if it were their own.

- She enlarged the number of breakfast insurance options. Some of the insurers maintained the managed breakfast options. Others offered a larger selection of restaurants, a greater range of covered items, and various levels of co-pays and deductibles. Some even targeted enrollees with special, frequently expensive, needs.

- She switched from insurance for covered items to a payment system in which restaurateurs named their own prices for meals. She thus rewarded chefs with an incentive to exercise their creativity. Those who provided good value for the money would succeed. Those who did not would fail.

- She provided extensive customer satisfaction data and more objective quality data about the insurance plans, restaurants, and the specific foods they served.

- She subsidized all insurers at the same rates. Employees' view of prices thus became entirely congruent with hers.

- She paid the insurers in accordance with the needs of their enrollees. Insurers who enrolled sick people with special nutritional needs received a higher price than those who enrolled individuals with average needs. Although her total costs remained the same, this payment formula encouraged insurers to innovate. After all, they were now receiving prices commensurate with their costs.

- She changed Bruce's role. He was no longer the poster child of the managed breakfast movement. Instead, he became the organizer of choice and information for newly empowered breakfast consumers.

Insurance for the Sick, the Self-Employed, the Poor, the Employers, the Chefs, the Insurers

A few years after the CEO made these changes, the breakfast situation improved. The skipping-breakfast problem abated; costs were controlled; people with serious nutritional problems were being served; and employees, chefs, farmers, the whole kit and caboodle, were happier.

Among the biggest winners were the restaurants and chefs who gave people the tasty, nutritious meals and courteous, efficient service they wanted. The most successful ones created guidelines for their menus, including how to scramble eggs. But these guidelines were devised by the chefs in response to their perceptions of their customers' needs, not by third-party breakfastologists.

The competition among restaurants moderated prices and enabled the poor and the self-employed to start eating breakfast again.

Zagat's issued a special *Breakfast* edition. And breakfasts were deluged with other reviewers' attention too. These evaluations enabled patrons to evaluate costs versus quality.

Breakfast suppliers who focused on people with special needs succeeded too because the new consumer-driven policies paid them more for these customers.

Breakfast insurers who responded to consumer demands were restored to profitability.

The CEO achieved these results with a simple change. *By switching to consumer-driven breakfast insurance, she restored choice and control to the employees, restaurants, and chefs.*

Although she did not cede control entirely, she created the elements of a real market by providing

- Incentives for consumers to choose intelligently—as if they were using their own money
- Incentives for providers to innovate by enabling them, and not a third party, to set the prices for the services they wanted to sell
- Incentives for insurers to offer innovative products with payments that reflected the users' needs
- Many distinctive choices
- Plenty of the good information that enables intelligent choice
- Transparent prices that reflected her costs, with equal subsidies for every option

There were a few losers. The breakfastologists' and breakfast economists' roles were much reduced. They returned to lauding the virtues of the European, government-controlled, universal breakfast system. And not all the chefs, restaurateurs, farmers, and other food industry breakfast participants succeeded. Those who could not respond to the demands of the consumer-driven sector failed. As for Bruce, he was no longer a star. He washed the mousse out of his hair and, clad in standard business garb, slipped back into corporate anonymity, along with millions of his peers. He mournfully donated the Armanis to the Salvation Army.

Pricing Breakfast Insurance Policies and Payments to Restaurants and Chefs

When the breakfast insurance companies required the employer to pay the same price for all enrollees, regardless of their nutritional needs, the results were not optimal. The insurers argued that this pricing makes insurance affordable to those with special needs. So, as illustrated in Figure 3.1, in the area labeled "One-Price-for-All," the bagel muncher and the person with severe food allergies are both priced at $3.86 per meal, even though the special eater's meal costs $25, and the other's meal costs only $1.90. At an average insurer price of $3.86 per person, the employer subsidizes each meal by $3.10 and the employees pay $.76.

How do these pricing policies affect the breakfast industry? Ironically, one-price policies motivate insurers to avoid those who really need the insurance. As the left-hand side of Figure 3.1 illustrates, under the one-price-for-all policy, insurers earn more when they serve the little eaters than when they serve the special needs individuals. After all, they make money, $1.96, on each of the bagel munchers and lose a hefty $21.14 on each of the others. One easy way to minimize the costs of serving these special needs people is to make it difficult for them to get the breakfast they need. For example, the insurer could require them to obtain approval for every slice of nonallergenic bread, limit their dining to hard-to-reach restaurants, and narrow the range of foods they can eat.

The insurers' incentives change, however, under a different-prices-for-different-needs policy (the right-hand side of Figure 3.1), where the employer pays more for the special needs person, $26.10, and less for the others. Insurers now have no reason to favor one enrollee or the other. Indeed, they earn more profit, $1.86, from the special needs eater than with the little eaters, whose profit is only $.81 per meal.

Further, the employers' and enrollees' costs and the insurers' profits remain the same under each form of pricing. Sure, the employer subsidy for the special needs person increases substantially with differential pricing, but the employer subsidies for the little eaters decrease commensurately.

Let us now turn to the impact of these two kinds of insurance pricing on chefs.

In one approach, the insurance companies generally pay every restaurant the same price for every covered breakfast item, regardless of the quality of the food or service. For administrative reasons, the insurers do not pay for meals, whose menus could differ significantly, but rather for a standardized set of individual items. This pricing penalizes innovative chefs, who once turned out creative breakfast menus. Instead of encouraging them to focus on a well-balanced breakfast, such as a heart-healthy one, this payment system forces them to focus on each of a breakfast's component parts. For example, if eggs are better compensated by the insurer than grain products, the restaurant will feature myriad egg concoctions; but if the reverse obtains, the menu will be crammed with cereals, French toast, waffles, and pancakes.

Further, the chefs have little incentive to improve quality because the insurers pay Joe's Diner and the Ritz Café the same. If prices rise, turf warfare breaks out. For example, when overall breakfast prices rose as described earlier, the dairy and poultry industries each fingered the other as the culprit. Under this supplier payment scheme, no one has a financial incentive to look out for the total welfare of the diner. Further, service quality and waiting times deteriorate because the customer does not pay the bill. The payer, the insurers, and the employer have little information about these aspects of quality. And even if such data were available, how can insurers adjust the prices they pay to the restaurants for the enormous variations in responses by customers?

	One-Price-for-All Pricing					Different-Prices-for-Different-Needs Pricing				
	Cost per Meal	Price Paid per Meal to Insurer by Employer	Price Paid per Meal by Employee	Total Cost to Employer, Enrollees	Profit (Loss) to Insurer, per Meal, Total	Cost per Meal	Price Paid per Meal to Insurer by Employer	Price Paid per Meal by Employee	Total Cost to Employer, Enrollees	Profit (Loss) to Insurer, per Meal, Total
Twenty little eaters	$1.90	$3.10	$.76		$1.96	$1.90	$1.95	$.76		$.81
One special needs eater	$25.00	$3.10	$.76		($21.14)	$25.00	$26.10	$.76		$1.86
Total cost to employer				$65.10					$65.10	
Total cost to employee				$15.96					$15.96	
Total profit to insurer					$18.58					$18.58

Figure 3.1. Breakfast Insurance Pricing.

Note: Actual numbers do not add precisely because of rounding.

In contrast, when employers pay the insurers different prices for people with different needs and when insurers permit the chefs to name their own prices and create their own menus, total costs are likely to fall. For example, if an innovative chef creates an excellent dietary regimen that costs only $21.60 per special needs meal, an insurer might sign the chef for an exclusive at $22.60, thus enabling the chef to earn a dollar per person. The insurer can then direct special needs clients to this chef, reduce its price to the employer from $26.10 to $24.80, and yet increase its profitability too.

Differential pricing thus motivates both the insurers and providers to compete for the people with special needs with cost effective products that are likely to reduce total expenditures.

Notes

1. Hargraves, J. L. "Patients Concerned About Insurer Influences." Data Bulletin No. 17. Washington, D.C.: Center for Studying Health System Change, June 2000.

2. Hargraves, "Patients Concerned About Insurer Influences."

3. Blendon, R. J., and Benson, J. M. "Americans' Views on Health Policy: A Fifty-Year Historical Perspective." *Health Affairs,* Mar.–Apr. 2001, *20,* 40–41.

4. Pear, R. "Gore's Intervention Restores Care for Ill Baby." *New York Times,* Feb. 29, 2000, p. A18.

5. Lewis, W. W., Palmade, V., Regout, B., and Webb, A. B. "What's Right with the U.S. Economy." *McKinsey Quarterly,* 2002, *1,* 31–40.

6. Mark Ulmer, DRI, personal communication to the author, Jan. 2003. The figures were obtained from DRI's Global Insight fourth-quarter 2002 forecast for its U.S. Industrial Analysis Service. Productivity is derived as a ratio of output per employee.

7. All quotations in the first part of this section about Aetna are from "Aetna Launches Aetna HealthFund™ to Expand Consumer Choice and Decision Making." Press Release. Hartford, Conn.: Aetna, Sept. 19, 2001.

8. Brady, D. "Aetna's Painful Recovery." *Business Week,* Dec. 8, 2003, pp. 86–88.

9. Trotter, C. "Don't Be So Sweet." *New York Times,* Mar. 21, 2001, p. D1.

CHAPTER FOUR

Consumer-Driven Health Insurance

What Works

Because defined benefit health insurance for employer groups is structurally flawed, it causes rapidly inflating costs; inadequate coverage and treatment for the sick; lack of quality incentives; and unhappy consumers, providers, payers, and insurers.

What are the root causes of these problems?

1. Employees have no incentive to trade off resources, as they do when they use their own money.

2. Employees are offered few differentiated health insurance and provider choices.

3. Employees have little useful information about their choices.

4. The prices employees face do not reflect the employer's cost. They are distorted by unequal subsidies to different health plans.

5. The prices paid to providers are determined by third parties. They generally pay efficient, effective providers in the same way as inefficient, ineffective ones. Innovations that integrate care are discouraged because insurers pay for fragmented episodes rather than a bundle of care.

The section of this chapter titled "Early Innovators in Consumer-Driven Health Care" was written by Howard Wizig, the founder of Vivius, Inc., the founding chairman of the Consumer-Driven Health Care Association, and a seasoned health insurance entrepreneur.

6. Insurers and providers are reluctant to innovate in care for the sick when they receive the same payment no matter who enrolls.

A cure requires remedies for each of these problems.

1. Provide Incentives to Shop Intelligently

Part of the cure is to enable employees to shop for health insurance as if they were using their own money. Employers can give employees a fixed sum or enable them to contribute their own funds on a pretax basis, require them to purchase an insurance policy that protects them against catastrophic events, and permit them considerable freedom in using the resulting savings for other health care needs.

For example, if my employer gives me $6,000, which I perceive as mine, to use for health insurance and care, I may opt for a $4,000 policy that insures me against catastrophically expensive events and accrue the remaining $2,000 in my health care savings account so I can purchase the new eyeglasses and the insurance policy that offers the long-term care and pharmaceutical benefits I want. The incentives guard against my overinsuring, and the requirement for catastrophic coverage guards against my underinsuring.

2. Provide Real Choice of Insurance Plans

Another part of the solution is to present employees with a menu of insurance options that differ from each other in the following five features:

- *Types of benefits.* Coverage for long-term care, health promoting regimens, and pharmaceuticals are but some of the new benefits that could be offered.

- *Out-of-pocket maximums.* Policies should enable the choice of higher out-of-pocket maximums in exchange for lower-cost insurance (subject to the requirement of buying a catastrophic insurance policy).

- *Term.* Multiyear policies that induce both the insurer and the enrollee to have a long-term relationship will support activities such as health promotion that pay off in the future.

These first three features will induce the creation of differentiated insurance policies.

- *Method of provider payment.* The providers who choose to offer bundles of care for diseases or procedures should be paid for the bundle, not for each individual item within it, and they should be free to name their own price.

- *Provider organization.* The provider organization can range from "any willing provider" to a tightly linked, small network.

These last two features will induce the kind of differentiated competition among providers that controls costs and improves quality.

3. Provide Relevant Information

It is essential to present two types of information—user ratings and objective data—about two aspects of health care—providers and health plans. This feature ensures transparency, so that Americans can shop for medical care on the basis of information, not rumor. As for the information they want, employees are much more interested in information about providers than about insurers.[1] And they want peer ratings as much as they want objective measures of quality.[2]

4. Provide Equal Subsidies for Each Plan

Each enrollee should be given the same financial contribution toward the cost of each plan and charged the actual price of the health plan to the employer. Currently, the prices enrollees are charged for health insurance rarely parallel the prices paid by their employers. In 2000, only 27 percent of employees were in firms that contributed the same amount to all types of plans. For more than 60 percent of the employees, the price of the plan to the employee reflected factors other than the price to the firm. And the employer's contribution was pegged at the price of the lowest-cost plan for only 57 percent of the employees.[3]

As a result, people may sign up for more insurance than they want because they do not see the real price, just as people who normally eat a bowl of corn flakes for breakfast might start consuming steak and eggs if they perceive them as free. And even if the steak and eggs were not entirely free, if their employer's contribution varied by plan, they might still choose the more expensive option. For example, if the employer subsidizes the $.20 cost of corn flakes by $.15 and the $5.00 cost of steak and eggs by $4.95, then employees perceive the two as equal in cost because they are required to pay only $.05 for each.

Why do employers distort prices in this way? Likely because their human resource (HR) people want enrollees to choose one option over the other for reasons other than current price. For example, if an HR benefit specialist believes that in the long run enrollees will receive better care in an HMO, she might subsidize its cost more than the cost of other options so that the enrollee thinks it is cheaper than the cost of other plans.

Differential price subsidization essentially replaces the enrollees' assessment of the cost effectiveness of different insurance plans with the agent's assessment. It reflects the views of HR personnel that nearly 80 percent of enrollees would have a "harder time" picking quality health insurance plans and "getting good prices" absent their guidance.[4]

Differential subsidization distorts resource allocation, especially in health care, where the purchase of health insurance is very sensitive to price. For example, when one employer switched to a policy of equal subsidization of all its health plans, many employees switched to lower-cost plans. Evaluators concluded that a 1994 price increase of $30 a month would have caused 34 percent of the enrollees to change plans.[5]

This equal subsidies feature ensures that the interests of employers and employees are squarely lined up. When employees choose, they will be looking at the same prices as their employers.

5. Do Not Determine Prices for Providers

Rather than determining prices for providers, enable providers to set their own prices for the bundles of care they select. Presently, providers generally cannot name their prices for a bundle of services. They usually are forced to accept the insurers' prices for episodic. The resulting fragmentation imposes devastating consequences on the health status of people with chronic diseases who require integrated care and, ultimately, on the costs of the health care system.

A consumer-driven health care system will naturally inspire the evolution of integrated teams. Individuals with chronic diseases or disabilities who can freely choose among many differentiated health insurance products will likely opt out of an everything-for-everybody system into one that provides the integrated, demonstrably excellent care they require, and at a lower cost to boot.

This insurance feature will motivate creativity and reward excellence. Innovative providers who give consumers good values for their money will succeed.

6. Adjust Payments for Each Enrollee to Reflect Enrollee Needs

The final element of the solutions is to adjust the payment to insurers and providers by the level of illness of the enrollee.

This will create incentives for insurers and providers to offer policies and services for the sick, such as multiyear policies that provide payment for health-promoting measures and medical programs tailored for specific needs.

PRICING HEALTH INSURANCE

The pricing of health insurance and providers is a critical part of any improvement because current insurance pricing practices suppress the consumer-driven health care innovations that can transform the sector.

Most large employers self-fund their health care costs. They hire insurance firms or third-party administrators (TPAs) primarily to design and administer the benefits provided to employees. Although some managed care plans offer insurance at a fixed price, the cross-subsidization of the costs of the sick—that is, the "insurance" function—is typically undertaken by the firm itself. Large employers find that self-funding is not only feasible but also frees them from various state government regulations, such as mandated benefits and special taxes.

To ease administration the features of the plans offered to employees are typically highly standardized. In contrast, consumer-driven health care rests on the creation of highly differentiated health insurance plans.

Self-funded employers can implement consumer-driven health insurance by engaging TPAs to administer differentiated insurance policies that the employers themselves or their consultants design. Some employers may prefer, however, to implement consumer-driven health care through a number of external insurers that offer their differentiated policies at a fixed price. These employers may reason that insurers are more capable of designing innovative products, that they are too small to provide the insurance function themselves, or that they can drive down costs by encouraging competition among insurance firms.

If a firm chooses to implement consumer-driven health care through insurers, it must assure them of adequate payment. Insurers are especially wary of designing policies that disproportionately attract the sick.

It was not always this way. Notes Stephen Hyde, an early managed care entrepreneur who founded Peak Health in the 1980s,

> [At] Peak Health getting a truly sick premature baby gave us the opportunity to provide such overwhelmingly great care . . . that our members and prospective members gained unmatched confidence that we would be there for *them* if they ever had such awful things happen to them. And it worked—we grew . . . made . . . money, and had extremely high member satisfaction. But we were *always* offered to employees in competition with other insurers. Had we not had to survive such a competitive environment, maybe we would not have been so magnanimous.[6]

In contrast to Hyde's experience, currently there is typically only one insurer per firm. And that insurer generally receives the same price for every enrollee in a group (at times adjusted for age, gender, and location). Similarly, most insurers reimburse every provider with similar payment policies and dictate the benefits for which they are willing to pay.

These pricing policies may sound innocuous, but they profoundly suppress innovation. How can innovators who focus on the care of sick people succeed economically if they are paid the same price for the sick as for the average person? And why should innovative, responsive providers be paid the same rate as sluggish, indifferent ones? Further, payment for individual benefits motivates turf warfare among different providers and undermines the creation of teams that focus on providing integrated care.

Most health policy theories stress the social aspects of uniform insurance pricing. They claim that average prices make health insurance affordable for the uninsured, because the high cost of insuring sick people is subsidized by the low cost of insuring the well. But the point is irrelevant for the self-insured market and causes dysfunctional behavior elsewhere. In the private, self-funded, employer-based insurance system, in which the employer pays for the actual cost of everyone in its group, the cross-subsidization argument is irrelevant. Elsewhere, the uniform pricing argument can reduce the total number of insured people. When every enrollee in a community is priced at the same rate, those who are well leave the market because they consider these averaged rates a bad value for their money. Insurers are thus forced to enroll a pool increasingly formed of sick people at the average community rate. Eventually, these insurers typically leave the market because they sustain huge losses. State governments that imposed uniform pricing in the individual market thus found that despite their good intentions, the numbers of insured and insurance companies willing to enroll them have decreased.[7]

Uniform pricing of providers similarly causes perverse motivational impacts, because it suppresses the provider innovations that would provide good care for the sick.

So how can we provide access to cost-effective care for all, including the uninsured?

We must address the issue of pricing separately from the issue of access. The pricing system should motivate insurers and providers to create the policies and care strategies that are appropriate for the sick. It should pay them more for the sick person than the average amount and commensurately less for the well person. And then, separately, we should ensure access to insurance for all through government payments for the poor.

As in the breakfast insurance example in the previous chapter, one-price-for-all health insurance policies motivate insurers that compete with others in an employer's pool to try to avoid the sick and limit risks. For example, a 2002 American Association of Health Plans' "White Paper" shows how to focus "plan features, benefits, and interventions . . . with a goal of minimizing risk (high use/claims risk . . .)."[8] These results are especially pernicious when it comes to health care. After all, it is the sick who most need access to care and who account for most of its costs. And payments for the fragmented components of care, rather than for integrated care, with similar, insurer-dictated prices for every provider, stop innovations that integrate care dead in their tracks and inhibit consumers from financially rewarding excellent providers.

For example, when Leo Henikoff, Rush Presbyterian–Saint Luke's Medical Center's visionary CEO, instituted a focused factory for AIDS—a comprehensive facility with primary care, diagnostic facilities, specialty services, complementary health care, and behavioral support—he confronted an irony that threatened his hospital: the healthier his patients, the lower their use of his hospital, and the worse his bottom line. In today's topsy-turvy insurance system that pays for fragmented episodes of care rather than an integrated bundle of care, Dr. Henikoff was forced to find other operating and capital sources to compensate for the losses he incurred from improving the health status of his patients. Only through a substantial endowment could his Core Center for Infectious Diseases attain reduced hospitalizations, emergency room admits, and lengths of stay without suffering a financial penalty.[9]

The pricing reforms illustrated in Figure 4.1 avoid these problems. When health insurers are paid differentiated prices for people with different medical needs, the incentives to care for the sick change profoundly. As demonstrated in Figure 4.1, employers' total costs will, at worst, remain the same under this system. But their total costs will likely decrease as the sick enrollees receive better care. For example, Merrill Lynch reduced the costs of its big-use enrollees by giving them ready access to specialist care. By focusing on the sick, it reduced its rates for large claims by 50 percent.[10]

With the different-prices-for-different-needs formula, enrollees' costs, whether an enrollee is sick or well, also remain the same.

As for the insurers, they can earn the same total profit under either pricing scheme. But they have a greater incentive to enroll the sick under the different-prices-for-different-needs formula because they earn a profit of $1,860 per sick enrollee, rather than losing $21,140 as in the one-price-for-all pricing.

Similarly, when providers are free to name their prices for bundles of services that they themselves create, the rewards for innovative, cost-effective care increase. Suppose a creative, competent provider group lowers the cost of treating the sick enrollee to $21,600 through better, integrated care. Under Policy B illustrated in Figure 4.2, an insurer could sign the group to an exclusive contract, and pay it $22,600 for this bundle of care, and charge the employer $24,800.

As shown in Figure 4.2, as a result of a system that rewards innovative providers, the employer saves approximately $2,100 on the sick enrollee ($26,864 – $24,800, rounded to the lowest hundred dollars). If the employer passes on these savings to her 21 employees, the employees' contributions to Policy B can be reduced by $100 per person, to $664 from $764, and the Policy B insurer can increase its profits by $300 (provider savings of $2,400 [$25,000 old cost less $22,600 new cost] less the fee reduction to the employer of $2,100 for the sick enrollee). And the providers under Policy B are likely to gain significant market share because they simultaneously reduce costs to the payer and increase the insurers' profits.

Thus, as illustrated in Figure 4.2, risk-adjusted prices motivate

1. Insurers to be interested in providers who innovate, especially in the care of the sick
2. Providers to innovate

The net result is lower cost to the enrollee and higher profits to both providers and insurers.

How does risk adjustment work in health insurance?

If it follows the pattern illustrated in Figures 4.1 and 4.2, employers' contributions to their enrollees' health plan reflect the risk-adjusted price of the health

	One-Price-for-All Pricing					Different-Prices-for-Different-Needs Pricing				
	Insurer's Cost per Enrollee	Price Paid to Insurer by Employer	Price Paid to Insurer by Employee	Total Cost to Employer, Enrollees	Profit (Loss) to Insurer, per Enrollee, Total	Insurer's Cost per Enrollee	Price Paid to Insurer by Employer	Price Paid to Insurer by Employee	Total Cost to Employer, Enrollees	Profit (Loss) to Insurer, per Enrollee, Total
Twenty healthy enrollees	$1,900	$3,100	$764		$1,950*	$1,900	$1,950	$764		$810*
One special needs enrollee	$25,000	$3,100	$764		($21,140)*	$25,000	$26,100	$764		$1,860*
Total cost to employer				$65,100*					$65,100*	
Total cost to enrollees				$16,040*					$16,040*	
Total profit to insurer					$18,060*					$18,060*

Figure 4.1. Health Insurance Impact on Employer and Employee Costs and Insurer Profits.

* Rounded to nearest ten dollars.

	Policy A—One-Price-for-All Pricing					Policy B—Different-Prices-for-Different-Needs Pricing				
	Price Paid to Insurer	Employer Contribution	Employee Contribution	Insurer's Cost per Enrollee	Total Cost/ Profit	Price Paid to Insurer	Employer Contribution	Employee Contribution	Insurer's Cost per Enrollee	Total Cost/ Profit
Twenty healthy enrollees	$3,864	$3,100	$764	$1,900		$2,914	$2,048	$664	$1,900	
One sick enrollee	$3,864	$3,100	$764	$25,000		$24,800	$24,136	$664	$22,600	
Employer, total cost					$65,100*					$65,100*
Enrollee, total cost					$16,040*					$13,940*
Insurers, total cost					$63,000*					$60,600*
Insurers, profit					$18,060*					$18,440*

Figure 4.2. Health Insurance Impact on Providers.

* Rounded to nearest ten dollars.

insurance they select, but the enrollees' contributions are not adjusted for their risk status. A neutral third-party intermediary or insurer implements risk adjustment for health insurers. Using a third-party risk adjuster or insurer is preferable to having the employer make the adjustment, for at least two reasons: first, it can protect the privacy of each enrollee's health status so it is not revealed to the employer unless the employee chooses to reveal it directly, and second, a firm that specializes in the process is likely to be more expert than individual corporate staff in performing the risk adjustment.

Firms like Minneapolis-based eBenX already perform this function for insurers. eBenX chairman Mark Tierncy reports that

> One of the largest retail department chains in Southern California has been paying the three health plans that serve their 10,000 members with our prospective risk-adjustment methodology.
>
> The idea of using prospective risk adjustment to create a business environment in which niche networks and consumer-driven concepts can flourish will not be initiated by the large insurers. It must be either demanded by large employers and employer coalitions of the health plans they choose to offer or be seen by a subset of health plans as a collaborative way to give employees choice and target the sole replacement carrier's market base. The latter strategy is being implemented by a start-up company, Benu (www.benu.com), in two markets, Ohio and Washington State.[11]

As for providers, those who feel that current risk-adjusted payments are inadequate should be free to name their own prices. After all, that is what suppliers in the rest of our economy do.

EARLY-STAGE CONSUMER-DRIVEN HEALTH CARE INSURANCE POLICIES

Although the consumer-driven health care movement is in its infancy, innovative firms have already created health insurance products that help both consumers and providers correct the problems produced by the present standardized products.

Different Coverage

Some consumer-driven health insurance policies enable consumers who face large, uninsured out-of-pocket expenditures to trade off the money now spent on insurance coverage they do not want for the things they do want. They also help the uninsured, including the growing percentage who decline their employers' present-day insurance policies, to obtain a policy that better suits their needs.

A few entrepreneurial insurers already offer policies that help enrollees obtain the benefits they want through a health savings account to which the employer contributes. In addition, the enrollee buys a lower-cost, high-deductible health insurance plan. In Medtronic's 2001 version of this plan, for example, the firm contributed $2,000 to the savings account for a family and additionally paid for 100 percent of preventive care. The account could be used for needs such as hearing aids and replacement batteries, prescription medications for weight loss and impotence, and smoking cessation programs. Unspent balances were rolled over to the next year. With a $3,000 deductible, this plan's $71 a month costs to the enrollee were nearly $1,000 a year less than many managed care plan options. The plan not only gave enrollees greater flexibility in their spending but also lowered their out-of-pocket maximums, in this example to $1,000 versus $2,000 to $3,000 for Medtronic's managed care options.[12]

David Ness, who oversees the plan for Medtronic, says:

> Approximately 10,500 employees were eligible for this plan when it was introduced in 2001 [and] 20 percent enrolled. The demographics of employees across the United States do not differ significantly between this plan and our other health plan offerings. The plan was rolled out to all major U.S. facilities in January 2002, which increased the total number of participants by 33 percent.
>
> Employee reaction to the plan during the first year of use was positive. They indicated a high level of satisfaction with their health plan and are paying more attention to their health care usage. For example, the use of the nurse line in this plan is several times greater than in other plans and generic drug utilization in this plan has been slightly higher than average. We expect lower costs as a result.[13]

Many large insurers—such as Aetna, Humana, and WellPoint—already offer variants of this plan. (Aetna's plans include long-term care insurance among the savings accounts options.) WellPoint Health Networks Inc. enrolls roughly eight million people in its health insurance plans. The publicly traded company, which merged with Anthem in late 2003, was widely regarded as a premium investment because of its history of steady earnings growth and excellent management.[14] In the year 2000, WellPoint's subsidiary, Blue Cross of California, introduced a series of low-cost health insurance plans for individuals.

How low cost?

Remember Sam, who paid $10,000 for a health insurance plan for his wife and himself with a $12,000 deductible? At his age, early sixties, Sam could buy a WellPoint plan with a $1,000-per-member deductible that capped his total out-of-pocket costs at $3,500 per person at the price of only $146 a month, or approximately $1,800 a year. If Sam wanted an HMO, he could obtain that too. With a $1,500-per-member deductible and a $3,000 per person out-of-pocket maximum, it would clock in at a price of roughly $4,500 a year.[15]

In 2001, WellPoint again innovated by offering defined contribution insurance to small companies. Employers can contribute as little as $80 a month and enable employees to pay for the remaining cost of the policy in pretax dollars.[16]

If the prices for these plans approximate those of the WellPoint individual plans, the employee could pay as little as $66 a month for protection against catastrophically expensive health insurance bills.[17] WellPoint also offers a wide range of other insurance plans and prices.

As WellPoint's CEO, Leonard Schaffer noted with some puffery but with well-earned pride too: "We pioneered the concept of choice."[18] Another variant on this theme, *tiered* plans, in which enrollees pay more for visiting more expensive providers, is also increasing in prevalence.[19] Rockwell Automation Inc. is tying these payments to the income levels of the enrollees.[20]

These innovations are not restricted to the United States. In Chapter Twenty-Two of this book, Shaun Matisonn describes South Africa's consumer-driven health insured system, in which 76 percent of the firms offer a high-deductible, major medical insurance policy and an accompanying savings account. The insurance policy covers all costly events, including drugs for chronic diseases. A comparison of the costs incurred by those covered by this insurance policy and a traditional insurance policy with a lower deductible, demonstrated a 50 percent reduction in expenditures for all age ranges. Of course, low users benefited from this system because it reduced their insurance payments, but interestingly, high users benefited as well because their major medical coverage was more extensive than that offered by a traditional policy.

Different Benefits

Destiny Health, the U.S. arm of a ten-year-old international insurance company, offers an unusual health-promoting program. As Ken Linde, the company's CEO, notes, "We do not just cover our members' medical needs, we are committed to helping them maintain and improve their overall health and wellness." The program includes the Integrated Personal Medical Fund™ (PMF), which covers the day-to-day health care services that are of the less costly, more frequent type and for which consumers have the most discretion in use. The employer, the employee, or both can fund the PMF, with posttax funds to ensure complete ownership of the funds by the employee, annual rollover, and distribution upon leaving the company. For higher-cost health care services for more severe health needs (hospitalizations, surgeries, and chronic medication), the plan provides comprehensive insurance protection.

Wrapped around the plan is an incentive-based wellness program that includes preventive care guidelines and health-promoting activities such as smoking cessation, weight maintenance, exercise, and public fitness events. Enrollees who follow the firm's health and wellness guidelines or activities earn points that can be used for higher interest in their Personal Medical Fund, mileage programs in participating major airlines, fitness club privileges, and hotel vacation packages. Members can also earn points by participating in public health activities such as donating blood or obtaining CPR and first-aid certification.[21]

Merrill Lynch and Union Carbide illustrate two variations on this theme of providing different kinds of benefits they focused on the sick.

In the early 1980s, Merrill's cash management accounts enabled customers to transfer their idle brokerage balances into interest-bearing accounts. This consumer-oriented account was so revolutionary that Merrill patented it.[22] The financial services superstar then brought its consumer-driven financial services vision to the health care benefits it offers its own employees. As in its financial products, the firm focuses on quality. It provides generous health care benefits that it regularly updates to accommodate employees' special needs. Unlimited home health visits and stays in mental hospitals and a $6,000 synthetic speech machine for a secretary whose illness made her mute—these are but some of Merrill's unusual health care benefits.

As with many other goods and services, higher quality translates into lower costs. Notes the *Wall Street Journal,* "adjusted for inflation, Merrill's health care costs have declined even while benefits have expanded." Its 1998 costs of $3,600 per employee were roughly 25 percent less than those of other comparable large employers.[23] How does Merrill control its costs? The cost savings occur largely because of the firm's information-based focus on high-cost events. Merrill's unusual systems identify employees who may suffer from serious illness and bring their problems to the attention of their physicians. Their database is consumer centered: it integrates the separate islands of information from laboratories, doctors, pharmacies, and hospitals that typically exist for each patient in the insurers' payment systems. Special algorithms trace "mistakes waiting to happen." While maintaining patient privacy, a third party then identifies these patients to their physicians, along with suggestions for improvements in their care.

As a result, Merrill's rates for large claims declined by 50 percent between 1995 and 1999. Although the rates of these large claims are low, 2.2 per 1,000 enrollees, the cost per claim is typically very high. Merrill's average cost per large claim of $100,000 remained stable over this time period.[24]

Similarly, as related by Robert Coburn, a consultant at Mercer Human Resources Consulting: "A pilot consumer-driven health care strategy by Union Carbide kept costs flat in 2000, following a 6 percent decrease in 1999. Meanwhile, employee satisfaction increased."

How were these results achieved? The company stressed that decisions were to be made by physicians and their patients. It empowered primary care physicians (PCPs) to refer patients to specialists as they deemed appropriate. The company then offered to share any savings realized with the PCPs. To help PCPs make referrals, the company conducted extensive cost analysis by episode of care and by individual specialist physician. The results showed astounding variability among specialists. For example, one physician exceeded total expected payments for treatment of his patients by 190 percent, whereas another treated clinically similar patients at 60 percent of expected payments.

Union Carbide shared these data with the PCPs, who were asked to place quality first and refer patients only to the specialists to whom they would send their own family members. Although not required to make referrals to lower-cost specialists, the PCPs obviously did. At the beginning of 2001, Union Carbide's costs were still below its cost levels at the end of 1998.[25]

Surprisingly, in a major break from European one-class systems, the Netherlands introduced an effort to offer different benefits by permitting the design of personalized health budgets that meet the needs of those who require long-term care and psychiatric services. One analyst forecasted that this concept will likely be extended to other services not covered by insurance for "necessary" care. In defense of this rupture with European one-size-fits-all plans, he said, "The health care system has gone too far in implementing solidarity: individuals have lost the ability to take personal initiative and to be responsible [for the use of] resources which society has put at their disposal."[26]

Different Groupings and Payments to Providers

The Buyers Health Care Action Group (BHCAG), a coalition of large employers in the Twin Cities, is an example of a consumer-driven health care innovation that permits providers to name their own prices. BHCAG contracts directly with twenty-five care systems, including world-famous institutions such as the Mayo Clinic and the Park Nicolette Hospital. Each care system, comprising primary care physicians, specialists, other health care professionals, and hospitals, determines its own policies (for example, requirements for a referral to a specialist) and independently governs its delivery of health care. The group also names its price for providing care. Through a risk-adjustment process, BHCAG adjusts the providers' prices in relation to the severity of illness of their enrollees, so that groups that wind up with more of the severely ill enrollees are not financially penalized. BHCAG hoped to combat the homogenization of care that the three large insurers in the area had caused. One local employee benefit purchaser said of these HMOs, "Doctors had no incentives to deliver outstanding performance or operate efficiently. Doctors can't shine through if they are good or bad."[27]

Ann Robinow, BHCAG's long-time executive director of care systems and finance, explains some of the personal influences that shaped the organization's provider orientation:

> I realized the perverse incentives of the old health insurance system in my prior job as the administrator of an obstetrics and gynecology IPA [independent practice association, which independent physicians organized to bid as a group for insurance contracts]. We were paid the same fixed rate for all our services by all our docs by our insurer.
>
> Our docs were great. So good, in fact, that they were sought out by high-risk mothers. Although the physicians performed high-cost work, they were very efficient in doing it.

But, because our contractual payments were not risk-adjusted, we lost our shirts.

What an irony!

The lack of adjustment in our payment for the riskiness of our patients forced us to fire excellent, efficient physicians. BHCAG employers realized that there were substantive differences among providers, but they were all being presented to consumers as one plan. There was no market incentive for good physicians to provide efficient, high-quality care because the health plan average would just be brought down by the poor performers.[28]

Under BHCAG, enrollees receive at least enough money from their employers to buy a care plan with the group that has the lowest total cost of care, and they also receive considerable information about their peers' perception of the different caregivers' quality. BHCAG's information enables enrollees to see that low cost does not necessarily mean low quality. For example, at one point, low-cost St. Croix Valley Healthcare outscored high-cost Health Partners Regional Affiliated on every dimension.

BHCAG's innovative plan thus contains a number of consumer-driven characteristics: enrollees have substantial choice and control of providers and considerable information about them. But BHCAG's primary innovations involve providers: they can quote their own prices, form their own systems, and enjoy protection from the economic penalties imposed by sick enrollees.

The plan has attracted excellent academic evaluations of its impact on enrollees, providers, and payers. These assessments reveal that enrollees responded strongly to BHCAG's price and information incentives—a 10 percent increase in enrollee costs reduced enrollment by at least 16.1 percent.[29] In 1996, 70 percent of members sought care from high-cost provider groups. In 2001, four years after the BHCAG value-purchasing initiative began, only 17 percent of members were enrolled in the high-cost care systems and 50 percent were in the low-cost systems. These shifts did not appear to affect the quality of care. Noted Robinow, "While there certainly has been significant consumer migration to low-cost plans, some of the care systems have also changed categories over the four-year period." Further, "the high-cost groups that have strong quality ratings" have experienced less migration than the other high-cost groups.[30]

As for providers, most applaud the plan.[31] These results are surprising. BHCAG should not have affected providers because it accounted for only a small slice of the market, about 130,000 enrollees in 2001. (Because the BHCAG plan supplanted insurers as intermediaries, it was subjected to ferocious opposition from the area's powerful managed care plans. This opposition and early-stage bumbles limited its market share.) Nevertheless, some providers responded by changing their costs. Park Nicolette, for example, was a high-cost system in 1997–1999, a medium-cost one in 2000, and a low-cost one in 2001.[32] A 2002 evaluation showed that providers increased the quality of care for some chronic diseases and health-promoting activities. Employers benefited too; their costs increased at lower rates for BHCAG enrollees.[33]

Vivius, a health care system based in Minneapolis, offers yet another variant. The Vivius Personalized Healthcare System (PHS) is a proprietary interactive system that allows consumers to build their own custom health plan with co-payments and provider networks that are unique to each family member. Under the Vivius plan, employers give employees a set amount of money to help them purchase medical coverage for themselves and their family members. Employees then enroll on-line to select their personal network of doctors and hospitals, co-payment levels for doctor visits and hospital stays, and the amount of their payroll deduction.[34]

Different Term

The consumer-driven portion of the Swiss health insurance system offers at least two innovative health insurance policies that reward health-promoting practices. After buying a compulsory set of insurance benefits, the Swiss may choose freely among different purveyors of health insurance products in the so-called supplementary market. To induce product differentiation, the Swiss system protects insurers against the costs of attracting the sick with risk adjustment of the insurers' prices. Switzerland is a relatively small country. In addition, the prices and rates of return of the Swiss insurers are reviewed by the government. Yet even under constrained circumstances in a small market, insurers have created two innovative products. These early-stage innovations suggest the creativity that will be unleashed in the large U.S. market under a consumer-driven health care system.

One innovation, created by an insurer that specializes in niche products, offers a nonsmoker option, which includes a 20 percent discount on the premiums. Since its introduction in 1995, this option has become relatively popular. Another innovation consists of a five-year, or more, bonus insurance model. Enrollees obtain progressive reductions in premiums for each year they do not use the insurance policy, thus aligning the interests of the insurer and the insured in maintaining the enrollees' health.[35]

EARLY INNOVATORS IN CONSUMER-DRIVEN HEALTH CARE

A Ferrari, a pickup, and a family sedan are all forms of transportation, but each has very different characteristics. Similarly, the attributes of the products from the consumer-driven health care companies vary from firm to firm, but all these attributes share the goal of injecting consumerism into health care.

The current products offer one or more of the following attributes:

Personal health care account (PHA). Typically offered in conjunction with high-deductible insurance coverage, the personal health care account is seeded with a combination of employer and employee dollars. Unused PHA dollars can typically be carried forward to future years. Once the PHA is exhausted, the member is responsible for medical claims until the insurance deductible (for example, $2,000) is met; therefore members are motivated to manage the PHA funds as if they were their own money. The IRS recently ruled in favor of *health-care reimbursement accounts* (HRAs), a type of PHA that is funded with employer dollars.

Decision support. Both on-line and off-line easy-to-use tools and information help members make health care and health coverage decisions. Decision support companies can help health care customers choose among multiple health programs, manage their health care decisions throughout the year, store their personal health information, and analyze where and how they are spending their health care dollars.

Benefit design. Traditionally, the trade-off between benefits and the employee contribution has been made by the employer. With benefit design, employees can customize their benefit levels to better meet their individual needs: for example, they might decide to pay a higher monthly contribution in return for lower copayments. Some programs offer a hybrid plan with PHA-style benefits for discretionary items and first-dollar coverage for nondiscretionary items.

Health plan catalogue. Some products give each employee a choice of multiple health plans. The employee's share of the monthly premium varies with the cost of the chosen plan.

Time of need network. Employees enrolled in these networks choose their health care providers at the time of service. Their share of the cost varies with the cost of their chosen physician or hospital.

Advance selection network. Employees enrolled in these networks choose their health care providers (or entire health systems) at the time of open enrollment. Their monthly share of the premium varies based on the cost of their chosen physicians and hospital.

Some start-up consumer-driven health care companies have become licensed insurance companies or have partnered with existing insurance firms. Others are targeting self-insured employers. The regulatory process that such companies must go through in each state in which they wish to offer insurance and the capital or reserve requirements they must meet have slowed the growth of those that have become licensed insurers, whereas those that target self-funded employers have recently seen more rapid growth.

Most of the early success has been with products that are easy to understand. Long-term success will come from the more complex products with the attributes described earlier in this section. Some existing carriers are now rolling out consumer-driven health care products too. New entrants that are trying to clone the existing consumer-driven health care products are finding that success is not as easy as it looks due to the robust content and programming needed to support these products. Table 4.1 presents some of the early-stage consumer-driven health care firms that incorporate the attributes discussed here.

Most of the consumer-driven health care activity has been in start-up ventures, which have already collectively raised over $300 million in capital. Leading venture capital firms, such as Acacia Venture Partners, Alta Partners, Clearstone Venture Partners, Delphi Ventures, Draper, Fisher Jurvetson, General Atlantic Partners, J. P. Morgan Partners, KBL Healthcare Ventures, Kohlberg Kravis Roberts, Liberty Partners, Merrill Lynch, Navis Partners, Psilos, Salix Ventures, Sapient Capital, and Whitney & Company, have invested in consumer-driven health care companies. These products already cover over 700,000 members. The early adopters include Aon, Budget Group, Medtronic, Novartis, Pharmacia, Raytheon, Scientific-Atlanta, and Textron.

Consumer-driven health care is receiving attention in the health benefits and insurance communities. Trade publications such as *Business Insurance* and *Modern Healthcare* regularly cover the topic and the emerging companies, as do other, more general publications, such as the *Wall Street Journal* and *Time.* The consumer-driven health care conferences are generally very well attended.

The key success factors are time, money, and talent. The consumer-driven health care entrepreneurs have created real companies with seasoned management, impressive clients, and significant capitalization. But because success does not happen overnight, undercapitalized firms have already exited the market, and consolidation among some of the remaining companies is likely. They are managed by seasoned health care and health insurance veterans, including Ken Linde, founding president and CEO of Principal Healthcare and now the founding president and CEO of Destiny Health; Tony Miller, formerly of UnitedHealthcare and Deloitte Consulting and now cofounder and CEO of Definity Health; and Lee Newcomer, former senior executive of UnitedHealthcare and now the chief medical officer and executive vice president of Vivius.

Large-scale adoption of consumer-driven health care will not happen overnight. It is now in its early stages. The health care system moves slowly, but it usually moves in the anticipated direction. Most people in the industry believe that consumer-driven health care is clearly the system of the future.

Table 4.1. Early-Stage Consumer-Driven Health Care Firms: Attributes and Focus.

	Major Product Attributes						Primary Marketing Focus		
	Personal Health Care Account	Decision Support	Benefit Design	Health Plan Catalogue	Time of Need Network	Advance Selection Network	Licensed Carrier	Partner with Carrier	Self-Insured Benefits
Aetna	X	X					X		
ChoiceLinx			X					X	
Definity Health	X	X							X
Destiny Health	X		X				X		
eBenX				X				X	
HealthAllies					X				X
HealthMarket	X		X					X	
Humana			X	X			X		
Lumenos	X	X							X
MyHealthBank	X			X				X	
Patient Choice						X		X	
UnitedHealthcare			X		X		X		
Vivius			X			X		X	

LESSONS FROM CONSUMER-DRIVEN
HEALTH CARE EARLY ADOPTERS

The successes and failures of early innovators of consumer-driven health care products suggest what others might emulate and what they might wish to avoid or redesign.

BHCAG

The early adopter that most closely mirrors the essential consumer-driven health insurance features is BHCAG. When BHCAG's plan features are compared to those that characterize today's failed defined benefit health care coverage market, they right many of the wrongs. The BHCAG plan provides

- Incentives for employees to think about their cost-coverage trade-offs because they pay out of their own pockets for care systems whose costs exceed those of the most cost-effective alternative
- Freedom for providers to set their own prices and to reap the financial rewards of their efficiency and effectiveness
- Risk-adjusted pricing
- Real choice at the provider level (as opposed to the health plan level)
- User satisfaction data
- Transparent pricing to enrollees

Yet the BHCAG system is not a perfect model of consumer-driven health insurance. For one thing, it does not pay providers in terms of bundles of care for the treatment of diseases or procedures. Instead, it uses a benefit-based payment system. Like the breakfast insurers, because it pays for each separate ingredient and not for a meal, it does not provide incentives for integrated care. Until recently, its benefits were standardized across care groups. And its information is currently restricted to users' satisfaction data.

Nevertheless, overall BHCAG is the best current example of consumer-driven health care coverage. Most of the other early adopters offer only partial consumer-driven health care solutions. Some, like Definity, Destiny, and WellPoint, focus on offering new insurance options in the form of a lower-cost catastrophic health insurance option. Others, like Merrill Lynch, focus on consumer-driven health care solutions that empower the sick via their providers.

To date, the results from the long-running experiences of BHCAG and South Africa's consumer-driven initiatives (see Chapter Twenty-Two) are positive. These plans have influenced enrollees to choose more cost-effective care with no apparent degradation in health status as a result. And the enrollees' decisions, in turn, appear to have influenced providers to become more cost effective.

Early Entrants to Consumer-Driven Health Insurance

A massive, multiyear experiment involving nearly 4,000 people, for example, convincingly demonstrated that those with $1,000 deductible insurance policies spent substantially less on health care.[36] Concerns that these savings were unwise and would ultimately lead to diminished health status were effectively disproven. The middle-class people in the study maintained their health status despite their reduced expenditures, as did the chronically ill.[37] The Destiny, WellPoint, and Definity consumer-driven plans have also met with market receptivity. Definity reported greatly increased use of generic drugs, and Humana substantial decreases in its consumer-driven health care plans cost trend rates relative to those experienced in other plans.[38] It reduced its medical cost inflation by 11 to 14 percent when 5,000 of its Louisville, Kentucky, associates used its SmartSuite products, which enable members to customize their plans. Behavior modification accounted for 67 percent of the reduction—through appropriate plan selection and utilization—and benefit reconfiguration for the rest.[39] MyHealthBank claimed annual decreases of $20 to $44 per member in administrative costs.[40]

An analysis of the 2002 results in a large firm that implemented a consumer-driven health care plan for all its employees in one location revealed the following:

- Reduced overall utilization
- No cost shifting by age
- Constant benefit values for those with high expenses
- Positive changes in drug usage (more generics), while high utilizers maintained their prior level of critical medications
- Chronically ill participants continued to receive routine and preventive care. For example, people with high blood pressure increased preventive visits while decreasing their visits to the hospital outpatient department and physicians' office.

Of course, these programs must be designed to ensure that enrollees do not skimp on critically needed care.

The Federal Employees Health Benefits Program

The Federal Employees Health Benefits Program (FEHB) is another example of a successful consumer-driven health care plan. This forty-year-old, $127 billion program, offers a large variety of insurance plans to nine million people, with the government contributing no more than 75 percent of the cost of the average plan. Extensive information, such as *CHECKBOOK's 2003 Guide to Health Plans for Federal Employees,* enables intelligent selection. As a result of these features, the FEHB has achieved better cost control than other plans. In 2002, for example, its premiums rose by 13.1 percent, compared to 15 percent for private sector plans.[41]

Although the FEHB illustrates the promise of choice, it suffers from the following non-consumer-driven health care features:

- Federally mandated benefits that all plans must offer inhibit product differentiation.
- Lack of risk adjustment means there are no incentives to create innovative programs for sick, high-cost enrollees.[42]
- Employees have little financial incentive to buy plans that cost less than 75 percent of the average plan cost.[43]
- Traditional payment methods are used for providers.[44]

For 2004, the program increased its options by 17 to a total of 205, while keeping its premium increases at a lower than natural rate of 10.5 percent.[45]

LESSONS FROM OTHER TYPES OF INSURERS

What can we learn about the characteristics of consumer-driven health insurance from other, longer-lived consumer-driven insurers, such as those in the automobile industry?

In health insurance the absence of risk-adjusted pricing is a critical problem. One-price-for-all-enrollees health insurance pricing causes insurers who compete with each other in an employer's insurance pool to try to avoid attracting the sick. Unrealistic pricing is not limited to health insurers. For example, after a scrupulous analysis of property and casualty insurers, McKinsey & Company concluded that careless practices led to "pricing [that] . . . is more or less random" and that insurers "manage profitability on the total portfolio rather than segment by segment." McKinsey warned the insurers that this careless pricing opened the door to more careful pricers of the risk attached to different segments of the market.[46]

Despite these observations about current practices, the success of the Progressive Corporation in providing insurance to high-risk drivers illustrates the feasibility of different-strokes-for-different-folks pricing. This firm achieves what many believe is impossible in dealing with high-risk clients—excellent profits *and* excellent service. In contrast to the opaque pricing of its competitors, Progressive's system provides the customer with a firm quote within ten minutes. An admiring Ralph Nader said, "It's the difference between a tricycle and a Boeing 747."

Steely-eyed data analysis, backed by years of analyzing the correlation between risk and the customer's characteristics, enable this swift and accurate pricing. Progressive has more risk categories and sets a wider variety of premiums than its competitors. For example, in pricing insurance for the high-risk motorcycle riders, the company classified the riders into eleven risk categories by age, whereas most of its competitors considered only two.

The firm also provides good service. CEO Peter Lewis says: "I think most people start out not trusting their insurance company; but if you are there right away, if you say I'm sorry this happened to you, and I'm here to help you, fewer people will get lawyers . . . and we wind up spending less. . . . In the end, this is a beautiful combination. We can be in the position of being both the low-cost and high-server provider at the same time." To implement Lewis's vision, the firm created an immediate response system whose aim was to have an adjuster at the policy holder's home or site of the accident within hours of the accident. The program achieved impressive results—an adjuster made personal contact within twenty-four hours for more than 75 percent of the claimants.[47]

DIFFERENCES BETWEEN CONSUMER-DRIVEN HEALTH CARE AND MANAGED COMPETITION

At one time the notion of *managed competition* was viewed as the savior of the health care system. As depicted by Stanford professor Alain Enthoven in many publications, including a 1989 article with the now ironic title "A Consumer Choice Health Plan for the 1990s," it would enable competition among managed care health plans for consumers. Employers would contribute the same amount toward each health plan, and managed care plans would then duke it out for the consumers' business. The resulting competition would control costs while increasing quality.[48]

Although the notion of managed competition was initially very appealing, as managed care fell into disrepute, its allure declined. As a result, physician Paul Ellwood's famed Jackson Hole conferences to debate the bells and whistles of managed competition ceased. However, some of the founders of managed competition now see the ascent of consumer-driven health care as an opportunity to resuscitate their idea. Ellwood, for example, has resumed the Jackson Hole meetings. They claim that they were consumer driven all along.[49] After all, they wanted competition, right? And is not competition at the core of consumer-driven health care?

Not so fast.

Do you note the adjective *managed* in the term *managed competition*?

Consumer-driven markets are not managed. They are driven by consumers.

So what is the "*managed*" part all about? Well, all the founders of managed competition want to do is to standardize benefits and coverage so you will not get confused. The managed health care plans that compete in the standardized arena they create will knock your socks off, they aver.

But as always, the devil is in the details.

The heart of consumer-driven health care lies in product differentiation among health plans—replete with variations in benefits, coverage, provider payments, terms, and other characteristics. Managed competition takes the very heart out of consumer-driven health care with its insistence on standardization of these features.

You want to trade off higher drug and long-term care coverage for a higher deductible?

Tough luck.

You want a network that highlights an integrated team of diabetes providers?

Sorry, friend.

The founders of managed competition think they know what is good for you better than you do.

But if managed competition is so wonderful, why did it bomb out? The fans of managed competition have many answers to this question:

- *Managed care did not bomb out.* It wrung fat out of our health care system. The double-digit inflation in costs between 2000 and 2003 occurred solely because profligate American consumers insisted on choice of providers and access to care. If Americans would just get out of the way, and let the real pros do their thing, cost increases could be easily controlled.

- *The wrong people got hold of managed care.* If the right people had run the HMOs, health care heaven would settle on earth.

- *As for the product differentiation that lies at the heart of consumer-driven health care, it is the root of all evil.* It will confuse consumers, end health insurance as we know it, and screw the sick.[50]

DOES CHOICE INSPIRE OR PARALYZE?

At its core, managed competition relies on technocrats to wring the fat out of standardized benefits. Consumer-driven health care, in contrast, relies on consumers and providers to create the health care services that best meet their individual needs through differentiated health plans.

The two concepts are as different as liberty and dictatorship, Jefferson and Hamilton, choice and monopoly.

So, does choice inspire or paralyze?

Psychology research articles reveal three interesting aspects of choice.

The first is that choice increases satisfaction, enhances motivation, and improves performance.[51] The second finding relates to the "tyranny of choice"—excessive choice undermines satisfaction and motivation.[52] The third indicates that the type of choice is key: increased market share is linked to increases in choices along a simple attribute—for example, the capacity of an oven—whereas decreased share is correlated with increases in noncomparable attributes.[53]

For those concerned about choice in consumer-driven health care, the implications are heartening:

- Because of the positive, consumer-satisfying aspects of choice, providers and insurers will increase it.
- They will not offer a paralyzing number of choices.
- They will likely increase choice among attributes that consumers consider important: for example, the amount of insurance and types of benefits rather than a large group of noncomparable characteristics.

IMPACT OF CONSUMER-DRIVEN HEALTH CARE ON THE FRAYED SAFETY NET

How will consumer-driven health care help those let down by the frayed safety net described in Chapter Two?

First, the differentiated insurance policies that characterize consumer-driven health care will enable people to obtain the coverage and benefits they want. In a consumer-driven health care system, Bea could have purchased long-term care insurance and Molly and Jacqui could have more easily accessed the providers they wanted, for example. Insurers will respond to consumer needs.

Second, the providers' ability to name their own prices for the bundles of services they wish to offer will help physicians such as Robert Monoson, who currently struggle to offer preventive or integrated care and support for patients with chronic diseases, such as Vivian.

Third, innovative policies inaugurated in the group insurance market will eventually migrate to the individual market and the wealthier uninsured, such as Sam.

Fourth, employees and their employers who lose work time and wages because of the fragmentation and perverse economic incentives in the present system will find consumer-driven health insurance policies that highlight convenience from the consumers' perspective.

Last, and most important, the innovations created by liberated consumers and providers will moderate costs and ease the financial burden on employers and governments (as will be discussed in Chapter Five) so that they can more readily broaden and strengthen the safety net for the poor uninsured.

Notes

1. Marshall, M. N., Shakelle, P. G., Leatherman, S., and Brook, R. H. "The Public Release of Performance Data." *Journal of the American Medical Association,* Apr. 12, 2000, *284,* 1866–1874.

2. KPMG. "A New Direction for Employer-Based Health Benefits." Publication No. 99-12-05. New York: KPMG, Nov. 1999.

3. Kaiser Family Foundation and Health Research Educational Trust (HRET). *Employer Health Benefits 2000.* Menlo Park, Calif., and Chicago: Kaiser Family Foundation and HRET, 2000.

4. Kaiser Family Foundation and HRET, *Employer Health Benefits 2000,* p. 172.

5. Buchmueller, T. C., and Feldstein, P. J. "Consumers' Sensitivity to Health Plan Premiums: Evidence from a Natural Experiment in California." *Health Affairs,* Spring 1996, *15,* 143–151.

6. Stephen Hyde, personal communication to the author, Apr. 2002.

7. See, for example, Ethan Allen Institute. *An Analysis and Response to the Report of the Governor's Bipartisan Commission on Health Care Availability and Affordability.* [www.ethanallen.org/index2.html], Jan. 2002.

8. Navarro, F., and Wilkins, S. *Using PATH to Increase the Profitability of Health Plan Member Acquisitions.* [www.pathorganization.com]. September 2002.

9. Leo Henikoff, M. D., personal communication to the author, 2002.

10. Gentry, C. "How Is Merrill Lynch Limiting Health Costs? By Expanding Benefits." *Wall Street Journal,* May 23, 2000, p. A1.

11. Mark Tierney, personal communication to the author, May 2002.

12. Herzlinger, R. E. *Consumer-Driven Health Care: Medtronic's Health Insurance Options.* Harvard Business School Case No. 302-006, Rev. Sept. 2002. Boston: Harvard Business School, 2001.

13. David Ness, personal communication to the author, Feb. 2002.

14. "WellPoint Health Networks." New York: UBS Warburg, Feb. 16, 2000.

15. Blue Cross of California. *Individual and Family Health Plans, Effective 1/01/01.* Newbury Park, Calif.: Blue Cross of California, Nov. 2000.

16. "Blue Cross of California Is First Major Health Plan to Offer Defined Contribution Plans to Small Business Owners." Press Release. Newbury Park, Calif.: Blue Cross of California, Feb. 28, 2001.

17. WellPoint's pricing was not available at the time I wrote this section.

18. Marsa, L. "Consumers Paying More for Their Prescriptions." *Los Angeles Times,* Sept. 24, 2001, p. S1; Wechsler, J. "Tiered Pharmacy Benefit Plans on the Rise." *Pharmaceutical Executive,* Oct. 2002, *22,* 35–37; Benk, L. B. "A New Level of Care." *Modern Healthcare,* Feb. 4, 2002, *32;* Greenwalk, J. "Taking Cost Control to Another Level." *Business Insurance,* Feb. 11, 2002, *36,* T3, T7.

19. Benko, L. B. "Loosening Their Grip." *Modern Healthcare*, Apr. 15, 2002, p. 34.

20. "Payers Refine Cost-Saving Technologies." *Managed Care Week*, Dec. 8, 2003, p. 7.

21. Ken Linde, personal communication to the author, Mar. 2002.

22. Lux, H. "Patent Spending." *Institutional Investor*, Mar. 2001, p. 140.

23. Gentry, "How Is Merrill Lynch Limiting Health Costs?" pp. A1, A16.

24. Gentry, "How Is Merrill Lynch Limiting Health Costs?" p. A16.

25. Robert Coburn, personal communication to the author, Apr. 2001.

26. Ter Meulen, R.H.J. "Limiting Solidarity in the Netherlands." *Journal of Medicine and Philosophy*, Dec. 1995, *20*, 607–616.

27. O'Reilly, B. "Taking On the HMOs." *Fortune*, Feb. 16, 1998, p. 100.

28. Herzlinger, *Consumer-Driven Health Care: Medtronic's Health Insurance Options.*

29. Christianson, J. B., and Feldman, R. "Evolution in the Buyers Health Care Action Group Purchasing Initiative." *Health Affairs*, Jan.–Feb. 2002, *21*, 76–88.

30. Herzlinger, *Consumer-Driven Health Care: Medtronic's Health Insurance Options.*

31. Herzlinger, *Consumer-Driven Health Care: Medtronic's Health Insurance Options.*

32. Ann Robinow, personal communication to the author, 2002.

33. Lyles, A., Weiner, J. P., Shore, A. D., and Christianson, J. "Cost and Quality Trends in Direct Contracting Arrangements." *Health Affairs*, Jan.–Feb. 2002, *21*, 89–102.

34. "Vivius, MMA to Provide Colorado with First-of-Its-Kind Consumer-Driven Health Plan." Press Release. [www.vivius.com], Aug. 15, 2002.

35. Herzlinger, R. E., and Parsa-Parsi, R. "Consumer-Driven Health Care: Lessons from Switzerland." Harvard Business School working paper, 2003.

    Note that despite its theoretical appeal, the longer-term product is not well accepted, likely because it offers no support for health maintenance and because its pricing makes it a poor value for the money. Although the discount can amount to as much as 45 percent, an enrollee who has no health care usage is still left paying 55 percent of the insurance costs.

36. Feldstein, M. S. "Economic Analysis for Health Service Efficiency: Econometric Studies of the British National Health Service." *Contributions to Economic Analysis* (vol. 51). Amsterdam: North-Holland Publishing, 1967; Brook, R. H., and others. "Does Free Care Improve Adults' Health? Results from a Randomized Controlled Trial." *New England Journal of Medicine*, Dec. 8, 1983, *309*, 1426–1434.

37. Lohr, K. N., Brook, R. H., and Kamberg, C. J. "Use of Medical Care in the Rand Health Insurance Experiment." *Medical Care*, 1986, *24* (Supplement), S1–S87; Wong, M. D., and others. "Effect of Cost Sharing on Care Seeking and Health Status." *American Journal of Public Health*, Nov. 2001, *91*, 1889–1894.

38. Tony Miller, CEO, Definity, personal communication to the author, 2002; Jim Boehm, CFO, Humana, personal communication to the author, 2002; "Humana Announces First-Year Savings." Press Release. Louisville, Ky.: Humana, Oct. 2002.

39. Jim Boehm, CFO, Humana, personal communication to the author, 2002.

40. Dave Sanders, CEO, MyHealthBank, personal communication to the author, 2002.

41. Martinez, B. "Health Benefits Post Highest Gain in Costs Since '90." *Wall Street Journal*, Dec. 9, 2002, p. A6.

42. U.S. Congressional Research Service. *The Federal Employees Health Benefits Program: Possible Strategies for Reform.* Washington, D.C.: U.S. Government Printing Office, 1989.

43. Francis, W. "Premium Costs and Taxes." In *CHECKBOOK's 2002 Guide to Health Plans for Federal Employees.* [www.retireehealthplans.org], Oct. 2002.

44. Moffit, R. "How Washington Can Improve Health Care Coverage for Federal Workers and Their Families." Heritage Foundation *Backgrounder* No. 1504. [www.heritage.org/library/backgrounder/bg1504.html], Nov. 19, 2001.

45. U.S. Office of Personnel Management. "2004 Federal Employees Health Benefits Program Premiums." [www.opm.gov/pressrel/eb-fehb4.asp], Oct. 30, 2003.

46. Maurstad, H. L., Riddergard, J., Vrolijk, C. "Insuring Profits." *McKinsey Quarterly*, 2001, *2*, 14–15.

47. Porter, M. *Progressive Corporation.* Harvard Business School Case No. 797-109. Boston: Harvard Business School, 1997.

48. Enthoven, A., and Kronick, R. "A Consumer Choice Health Plan for the 1990s." *New England Journal of Medicine*, Jan. 5, 1989, *320*, 29–37.

49. Ellwood, P. "Heroic Pathways: The American Healthcare System at the Frontier: Jackson Hole Group." [www.chsm.org/presentations/ellwood.ppt], Nov. 14, 2002.

50. Fuchs, V. R. "What's Ahead for Health Insurance in the United States?" *New England Journal of Medicine*, June 6, 2002, *346*, 1822–1824.

51. See, for example, Iyengar, S. S., and Lepper, M. R. "When Choice Is Demotivating." *Journal of Personality and Social Psychology*, 2002, *79*, 995–1006.

52. Iyengar and Lepper, "When Choice Is Demotivating," p. 1003; Dhar, R. "Consumer Preference for a No Choice Option." *Journal of Consumer Research*, Sept. 1999, *24*, 215–231.

53. Gourville, J. T., and Soman, D. "Consumer Choice Behavior Among Wide Assortments: Is More Choice Always Better?" Working Paper No. 99-102, Harvard Business School, 1999.

CHAPTER FIVE

Health Care Productivity

How does consumer-driven health care work? How do differentiated health insurance products cause health care to become both better and cheaper? After all, key to the efficacy of consumer-driven pension plans was the revolution in the financial industry. In response to the demands consumers unleashed with their 401(k) purchasing power, the industry introduced differentiated mutual funds and reliable information sources that enabled average people, like you and me, who were not financial wizards, to achieve good returns and drive transaction costs down.[1]

Can consumer-driven health care achieve similar results?

The 800-pound gorilla here is the existing health care system. Can consumer-driven health care insurance products motivate it to become more productive?

Many of the traditional explanations of the efficacy of consumer-driven health care are unconvincing or incomplete in this regard.

The most common explanation is ideological, replete with frequent, fervent, but vague invocations of the efficacy of the market.[2] These explanations, though sincere, are unsatisfactory because they fail to connect the dots between consumers' payment for health insurance and the re-creation of the sector.

The next most common explanation equates consumer-driven health insurance with catastrophic policies that feature high deductibles and low premiums.[3]

The section titled "Focused Factories and the Public Interest" is based on Regina E. Herzlinger and Peter Stavros, *MedCath Corporation*, Harvard Business School Case No. 303-041 (Boston: Harvard Business School, 2002).

102

It asserts that a considerable fraction of present-day insurance is wasted—used to cover health care expenditures of low marginal utility. When people shop for these services using their own funds, they will restrict their usage without damaging their health status.

This explanation of the cost-reducing impact of consumer-driven health care is somewhat more compelling. Decreased levels of insurance unquestionably lead to lower health care expenditures.

Nevertheless, this explanation also fails to provide fully compelling reasons for the productivity-enhancing power of consumer-driven health insurance. For one thing, high-deductible insurance may not be the most popular consumer-driven health care innovation. For example, in 2002, when University of Minnesota employees were first offered high-deductible insurance, only 4 percent chose it.[4] Then too, the societal effects of high-deductible health insurance are unsettling. If the deductibles are not adjusted for income, some Americans would be hard-pressed to pay them. The average U.S. household, whose after-tax 1999 income was $41,000, might well struggle to pay a $2,000 deductible[5] (although the health savings account feature of some high-deductible policies will enable lower-income people to accumulate much-needed assets for uninsured care[6]). Further, because most health care costs remain fully insured, the impact of even the highest deductibles will be limited. Thus the Commonwealth Fund concludes its review of consumer-driven health care initiatives by noting that "any long-term savings are limited since none . . . address the underlying factors that raise health care costs, especially the demand for new technologies and the aging of the population."[7]

So, how will consumer-driven health care improve the productivity of health care?

Consumer-driven innovations in insurance products will cause a massive restructuring of the health care sector that will reduce costs by improving the quality of care.

In response to consumer demands, health care providers will create three new types of important innovations: *focused factories* that integrate formerly fragmented providers around the patients' needs for care in ways that improve long-term health status; *integrated information records* that consolidate the many dribs and drabs of medical information that exist for each individual into a cohesive system; and *personalized medical technologies* designed for individual needs. These innovations will be bundled by consumer-driven health insurers. For example, multiyear policies that feature focused factories supported by integrated information records and personalized medical technologies may be offered to people with genetically linked diseases, such as diabetes. These consumer-driven innovations will create better-quality, lower-cost health care.

Yet many health care policy experts disagree with these views. To them, nothing in the consumer-driven health care system can make health care better and cheaper. They think that the only way to control health care costs is for experts to ration care under the aegis of a universal, government-controlled health care system.

Such views ignore the promise of innovation in health care and the miracles innovation has created elsewhere in the economy. Consider the Model T Ford, for example. According to the British magazine *The Economist*, when Henry Ford introduced the Model T in the early 1900s, he promised to make his car the best *and* the cheapest. He aimed his innovative automobile at the middle class, not at the rich who accounted for most of the automobile ownership at the time. In his words, it was "for the greatest multitude, constructed of the best materials, . . . so low in price that no man making a good salary will be unable to own one."

As with health care today, most of the experts scoffed at Ford's promise to improve *both* costs and quality. After all, at that time in Great Britain, a car cost more than most houses. Yet over the next twenty years, Ford's good car at a good price—35 percent lower in 1914 than in 1908—resulted in volume that soared from the 17,700 cars built the year he founded his company to 202,000 five years later, for the whole company. How did Ford make cars that were both cheaper and better? His innovations focused on production, with an early-stage focused factory and an integrated system. Ford was appropriately modest about his skills—he assembled purchased components rather than manufacturing them himself—yet visionary in the integration of these components, bringing the assembly line to the worker, rather than forcing the worker to go to it.[8]

Ford's ultimate failure was in ignoring the third important source of innovation, the consumer's desire for personalization, with his rigid adherence to the one-size-fits-all Model T. He thus opened the door for General Motors, whose multiple brands responded to this desire.

Will consumer-driven health care motivate these kinds of innovations in the health care sector?

The BHCAG experience indicates that it will. Some of the Twin Cities providers changed their cost structure in response to consumer demand. But BHCAG is only one experience, a mere pebble in an ocean of inefficiency. Can its results be widely replicated?

Many economists feel that it is simply impossible to enhance the productivity of health care services. As Princeton economist William Baumol famously notes about attempts to increase the productivity of live artistic performances: "It requires about as many minutes for Richard II to tell his 'sad stories' (today) as it did on the stage of the Globe Theater."[9]

In one sense, Baumol is correct. Speeding up artistic performances is surely not an effective way to increase productivity.

But this view of the range of productivity-enhancing techniques is excessively narrow. There are many possibilities for increased efficiency, even for live performing arts organizations. For example, a repertory company whose members jointly hone their craft is likely more efficient than a group of performers who are newly assembled for every production. A traveling company that visits many different sites with the same production can spread the fixed costs of mounting a production, such as sets and costumes. A company composed of veteran Shakespearean actors, directors, and producers will obviate the training costs for novices. And so on.

HOW CONSUMER-DRIVEN HEALTH INSURANCE LOWERS COSTS AND RAISES THE QUALITY OF HEALTH CARE

When it comes to health care, the three innovations discussed in more detail below hold special promise.

Integrated Information Records

The need for integrated information records is widely acknowledged. I first urged this innovation in a 1978 *Harvard Business Review* article, for example.[10] But some twenty-five years later such records still do not exist, resulting in errors of commission—for example, adverse interactions among drugs prescribed by physicians who are unaware of each other's recommendations—and omission—lapses in appropriate medical intervention. The National Institute of Medicine has documented the dreadful consequences of their absence on the quality and costs of health care. Its 2001 report, *Crossing the Quality Chasm,* stated: "The 21st century will require . . . far greater than [the] current investments in information technology by most health care organizations."[11]

The lack of integration arises because individuals' medical data are stored in the warehouses of those who pay for them—providers and insurers—and there is no incentive for overall integration. The best overall drivers of integration are the consumers themselves. In a consumer-driven health care system, consumers will demand such records as tools to help them manage their health and their insurance. Innovative providers will respond, just as firms such as Intuit, which makes Quicken software, and Fidelity Investments responded to consumer demands for integrated financial records.[12]

Focused Factories

The support for the second innovation, focused factories,[13] is more diffuse. Although most of the critics of the health care delivery system acknowledge the problems caused by fragmentation of care, especially in the treatment of chronic diseases and disabilities,[14] their standard solutions differ in scope from the focused factory one.

The need for some form of integration arises because the health care system is organized around the providers of care and not around the needs of users of care. The mismatch can lead to devastating results, especially for those with chronic diseases or disabilities and for underserved groups with special needs, such as American Indians and women.

To gain more perspective on this problem, consider chronic diseases. Debilitated patients, who typically require the service of many different kinds of health care providers, vainly struggle to patch together an integrated system of care.[15] More than half of the individuals with asthma, depression, and hypertension who have been surveyed on this topic have complained that they do not have a helping hand—someone to assist them in coordinating care when more than one provider is involved.[16] The economic consequences of this lacuna are suggested by the magnitude of the financial expenditures and opportunity costs caused by chronic diseases. Employers in one Florida region lost an estimated $7,000 in work days for each employee who suffered from chronic problems.[17] On the national level, five chronic diseases—mood disorders, diabetes, heart disease, hypertension, and asthma—accounted for 49 percent of total 1996 health care costs and an additional $36 billion in lost work.[18]

For an example of the difficulties encountered by those with chronic diseases, consider the seventeen million people with diabetes. Comorbidities are frequent—46 percent of those with diabetes also suffer from high blood pressure and 4 to 11 percent, depending on the illness, from asthma, heart disease, and behavioral problems.[19] They require a team of health care professionals to help them manage this complex, insidious disease—endocrinologists, cardiologists, nephrologists, dermatologists, podiatrists, and behavioral support specialists, among others, who will encourage them in the taxing regimens required for the best management of the disease. Where do they find a team to provide the integrated care they need? Virtually nowhere. As a result, many get lousy care—for example, in one study only 36 percent of fully insured, elderly people with diabetes received a biannual glycosylated hemoglobin test, a must-do exam for these individuals. These abysmal results were worse among African Americans and poor people.[20] In another analysis, over 42 percent of diabetic individuals felt they were not effectively counseled about appropriate self-management of their disease.[21]

The fragmentation of the health care system imposes serious, long-term consequences for those coping with chronic diseases because no one person or group is ultimately responsible. The consequences are financial as well as medical. Sustained, integrated care has been shown to reduce the heart attacks and circulatory complications that plague those with diabetes by 14 percent and 37 percent respectively, for example.[22] These improvements in health status would likely significantly reduce the direct costs of diabetes, $54 billion in 1996, the billions more wasted in lost days of work,[23] and the additional $54 billion lost through premature death and disability.[24] Even moderate short-term improvements in diabetes markers through an integrated regimen of diet and drugs achieve impressive results—greatly reduced absenteeism, restricted activity days, and hospital stays.[25]

For an example of the efficacy of a focused factory that integrates provider care, consider Georgia's Comprehensive Sickle Cell Center, housed at the Grady Health System. It provides round-the-clock comprehensive care in facilities focused on those with sickle cell anemia. "We really do everything—one-stop shopping—so [patients] don't have to run to three or four places," explains the program's coordinator. "[We also] provide the whole patient with psycho-social support. . . . We see that this is a life-long disease, so we try to hit (all) the problems."

The results? In eight years this focused factory halved hospital admissions and cut emergency admissions among its patients by roughly 80 percent. The net financial savings were $1.2 million per one hundred patients, and the impact on the quality of life of the individuals dealing with sickle cell anemia is incalculable.[26]

The problem is not with the individual providers; we are blessed with excellent doctors, caring nurses, extraordinary researchers, and outstanding hospitals. But, as the authors of a marvelous *Milbank Quarterly* article reviewing the quality of care in the United States put it, "we can do much better."[27] In the absence of a system for integrated care, all too many patients fall through the cracks. The creation of focused factories for victims of chronic diseases and disabilities, such as back pain, and the needs of other undertreated populations, such as African-Americans, Native Americans, and women, will lead to a better, lower-cost health care system.

The conventional solutions suggested for the problem of fragmentation differ in scale from the focused factory one. Rather than an organization focused on the patients' needs for a team that contains all the resources required for one disease or disability or underserved group, most experts favor massive consolidation of the delivery process, through large physician group practices[28] or hospitals vertically integrated with physicians and insurers.[29] Some have even grander visions for population-based medicine.[30]

All these ideas rest on the fervent belief that big is beautiful.

There is nothing wrong with them but for the fact that they are unlikely to work.

As many businesspeople have discovered, the simple fact is that vertical integration is immensely difficult to pull off: the larger the scale, the larger the problems encountered.[31] For that reason, brand-name products, such as Dove soap, Calvin Klein jeans, and Coca-Cola, are not manufactured by the companies that design and market them.[32] The executives think their skills lie in marketing, not in manufacturing, and they have organized themselves accordingly. Similarly, companies like Dell choose to rely on external suppliers, rather than to manufacture their product themselves. Their excellent information systems enable them to deliver a customized product, integrated from outsourced components.[33]

My analysis of the failures in vertical integration in other industries led me to predict in my 1997 book, *Market-Driven Health Care*, that the then prevalent vertical integration of notoriously inefficient institutions like hospitals and insurers with physicians in order to provide everything-for-everybody health care was a recipe for disaster. I worried as the number of physician practices purchased by hospitals jumped from 6,600 in 1995 to 19,200 in 1998, growing at a 30.5 percent annual rate. The results? Unfortunately, the disaster I predicted. In 1998, for example, these integrated hospitals incurred $1 billion in losses, or an average loss of $80,000 per physician.[34]

The reason? Vertical integration is such a notoriously difficult strategy to implement that most other industries spurn it.[35] It is hard enough to manage a hospital. It is harder still to manage doctors. When the two are combined, the complexity multiplies. It is no wonder that productivity of the physicians decreased by 15 to 20 percent two years after acquisition. And the low growth of their patient referrals to the acquiring hospitals failed to offset these productivity losses.[36] Most of these everything-for-everybody vertical integrations also failed to deliver integrated management of chronic diseases.

The hospitals that integrated with health plans experienced difficulties too. In *Market-Driven Health Care* I spotlighted the conflict of interest and loss of focus that the then hospital firm Humana encountered when it created an insurance division. Humana's hospital division wanted to maximize occupancy, but the insurance division wanted to minimize it. Ultimately, the firm shed its hospital division to resolve this paralyzing conflict.[37] By 1999, many of the hospitals that had ignored Humana's experience replicated these problems and were forced to purge their health maintenance organizations.

In 2002, a leading industry journal, *Modern Healthcare*, reported: "Healthcare organizations spent a good deal of 2001 taking apart what they had previously pieced together. Many health systems . . . that acquired physician practices and HMOs retreated from these businesses as costs rose and income fell."[38] In a 2000 survey of integrated delivery systems, 41 percent of the respondents were engaged in disintegration, spurred by the mounting operational losses encountered by 34 percent of them and the anemic 0 to 1.9 percent profits earned by 31 percent of them.[39] The venerable Moody's debt rating service applauded these trends with the heading, "dismantling of vertical integration strategies heralds the "back-to-basics" theme."[40]

Population-based medicine, even more grandiose in scope, offers commensurately lower promise for success. Population-based medicine was to be achieved through providers' offering all the care a population required at a fixed price. Encouraged by academic cheerleaders, many physician groups, especially in California, undertook *capitation,* as this fixed payment practice is called.[41] But capitation rapidly fell into disfavor when many of these groups were forced into bankruptcy or to close their doors. Some blamed the low per-patient payments these groups received for this situation, but one report found that groups that received higher fees were not necessarily better off than the others. More likely, the executives of many medical groups found the managerial requirements of everything-for-everybody population-based health care difficult to fulfill.[42]

Because focused-factories are more modest in scale, they present a much more feasible solution to the problem of fragmentation. They resemble the mass-customization factories of today that achieve higher-quality, lower-cost results by turning conventional notions of manufacturing excellence upside down. In the old economy, manufacturers reduced costs by producing huge volumes of goods in cavernous, assembly-line factories. Each worker created small components of the end product. None had a vision of the whole. These products were manufactured for an unknown customer and held in inventory or on a showroom floor until they were finally sold. New-economy, mass-customization factories, in contrast, tailor the product to the needs of a specific customer or customer group in small, flexible factories designed so that workers can see the whole product before their eyes. Maytag's mass-customization dishwasher factory exemplifies the virtues of this approach; it increased quality by 55 percent, while work space and capacity were reduced by 50 percent or more.[43] The key to mass customization is its focus on the customer. Notes one analyst, "Customers are no longer passive recipients of a message. They tell you what they want. You stay with me because we have a learning relationship."[44] Health care–focused factories resemble these mass-customization organizations in their modest scale, integrated view, and focus on the whole customer.

Yet, under the present fragmented insurance reimbursement system, health care–focused factories are not economically feasible. Recall, for example, the discussion in Chapter Two of Duke University's integrated program to manage congestive heart failure (CHF), a complex, costly health care problem. CHF victims have 50 percent five-year mortality rates and account for seven million hospital days and $22.5 billion of direct costs. Suspecting that fragmented care exacerbates these statistics, Duke's program integrated care providers from the hospital to the home; developed best-practice protocols for medication, symptom management, and self-care support; and provided patients with continuous access to clinicians. The care was as focused as focused could be. The results? Significant decreases in hospitalization days and increases in adherence rates for medications. The costs per patient year dropped by 32 percent because the health status of the enrollees increased.[45] But Duke University was not rewarded for increasing productivity. Because its cost decreases were caused primarily by reduced hospitalizations, the medical center ate virtually all the savings. It paid for the program in the form of decreased hospital revenues.

Unlike the present system, a consumer-driven health care system will support the evolution of these integrated teams. First, users will demand them. For example, a woman with diabetes who can freely choose among many differentiated health insurance products will likely opt out of an everything-for-everybody system into one that provides the integrated, demonstrably excellent care she requires, and at a lower cost to boot. Then too, some consumer-driven health insurance policies will no longer pay every provider at the same price for a limited range of covered services. Instead, a team of providers will quote its own price for the bundle of services that its members have jointly determined as appropriate. This switch in reimbursement methods for providers will enable those who want to offer focused factory services to do so without suffering the devastating economic consequences imposed by the current reimbursement system. With the risk-adjusted pricing described in Chapter Four, providers will be rewarded for serving sick patients.

Consumer-driven competition and reimbursement policies that reward efficient focused factories will thus cause focused factories to flourish.

Personalized Medicine

The most controversial innovation for increasing productivity is personalized medicine—genome-derived diagnostic tests, drugs tailored to genetic code variations that cause or contribute to diseases, and devices that enable us to monitor the functioning of our bodies.

The innovations of Millennium Pharmaceuticals, a Cambridge, Massachusetts, firm, illustrate the promise of personalized medicine. One is Melastatin, a gene that produces a marker for skin cancer. Because the level of the marker appears to be linked to the aggressiveness of the cancer, it could be used to tailor individualized therapeutic regimens. The firm's pharmacogenomic tools, a mouthful used to describe genetic indicators for the therapy that best suits our individual responses and metabolic rates, will likely improve, for example, the current painful, debilitating chemical therapies for breast cancer by eliminating regimens that have no impact and optimizing the dosage of those that do.[46] In 2003, two drugs for genetically linked cancers were marketed.

Few would quarrel with the view that the "right drug for the right person" will not only improve health status but also reduce the costs resulting from ineffectual and possibly injurious medications, the wrong drug for the wrong person. One study revealed, for example, that 59 percent of the twenty-seven drugs frequently cited for causing adverse drug events were linked to genetic variations in patients' ability to metabolize the drugs.[47] Nevertheless, most health policy experts essentially dismiss these benefits; in their eyes, personalized medicine and other new technologies will primarily create unsustainable strains on health care costs.[48] One study dourly concluded, for example, that "[in] an era of finite resources, the question is how to balance providing access to as many of these innovative, life-saving drugs as possible without increasing premiums beyond ability to pay."[49]

Predictions like this are based on a blinkered economic framework that ignores the systemic effects of increasing costs in one sector on the overall costs of health care and the productivity of the economy. These narrow views of productivity are largely absent for other sectors of the economy. For example, most people readily acknowledge that increased computerization expenditures increase overall productivity. But when it comes to health care, views like these, no matter how illogical, are unlikely to disappear. Luddite-like suspicions of science persist, from the repudiation of Galileo's astronomical views to today's denials of the economic efficacy of medical innovators.

Nevertheless, an increasingly large, impressive body of evidence refutes them. An evaluation of the impact of medical technology on medical conditions, for example, illustrated the importance of a broad framework that examines the impact of medical technology innovations on the economy as a whole. It documented productivity and quality-of-life benefits that exceeded the additional costs of new technologies for medical problems such as heart attacks, low-birthweight infants, depression, and cataracts.[50] Similarly, studies of the impact of cost increases in pharmaceuticals on total health care costs have demonstrated that they frequently cause overweening reductions in hospital costs.[51] That is not to say that every new technology is cost effective, but rather that, taken as a whole, new medical technologies create benefits in excess of their costs. Newer medical innovations appear to be increasingly cost effective: new drugs have caused greater improvements in well-being and more reductions in work loss than older ones.[52]

Americans persist in what the health care policy experts who survey them believe to be the muddle-headed view that payment for all this new technology is feasible.[53] They are unlikely to accept the experts' doubts. Americans are staunch supporters of new technology and consider themselves very knowledgeable about it. To meet their expectations, consumer-driven health insurance policies will surely incorporate the personalized medicine that will significantly improve the productivity of our health care system and our economy.

PRODUCTIVITY IMPROVEMENTS AMONG ATHLETES: THE LESSONS FOR HEALTH CARE

Athletes, the ultimate service providers, present evidence of the possibilities for productivity in the service sector. Over the years athletic performance has continually improved; athletes became stronger, faster, and more accurate. Yet in 1934, when Brutus Hamilton, a college track coach, predicted twenty-seven goals that athletes would eventually attain, such as running a four-minute mile, Baumol-minded colleagues found his predictions preposterous. Today, every one of his twenty-seven goals has been not only attained but surpassed.[54] Current athletes and their publics would find the observation that they cannot improve laughable. Try telling that story to Tiger Woods, the Williams sisters, or their adoring golf and tennis fans.

Athletes bettered their performance through improvements in nutrition, technique, and athletic gear from shoes to vaulting poles. Each of these improvements belongs to a general class of economic activities that increase productivity. They can increase health care productivity too.

Personalized medical technologies are an obvious analogue to better athletic gear, and integrated medical records are the health care equivalent of better nutrition. Helping people to take care of their own health, one outcome of complete medical records, is enormously cost effective. In a consumer-driven health care system, consumers will be able to purchase the support they need and want, including information support. In the present third-party-controlled health care system, in contrast, successful purveyors of health promotion struggle against the indifference of insurers. Some insurers may doubt the efficacy of health promotion. Others may not want to invest now in a remedy whose cost savings will become apparent only years in the future, when the enrollee may no longer be with their plan.

Dean Ornish vividly illustrates this problem in Chapter Forty-Seven of this book. Despite mountains of scientific evidence about the efficacy of his diet and exercise regimen for reversing heart disease, Ornish was forced to lobby the U.S. Congress and president to obtain a trial run of it for Medicare recipients. A successful and energetic medical entrepreneur, Ornish marshaled his many talents to change the Medicare bureaucracy's mind. Many other health-promoting specialists would doubtless back off from such a gargantuan challenge. In contrast, under a consumer-driven health care system, people could easily select or avoid his regimen, as they chose. And insurers could offer multiyear contracts that would enable them to earn the rewards, in the form of cost reductions, for the investments they made to promote enrollees' health years before.

Last, improving the management of health care enterprises through focused factories is the health care equivalent of better athletic techniques. The ergometer, a training tool that simulates rowing, is an example of a new productivity-enhancing technique. It caused Olympic rowing times to plummet by nearly 10 percent in the first games after its introduction.[55] In health care, focused factories that integrate the many diverse or segmented providers involved in caring for particular diseases or categories of care into a cohesive system hold special promise, especially when coupled with the *horizontal integration* of the cottage health care industry. As described in Chapters Fifty-Four, Fifty-Six through Sixty, and Chapter Sixty-Four of this book, focused factories simultaneously improve quality and lower costs. Chapters Sixty-One and Sixty-Two, among others, describe how horizontal integration achieves similar results.

FOCUSED FACTORIES: BETTER CARE
FOR THE POOR AND THE SICK

Elsewhere in the economy, the arrival of a new firm is celebrated. The premise is that new entrants will increase competition: they will improve quality and/or control costs. Government laws focus on antitrust and other corporate maneuverings to reduce competition for this reason. In health care, however, new entrants that are demonstrably more efficient and provide higher quality face an uphill battle, as demonstrated in the MedCath case that I discuss in this section.

Why?

Although most entrenched competitors try to protect themselves against powerful new rivals, their arguments typically fail, viewed as transparent, self-serving attempts to reduce competition. Why are such appeals more sympathetically received in the health care sector?

Because the *financing* of health care is confused with its *production.*

Most people agree that our financing system should provide for the care of the sick and the poor. Similarly, virtually everybody would agree that health care services should be produced by the most cost-effective organizations. In our present financing system, the two are inextricably intertwined, enabling entrenched providers to argue effectively against new competitors.[56] In contrast, consumer-driven health care appropriately decouples financing and production decisions. As a result, these goals can be met simultaneously:

1. If focused factories can demonstrate that they are the most cost-effective providers of care, consumers will choose them and they will prevail.

2. Sick people will be assured of receiving care in any facility through risk-adjusted pricing of consumer-driven insurance policies. They will likely choose quality-enhancing focused factories.

The poor will thus have a better chance of receiving care through the broadening of the safety net that cost-controlling consumer-driven health care innovations will induce.

Focused Factories and the Public Interest

Multipurpose hospitals generally oppose free-standing focused factories. They claim that the latter undermine the health care system by skimming off the healthier patients and profitable care that the hospitals rely on to subsidize sicker patients and unprofitable services and that they offer no compensating benefits.

The case of the MedCath Corporation, a publicly traded operator of heart hospitals, illustrates these complaints and management's responses to them. When MedCath tried to open a heart hospital in Wisconsin, the president of an existing hospital system said, "If businesses are concerned about premiums going up, here is $30 million being spent with no incremental benefits to the community."

MedCath noted three benefits in its response. First, its management countered that its operational focus improved quality, as demonstrated by lower mortality and morbidity rates and a lower average length of stay among its patients compared to patients who received care at general hospitals. (An analysis of Medicare discharge data provided by Solucient, an independent health care consulting firm providing strategic information, market intelligence, and clinical and financial analysis, showed that MedCath had lower mortality rates than competing traditional hospitals for cases of comparable severity.) Management credited the improved outcomes to the fact that physicians, nurses, technicians, and other staff members concentrated all of their professional care on a single type of patient. This operational focus was especially beneficial for staff training. Whereas a general hospital often could not afford to train all staff members in each of the clinical areas in which the staff members were involved, MedCath focused all its training around one disease. Management believed that this intense training allowed heart hospitals to recognize warning signs and take corrective action earlier.

Second, whereas MedCath could invest its available funds exclusively in equipment and technology for cardiovascular care, traditional hospitals needed to allocate their funds among many different specialties. Third, patient satisfaction data indicated that patients preferred MedCath heart hospitals to larger full-service hospitals. In an independent study by National Research Corporation that rated California hospitals on seven dimensions through mail surveys of recent patients, MedCath's Bakersfield Heart Hospital received the highest rating—three stars—in all seven categories.

MedCath's management attributed some of these high ratings to the unique design of MedCath facilities, which afforded all patients private rooms and also allowed care to be provided in a single room (the Universal Patient Room). In contrast, in traditional hospitals patients were moved through a series of different rooms where equipment and the nurse-to-patient staffing ratio increased with the patient's acuity level.[57] Management believed the Universal Patient Room design led to a less stressful experience for patients and their families. According to a recent patient in MedCath's Heart Hospital of South Dakota: "Giant hospitals are a scary experience for patients and their families. If you can be close to everything you need in a small [building], [where] it is easy for visitors to find you, that's a major improvement."[58]

Most general hospitals do not accept these points. Their perspective is outlined in the debate that surrounded the establishment of the Heart Hospital of Milwaukee, which is summarized here:

Criticism 1: A New, Focused Facility Will Lead to Excess Capacity. Local hospitals claimed that by opening a stand-alone heart hospital, MedCath was duplicating resources and expanding capacity beyond that required by the Milwaukee area. A 1999 study found that utilization of open-heart surgery and angioplasty among Milwaukee Medicare enrollees was 19 percent and 50 percent higher, respectively, than the national averages for these two procedures. Milwaukee ranked forty-seventh (eightieth percentile) and thirty-third (eighty-fifth percentile) in utilization of open-heart surgery and angioplasty, respectively, among 306 major cities surveyed by the study. (The study adjusted for geographical differences in age and relative heath).[59] Local hospitals argued that MedCath had chosen to operate in non-certificate-of-need states (such as Wisconsin) precisely because it could not justify the need to regulators.

Further, when MedCath pulled volume out of the local hospitals, these hospitals' cost per treatment increased because of their high percentage of fixed costs. With roughly 70 percent of cardiac care paid for by the government via Medicare and Medicaid, the public would eventually foot the bill through higher taxes.[60]

MedCath's management disagreed with the assertion that there was excess cardiac care capacity in the Milwaukee area. MedCath argued that one had to distinguish between general medical-surgical (med-surg) beds and cardiac beds when drawing any conclusions regarding capacity. Because of the high level of disease acuity in a cardiac care setting, cardiac beds needed special monitors (for blood pressure, heart rate, and so forth) and equipment (for renal dialysis, for example) that ordinary med-surg beds lack. According to MedCath, Milwaukee had insufficient capacity in cardiac beds. Given the demographic trends in the area (and the country as a whole), this capacity shortage would only worsen with time.

In addition, many local Milwaukee hospitals were simultaneously adding to their own cardiac care capacity while fighting the addition of MedCath's capacity. For example, St. Luke's Hospital was building a $180 million, 280-room cardiac care center, and Community Memorial hospital, another local competitor, a $40 million heart and vascular center.[61]

Criticism 2: It Will Skim the Cream. The most common criticism of MedCath made by local incumbent hospitals was that MedCath was doing nothing more than "skimming" hospitals' most profitable line of business, cardiac care. According to the American Hospital Association (AHA), a typical full-service hospital generated 20 percent of its revenue and 50 percent of profits from heart care. A 2002 report found that cardiac surgeons topped the list of revenue generators for a hospital, at $3.1 million per year each.[62] By reducing the local hospitals' cardiac care volume, therefore, MedCath threatened the very viability of these community hospitals, which were expected also to provide such money-losing activities as burn units, trauma facilities, and drug and alcohol treatment centers.

Large general hospitals around the country, not only those in the Milwaukee area, were preparing to use this claim in petitioning politicians to fight the spread of hospital specialization. In the words of Rick Wade of the AHA: "We are very concerned about the future viability of community hospitals under a scenario in which all of the profitable services are provided by these entrepreneurial firms. We aren't just concerned about cardiac care, but also the freestanding surgery centers, orthopedic centers, birthing centers, diagnostic imaging centers, etc. Simply put, there are some services and some people that will never be profitable. As a society, we need to decide whether it's important that these services are provided and these people are cared for."[63]

A cardiac surgeon who was closely affiliated with a general hospital expressed a similar viewpoint: "It should come as no surprise that if you take a profitable hospital service, and then move it outside of the hospital—thereby removing the entire overhead associated with providing the entire range of necessary services—it will be extremely profitable."[64]

MedCath disagreed with the notion that a local community hospital needed its share of cardiac care services in order to subsidize other, unprofitable services. Using open heart surgery as a proxy for cardiac care, management pointed to the fact that only 921 of 4,556 (20.2 percent) acute-care hospitals in the United States even had open heart programs, and only 160 of those 4,556 (3.5 percent) hospitals had "major" (defined as 250 cases or more per year) open heart programs, yet most were profitable.[65]

MedCath believed that in no other industry would the high-cost incumbent be allowed to maintain its position and bar new entrants because of concern that the incumbent's costs might increase further. In other industries incumbent full-service providers respond to focused, niched competitors by reducing their overhead. (Costs are "fixed" only if capacity remains unchanged as competitors successfully reduce the incumbent's market share.) Resourceful incumbents reduce their capacity, if needed. Hospitals' per-patient fixed costs would increase only if they refused to slim down in response to loss of volume.

As for cross-subsidization, the appropriate response is to bring up the prices of money-losing services, rather than to suppress efficient competitors. After all, inefficient everything-for-everybody providers raise the costs of health care and consume funds that should be used instead for undercompensated care.

Criticism 3: It Will Be Unsafe for Patients. Finally, local hospitals warned that it could prove unsafe to perform open-heart surgeries without the support available in a full-service hospital. One reason for this opinion is that many comorbidity problems are associated with cardiac care, such as diabetes and pulmonary disease.

But MedCath management believed this was more criticism of a misunderstanding than anything else. MedCath facilities are licensed as general acute-care hospitals and therefore must meet all accreditation, state licensing, and Medicare requirements and have all of the equipment, staff (ER, orthopedic, trauma, general surgery, obstetric, and so forth) and training required of such hospitals. MedCath heart hospitals also contain the equipment and staff needed to treat the comorbidities commonly associated with cardiac care. As a result, only about 10 to 20 percent of the medical staff in a MedCath heart hospital were cardiologists or cardiac surgeons.[66]

Management also pointed out that MedCath's severity index was comparable to or higher than those of competing local hospitals at the same time as MedCath was providing lower mortality, shorter length of stay, and lower postdischarge expenses than other hospitals offering cardiology services. MedCath's lower mortality and morbidity rates, despite comparable severity indices, attested to its ability to take on even the most challenging and difficult cases. MedCath facilities treated patients with a higher level of acuity and case complexity and achieved superior clinical outcomes.

Focused Factories: The End of Turf Warfare?

The present reimbursement structure of the health insurance sector motivates turf warfare because it pays for inputs—for example, drugs, doctors, and hospitals—rather than outcomes—such as a complete bundle of care for diabetes. When health care costs rise, various input factors finger each other as the prime culprit. In 2002, for example, pharmaceuticals were largely blamed for the rise in health care costs.[67] Such turf warfare is ultimately self-serving. As its name indicates, this war is motivated by its participants' desire for control over more territory. Unlike World War II, whose purpose was to save humanity, turf warfare is not noble. In its health care incarnation, it is singularly pointless. After all, no matter who the culprits are said to be—doctors, hospitals, or pharmaceutical companies—they are a necessary component of the health care system. Attempts to minimize the cost or quantity of the demonized component may result only in diminution of quality or an increase in total cost. For example, if a drug that reduces the need for hospitalization is demonized and as a result is either used less or encounters pricing pressures that force its manufacturer to cease improving it, overall costs may well rise as more people are admitted to costly hospitals.

With a focused factory reimbursement system, in contrast, the blame or praise for price movements belongs to the focused factory rather than its component parts. The leaders of the focused factory are rewarded or punished for the aptness of their combination of different components. This kind of reimbursement generally advances the public interest.

To gain a clearer picture of the impact of a switch from reimbursement for components to reimbursement for a total, imagine a system that pays for the various ingredients used in a loaf of bread rather than the bread itself. Under the ingredient reimbursement system, when the price of the loaf goes up, the wheat farmers blame the egg farmers and the yeast manufacturers. If the yeast manufacturers are politically inept, their reimbursement for their contribution to the bread will be reduced. I hope you like flat breads, hard as a piece of wood.

If, instead, the bread bakers are paid for the loaf, they will be blamed when prices rise. They will then have to figure out for themselves how to recombine the ingredients needed to make a more cost-effective loaf of bread. No one will force them to reduce the amount of any one ingredient. If the bread bakers inflict a flat, hard bread on their customers, all of them will be appropriately pilloried until an innovator who can produce a fluffy, low-cost bread emerges, the Henry Ford of the bread industry.

Currently, the pharmaceutical industry is the component most frequently blamed for the double-digit rise in health care costs.[68] The allegation is dubious. The consumer price index for all medical care increased by 4.4 percent from 2001–2002, and the pharmaceutical industry index grew by about 5.5 percent.[69] Simple algebra indicates that pharmaceuticals could thus account for all of the increase only if the costs of the other components of the system had shrunk. A more realistic assessment pegged the impact of retail prescription drug spending on the 13 percent increase in premiums in 2001–2002 at 12.1 percent. This was exceeded by provider increases in costs (18 percent), with costs related to government regulations close behind (15 percent).[70]

Nevertheless, drug manufacturers are the current culprit of choice—demonized for activities such as spending $2.8 billion on informing consumers and $13.2 billion on informing doctors.[71] Left unexplained in these criticisms is how consumers and doctors would learn about these new products in the absence of these expenditures. Do not get me wrong. The pharmaceutical companies are like the rest of us: they are not saints. In the twelve-year period from 1989 to 2000, only 35 percent of the new drugs approved by the U.S. government contained new active ingredients. The remaining 65 percent differed from existing drugs only in their dosage or delivery or in the way they were combined with other, already approved ingredients.[72] But many of the new drugs were substantially important for treatment of cardiovascular disease, osteoporosis, and impotence. As genomics substantially increases the number of drug targets and the quality of new drugs, drugs will increasingly become frontline therapies. Attempts to contain drug costs may only slow down the introduction of these important innovations.

We can continue to fight expensive, self-serving turf battles.

Or we can rely on focused factories to figure out the appropriate balance of each component part in the total package of care they offer.

To my mind, the latter approach is unquestionably better. Consumer-driven health care will help to advance it.

Can We Afford Focused Factories?

Those who argue against focused factories because they are "so expensive" miss the point. We already spend vast sums on the problems that focused factories are designed to treat: chronic diseases and disabilities and the needs of underserved populations. Focused factories will provide more cost-effective care for these needs. Indeed, the very magnitude of the sums misspent on fragmented care is the reason for the focused-factory innovations.

For example, the $54 billion spent in 1996 on the care of people with diabetes could support, in each of the fifty states, one 500-bed hospital, five 200- to 299-bed hospitals, and thirty community facilities at a cost of $10 million each that are entirely devoted to diabetes and its comorbidities. They could largely supplant the current, ineffectual patchwork quilt of care for diabetes.[73] And these impressive figures do not include the massive economies that focused factories will create in the delivery of health care.

THE SICK: THE EIGHT-HUNDRED-POUND GORILLA

The image of an eight-hundred-pound gorilla is frequently invoked to indicate that an obvious factor is being ignored in a discussion. For example, a Boston columnist once critiqued the process for selecting the head of a major community service organization by noting that because the process took place within an old-boys' network, it evaluated "candidates without acknowledging the eight-hundred-pound gorilla in the room: race, gender, age, fill in the missing blank."[74]

Sick people are the eight-hundred-pound gorilla in health care. They consume most of the health care and account for most of the expenditures. National data indicate that the top 1 percent of users accounted for 27 percent of costs in 1996, the top 10 percent accounted for 55 percent,[75] and the top 20 percent accounted for 83 percent.[76]

The best way to control health care costs is to focus on improving care of the sick. Voluminous evidence indicates that their care is less than ideal: it is delivered episodically and does not adequately support self-care, especially monitoring and scrupulous adherence to complex regimens.

Improved care typically leads to reduced costs. Yet despite all the talk about managing care, the care of the sick has not improved. In 1928, the top 5 percent of users accounted for 52 percent of all health care costs. That percentage remained steady through 1996.[77]

Three obvious strategies can improve the quality of care to the sick:

- Integrate the many diverse sources of care around organizations focused on their needs
- Support patients' ability to promote their health status and to care for themselves
- Ensure use of the technological advances in treating chronic illness

Consumer-driven health insurance will advance all three strategies by offering enrollees options that include focused factory providers and long-term, health-promoting, health insurance policies; personalized medicine; and integrated medical records.

Consider diabetes again as an example of the causes of the health care system's problems and their likely cures. One way this disease wreaks havoc is by destroying blood vessels. As a result those with diabetes frequently suffer degradation in the organs heavily perfused by blood vessels: the heart, kidneys, and eyes. The damage sustained by these organs also causes collateral consequences elsewhere in the body—neuropathy in the feet and associated gangrene and open wounds that do not heal on the legs, the parts of the body farthest from the ailing heart. Diabetes exacts high tolls. It is the leading cause of blindness in people twenty to seventy-four years of age, end-stage renal disease, and amputation of lower limbs. And individuals with diabetes are at least twice as likely as others to suffer from heart disease or a stroke.[78] Unfortunately, the prevalence of the disease is growing, increasing by 33 percent from 1990 to 1998.[79]

Diabetes exacts substantial economic costs as well as personal ones. The costs of diabetes clock in at $100 billion.[80] One survey of employers' medical expenditures revealed that people with elevated blood glucose levels accounted for about 7 percent of employers' total costs for all illnesses.[81] In one region in Florida, diabetes caused about twenty-four days of decreased productivity per four-week period and $160,000 in lost wages per 1,000 employees.[82] Another, extensive study documented the excess costs for treatment of 85,209 people with diabetes at $282 million relative to the costs for a matched set of nondiabetic individuals. The excess costs were most pronounced for hospitalizations and outside referrals. Complications accounted for 38 percent of the excess. The authors concluded that "programs [that] can reduce the occurrence of these complications" would generate substantial savings.[83] Diabetics who had not yet been diagnosed with the disease required $1,200 more in medical care costs per person than did people with similar characteristics but without undiagnosed diabetes.[84]

Management of diabetes requires scrupulous monitoring and control of the level of sugar in the bloodstream. Sugar concentration can be affected by many factors, including nutrition, exercise, emotional state, and the time of day. Programs can support self-care to monitor blood sugar levels and adjust drug dosages and personal habits. The more tightly blood sugar levels are controlled, the better the long-term outcomes of the disease.[85] The Diabetes Control and Complications Trial, a major study published after ten years of observation, demonstrated that control of blood sugar levels significantly reduced the risks of eye, kidney, neurological, and cardiovascular disease.[86] The greatest benefits accrued to those with less advanced cases of the disease.[87] Programs that support self-care have shown effective results.[88] However, ideal management requires frequent blood sampling to measure sugar levels and taxing self-control. These requirements are so onerous that many patients, understandably, fail to achieve them. One survey revealed that one-third do not test their blood sugar at all or not as often as needed.[89]

Why? Likely because they are not sufficiently supported in these diagnostic tasks by their providers. Even among those insured by Medicare, only 36 percent were tested for glucose levels every six months and only 43 percent had annual eye examinations.[90] Those cared for by doctors whose appointments were classified as "fast" had markedly lower levels of testing than these. Among those taking insulin, for example, only 25 percent received retinal screening.[91]

Dramatic improvements in adherence to necessary regimens occur when people with diabetes receive integrated care that focuses on their disease and supports the repetitious tasks they must do themselves. For example, those treated in the Diabetes Center of the world-famous Massachusetts General Hospital had significantly better diagnostic screening than those treated in the same hospital's Internal Medicine Clinic: eye exams, 70 percent versus 42 percent; foot exams, 85 percent versus 42 percent; and home glucose monitoring, 91 percent versus 53 percent. Moreover, even though the Diabetes Center treated more severely ill individuals, diabetics, health care utilization costs were no higher than those in the Internal Medicine Clinic.[92]

Technology helps too. For example, implanted pumps that match insulin and sugar levels have significantly reduced patients' blood sugar levels, without the side effects that can accompany tight sugar control.[93]

To achieve results like these, the American Diabetes Association advises those with diabetes to build "Your Health Care Team," consisting of a general physician, nurse educator, registered dietician, ophthalmologist, behavioral therapist, podiatrist, dentist, and exercise physiologist, all trained in working with people with diabetes.

The association's article also notes, "if you build it, they will come."[94]

I do not think so.

Indeed, advice, however well intended, that asks debilitated people coping with diabetes to stitch together their own team borders on the ludicrous. It is akin to asking individuals with paraplegia to build their own wheelchairs. Provider-led focused factories are much better candidates for building the teams that the victims of our fragmented U.S. health care system need.

The best way for the sick to obtain the focused, health-promoting, integrated team they require is through a consumer-driven health care system that motivates and rewards the providers who develop it.

Notes

1. Johnson, B. C. "Retail: The Wal-Mart Effect." *McKinsey Quarterly*, 2002, *1*, pp. 40–43.

2. See, for example, Turner. G.-M. "Two Visions of Health Reform." [www.galen.org], Feb. 14, 2002.

3. Conlin, M. "Workers Beware of Brave New Health Plans Delivering Less." *Business Week,* Sept. 9, 2002, p. 128.

4. Howatt, G. "New Health Plan Fares Poorly at 'U': Workers Pick Old Favorites over Newcomers." *Star Tribune,* Dec. 15, 2001, p. 1D.

5. U.S. Bureau of the Census. *Statistical Abstract of the United States: 2001.* Washington, D.C.: U.S. Government Printing Office, p. 435, table 664.

6. Gokhale, J., Kotlikoff, L. J., and Warshawsky, M. J. "Life-Cycle Saving, Limits on Contributions to DC Pension Plans, and Lifetime Tax Benefits." Working Paper 0102, Federal Reserve Bank of Cleveland, Apr. 2001.

7. Silow-Carroll, S., and Duchow, L. *E-Health Options for Business: Evaluating the Choices.* New York: Commonwealth Fund, Mar. 2002.

8. "Putting America on Wheels." *The Economist,* Dec. 31, 1999, p. 82.

9. Baumol, W. J., and Bowen, W. G. *Performing Arts: The Economic Dilemma.* New York: The Twentieth Century Fund, 1966, p. 164.

10. Herzlinger, R. E. "Can We Control Health Care Costs?" *Harvard Business Review,* Mar.–Apr. 1978, *56,* 102–113.

11. Institute of Medicine. *Crossing the Quality Chasm.* Washington, D.C.: National Academy Press, 2001, p. 174.

12. Barrett, M. J., and others. *Personalized Medicine.* Cambridge, Mass.: Forrester Research, Aug. 2000.

13. The concept of focused factories was first applied to industry by Harvard Business School professor Wickham Skinner. It is an apt analogy for focused health care, first popularized as focused factories in my book *Market-Driven Health Care.*

14. Institute of Medicine, *Crossing the Quality Chasm.*

15. Herzlinger, R. E. *Market-Driven Health Care: Who Wins, Who Loses in the Transformation of America's Largest Service Industry.* Cambridge, Mass.: Perseus Books, 1999.

16. Robert Wood Johnson Foundation. *A Portrait of the Chronically Ill in America, 2001.* Princeton, N.J.: Robert Wood Johnson Foundation, 2002, p. 39.

17. Brocato, F. M., Borden, S., Barnes, J., and Allen, H. "Disease Impairment at Work: Year 2 Update," *Healthy People, Productive Community Survey.* Tampa, Fla.: Employers Health Coalition, 2000, p. 5.

18. Druss, B. G., Marcus, S. C., Olsfson, M., Tanielian, T., and others. "Comparing the National Economic Burden of Five Chronic Conditions." *Health Affairs,* Nov.–Dec. 2001, *20,* 233–241.

19. Druss and others, "Comparing the National Economic Burden of Five Chronic Conditions," p. 235.

20. Asch, S. M., and others. "Measuring Underuse of Necessary Care Among Elderly Medicare Beneficiaries Using Inpatient and Outpatient Claims." *Journal of the American Medical Association,* Nov. 8, 2000, *284,* 2325–2333.

21. Robert Wood Johnson Foundation. *A Portrait of the Chronically Ill in America, 2001,* p. 47.

22. Turner, R. C., Holman, R. R., Stratton, I. M., Cull, C. A., and others. "Effect of Intensive Blood-Glucose Control with Metformin on Complications in Overweight Patients with Type 2 Diabetes (UKPDS34)." *Lancet*, Sept. 12, 1998, *352*, 854–865.

23. Cunningham, R. "Old Before Its Time: HIPAA and E-Health Policy." *Health Affairs*, Nov.–Dec. 2000, *19*, 231–238.

24. Ray, N. F., Thamer, M., Gardner, E., and Chan, J. K. "Economic Consequences of Diabetes Mellitus in the U.S. in 1997." *Diabetes Care*, Feb. 1998, *21*, 296–309.

25. Testa, M. A., and Simonson, D. C. "Health Economic Benefits and Quality of Life During Improved Glycemic Control in Patients with Type 2 Diabetes Mellitus: A Randomized, Controlled, Double-Blind Trial." *Journal of the American Medical Association*, Nov. 4, 1998, *280*, 1490–1496.

26. National Health Information. *Disease Management Advisor.* [www.nhionline.net], Mar. 2001.

27. Schuster, M. S., McGlynn, E. A., and Brook, R. H. "How Good Is the Quality of Health Care in the United States?" *Milbank Quarterly*, 1998, *76*(4), 517–563.

28. Robinson, J. C. "Financial Capital and Intellectual Capital in Physician Practice Management." *Health Affairs*, July–Aug. 1998, *17*, 53–74.

29. Shortell, S., Gillies, R., and Anderson, D. "The New World of Managed Care: Creating Organized Delivery Systems." *Health Affairs*, Winter 1994, *13*, 46–65.

30. See, for example, Budetti, P. P., and others. "Physician and Health System Integration." *Health Affairs*, Jan.–Feb. 2002, *21*, 203–210.

31. Gulati, R., Nohria, N., and Zaheer, A. "Strategic Networks." *Strategic Management Journal*, Mar. 2000, *21* (Special Issue, "Strategic Networks"), 203–215; Gulati, R., and Singh, H. "The Architecture of Cooperation: Managing Coordination Costs and Appropriation Concerns in Strategic Alliances." *Administrative Science Quarterly*, Dec. 1998, *43*, 781–814.

32. "Ghost Cars, Ghost Brands." *Forbes*, Apr. 30, 2001, p.109.

33. Andrews, F. "Dell, It Turns Out, Has a Better Idea." *New York Times*, Jan. 26, 2000, p. C12.

34. Herzlinger, *Market-Driven Health Care.*

35. Figluilo, M. L., Mango, P. D., and McCormick, D. H. "Hospital, Heal Thyself." *McKinsey Quarterly*, 2000, *1*, 91–97.

36. Figluilo and others. "Hospital, Heal Thyself."

37. Herzlinger, *Market-Driven Health Care.*

38. "Hitting the Brakes." *Modern Healthcare*, Jan. 14, 2002, p. 22.

39. Arista Associates. *2000 Survey of Integrated Delivery Systems.* Northbrook, Ill.: Arista Associates, July 15, 2000.

40. Moody's Investor Service. *Not-for-Profit Health Care.* Report No. 58944. Boston: Moody's Investor Service, Aug. 2000, p. 7; Dixon, R., and Coye, M. J. "Strategies to Improve Clinical Care Management for Chronic Illnesses: A Critical Assessment Project." Unpublished manuscript prepared by the Lewin Group for the Robert Wood Johnson Foundation, May 2002.

41. See, for example, Robinson, J., and Casalino, L. "The Growth of Medical Groups Paid Through Capitation in California." *New England Journal of Medicine,* Dec. 21, 1995, *333,* 1684–1687.

42. For an exception, see Chapter Fifty-Nine in this volume; Robitaille, S. "Are IPAs Dead?" *Health Leaders,* Feb. 2002, *5,* 40–45. See also Hurley, R., Grossman, J., Lake, T., and Casalino, L. "A Longitudinal Perspective on Health Plan Provider Risk Contracting." *Health Affairs,* July–Aug. 2002, *21,* 144–153.

43. "The Long March: Mass Customization." *The Economist,* July 14, 2001, p. 63.

44. "All Yours." *The Economist,* Apr. 21, 2000, p. 58.

45. Snyderman, R. "New Approaches to Chronic Disease Management," talk at the Medtronic CEO Summit, Minneapolis, Aug. 23, 2000; Conway, K. J. "Millennium Predictive Medicine." *Wall Street Transcript,* Feb. 21, 1999, pp. 82–85.

46. "Millennium Predictive Medicine."

47. Phillips, K. A., and others. "Potential Role of Pharmacogenomics in Reducing Adverse Drug Reactions: A Systematic Review." *Journal of the American Medical Association,* Nov. 14, 2001, *286,* 2270–2279.

48. Fuchs, V. R., and Sox, H. C. "Physicians' Views of the Relative Importance of Thirty Medical Innovations." *Health Affairs,* Sept.–Oct. 2001, *20,* 30–32.

49. Mullins, C. D., Wang, J., Palumbo, F. B., and Stuart, B. "The Impact of Pipeline Drugs on Drug Spending Growth." *Health Affairs,* Sept.–Oct. 2001, *20,* 210–215.

50. Cutler, D. M., and McClellan, M. "Is Technological Change in Medicine Worth It?" *Health Affairs,* Sept.–Oct. 2001, *20,* 11–29.

51. Kleinke, J. D. "The Price of Progress: Prescription Drugs in the Health Care Market." *Health Affairs,* Sept.–Oct. 2001, *20,* 43–60.

52. Lichtenberg, F. R. "Are the Benefits of Newer Drugs Worth Their Cost? Evidence from the 1996 MEPS." *Health Affairs,* Sept.–Oct. 2001, *20,* 241–251.

53. Kim, M., Blendon, R. J., and Benson, J. M. "How Interested Are Americans in New Medical Technologies? A Multicountry Comparison." *Health Affairs,* Sept.–Oct. 2001, *20,* 194–201.

54. Litsky, F. "On the Playing Field the Best Is Yet to Come." *New York Times,* Jan. 1, 2000, p. 10.

55. Litsky, "On the Playing Field . . ."

56. For more on this topic see *Developments in Antitrust Health Care Law.* Chicago: American Bar Association, 1990.

57. Bill Moore, president, Hospital Division, MedCath Corporation, personal communications to the author, Mar. 2002.

58. Dobbs, K. "Compact Size Yields Efficiency, Officials Say." *Argus Leader,* Mar. 11, 2001, p. 1A.

59. Dartmouth Medical School, The Center for the Evaluative Clinical Sciences. *The Dartmouth Atlas of Healthcare.* (J. Wennberg and others, eds.) Chicago: AHA Press, 1999, pp. 154–174.

60. Bourna, C. "Local Hospitals: How Many Are Too Many?" *New Orleans City Business,* Nov. 11, 2001.

61 Manning, J. "For Anyone with a Heart." *Milwaukee Journal Sentinel,* July 22, 2001, p. 1D.

62. "Survey Puts a Price Tag on Doctors' Value to Hospitals." *American Medical News,* Apr. 15, 2002, p. 20.

63. Rick Wade, vice president, public affairs, American Hospital Association, personal communications to the author, Mar. 22, 2002.

64. Denton Cooley, M.D., surgeon in chief, Texas Heart Clinic, personal communication to the author, Mar. 25, 2002.

65. MedCath internal documents, based on data from the American Hospital Association.

66. Goldberg, S. "Provider of Cardiovascular Services Perceives Growing Need for Heart Hospitals as 55-and-Older Population Burgeons: An Interview with David Crane, Chief Executive Officer and President of MedCath." *Deloitte & Touche Healthcare Review,* Sept. 2001 (entire issue).

67. National Public Radio, Kaiser Family Foundation, and Harvard University's John F. Kennedy School of Government. *National Survey of Health Care.* [www.kff/content/2002/3238/NPR_Chart_Pack_FINAL2.pdf], June 2002.

68. National Public Radio, Kaiser Family Foundation, and Harvard University's John F. Kennedy School of Government. *National Survey of Health Care.* June 2002.

69. U.S. Bureau of Labor Statistics. "Medical Care." In *Consumer Price Index.* [www.bls.gov/data/home.htm], Apr. 2002.

70. PricewaterhouseCoopers. *The Factors Fueling Rising Health Care Costs.* [www.aahp.org/InternalLinks/PWCFinalReport.pdf], Sept. 2003.

71. Kaiser Family Foundation. *National Survey of Physicians, Part II: Doctors and Prescription Drugs.* [www.kff.org/2002/200204156], 2002.

72. National Institute for Health Care Management Research and Educational Foundation. *Changing Patterns of Pharmaceutical Innovation.* [www.nihcm.org/innovations.pdf], May 2002.

73. National Center for Health Statistics. *Health, United States, 1999.* Washington, D.C.: U.S. Government Printing Office, 2000, p. 334: 500-bed hospital cost = $75 billion ÷ 250 hospitals; 200–299 bed hospital = $56.5 billion ÷ 692 hospitals.

74. Bailey, S. "Elephant in the Room." *Boston Globe,* Mar. 30, 2001, p. E1.

75. Berk, M. L., and Monheit, A. C. "Concentration of Expenditures Revisited." *Health Affairs,* Mar.–Apr. 2001, *20,* 12.

76. Mark L. Berk, personal communication to the author, 2001.

77. Berk and Monheit, "Concentration of Expenditures Revisited," p. 12.

78. American Diabetes Association. *Diabetes Facts and Figures.* Washington, D.C.: American Diabetes Association, 2000.

79. Mokdad, A. H., and others. "Diabetes Trends in the U.S.: 1990–1998." *Diabetes Care,* Sept. 2000, *23,* 1278–1283.

80. American Diabetes Association. "Economic Consequences of Diabetes Mellitus in the U.S. in 1997." *Diabetes Care,* Feb. 1998, *21,* 296–309.

81. Anderson, D. R., and others. "The Relationship Between Modifiable Health Risks and Group-Level Health Care Expenditures." *American Journal of Health Promotion,* Sept.–Oct. 2000, *15,* 45–52.

82. Brocato, F. M., Borden, S., Barnes, J., and Allen, H. "Disease Impairment at Work." Tampa, Fla.: Employers Health Coalition, May 2000, pp. 5, 9.

83. Selby, J., Ray, G. T., Zhang, D., and Colby, C. J. "Excess Costs of Medical Care for Patients with Diabetes in a Managed Care Population." *Diabetes Care,* Sept. 1997, *20,* 1396–1402.

84. Nichols, G. A., Glauber, H. S., and Brown, J. B. "Type 2 Diabetes: Incremental Medical Care Costs During the 8 Years Preceding Diagnosis." *Diabetes Care,* Nov. 2000, *23,* 1654–1659.

85. Marwick, C. "Development of Noninvasive Methods to Monitor Blood Glucose Levels in People with Diabetes." *Journal of the American Medical Association,* July 22–29, 1998, *280,* 312–313.

86. Diabetes Control and Complications Trial Research Group. "The Effects of Intensive Treatment of Diabetes in the Development and Progression of Long-Term Complications in Insulin-Dependent Diabetes Mellitus." *New England Journal of Medicine,* Sept. 1993, *329,* 977–986.

87. Diabetes Control and Complications Trial Research Group, "The Effects of Intensive Treatment of Diabetes . . ."

88. Berger, M., and Muhlhausen, I. "Diabetes Care and Patient-Oriented Outcomes." *Journal of the American Medical Association,* May 12, 1999, *28,* 1676–1678.

89. Edlin, M. "Personalized Web Sites Help Keep Diabetes in Check." *Managed Healthcare,* Sept. 2000, pp. 47–48.

90. Asch, S. M., and others. "Measuring Underuse of Necessary Care Among Elderly Medicare Beneficiaries . . ."

91. Streja, D. A., and Rabkin, S. W. "Factors Associated with Implementation of Preventive Care Measures in Patients with Diabetes Mellitus." *Archives of Internal Medicine,* Feb. 8, 1999, *159,* 294–302.

92. American Diabetes Association. "Article Title Will Go Here." [www.diabetes.org/am99/a100105.html)]. Month date, YEAR.

93. Scavini, M., and Schade, D. S. "Implantable Insulin Pumps." *Clinical Diabetes,* Mar.–Apr. 1996, *14,* 30–36.

94. American Diabetes Association. "Your Health Care Team." [www.diabetes.org/main/info/facts/healthcare/jsp], Aug. 2002.

CHAPTER SIX

The Silent Revolution

No wonder I feel weak and dumb in the health insurance selection process. *When it comes to health insurance choices, consumers are weak and dumb.* In the pension area, investors were aided by extraordinary, effective entrepreneurs. Do such people exist in health care?

Where are the John Bogles of health insurance, the brilliant, out-of-the-box thinkers who would empower consumers with a plethora of innovative, efficient products, who would provide Bea, Jacqui, and Sam with the consumer-driven health insurance that best met their needs?

Where are the Morningstars that would rate health insurers and providers in powerful, yet simple-to-understand ways, that would warn Molly about Dr. Scar, and guide Vivian to empowering physicians like Dr. Monoson?

Where are the Harry Moskowitzes to devise measures that adjust the performance results of providers by the riskiness of the activities they undertake?

If choice and information were widely available, the health care sector would improve. Like the financial markets, it too would become better and cheaper.

How do we get there?

As always, we get there because people who can make what we want happen are interested in doing so.

Who are these people?

THE SILENT REVOLUTION

Across the United States a silent revolution is creating a new kind of health care. Its creators are largely unaware of each other's existence. Their methods and ways differ considerably. But they breathe the same air—the zeitgeist of consumerism. They long to bring the consumerism that reshaped our economy when assertive, picky consumers denied companies the ability to raise prices easily to health care. This revolutionary consumerism, that demanded better products without price increases, led to a new phrase among managers, *pricing power*. Noted one economist, "Raising prices was just an easier way of making money [but]—now . . . that you do not have pricing power—you have to do something else to make money."[1] That "something else" was to cut costs and improve quality.

Thus, when consumers demanded better, cheaper cars, they got them: the Consumer Price Index (CPI) for new vehicles did not inflate from 1995 to 1998.[2] When consumers asked for better services and lower costs from retailers, they got them too: the CPI for apparel and house furnishings also remained flat from 1995 to 1998,[3] and productivity for various retailers grew at a minimum of 2.3 percent per year from 1987 to 1997.[4] This consumerism democratized our financial system and brought prosperity to the American people.[5] When U.S. manufacturers finally internalized customer preference as their lodestone, quality zoomed while costs fell. When they denied customer primacy—in effect saying, "we are smarter than our customers"; "they cannot tell the difference"—quality deteriorated and costs swelled.[6]

The creators of the new kind of health care believe that the consumerism that helped to boost the productivity of the U.S. economy by 2.3 to 4.2 percent a year in the period from 1996 to 2000, after years of substantially lower growth, will do the same for health care.[7] In their view, consumerism will control health care costs while increasing health care quality.

In this belief they are revolutionary.

Their views fly in the face of the health care policy experts who stoutly contend that costs can be lowered only by rationing quantity. To these experts, health care cost inflation is fueled by *excessive* consumerism. People simply use too much health care: too many tests, too many doctor's visits, too many days in the hospital. The people are not bad, merely ignorant.

The experts' solution? In all modesty they offer themselves up as those who can lead consumers onto the path to righteousness, guiding them to appropriate health care usage and gently dissuading them from inappropriate ways.[8] It is not power, wealth, or fame that motivates them. Their sole interest is to help those who are not as smart as they. For example, one says that "artificially limiting the capacity of the health care system and then . . . rationing . . . by administrative or clinical algorithms is a more civilized method of reining in . . . health services" than are various consumer-choice options. But "unfortunately, non-economists would be unlikely to understand these semantic fine points."[9]

Some call this strategy managed care, others more openly call it what it is— rationing of health care.[10]

Reform health care by *responding* to the consumer?

No way.

To these experts, health care can be reformed only by *managing* the consumer.

But the creators of the new, consumer-driven health care system are unde-terred by these views and perhaps inspired by their very wrong-mindedness. They know that American consumers are smart, knowledgeable, assertive. All they need are the tools to drive the health care system.

Revolutionary Strategies

All these revolutionaries intend to reform health care by turning the reins of control over to consumers, although their strategies vary.

Some aim to revolutionize *health insurance*—to enrich the choices of health insurance policies so that consumers can buy the policies that best meet their needs, just as they buy mutual funds. Some aim to revolutionize *information about health care prices and quality* so that health care consumers are armed with the same kind of information that enables them to shop intelligently for everything from financial instruments to cars to tomato sauce. Some aim to revolutionize *health care services and technology* so that like other sectors of our economy, such as computers, cars, and food, they too become simultaneously better and cheaper by responding to consumers' needs. Last, some aim to revolutionize the *role of government in health care* away from a micromanaging, hectoring presence that *manages* health care to one that *protects* consumers by providing access, information, and oversight.

The Revolutionary Mosaic

The new consumer-driven health care mosaic is composed of many individuals across the United States, following their own guiding star with their own iconoclastic activities. Viewed one at a time, they represent merely themselves. But when their activities are juxtaposed, they form the pattern of the new, consumer-driven health care system.

Out of the heartland of the United States, two health insurance revolution-aries emerge: one the reserved, gray-suited, revered CEO of a revered *Fortune 500* firm, the other a clog-wearing, body-building, ardent liberal, a 2003 incar-nation of the 1960s' hippie.

From the coasts of the United States, both East and West, come health information revolutionaries. The one on the West Coast, a fashionably stubbled

McKinsey graduate, publishes health price information for consumers. The East Coast houses a pair of Pulitzer Prize–winning, Harvard-trained lawyers who provide easy access to the country's best doctors.

Riding out of the Southwest comes an entirely different type of revolutionary: a distinguished surgeon who provides consumers with low-cost, high-quality cardiovascular procedures. Complementing him, in the Northeast, is a genomics revolutionary, the hula-shirt clad CEO of a leading company who is determined to use the rapidly unraveling knowledge of the genome to bring the right drug to the right person.

The health care policy community is not entirely blind to these revolutionaries. Missoula, Montana, is the home of a lifelong Democrat who has single-mindedly championed the kind of tax reform that would provide a more level playing field for the uninsured. And Virginia is the home of yet another revolutionary, an African American Republican, who for years has brought consumer-driven health care to the nation's poor.

They and many others are the pieces in a mosaic. Each has a different shape, texture, and color. But taken together they form the consumer-driven health care system.

Parts Two through Five of this book contain the stories of many of these individuals in their own words. The chapters in Part Two impart the visions and models of the U.S. and European revolutionaries who are creating a consumer-driven health insurance system; the chapters in Part Three tell the stories of the new intermediaries who provide consumers with the information and support they need to act as effective leaders of the new consumer-driven system; the chapters in Part Four delineate the models of the health care service and technology revolutionaries who are simultaneously increasing quality and decreasing costs; and the chapters in the final section expand on the important ideas of the health care policy revolutionaries who are transforming the role of government so it can better meet the societal needs of a consumer-driven health care system.

HEALTH INSURANCE ENTREPRENEURS: VISIONS AND MODELS

Bill George, a Fortune 500 CEO, and Ray Herschman, an entrepreneurial iconoclast, are both restructuring our health insurance system, each in his own way.

Straight from the Heart, I: The Heartland

Suddenly, William W. "Bill" George's picture was everywhere—or everywhere in the kinds of things I read—*Fortune, Forbes,* and the like. The pictures showed a thinnish, handsome man in a dark, well-tailored, conservative suit. George is smiling, sincerely, but not broadly, into the camera, his lids half-masking his eyes. They capture George's essence—his sobriety, intellect, and reserve. They reflect a corporate guy. A soccer-coach-dad, devoted-husband, community-leader kind of guy. The stories that accompanied the pictures all bore roughly the same headline: "The 100 Best Companies to Work For." "The 400 Best Big Companies in America."[11]

Medtronic, the legendary Minneapolis company that Bill George until recently headed as the CEO, is usually included in these lists—for good reasons too. Medtronic is a leader in the medical device sector. It creates instruments, such as pacemakers, that keep people alive. It builds them well. It earns a lot of money for its shareholders in the process. And it accomplished all this without raising prices.

Bill George has much to do with Medtronic's excellence. Under his watch, Medtronic's sales quintupled, its product portfolios blossomed, and its market capitalization grew from $3 billion, in 1991, when he became the CEO, to $72 billion in 2001.

He does not fit your typical revolutionary profile. Nevertheless, under the business veneer, Bill George *is* a revolutionary. He is the first, big-time CEO to trust his employees to choose the health care that is right for them. He gives them the money to buy health care, he gives them many choices, he gives them information so they can shop smartly, and then he gets out of their way.

And what choices they are. As but one example, Medtronic is among the few big firms that enable their employees to choose complementary health care: the acupuncture and meditation kind of health care that is not offered by the traditional medical system. Some might think that complementary health care is an unusual benefit for a firm that develops very high technology medical devices. But any irony here is lost on Bill George. His wife, Penny, uses complementary health care to wage her brave battle against breast cancer, and Bill meditates daily. (For George's discussion, see Chapter Nine.)

The Hippie Actuary

Also in the heartland, in Ohio, lives yet another revolutionary. He looks more like a revolutionary than George: short and body-builder wide, with a backpack, clogs, and an ear lobe pierced for the earring he wears when he is not talking to people like me. Born to liberal, activist parents, he attended the University of Wisconsin because he was attracted to the progressive ideas many of the school's faculty espoused.

This revolutionary, Ray Herschman, is a health actuary. A revolutionary actuary? It is no oxymoron. Herschman believes that health care can become better and cheaper through consumer-led competition. But, to him, you cannot have competition without choice.

Had all the automobile manufacturers followed Henry Ford's lead, every car today would likely still resemble a Model T and come in any color, as long as it was black. But Ford's rivals saw opportunity in his rigidity. They offered choices: coupes, unique transmissions and engines, more comfortable body types, elegant styling, and yes, loads of colors. The many different choices led to ferocious competition. And the competition produced better, cheaper cars. Today's cars are not only safer, more fuel-efficient, and more reliable but also cost relatively less as a percentage of income.[12] In contrast, most defined benefit health insurance policies provide little choice. They all cover the same benefits and give access to the same providers. In these ways they are all more or less Model T Fords.

As a revolutionary, Herschman wanted to bring the automobile industry's kind of competition to health care. As an actuary, he understood why health care insurers do not compete with each other by offering different products. They are hamstrung by three significant characteristics that make them different from other businesses, all discussed in the previous chapters. First, insurers receive the same payment whether their enrollees are sick or well. You do not need to be an actuary to understand the economic incentives created by this payment system. Health insurers want to sell health insurance policies that attract healthy people and deter sick ones. After all, with uniform pricing for all enrollees, they can earn profits by insuring the well and lose their shirts by insuring the sick. *Adverse selection* is the term insurers use to describe the process of losing their shirts by enrolling sick customers. Thus, ironically, they would prefer to sell health insurance to those who do not need it.

And that is not the whole story. Health insurance differs from other businesses in yet a second important way. Unlike virtually every other good or service, it is not selected directly by its users. Instead, most employed people find their health insurance options are selected by the health care human resource (HR) specialists in their firm. These specialists narrow the range of health insurance options to a handful in the belief that big is beautiful. In 2000, the workers in 50 percent of firms could "choose" from one plan.[13] The specialists reason that insurers that control a big chunk of the health care providers' income can muscle down providers' prices much more effectively than insurers that accounted for only a small fraction of this income. To direct enrollees to the health plans they consider the best, they subsidize the employees' costs for different plans at different rates. Only a few workers receive equal company contributions for each plan.[14] As a result, the insurance prices seen by the enrollees differ from those paid by their employers.

Finally, to ease their own selection process, the HR specialists have forced health insurers to differ from other businesses in a third significant way. They frequently require that all the health insurance options offer more or less identical benefits.[15] Their desire for uniformity is understandable: With all health insurers offering the same options, the HR specialists can more easily compare the costs of the different policies. But the requirement carries a significant downside: it stops health insurers from differentiating their products in order to compete.

As a result, there is little real product competition: the few health insurance policies that are offered generally cover the same benefits. Further, because insurers are paid the same price for all their enrollees, they live in deadly fear that if they alter their policies—changing, say, the employees' level of payment or provider network—they will attract the sick or deter the well from enrolling. Last, consumers have little voice in shaping the content of the policies or affecting price by their choices. In classic economic terms this market suffers from several fatal flaws: the absence of differentiated products, distorted prices, few competitors, and an agent acting for the consumer.

Herschman the actuary understood those problems well.

Herschman the revolutionary thought he could solve them with a system that provided consumers with many choices and protected insurers from adverse selection.

To promote choice and consumer involvement, he envisioned a market in which consumers could choose directly from a wide variety of health insurance options—a health insurance supermarket, which he called HealthSync. (Herschman is a very smart guy; but, like all of us, he is not infallible. I would not include naming companies among his major strengths.) Employers who wanted to outsource their health care benefits process could contract with HealthSync to provide its health insurance supermarket to their employees. To encourage the development of different kinds of health insurance products, HealthSync did not constrain the insurers' policy design. Insurers were free to create any product they like. And to protect the insurers against adverse selection, HealthSync's system prospectively paid insurers more for enrolling sick people and less for well ones.

For an example of the workings of the HealthSync system, imagine an employer who has only two employees—one a sixty-year-old woman, the other a thirty-year-old man. The employer's annual health care costs are $13,000. Although the average insurance price for this employer is $6,500 per person, the $13,000 in costs is actually composed of $12,000 for the older woman and $1,000 for the younger man. (These amounts are only illustrative.)

In today's system an insurer will jump through hoops to attract the thirty-year-old and will try to deter the older person. But with HealthSync, an insurer that attracts the older person would be paid more; the one that attracts the younger person would be paid less. Imagine, for example, that HealthSync had determined that a sixty-year-old woman costs 1.85 of the average payment and that a thirty-year-old man costs .16 of the average. The insurer that priced a policy at $6,500 would receive roughly $12,000 for the sixty-year old ($6,500 × 1.85) and $1,000 for the thirty-year old ($6,500 × .16). With this system, the employer's total costs remained the same at $13,000, but the insurance company was now appropriately rewarded for enrolling an older person and not excessively rewarded for enrolling a younger one. To avoid bias and invasion of privacy, HealthSync's risk-adjustment weights were built on generic data such as age and illness, not personal data such as level of illness.

Herschman believed that HealthSync's system would unleash the insurers' creativity and reward them for designing products that meet consumers' needs. For example, sick people could find policies that enabled them to use providers who specialized in the treatment of their disease or disability. Conversely, younger people could find policies that concentrated on the superb maternity, pediatric, and wellness services they are most likely to use.

I use the past tense here because HealthSync was forced to close its doors when the venture capital markets collapsed in 2001. But you cannot keep a good innovator down. Herschman still ardently pursues his vision as a consultant with a major health benefits firm.

More Health Insurance Revolutionaries

Of course Bill George and Ray Herschman are not the sole heartland entrepreneurs. As described earlier, Minnesota's Buyers Health Care Action Group (BHCAG) is another supporter of revolutionary consumer-driven health insurance products. BHCAG has already established that consumerism pays off. And Definity and Vivius, both Minneapolis firms, also offer a different kind of health insurance plan.[16]

The U.S. government's Federal Employees Health Benefits Program (FEHB, pronounced "feeb") is yet another partially consumer-driven health care health insurer. The federal government has provided its employees with plenty of choice—more than three hundred plans nationwide and at least ten in most regions.[17] The choices are priced on two bases: the insurers' experience with the group (experience-rated) or their experience with the community (community-rated). In 1998, the federal government paid 75 percent of any plan's price up to a maximum amount that is determined by the U.S. Congress. Enrollees receive comparative information about the quality of the insurance plans, including the results of satisfaction surveys.

For much of its forty-year history, these three features, information, choice, and a dollar maximum for the employer's contribution, created competition that moderated the program's cost increases and swelled consumer satisfaction. Between 1992 and 1999, the program's cost grew by 3 percent as private sector premiums grew by 5 percent.[18] Nevertheless, the failure of the FEHB to create an incentive for consumers to save and to risk-adjust its insurers' premiums and its standard benefits, has created some problems. One analysis found that enrollees overinsure in order to obtain the maximum 75 percent matching funds from the federal government. (The matching option reduces the enrollees' share of the cost for incremental benefits to $.25 per $1.00 of benefits.) Not surprisingly, the prices of plans above the maximum dollar contribution grew more slowly than the prices of the others.[19] And the absence of risk adjustment has inhibited product differentiation in the program. As one insurer noted: "The trick is to structure benefit packages with extreme precision to attract the widest possible mix of ages and conditions. You don't want to appeal overly to groups looking for specific benefits, such as generous drug coverage." (In the absence of risk adjustment, plans that attract the sick have gone bust.[20]) Last, the standardized benefits have limited competition through innovation.[21] (For the history of the FEHB, as described by its long-term director James Morrison, see Chapter Seventeen.)

Other health insurance revolutionaries offer their services for both large and small businesses. Some even cater to individual consumers. For example, Quotesmith.com, a firm that maintains an insurance quote Web site for individuals and small businesses, offered quotes from more than forty firms. It thus decreased the complexity of comparison shopping for health insurance and likely the time required as well.[22] Using the services of this firm could also substantially reduce the typical brokerage commission.[23] Ins.Web.com, a similar firm, charged transaction fees of only $9 for an on-line search session.[24]

Some nonprofits also serve this sector. Health marts are nonprofit markets that offer a large selection of health insurance policies to individuals. These policies are free of legislated benefit mandates—the more than 1,000 state laws that require coverage of special benefits and providers by health insurers.(For further discussion of this topic, see Chapter Seventy-Two.)

Although these intermediaries have only a brief organizational history, and may not have a long future, some already provide compelling evidence of their impact. For example, an astonishing 44 percent of the Ins.Web customers switched carriers after completing a shopping session.[25] As this statistic also indicates, however, the relationship between the edgy health care consumer and the new intermediaries is not all sweetness and light. Consider the tale of Healthaxis, Inc. In typically grandiose PR prose, the company described itself as "the leading provider of Internet solutions for health care insurance."[26] But *SmartMoney* begged to differ: "Healthaxis.com will 'guide you to the insurance you need'—unless you live in the wrong state, want a decent selection of products, or to compare price. As of now, the site offers just a few types of insurance . . . and the level of choice is, well, dismal," said this magazine's scathing review.[27] Not surprisingly, the market value of Healthaxis fell from $464 million in 1999 to $8.6 million in 2001.[28]

Innovative Services for the Poor

Can insurance products be sold efficiently and effectively to the poor?

Innovative firms in South Africa have achieved remarkable market penetration selling both insurance and banking products to this population and have done so profitably. One of them, Old Mutual, sells death, disability, and savings products to almost one million people. Its minimum monthly premiums are 25 percent of those charged by "more-upmarket mutual distribution companies." Another, Standard Bank of South Africa, has 26 million low-income consumers, nearly a quarter of the country's working population. Their average account balance has doubled in the past two years.[29]

The key to their success?

Consumer-driven financial products. These firms tailor their products to the population: clearly defined products, pricing transparency, education, and ease of access provide the keys to success. Old Mutual holds local seminars on financial planning. Its sales staff is recruited from the community and its marketing techniques are focused on local schools and media outlets. Standard Bank uses automatic teller machines (ATMs) to enhance access and cut costs. The ATM centers are located on main streets and malls and open at hours that respond to the population's needs. As a result, its costs per outlet are 30 to 40 percent lower than those of traditional banks, and its salespeople's productivity is as much as 400 percent higher. The bank also fulfilled the need to educate low-income users about the benefits of saving by targeting low-income affinity groups.

These two firms provide substantial benefits to the low-income population. Many of the clients are new to banking and insurance. And they receive education, transparent pricing, and easy access as a bonus. (For Shaun Matisonn's description of a similar health insurance innovation in South Africa, see Chapter Twenty-Two.)

NEW INTERMEDIARIES: INFORMATION IS GOOD FOR YOUR HEALTH

Who will provide the information that consumers need in a consumer-driven health care world? The insurance revolutionaries in the heartland of the United States are joined by information revolutionaries on both coasts.

The East Coast Matchmakers

On the East Coast, in Aiken, South Carolina, Gregory White Smith and Steven Naifeh conduct a matchmaking service, Best Doctors, that enables sick people to find the best doctor for their problem. Their database consists of more than 30,000 doctors who have been named by their peers as the "best" in their fields.

There is considerable demand for this information. In the few years that I have known Greg and Steve, I invariably wind up referring many of the people I meet to them. One was a friend searching for the best doctor to operate on his prostate cancer. Another was a mother, deeply concerned about the rate of development of her children, who was looking for the best genetic counselor.

Most of those who used their service raved about it. After all, it not only short-cuts the search process but also, and more important, it gives desperately ill and despondent people the power and control they seek.

Like many of the other consumer-driven health care revolutionaries, Smith and Naifeh are unusual people who tailor the world to their needs. Educated as lawyers at Harvard University, they chose to become authors instead. They succeeded wildly in their new profession, winning a Pulitzer Prize for their biography of Jackson Pollock and earning sufficient capital to renovate a magnificent, art-filled mansion along the way.

But life is rarely totally wonderful. Tragedy struck when Greg Smith was diagnosed with a brain tumor. A distinguished doctor gravely informed him that he had but a few months of life left.[30]

Did Smith politely comply with his death sentence?

No way.

Instead, he searched ferociously for the best doctors, those who would keep him alive. On his journey he found all too many nonbest doctors who patronized, insulted, and mistreated him. The success of his quest is evident in his robust, immaculately groomed self, some twenty years after he received his death sentence. The concept of Best Doctors was born as a result of his search. Smith and Naifeh created it to spare other sick people the prolonged, circuitous, costly, demeaning process they endured to find the best doctors. (For Smith and Naifeh's description of their work, see Chapter Forty.)

The California Roll

Superficially, Andy Slavitt, Smith's and Naifeh's West Coast information-providing partner, is a polar opposite to them. Slavitt is a midthirties California type whose fashionably stubbly beard and rumpled khaki pants contrast with Smith's and Naifeh's meticulous Southern grooming. He is intensely focused on business, in contrast to their broad-based interests. Last, unlike the visual, writerly, painterly Smith and Naifeh, Slavitt is an MBA all-star, with Wharton and Harvard Business School degrees and a spell at McKinsey's famed Los Angeles health care practice.

But like many other revolutionaries in the consumer-driven health care world, Slavitt, Smith, and Naifeh are soul mates. The superficial differences are unimportant and misleading.

Like Smith and Naifeh, Slavitt was propelled by a personal loss into founding a firm that empowers health care consumers with information. His inspiration came when a friend's wife turned to him for help after her husband died of cancer. She was surrounded by mounds of medical bills, whose bulk was matched only by their incomprehensibility. Slavitt the MBA all-star was a sensible choice to help her plow through the paper. But Slavitt the social activist was an even better choice. He is as intense about his societal interests as his business ones. Slavitt serves on the board of directors of the Special Olympics and the board of advisors for Habitat for Humanity and has traveled to El Salvador to help build housing in that war-ravaged country.

These two sides of his being meshed as he organized her medical bills. On the social side, Slavitt wondered if the bills' lack of transparency and sheer volume were designed to take advantage of a vulnerable, grieving person. On the business side, he was outraged by charges to an individual that vastly exceeded the charges for the same services to large groups. And try as he might, Slavitt could not link the charges to the actual care received. Did a radiology charge represent diagnostic procedures or a dose of x rays to kill wildly proliferating cancerous cells? Did the patient actually receive the care in the charges? Was it fairly priced? Was it a necessary part of his therapy?

If Andy Slavitt, all-star MBA and health care analyst, could not answer these questions, who could?

HealthAllies, the firm Slavitt created to serve uninsured or underinsured people, helps answer these questions. The firm's Web site empowers its users by providing information about the prices for medical care alongside the credentials of those providers. The firm also offers them discounts on health care prices that are similar to those obtained by large groups. And consumers can obtain prices for bundles of care, rather than a la carte services. For example, a pregnant woman can obtain a discounted fee for the entire maternity and birth process from her choice of providers through HealthAllies.

Had the HealthAllies site been available to the wife of Slavitt's friend, she would have received one bill for the bundle of care given to her husband rather than hundreds of individual ones; she could have easily compared her price to prices charged by other providers; and she could have obtained the same discounted rate as large-group buyers.

Consider the following illustrative case:

A woman who needs a hip replacement inquires about the charge at an academic medical center. She is quoted a price of $35,000. (In hotels, this kind of price is known as the *rack rate,* the rate quoted to individual customers who lack the bargaining power of a group.) She then logs onto the HealthAllies site to search for a better hip replacement price. In response to her specifications about the type of providers she wants (for example, a surgeon who performed more than 75 hip replacements last year and who operates in an academic medical center that performed more than 500 hip replacements last year and that is located within thirty miles of her home), she chooses a hospital that quotes a price of $25,000. Ironically, it is the same hospital that initially quoted the $35,000 price.

To ensure that its interests are squarely lined up with those of the user, HealthAllies' revenues are derived from the savings it creates for the consumers and their employer.[31] (In 2003, United Health, a large insurer, acquired Health Allies.)

More Health Care Information Services

Many other sources of consumer-driven health care information exist. Indeed, clinical health information sources are so easy to find that they are virtually unavoidable. They appear regularly on radio and television, typically in the form of patronizing lectures from reading-off-the-TelePrompTer "Health Beat"–type announcers (not so good); in newspaper features (good); and in magazines devoted solely to the topic (better still). For example, more than three million copies a month of *Prevention* magazine were sold in outlets such as supermarket checkout areas in 2001.[32] Many authoritative health care books are available as well, including best-sellers such as the *Mayo Clinic Family Health Book* (in my view, the best).[33]

Some organizations even help consumers to evaluate their doctors' advice. For example, Consumer's Medical Resource (CMR), a Massachusetts firm, provides medical decision support services via a team led by a practicing Harvard Medical School physician. The team assembles a customized report and provides telephone counseling. In one case, CMR concluded that a member had been mistakenly diagnosed with Parkinson's disease. Its counsel not only saved the cost of needless medication but also, and more important, spared the client considerable anguish.[34] One of CMR's corporate clients saved $280 for every $1 spent on the program and found quality improvement in 66 percent of the cases. (For further discussion of CMR, by its president and founder, David Hines, see Chapter Forty-Six.)

The Web is a major source of health information. It not only enables mass customization of information but also facilitates consumers' feedback about the quality of their health care experiences. This kind of information is much valued. For example, a KPMG survey of almost 15,000 employees of the Fortune 1000 revealed that they placed the highest trust in information received from friends and family.[35]

Nevertheless, substantial market needs still remain largely unserved. A 2000 survey revealed that the information that consumers sought most was largely unavailable. Most of the available information focuses on diseases; however, over 50 percent of respondents wanted additional information: evaluations of doctors, hospitals, and insurers; e-mail reminders; and personal medical reports.[36] A 2002 review of forty physician directory Web sites found many were incomplete, inaccurate, and out-of-date.[37]

Although consumers overwhelmingly prefer their own doctor or national medical experts as the source of on-line health information,[38] physicians have been slow to get on-line. In 1998, only 37 percent of physicians were using the Internet, according to an American Medical Association survey, and only 41 percent of office-based doctors used a computer. In contrast, 52 percent of U.S. households owned computers in 1999, and 72 percent of them had access to the Internet. Physicians are understandably reluctant to join the Internet revolution. They fear a flood of e-mail from their patients. States one, "I just don't have the time . . . I'm in the car . . . on the telephone, seeing patients, making rounds at the hospital. [I'm] never sitting at my desk." Nevertheless, he noted, "I'm getting nervous that I'm getting archaic. I've got to do something with the Internet, no question."[39]

The new intermediaries who offer to set up "free" Web sites for physicians hope to attract clients like him.[40] Although demand exists, how quickly it will develop is unclear. Says one physician, speaking for many: "I think Web sites are the wave of the future, but I'm not sure how quickly I'll jump on."[41] The new, consumer-driven reimbursements offered to some physicians for on-line interaction will surely accelerate the transition.[42]

Information that rates the quality of providers and insurers is also currently sparse, but ample evidence of its imminent arrival exists. As an example of the depth of desire for such information, consider three full-page stories in the New York City tabloid the *Daily News.* The first tells the tale of two mothers whose young children died after treatment by physicians who had had numerous malpractice suits filed against them. The two joined forces to require public disclosure of physicians' malpractice histories.[43] The extent of their consumer-driven success is attested to by two other stories in the same issue of this paper. Both feature politicians who agree that the public has a right to information about doctors' performance history. One features your typical politician—silver-haired, meticulously coiffed, toothy: "We're trying to get as much disclosure out there to help people. . . . People have a right to know what a doctor's medical history is." He is a Johnny-come-lately to the cause, as the second story, featuring a more cerebral type of politician, built on an academic model, replete with overgrown hair, a bushy beard, and glasses, makes clear. He had sponsored a bill requiring public disclosure of physician malpractice but got nowhere until the *Daily News,* responding to the interests of its blue-collar readership, identified New York's fifteen most-sued doctors[44] and Governor Pataki signed the bill.[45]

A number of Web sites already serve the general market that seeks consumers' ratings. For example, consumers can post their reviews of products and retailers on Epinions.com, BizRate.com, and ConsumerReview.com. There are even professional raters of the raters. For example, a *New York Times* article critically evaluated the sites that rated cars, including the Web site of the *Kelley Blue Book,* the lycos.com Auto Section, and the ultimate winner of that evaluation, consumerreports.org.[46]

The felicitously named Quackwatch.com performs this review function for health care. Quackwatch was formed by a retired psychiatrist and features more than one hundred doctors on its board. The organization cooperates with the National Council Against Health Fraud and *Consumer Reports.*[47] The U.S.

government has jumped into the rating fray too. Responding to findings of questionable Internet information by the Federal Trade Commission and the Food and Drug Administration, the private firm Hi-Ethics (or Health Internet Ethics) was formed to promulgate principles to improve the accuracy of health care information, and the nonprofit organization URAC (also known as the American Accreditation Health Care Commission) was started to provide independent accreditation of Web sites.[48]

HEALTH CARE SERVICES AND TECHNOLOGY REVOLUTIONARIES

Bill George, Ray Herschman, Greg Smith, Steve Naifeh, and Andy Slavitt represent important components in the pattern of the consumer-driven health care mosaic. George's and Herschman's innovations provide consumers with money and choice. Smith's and Naifeh's and also Slavitt's innovations provide consumers with the information that can help them make good choices.

But the health care system is not primarily composed of money, choice, and information. Its core lies in the blood, sweat, and tears of those who provide the services and create the technology—the devoted doctors and nurses who may sport balloonlike ankles as mementos of a day spent standing on their feet to perform arduous surgeries, the brilliant scientists who may display a pallor testifying to years cooped up in labs in the hope of devising new ways to conquer disease, and the many other often underpaid, overworked people who produce health care services and products.

They account for the bulk of health care costs and most of the quality of care. If they do not respond to consumers with better, cheaper health care, all the choice and information innovations will be largely for naught.

Can they respond?

Will they respond?

Many of those who espouse health care markets are stopped dead in their tracks by this point. Sure, they preach competition, but if the health care providers and scientists do not cooperate in innovating health care, the competition that really matters will never materialize.[49]

After all, the competition among health insurance products that the market ideologues advocate cannot materially affect health care. The costs of administering insurance are relatively small—an average of $19.20 per member per month among Blue Cross Blue Shield plans in a 2002 report.[50] The program administration and net cost of private health insurance in 1998 accounted for only 6 percent of health care expenditures. Although this percentage amounts to a hefty $82 billion, it is a mere pimple on the massive body of the U.S. health care system.[51] Most health care costs are consumed in delivering health care services and technology, not in administering insurance. And these costs accounted for $1.2 trillion in 1999,[52] growing at a rate substantially higher than that of nonmedical inflation as a whole.[53]

Unless consumer-driven health care convinces the folks behind these costs to do things in a better, cheaper way, it cannot possibly succeed.

Are they interested?

Can they do it?

Two consumer-driven health care revolutionaries—one a silver-haired, reserved Texas surgeon, the other a CEO incongruously clad in a Hawaiian shirt in chilly Cambridge, Massachusetts—illustrate the interest of both doctors and scientists in creating a consumer-driven health care system and their abilities to do so.

Straight from the Heart, II: The Texas Heart Institute

Denton Cooley, one of the world's leading cardiovascular surgeons, moves with the grace of the natural athlete that he is. His soft Texas drawl is gentlemanly and cadenced. But as with many revolutionaries, the exterior masks the interior—the daring, ferociously competitive innovator that resides within.

The litany of Cooley's surgical firsts is staggering: the first in the world to implant an artificial heart, the first to perform a successful heart transplant in the United States, and a member of the first surgical team to correct the heart defect that leads to the now seldom heard of blue baby syndrome.[54] It takes considerable courage to amass such a list. Imagine yourself peering deep within the exposed cavity of the human body, staring at a heart ensnared by a tangle of veins and arteries, bathed in blood, layered in fat, and guarded by a fence of spikey ribs. Would you, like Cooley, have the courage to disentangle that heart, remove it, and sew in a new one? Count me out!

Cooley's courage is not restricted to medicine. His business ventures are as daring on their own terms as his medical ones. He invested millions in Texas real estate, oil, and gas. His kind of investing is not for the novice or the faint of heart (excuse the pun). His investing is for the high-flyer, the boomer and the buster. Not surprisingly, Cooley's early sport of choice was basketball— a body-contact team sport played with the elbows and shoulders as much as the hands and eyes, a game that calls for spontaneity and courage as much as skill and discipline.

As befits such a courageous man, Cooley's highs are almost equaled by his lows. Some of his surgical firsts were accompanied by ethical challenges to the medical aggressiveness of his procedures.[55] And his high-flying business ventures collapsed in a 1988 bankruptcy with personal liabilities of nearly $100 million.[56]

So what is this skilled daredevil doing today, now that he is in his eighties?

Denton Cooley is devoted to improving the quality and lowering the cost of open heart surgery and a few other cardiovascular procedures. His thesis is that focus and repetition can achieve this goal. Cooley leads a team of people in well-orchestrated procedures for performing surgery. This is no pickup basketball game. Every move is drilled; every member of the team knows his or her role; every piece of equipment is chosen with care and thought. Victories are celebrated; failures are analyzed. His is a learning organization.

In a sense, Cooley's attention to increasing the productivity of health care is not surprising. He is, after all, both a physician and a businessman. But as is his wont, this venture too is controversial. It flies in the face of the conventional medical dogma that quality and cost are inevitably correlated. Speaking for many surgeons, Michael DeBakey, Cooley's archrival, says: "Sure, you can cut costs. But you get what you paid for."[57]

However, Cooley's results have shown him, once more, to be correct. He has *simultaneously* lowered costs and improved quality. While his open heart surgery costs declined by as much as 16 percent, his patients' satisfaction rates and outcome statistics exceeded those of a general purpose hospital. And Cooley rebuts accusations that he achieved these results by avoiding sick patients: "Our patients are sicker than the average because we are a tertiary care center and take many patients who have been turned down elsewhere."[58] (For further views of this topic, by Denton Cooley and John Adams, see Chapter Fifty-Six.)

The Right Drug for the Right Person: Consumer-Driven Pharmaceuticals

You have probably heard of designer drugs as mood-altering, illegally obtained drugs for people with more money than brains, more ego than charity. Well, Mark Levin, CEO of the Cambridge, Massachusetts, genomics firm Millennium Pharmaceuticals, does designer drugs. But in his case the designer drugs are not illicit. Nor are they mood altering. His drugs are designed to ameliorate diseases by matching their characteristics to those of your genetic structures.

Seemingly minor genetic variations among us can lead to certain diseases or a predisposition to them and to differences in our receptivity to the drugs meant to cure them. Some of us may not respond at all to some drugs. Only an estimated 60 percent of drugs effectively treat the condition for which they were prescribed.[59] And then again, we may respond very badly to the drugs we are prescribed. A 1994 study indicated that more than two million adverse drug events had occurred among hospitalized patients, and in 1997, such events were rated fifth among the leading causes of death.[60]

How can designer drugs correct these problems?

For one example, consider the genetic variation that appears to cause differential responses to chemotherapy treatment for an aggressive form of brain cancer. Designer drugs could be tailored to the patient's likely receptivity to chemotherapy. Or consider the fact that we metabolize drugs at different rates that can be roughly categorized as fast, normal, and slow. Designer drugs that deliver dosages tailored to our metabolic rates would minimize possibly toxic build-ups in slow metabolizers and ineffective doses in fast ones.[61]

Designer drugs can not only increase the effect of useful drugs and decrease the costs of ineffective or harmful ones but are also inherently more efficient to discover and commercialize than the traditional everything-for-everybody types. Drugs precisely designed to intervene with the proteins produced by an errant genetic structure may well reduce the funds and time required for drug discovery by roughly 50 percent by reducing the number of wild-goose chases. These savings could be substantial. Currently, every successful new drug requires an investment of $800 million and up to ten to twelve years of research prior to its commercialization.[62]

Early in the genomics revolution, Mark Levin understood the potential of designer drugs. Back in 1991, Levin's firm was a wee, small thing, a glimmer in his eye. By 1993, he counted himself lucky to have raised $8.5 million in financing.[63] But by January of 2002, Millennium's market capitalization had grown to $5.4 billion. Many factors have contributed to the firm's remarkable success. Levin's keen grasp of the medical and financial prospects of the genome were key, but as important, and perhaps more important, was his keen sense of humanity. "I know how important it was to hire the best people and create a culture where those people could do greater things,"[64] he says. And the soft-spoken Levin practices what he preaches. He works hard to maintain an intense but irreverent business culture in the firm. Millennium's motto, "Nothing is impossible," is exemplified by Levin's appearance in drag at the firm's annual Halloween party, in costumes ranging from the genie Jeannie to a French maid.

Levin says that

> The personalized medicine vision developed over a several-year period. It was clear as we started the company that the genomics revolution would have a major impact on our ability to identify genes and targets that were at the root cause of human disease and that this would lead to breakthrough products never seen before—attacking the cause, not the symptoms. Over the next couple of years, I began to understand that this same revolution was not limited to the therapeutic but would allow us to identify the right drug for the right disease for the right person at the right time. Whether it was diabetes or schizophrenia or asthma or cancer or heart disease, all human disease has a major genetic component, five to ten major genes and many modifier genes that may cause/influence the disease. This meant that each person would have a different combination of these that would present as a particular disease.
>
> It then became clear that we could use the same technologies we were using to look inside the diseased cell or diseased animal to analyze a particular diseased person and identify which genes were involved in the cause of their disease. This would then allow us to administer *personalized medicine*, by giving the patient the *right drug* that would most effectively treat their genetic presentation of the disease.[65]

Levin's sense of humanity shaped one of Millennium's key strategies—a predictive medicine unit aimed at early identification of genetically based diseases. In a sense, the unit is incongruous in the drug firm because it may well reduce the quantity of pharmaceuticals a patient needs. Lifestyle modification is more effective than drugs in altering the course of many diseases that are diagnosed at an early stage. For example, genetic testing of individuals for a variation of the apolipoprotein gene, E, that is linked to heart disease because it affects the fat-transporting ability of the blood, is much more likely to result in counseling individuals into a low-fat diet, high-exercise regimen than in a drug prescription.[66]

Although predictive medicine appears antithetical to the firm's bottom line, Levin's reason for creating the unit is clear. The group that is most interested in preventing diseases and in using designer drugs for cures consists of consumers. The closer he can bring the arcane products of the company to the consumer, the better for him—and the better for society. (For Levin's discussion of these concepts, see Chapter Sixty-Nine.)

HEALTH CARE POLICY REVOLUTIONARIES: THE ROLE OF GOVERNMENT

Continuing the pattern found among the other innovators discussed here, two of the consumer-driven health care policy revolutionaries could not differ more, at least on a superficial level. One is an intense, voluble African American who was a welfare recipient when he was growing up in Brooklyn, New York. The other has the manner and appearance of a classic WASP. He grew up in sylvan, middle-class Downers Grove, Illinois. His clipped speech epitomizes his reserve, and his thin, blond appearance attests to his heritage.

Yet once again, outward appearances are deceptive. Running across the grain of stereotypes, the reserved WASP, David Kendall, is an ardent Democrat, and the voluble former welfare recipient, Tony Welters, is an equally ardent Republican. More important, despite their superficial differences, both share a passion for using the instruments of government to support a consumer-driven health care system.

Care for Those with the Greatest Needs

Like many other consumer-driven health care revolutionaries, Kendall's and Welters's consumer activism was shaped by profound personal losses.

Tony Welters's beloved mother had asthma and died when he was nine years old from an adverse reaction to a drug inappropriately injected for her disease. The idea Welters took away from this loss was that the more consumers manage their own health care, the better their health status. Whether rich or poor, consumer-driven health care is the key to better health. Welters became a lawyer and was drawn to government service. He served as an aide to the late Senator Jacob Javits (R-NY), but the reflective nature of legislative work did not satisfy his activist character. Not surprisingly, he became the CEO of an entrepreneurial firm, AmeriChoice.[67]

AmeriChoice serves those whose health insurance is paid by the government, those on Medicare or Medicaid, and the uninsured. It actualizes Welters's vision of consumer-driven health care for those with the greatest needs through its *personal care model.* The model first identifies high-risk enrollees. Typically, these are individuals with chronic diseases and disabilities and those who lack the support structure to manage acute needs, such as a pregnancy. The firm then empowers these consumers by providing them with the resources that help them manage their needs. Welters's firm recognizes that its enrollees may lack support structures—such as a telephone, adequate housing, family, or close friends—and provides practical solutions that deal with the reality of their situations. For example, the firm's personal care manager may aid a pregnant teen by providing her not only with traditional prenatal, pediatric, and birth care but also with transportation, help in acquiring parenting skills, and assistance in obtaining government-subsidized housing. The firm's 24/7 call center enables around-the-clock accessibility.

The potential impact of Welters's consumer-driven approach is substantial. Medicaid, the U.S. health insurance for the poor, consumed $172 billion in 1999. Welters estimates that as many as 10 to 15 percent of his Medicaid members suffer from chronic diseases. If his consumer-driven approach reduced costs by only 10 percent, the savings would amount to many billions of dollars. In a pre- and post-AmeriChoice study of 1,755 Medicaid beneficiaries, the firm found that its strategies, which included appropriate primary care and medication, lowered total per-member costs by 19 percent.[68] (For Welters's discussion of AmeriChoice, see Chapter Seventy-Five.)

Leveling the Playing Field

David Kendall's consumer activism was fueled by his first wife's death from a brain tumor when he was only thirty-one years old. At the time, Kendall's position as the health care aide to a powerful U.S. Congressman helped his wife to enroll in a clinical trial for a new therapy to treat her tumor. Although the trial prolonged her life by a few joyous months, Kendall recoiled from a *1984*-ish system in which some were more equal than others. His participation in a support group after her tragic death reinforced for him the importance of consumers in the health care system. "I would have been lost without their support," he notes.

These experiences shaped a consumer activism that attempts to, as Kendall says, *uncentralize* the government and use its power to provide money and support for those in greatest need of health care. Kendall's choice of language reflects his brand of consumerism. To him, *decentralization* of government implies that a central controlling authority remains. *Uncentralization* more appropriately reflects the completeness of the transfer of power to the consumer.

What stands in the way of those in need?

The U.S. federal income tax code serves as one of the formidable barriers they face. It allows employers who provide health insurance benefits for their employees to deduct their full expenses from their revenues in computing their income and payroll tax payments. But most uninsured people who purchase health insurance must do so primarily with their after-tax income, because the tax code does not permit their expenses to be fully deducted for income tax purposes.

The differential income tax treatment of corporations and individuals in the purchase of health insurance represents a substantial, if somewhat incomprehensible, barrier. To clarify it (says the old teacher hopefully), consider the situation of individuals whose annual health insurance policy costs $2,400. If they were to purchase their own health insurance policy, and if they are in a 50 percent federal tax bracket, they will need $4,800 in income to pay for their $2,400 insurance policy [$2,400 = $4,800 in earnings – $2,400 in taxes]. In contrast, an employer who can deduct health insurance expenses from revenues for income tax calculations can earn as little as $2,400 in revenues, purchase a $2,400 health insurance policy, and still break even.

Kendall the ardent Democrat is appalled by the inequity created by this differential tax treatment of individuals and corporations.

But Kendall the consumer-driven activist does not wish to correct this inequity merely by doling out to individuals the funds that would equalize their tax status and that of corporations. Instead, he proposes a tax credit against earned income—which in the case of the poor would become a voucher for the purchase of health insurance.[69]

If adopted, Kendall's proposal would substantially reduce the number of uninsured, although not by forcing them to join a government health insurance program. Instead, his proposal would create empowered members of a consumer-driven health care system.

Designing Government Initiatives

Politicians of virtually all types are coalescing around consumer-driven health care. The Republicans have generally favored market-oriented health care, but even centrist Democrats now favor it. The cover of a recent issue of the Progressive Policy Institute's *Blueprint* journal featured the headline, "Health Care: Igniting a Consumer Revolution," for example.[70] (The institute is a think tank formed by then governor William Clinton.) As further evidence that politics does indeed make for strange bedfellows, former U.S. Senator Bill Bradley, who received an 85 percent rating from Americans for Democratic Action while he was in office,[71] ran for the Democratic nomination for U.S. president on a platform favoring a consumer-driven type of health care plan.

The political reason for supporting consumer-driven health care is simple: the American people want empowerment.

They do not want government to provide services; they want government to provide money.

Increasingly, the American people do not want public housing; they want government to provide money to the poor so they can select their own housing.[72] And when it comes to health care, empowerment—choice and control—is what the people want.

Americans want the government to enable them to purchase the health care they choose. A 2000 survey revealed that 40 percent of respondents lacked confidence in their ability to afford the health care they need, and 30 percent worried about having "enough choice about who provides your medical care." Their favorite solution? The respondents overwhelmingly favored a contribution from the government that allows Medicare beneficiaries to choose among many private health plans. They also want the government to provide oversight of the health insurance and health care sectors.[73]

But consumers want still more from the government—they want protection against loss of privacy and prevention of medical errors. Their solution for medical errors? Not regulations and not lawsuits. More than 70 percent of respondents thought that required reporting of all medical errors was the most effective remedy for protecting public safety.[74]

I have long favored the creation of a government agency that requires dissemination of such information. In Chapter Seventy-Eight, I discuss how this agency could be modeled on the U.S. government's Securities and Exchange Commission (SEC). Like the SEC, this proposed government agency would require performance disclosure from providers and insurers and carry substantial punitive powers. But the promulgation of the standards of measurement would be left up to a private organization that represents health care interest groups—consumers, providers, payers, and insurers. This organization would be modeled on the FASB (Financial Accounting Standards Board), a private sector, nonprofit organization that establishes generally accepted accounting principles.

I contend that the health care analogue to the SEC-FASB will bring the same benefits to health care as the SEC-FASB has brought to the finance industry: transparency and efficiency. Like most the other authors writing in Part Five, I am a long-standing, consumer-driven health care policy revolutionary who seeks to use government to protect consumers with oversight and not with micromanagement of the health care sector.

Notes

1. "Cost-Consciousness Beats 'Pricing Power.'" *Wall Street Journal*, May 3, 1999, p. A1.

2. U.S. Census Bureau. *Statistical Abstract of the United States, 1999.* Washington, D.C.: U.S. Government Printing Office, 2000, p. 497, table 778.

3. U.S. Census Bureau, *Statistical Abstract of the United States, 1999*, p. 441, table 664.

4. U.S. Census Bureau, *Statistical Abstract of the United States, 1999*, p. 441, table 664.

5. Vatter, H. G., and Walker, J. F. "Did the 1990s Inaugurate a New Economy?" *Challenge*, Jan./Feb. 2001, *44*(1), 90–116.

6. Cole, R. E. "Learning from the Quality Movement: What Did and Didn't Happen and Why." *California Management Review*, Fall 1998, *41*, 43–73.

7. U.S. Census Bureau, *Statistical Abstract of the United States, 2001.* Washington, D.C.: U.S. Government Printing Office, 2002, p. 399, table 613.

8. Buchanan, R. "Managed Care: Rationing Without Justice, But Not Unjustly." *Journal of Health Politics, Policy and Law*, Aug. 1998, *3*, 617–634.

9. Rice, T. *The Economics of Health Care Reconsidered*, 2nd ed. Chicago: Health Administration Press, 2002, p. xxi.

10. Mechanic, D. "Muddling Through Elegantly: Finding the Proper Balance in Rationing." *Health Affairs*, Sept.–Oct. 1997, *16*, 83–92.

11. Whitford, D. "A Human Place to Work." *Fortune*, Jan. 8, 2001, pp. 108–119; Zajac, B. "The 400 Best Big Companies in America." *Forbes*, Jan. 8, 2001, pp. 96–143.

12. Mauss, D. W. "Detroit Updates Its Economic Models Amid Latest Boom." *Los Angeles Times*, Sept. 19, 1999, p. C1.

13. Kaiser Family Foundation and Health Research and Educational Trust (HRET). *Employer Health Benefits 2000.* Menlo Park, Calif.: Kaiser Family Foundation and HRET, 2000.

14. Kaiser Family Foundation and HRET, *Employer Health Benefits 2000.*

15. Kaiser Family Foundation and HRET, *Employer Health Benefits 2000.*

16. Definity Health. *Definity Health.* Minneapolis, Minn.: Definity Health, Oct. 2000.

17. Murray, S. "Why Health Insurance That Works Still Fails to Catch on Broadly." *Wall Street Journal*, Jan. 18, 2000, pp. A1, A8.

18. "Structure of Employer Contributions in the FEHB." HCFO [Changes in Health Care Financing and Organization]. *News & Progress*, Nov. 1999, p. 6.

19. Thorpe, K. E., Florence, C. S., and Grey, B. "Market Incentives, Plan Choices, and Price Increases." *Health Affairs*, Nov.–Dec. 1999, *18*, 195–202.

20. Murray, "Why Health Insurance That Works . . .," p. A8.

21. Moffit, R. "How Washington Can Improve Health Care Coverage for Federal Work-ers and Their Families." Heritage Foundation *Backgrounder* No. 1504. [www.heritage.org/library/backgrounder/bg1504.html], Nov. 19, 2001.

22. Stephens Inc. "Quotesmith.com." Little Rock, Ark.: Stephens Inc., Jan. 18, 2000.

23. PaineWebber. "Quotesmith.com." New York: PaineWebber, Dec. 15, 1999, p. 3.

24. SalomonSmithBarney. "InsWeb.Corp." New York: SalomonSmithBarney, Feb. 3, 2000, p. 5.

25. SalomonSmithBarney, "InsWeb.Corp."

26. See [www.healthaxis.com], Jan. 2003.

27. Andrews, M. "Healthaxis.com: An Online Health-Insurance Broker." *SmartMoney,* Feb. 15, 2000, p. 90.

28. Market cap information for Healthaxis.com from Datastream International.

29. Moore, D. "Financial Services for Everyone." *McKinsey Quarterly, 2000, 1,* 125–131.

30. Smith, G. W., and Naifeh, S. W. *Making Miracles Happen.* Boston: Little, Brown, 1997.

31. Sherman, M., and Herzlinger, R. E. *Health Allies.* Harvard Business School Case No. 302-019, Rev. Sept. 2002. Boston: Harvard Business School, 2001.

32. Audit Bureau of Circulations (ABC). [www.AdAge.com], Jan. 2003.

33. Larson, D. E. *Mayo Clinic Family Health Book.* New York: Morrow, 1996.

34. Kochaniek, J. W. "Patients as Gatekeepers." *Business Insurance,* Feb. 21, 2000, pp. 1, 44.

35. "A New Direction for Employer-Based Health Benefits." Publication No. 99-12-05. New York: KPMG, Nov. 1999.

36. Reents, S. *Impact of the Internet on the Doctor-Patient Relationship: The Rise of the Internet Health Consumer.* New York: Cyber Dialogue. [www.cyberdialogue.com/pdfs/wp/wp-cch-1999-doctors.pdf], 1999, p. 5.

37. Commonwealth Fund. *Accessing Physician Information on the Internet.* New York: Commonwealth Fund, Jan. 2002.

38. Miller, T. E., and Reents, S. *The Health Care Industry in Transition: The Online Mandate to Change.* New York: Cyber Dialogue. [www.cyberdialogue.com], 1998, p. 7.

39. Chin, T. "More Doctors Are Catching Web Fever." *American Medical News,* Jan. 17, 2000, pp. 18, 20.

40. Reents, S. *Impact of the Internet on the Doctor-Patient Relationship,* p. 5.

41. Chin, "More Doctors Are Catching Web Fever," p. 20.

42. Chin, T. "Healthcom/Web MD Eyes Online Dominance." [www.ama-assn.org/sci-pubs/D1590306.htm]. Mar. 6, 2000.

43. "Push Paying Off for Two Moms." *New York Daily News,* Mar. 13, 2000, p. 4.

44. Buettner, R., and Sherman, W. "No More Hiding for Bad Docs." *New York Daily News,* Mar. 13, 2000, pp. 4, 5.

45. Hernandez, R. "Pataki Orders State Records on Doctors to Be Posted," *New York Times,* Oct. 7, 2000, p. B2.

46. Slatalla, M. "Turning the Tables to Rate the Raters." *New York Times,* Mar. 23, 2000, p. D4.

47. "Quack Patrol At Your Service." *Los Angeles Times,* Mar. 23, 1998, p. S1.

48. Carey, M. A. "The Internet Healthcare Coalition: E-Health Ethics Initiative." *Journal of the American Dietetic Association,* Aug. 1, 2001, *101,* 878. URAC originally stood for Utilization Review Accreditation Commission.

49. Butler, S. M. *Health Care Tax Credits and the Uninsured.* Testimony No. 021302. Washington, D.C.: Heritage Foundation, Feb. 13, 2002; Pauly, M. "Expanding Coverage Via Tax Credits: Trade-Offs and Outcomes. *Health Affairs,* Jan.–Feb. 2001, *20,* 9–26.

50. Sherlock Company, "Administrative Expense Benchmarks," PR Newswire, Aug. 14, 2002.

51. U.S. Bureau of the Census, *Statistical Abstract of the United States, 1999,* p. 121, table 171.

52. Cowan, C. A., Lazenby, H. C., Martin, A. B., and others. "National Health Expenditures, 1999." *Health Care Financing Review,* Summer 2001, *22,* 108.

53. "All Medical Care—CPI Less Medical Care." In National Center for Health Statistics, *Health, United States, 1999.* Washington, D.C.: U.S. Government Printing Office, 2000, p. 344, table 118.

54. Fenley, L. "The Glamour's Gone: But Pioneer Surgeon Keeps Pumping." *San Diego Union-Tribune,* Sept. 6, 1989, p. E1.

55. Nichols, B. "Heartfelt Rivalry." *Dallas Morning News,* Sept. 5, 1993, p. 31A.

56. Fenley, "The Glamour's Gone . . .".

57. Myerson, A. R. "Two Rival Doctors, Two Rival Reactions." *Medical Economics,* May 23, 1994, *71,* 130–136.

58. Denton Cooley, personal communication to the author, 2002.

59. Goldwasser, R., and Ulrich, B. *Genomics: Concept to Reality.* New York: UBS Warburg, Jan. 18, 2001, p. 54.

60. Goldwasser and Ulrich, *Genomics,* p. 29. Of course, not all drug-related adverse events are caused by genetic variations. Some are caused by good old-fashioned incompetence, laziness, or lack of systematic checks of the appropriateness and accuracy of hand-written prescriptions.

61. Goldwasser and Ulrich, *Genomics,* pp. 29, 54; "Brain Cancer," *Cancer Weekly,* Sept. 2, 2003, p. 18.

62. Herzlinger, R. E. *ABC Pharmaceuticals.* Harvard Business School Case No. 193-168, Rev. Dec. 2002. Boston: Harvard Business School, 1993.

63. Rosenberg, R. "Biotech Thrives on the Hot Idea." *Boston Globe,* Apr. 10, 1994, p. 77.

64. Stipp, D. "Hatching a DNA Giant." *Fortune,* May 24, 1999, pp. 179–187.

65. Mark Levin, personal communication to the author, 2002.

66. Ridley, M. *Genome.* New York: HarperCollins, 2000, pp. 259–261.

67. Anthony Welters, personal communication to the author, 2002.

68. Cowan and others. "National Health Expenditures, 1999."

69. See Kendall, D., Lemieux, J., and Levine, S. R. "Covering the Uninsured." *Blueprint,* Winter 2001, *209,* 26–31.

70. *Blueprint,* Spring 2000, *6* (Entire issue).

71. Kranish, M. "On The Trail." *Boston Globe,* Nov. 28, 1999, p. A1.

72. Swope, C. "Rehab Refugees." *Governing,* May 2001, *14,* 40–44.

73. Employee Benefit Research Institute (EBRI). *2000 Health Confidence Survey.* Washington, D.C.: EBRI, June 2000, pp. 8, 15, 21.

74. Employee Benefit Research Institute, *2000 Health Confidence Survey,* p. 20.

CHAPTER SEVEN

Scare Stories, Opponents, and the Role of Government

Whenever we contemplate something new, we stamp it with a unique face and shape in our mind's eye. When I read a book that interests me, for example, I picture the protagonists clearly. So vivid is my personal portrait that I am typically disappointed when I see or hear a media version of the work. The actors rarely conform to my vision.

Joseph Fiennes as Shakespeare in the film *Shakespeare In Love*? The slim, darkly handsome Fiennes is a beauty, no question, but Shakespeare? Forget about it. My William Shakespeare is a stocky fellow, sensuous and sly, with a reddish beard, gold glints within it, who manipulates his identity, toying with his public. He cloaks his brilliance under the guise of a common man, whereas Fiennes, like all actors, is ultimately an exhibitionist.

Somebody chose former U.S. Senator Paul Simon to dub Abe Lincoln's voice on the 2000 public television series *The American President*. Surely you jest. My Lincoln is a dark, brooding presence, with a lumbering, sonorous voice. It hints at his hidden turmoil, the brew of ambition, depression, brilliance, and idealism that tormented and shaped the man. Yes, both Paul Simon and Lincoln came from the State of Illinois; but Simon is a neat, bow tie–wearing man—light and transparent—an unlikely representative for the powerful, tormented Lincoln.

In truth I have no idea what Shakespeare looked like and little notion of Lincoln's voice. But my mind has cut a picture about how the world's greatest wordsmith and our country's greatest leader would look and sound. To me, great poets, like Shakespeare, are sly and secretive. Think T. S. Eliot. And great politicians, like Lincoln, are tortured and brooding. Think Jefferson.

So it is with consumer-driven health care.

The vision is shaped by the viewer's preconception.

Many who oppose or fear consumer-driven health care visualize it through a filter woven by their preconceived notions. One filter is used by technocrats who simply cannot accept the idea that consumers can function without their oversight. Viewed through their filter, solo consumers in the market are vulnerable and timid. They must be protected and informed by the technocrats' superior knowledge and strength. Another filter is used by status quo advocates, among them many of those who maintain the present, employer-based system. Although their motives are professional, they understandably worry that consumer-driven health care will upset their apple cart. Yet another filter is that of the universal health insurance ideologues, who typically pair access to care with control by a central government. Looking through this filter they likely fear that decentralization of health insurance purchasing to individuals will undermine their goals. In their worldview, the ideal purchaser of health insurance is a government; large employers are next best; and a decentralized market is the nightmare that keeps them up at night.

In this chapter I discuss the widely promulgated consumer-driven health care scare stories that result from these three filters. I also detail the views and beliefs of those who use these filters, and respond to their concerns. I conclude with further observations on the appropriate role of government in health care.

HEALTH CARE SCARE STORIES

The consumer-driven health care movement's many powerful enemies have promulgated a number of scare stories intended to diminish its adoption.

The Haunted House Story

The misleading "moral" of what I call the haunted house scare story is that *consumers will be forced to shop for health insurance by themselves in the open market and lose the tax-advantaged status of their current health insurance payments.* A frequent image painted by critics of consumer-driven health care is of a consumer cast out into a mystifying health insurance market, like a small child innocently entering a haunted house. Fierce creatures jump out—health insurance policies offered by venal, fraudulent vendors. Consumers lose their tax protection and wander about without a map or a sense of direction—aimlessly, futilely—only to emerge diminished by the experience: their health insurance threatened, their confidence shaken, and their health broken.

This image was invoked, for example, when, in December of 1999, Xerox announced that it hoped at some time in the future to give each of its employees

$5,000 to $6,000 to buy health insurance. "This could totally unravel American health care," noted one booster of a government-controlled model in response to the proposal.[1] A chastened Xerox hastily retracted its tentative plans.

These views misrepresent the consumer-driven health care movement in two ways. First, they set up the frightening prospect of hundreds of millions of individuals futilely shopping for health insurance in a small market that is not prepared to handle them.[2] Second, they assert that consumer-driven health care will cause the loss of the tax-advantaged status of corporate health insurance purchases.[3]

Neither view is valid.

Consumer-driven health care is implemented primarily under the employers' umbrella. The corporate umbrella is the appropriate home for consumer-driven health care initiatives because employers can nourish and support the small, innovative health insurance offerings that would otherwise easily get lost in the vast consumer ocean. As these products and the measures of their performance mature, they will be offered to individual consumers as well. Says Peter Lee, the CEO of the Pacific Business Group on Health, a consortium of forty-five large employers: "Virtually none of our members is looking at [consumer-driven health care] in terms of capping financial contributions and walking away."[4] Similarly, a 2002 *Health Affairs* report on consumer-driven health care says, "We talked to no benefit consultant, health plan, or employer seriously considering the possibility [of handing] their employees a voucher to purchase health insurance in the individual market."[5]

The history of mutual funds, the innovations that enabled consumer-driven investment in financial assets, is instructive in projecting the likely dissemination of consumer-driven health insurance. The employers who adopted 401(k) plans were a key element in the initial success of mutual funds. For example, in 1976, when the first indexed, consumer-oriented mutual fund was introduced for investors on the New York Stock Exchange, it met with a poor reception and its founder was portrayed as a wild-eyed zealot.[6] But as 401(k)s become widespread and as excellent evaluations of mutual fund performance became widely available, mutual funds eventually grew in the $1.8 trillion 401(k) market.[7] By 2001, 52 percent of U.S. households owned mutual funds. Although most of them were introduced to these investments through an employer-backed defined contribution (DC) plan, nearly 70 percent now own mutual funds purchased in the open market.[8] As for the consumer-oriented fund company that introduced the first index fund, its name is Vanguard. By 2001, it controlled about $600 billion of assets and its brilliant founder, John Bogle, was appropriately lionized.[9] (In 2003, a number of mutual funds were found to have permitted special trading privileges to large investors, such as union managers. I view these discoveries as an indication of the vigor of a consumer-driven industry. No doubt special privileges to the wealthy and powerful are granted in health care, too, but we do not hear of them.)

Consumer-driven health insurance will likely follow this pattern. Consumer-driven health insurance plans will be introduced under the corporate umbrella. With time, as the industry matures, highly differentiated insurance products will migrate from the corporate to the individual consumer market, along with reliable evaluations of their performance. These new health insurance products will likely appeal to those who are now uninsured.

As for the assertion that consumer-driven health care will cause corporate health insurance payments to lose their tax-advantaged status, that is simply a canard. Employees are currently exempted from income taxes on their health insurance payments because the tax code does not consider them to be income. If the employer continues to pay for the employees' choice of health insurance, consumer-driven health care will not affect this situation. A 2002 Treasury Department ruling affirms that health savings accounts are sheltered from income taxes (for further discussion of these tax issues, see Chapter Fifteen in this volume).

A variant on the haunted house story is that consumer-driven health insurance will cause individuals to lose the negotiating clout of big groups in determining insurance prices. Of course, in the real-life version of consumer-driven health care, the selection of health insurance options will continue to occur under the employer's umbrella. (But if the clout of group purchasing were actually so powerful, every consumer product—cars, homes, and food—would be purchased under the employer's group-purchasing models. The Achilles heel of group purchasing is that it inhibits product differentiation. The fundamental tenet of a market-based economy is that competition among differentiated products is much more effective in controlling costs than is the clout of group purchases.)

The Wrong Time and the Wrong Place Story

The message of the wrong time and the wrong place story is that *consumers will be forced to negotiate the price for their health care when they are at their weakest—at the point of care.* To dramatize this point, some paint the picture of a bullet-riddled person, perhaps the unlucky passerby to a gang war, being forced to negotiate the price of admission at the emergency room desk.

But they have the plot wrong.

In a consumer-driven health care system, consumers make their choices when they buy insurance, not when they use health care. In the quiet of their homes, people review helpful information to select the policy that best meets their needs. At a time of emergency they use the insured providers they have specified. Even those who have selected high-deductible plans, like Definity's, under which they can shop for any provider, can find ready access through the network of doctors and hospitals that the firm has assembled. And the high-cost emergency situations depicted by the writers of the wrong time and wrong place plot are almost fully insured even under plans like Definity's.

The Screw the Sick Story

The screw the sick story would have us believe that under consumer-driven health insurance *sick employees will no longer be able to buy affordable health insurance.* This contention defies simple mathematical reasoning. The underlying pool of self-funded employer health care costs is unaffected by the insurance pricing formula. Whatever their insurance pricing policies, self-funded employers who pay for the care of their employees will continue to do so under consumer-driven health care. (Figure 4.1, in Chapter Four, provides an example, illustrating that the employers' total costs and employees' payments can remain the same under different insurance pricing formulas.)

This tale is favored by advocates of universal, government-controlled health care and those who worry about competition from innovative, consumer-driven health care insurers that offer differentiated products.[10] Insurers that would prefer to avoid the perils of different-strokes-for-different-folks pricing of highly differentiated products disseminate the screw the sick story to maintain their position as the sole providers of barely differentiated health insurance for all the employees in each employer's pool. As one industry journal notes, "Several large insurers have reconsidered contracting with purchasing groups that sign multiple plans, because it's costly for an insurer to market to thousands of employees in one group and then enroll very few of them."[11] In 2002, the insurer Humana refused to sell any consumer-driven products that would be selected by only a slice of the employer's pool.[12] And insurers have even more fundamental reasons to fear consumer-driven health insurance: it will require them not only to offer sharply differentiated products to niche groups but also to open the market to the kinds of new, entrepreneurial competitors who play hard ball.

Presently, non-HMO insurers face only a small risk of unanticipated costs because they are paid by most large employers for the actual costs incurred by their enrollees.[13] Even when insurers are forced to accept a fixed price for their policies, their barely differentiated insurance packages are unlikely to cause the sort of unanticipated enrollment or usage patterns that could adversely affect their medical costs. But these cozy conditions will change in a consumer-driven health insurance world. There, insurers will have to offer all sorts of innovative packages for new types of narrow-niche enrollees, including the sick, at a fixed price. In this new world, although the employers' costs will be limited to payment of the insurers' price, the insurers will be liable for the actual expenses of new types of services to new groups of enrollees. At the same time, consumer-driven health care will limit the insurers' ability to jack up their prices. After all, consumer-driven health insurance is competitive, and the ultimate buyer is the highly cost-sensitive consumer, not an agent. Not surprisingly, some insurers vastly prefer the status quo.

Perhaps more frightening to them is the prospect of competition with entrepreneurial providers of consumer-driven health insurance, including some that have already entered the field. Notes Mark Tierney, a veteran health insurance executive, "Large insurers do not see risk adjustment as being in their best interest because it encourages the offering of side-by-side competitors. The natural desire is to be the sole carrier that the employer offers. With risk adjustments, small, innovative plans can get a toehold and chip away at the large insurers' market share."[14]

The present crop of health insurance companies consists of battle-scarred survivors of the 1990s war for market share waged with entrepreneurial managed care firms. Presently, the health insurance industry is highly concentrated, with three of the largest insurers accounting for more than half the large-group business in thirty-three states and 23 percent, or more, in the rest.[15] But it was not always so. In the 1990s, feisty, entrepreneurial managed care firms invaded and won market share from traditional insurers. In response, members of the old-boys' insurance network either consolidated with or purchased their competitors, at exorbitant prices.

The saga of U.S. Healthcare exemplifies how worrisome these entrepreneurial firms can be. Formed in 1976, as a nonprofit organization funded by a government loan, it did not take long for the CEO to figure out that there is gold in them thar managed care hills. By 1983, it was a publicly traded company, renowned for its low prices, allegedly attained with the brass knuckles it wore when reimbursing providers. Its low prices so worried Blue Cross in the key Philadelphia market, that it took out ads to decry U.S. Healthcare's stringent referrals to emergency rooms and specialists. Bad mistake. When U.S. Healthcare sued, guess who won?

By 1996, the old-time insurer Aetna, worn down by competition with entrepreneurial start-ups, had purchased U.S. Healthcare for $9 billion. Aetna was so confident that the purchase would enable it to emulate U.S. Healthcare's success, that it exited all other product lines.[16] Public policy fans of managed care thought this was a great move. In November of 1999, a leading health care public policy journal, *Health Affairs,* published a long interview to share the wisdom of Aetna's CEO with its audience.[17] But the public markets were not nearly so impressed with Aetna's financial performance, and its hard-ball managed care practices were widely excoriated by its patients and providers. As Aetna's reputation soured, along with those of other managed care players, its share price tumbled. In December of 1999, the company's CEO was forced to resign.[18] Current health insurance executives, who know this story all too well, understandably are not looking forward to competition with yet another crop of entrepreneurs.

To increase the palatability of the screw the sick scare story, it is sometimes packaged with the haunted house scare story. If we set aside for a moment the low likelihood of the haunted house scenario and accept the allegation that employers will force their employees to shop for insurance in the outside market, sick people will undoubtedly have difficulty in purchasing insurance, *if the employer funds each employee at the same average rate.* But why would a caring employer fund the well at the same rate as the sick? You do not need a CPA to figure out that if all enrollees receive the same amount of money from their employer, insurers will rush to insure the well and stampede to avoid insuring the sick.

Contrary to the message of the screw the sick scare story, when consumer-driven health insurance is offered under the employers' umbrella, it will *help* the sick with innovative products that are designed for their special needs. Currently, as I have discussed, health insurance fosters a system that is *not for the sick.* This fault can be traced directly to the absence of risk-adjusted payment. The risk adjustment of insurance prices and provider payments that is inherent in instilling competition through consumer-driven health insurance will correct this failure rather than exacerbate it. It will reward those who attract sick enrollees by paying them more and paying those who attract well enrollees less. It is precisely by this undermining of the homogenized pricing of the present insurance system that the sick will, finally, receive the excellent, focused care they deserve. (Of course, risk adjustment of prices increases the risk of invasion of the enrollees' privacy and heightens the urgency of the need for federal oversight of health information, as discussed later in this chapter.)

The Disappearance of Health Insurance Story

The disappearance of health insurance story argues that *consumer-driven health care is a wolf in sheep's clothing. Employers will use it to back out of paying for health insurance benefits. And employees will opt out of it, preferring cash payments to health insurance. They will insure themselves only if they are sick.*

Some essentially ask of consumer-driven health care initiatives, "Are they just sugar-coating a disappearance of benefits?" This scare story is promulgated mostly by those who worry that consumer-driven health care will undermine access to health insurance. As the authors of a Commonwealth Fund analysis note, "[Consumer-driven health care] could lead to more effective and efficient health care, or it could simply shift costs to the individual."[19] Ironically, labor unions, the purported champions of the workers, are among the most ardent advocates of the disappearance of health insurance scare story.[20]

But this scare story too is dubious because most employers do not want to back out of providing health insurance. For example, a detailed analysis of the correlation between the returns of small business owners and their health insurance benefits concluded: "The business's owner and the employees are in the venture together . . . they jointly prosper and they jointly fail."[21] Employers understand that health insurance is a highly valued corporate benefit. For example, as one expert notes, a Generation Xer "who believes that the employer is not making a commitment to him, will leave."[22]

Employers' willingness to offer insurance is influenced primarily by their economic situation. Notes one authority, "As long as the economy is strong, employers do not cut back on benefits."[23] Indeed, since 1993, as the U.S. economy prospered the number of workers who received health insurance through their employers steadily increased, and the employers' share of premiums increased from 69 percent in 1987 to 76.4 percent in 2000.[24] The employers who did not offer health insurance typically could not afford it. By far the lowest insurance rates were in the trade and personal service sectors, whose paltry profit rates ranged from negative to a maximum of 2 percent in 1998.[25] But, as the U.S. economy worsened, from 1987 to 2001, the share of uninsured workers in large firms increased from 25 percent to 32 percent.[26] Indeed, in tough economic times, employers are more likely to offer consumer-driven health insurance products than conventional ones because of their lower costs. The availability of this lower-cost option may even keep them from giving up the health insurance benefit.

A variant on the disappearance of insurance theme is that employees will no longer insure themselves under consumer-driven health care. Instead, they will prefer to take the money over the insurance and will insure themselves only when they are sick.

But once again, the allegation defies logic. Most people want to buy health insurance. The main obstacle is its high cost. Not surprisingly, the lowest rates of acceptance of employers' offers of insurance occur in the low-earning sectors, such as agriculture, trade, and personal service. In 2001, for example, only half of the workers in personal service firms, whose hourly pay hovered around $9 in 1998, took up their employers' offer of insurance, in contrast to 79 percent in the manufacturing sector, whose hourly wages averaged 50 percent more.[27]

The popularity of Blue Cross of California's plans for individuals—800,000 enrollees in one year alone—illustrates the positive response when health insurance prices dip, as low as $1,400 a year for a mother and her children in Los Angeles in 2000. Consumer-driven health care models also expand the opportunities for the previously uninsured in the small-group employer market (two to fifty employees). Blue Cross of California's innovative FlexScape program offers a good example. Through a defined contribution feature, small employers can pay a fixed $80 per employee per month ($960 a year). This feature creates budget predictability and an affordable price for employers who might otherwise hesitate to offer insurance. Employees can then select the plan design that best fits their budget and health care needs. Depending on plan choice, an employee's portion of the health care premiums can drop as low as $80.[28] Perhaps for this reason, the share of the uninsured working in small firms dropped from 61 percent in 1987 to 51 percent in 2001.[29]

As these examples suggest, rather than *diminishing* the number of people with insurance, consumer-driven health care will likely *increase* that number by offering innovative, lower-cost insurance policies.

The Class Warfare Story

According to the class warfare story, *consumer-driven health care will stratify the market so that poor people will receive much worse health care than the rich and powerful.* Exponents of the class warfare story typically espouse a classic centrist solution for achieving equality—a government-controlled system with standardized benefits that is overseen by selfless, superbly able elites whose sole interest is in protecting us.[30]

The class warfare story is based on two assertions. The first is that good-quality health care is more expensive than poor-quality health care and the second is that suppliers are interested in serving only the rich and will not innovate to reach the other, much more numerous part of the population.

And all of these assertions are mistaken. As discussed earlier, good-quality health care—integrated, wired, and personalized—costs *less* than poor-quality health care. As consumer-driven health care increases quality, more health care will be available at a better price. Further, suppliers are vitally interested in serving the consumers who are not rich but are very numerous.

As before, the automobile industry provides a good example of all these points. First, consumer pressures forced continuous improvements in automobile quality. In 2001, for example, problems in five year old cars diminished by 9 percent.[31] As cars became better, they also became cheaper. Quality improvements in the manufacture of cars reduced their production costs. Automobile manufacturers also reduced car prices to reach the enormous nonrich market. Paralleling these quality and price improvements was a narrowing of the gap between the best car and the average one. For example, in 2000, 88 percent of the cars tested for safety by the government were in the top two categories, versus only 31 percent in 1979.[32] So even though a top-of-the-line Mercedes costs substantially more than a Toyota, the quality differences between the two have continually narrowed.

When health care is consumer driven, it too will produce better, cheaper services, and the quality differentials between the best and the average will narrow. All the options will deliver safe, effective health care services, just as all of today's cars meet basic consumer and societal needs for safety, reliability, and fuel efficiency. This is not to say that all differentials will be eliminated. To the contrary, distinctive features will fulfill different consumer preferences. For example, although the retail stores Wal-Mart and Target both successfully serve the discount market, they serve it in different ways. Wal-Mart caters to the rock-bottom-price crowd, and Target serves those who are willing to pay a little more for cutting-edge style.[33] Similarly, as quality improved and costs dropped in the automobile market, choice increased from 140 models in the early 1970s to 260 in 1999.[34] Similar differentiation will occur in consumer-driven health care.

The Limited Access Story

The limited access story tries to tell us that *consumer-driven health care will reduce choice. For example, we cannot afford a large number of focused factories, so the handful that exist will be difficult for many to access.*

The first of these choice-limiting tales is propagated by those who view health care through a managed care, one-payer lens. In their eyes, costs and quality are best controlled through one payer, preferably a government, who can end fragmentation of the risk pool (mentioned also in the screw the sick scare story). The one payer will use its clout to wring price concessions out of fat and lazy providers, just as managed care does. After all, what provider can stand up to an 800-pound gorilla? Therefore, these critics question the explosion of choice under consumer-driven health care. In the words of a Commonwealth Fund report, "As the choices offered to workers grow, patients are likely to be spread out more thinly across providers, meaning less volume for each. . . . There may not be enough volume to allow providers to continue offering discounts and they may not be willing to participate at all in health plans that have large provider networks."[35] The logical outcome in this view is that employers will inevitably limit choice to control costs. Hence the limited access scare story.

But we have already tried limited choice. It forms the basis of our present, failed system in which costs are again rapidly inflating. Consumer-driven health care will create *more* choice because choice promotes competition and competition promotes innovation. It is through innovation that productivity increases can best be achieved.

The parallel allegation that consumer-driven health care will limit access to providers is promulgated primarily by those who are fixated on a bricks-and-mortar version of health care delivery, one that is anchored by a megalith hospital. In a consumer-driven health care system, in contrast, focused factories for chronic diseases will integrate different providers in many different locations—ranging from the home, for continual support, to the community, for checkups, to a centralized tertiary care facility, for complex, high-end care.[36]

The allegation that we cannot afford this decentralization of care is belied by the magnitude of the expenditures on chronic diseases. They are so enormous per person that a relatively small number of chronically ill individuals can justify extensive decentralization. Recall for instance, the example in Chapter Five that pointed out that the $54 billion spent in 1996 on the care of individuals with diabetes could support, in each of the fifty states, one 500-bed hospital, five 200- to 299-bed hospitals, and thirty community facilities at a cost of $10 million each that would be entirely devoted to diabetes and its comorbidities and that would largely replace the current inadequate system in which patients must assemble their own care teams.

CONSUMER-DRIVEN HEALTH CARE OPPONENTS

Technocrats favor systems centrally controlled with the complex algorithms they devise. They are highly skeptical of the intellectual prowess of anyone other than themselves.

The Technocratic Naysayers

As I personally experienced in higher education with those who opposed student ratings, a technocratic mentality fundamentally opposes consumer control. Technocrats feel obligated to oversee consumers because in their eyes consumers are too weak-minded to respond appropriately to information and to help themselves. The technocratic mentality recoils against mechanisms that create consumer-driven markets. For this reason educators opposed consumer ratings. And when Medicare's administrators first proposed to become more marketlike by changing from reimbursing providers for their costs to reimbursing providers via preset prices, a technocratic storm erupted. Medicare would simply not set appropriate prices, it would bankrupt the providers, the new price-based system would reduce the quality of care, and so forth and so on.[37]

The overall ethic at work here is articulated through two technocratic objections to consumer-driven health insurance:

- Consumers will not, cannot, use information intelligently. In a consumer-driven system they will make disastrous choices that technocratic oversight would have avoided.

- The risk adjustments needed to avoid adverse selection cannot be accurately computed. We must maintain risk pools that do not differentiate payments for the sick and the well.

I will address each of these concerns separately.

Information Is Not Good for Your Health. We live in an information age, surrounded by newspapers, televisions, telephones, computers, radios, magazines, and books that are available worldwide and round-the-clock and that address three of our senses—sound, vision, and for the vision- and hearing-impaired, touch. The ubiquity of information clearly responds to people's desires. When there is no demand, there is no supply.

People use information to inform and amuse. The best information sources combine the two. Morningstar's stars help individuals buy mutual funds. The pithy reviews in Zagat's restaurant guides help them find restaurants. J. D. Power's powerful brand name helps them select automobiles and airlines. And *Consumer Reports* magazine's accurate, comprehensive ratings help them buy virtually everything.

If consumers do not like these sources, many others exist. If they find Morningstar excessively terse, the SEC's EDGAR system[38] contains much more information about publicly traded corporations. If they find Zagat's too trendy, they can turn to the *Boston Globe*'s "Cheap Eats" section or its equivalent in their hometown paper. If they question J. D. Power's objectivity, they can turn to the federal government's data about cars and airlines, such as those provided by the National Highway Traffic Safety Administration and the Federal Aviation Administration.[39] And if they feel *Consumer Reports*' articles are biased against American cars, they can turn to other sources of consumer information, such as *Car & Driver* magazine and *Consumer's Digest.*

People use information to improve themselves too. In 2002, Bill Gates was the world's richest man because he helped people to become more productive by organizing and processing their information easily and efficiently. Michael Bloomberg became a billionaire because his information services, news, and media company provided data that helped people invest in financial instruments with confidence.[40] Martha Stewart gained fame because her publications and TV shows helped people attain the elegant, easy lifestyle they wanted.[41] The endless lineup of self-help gurus, from Dale Carnegie, author of *How to Win Friends and Influence People,* to Stephen Covey, of *The Seven Habits of Highly Effective People* fame, helped themselves to a tidy fortune too as they helped people to help themselves become more effective.[42]

When it comes to health care, the health care-equivalents of J. D. Power and Zagat's can provide the useful ratings that people crave. And health care entrepreneurs in the Stewart, Bloomberg, and Gates mold can help people to help themselves.

But some of the health care policy crowd have their doubts. They question whether average Americans can use health care information to help them help themselves.

The reason?

Well, to put it bluntly, the average American is not nearly as smart as they.

Then, too, they doubt that good information can be provided. To them, the effect of health care, unlike the effects of all other human activities, cannot be adequately measured.

In their critiques these experts misunderstand how markets work and information is produced and disseminated and misjudge the aptitude of the average person.

Why the Health Care Market Does Not Currently Work Like Other Markets. As I have discussed, the current health care market does not work at all like other markets. Unlike cars, for example, health care services have not become better and cheaper over time. Instead, they have become more costly, and people are worrying about quality too. Why? Because the health care market lacks the two essential ingredients of other markets: its consumers have little of the information that interests them, and they cannot express their feelings about the price because they rarely see the real cost of their health insurance, have a narrow range of choices, and pay only a portion of its price.

Consumer-driven health care insurance aims to provide the second ingredient: a fixed sum of money, a large array of choices, and prices that reflect costs. But absent information, the market cannot work. How can people choose effectively if they lack the information needed to make intelligent choices? And yet many technocrats believe that information will not help consumers. Some question the consumers' ability to interpret information and use it effectively. Others question whether reliable information can be produced in health care.

An example of this train of thought is provided by a professor of public health who notes the following problems with consumers' use of information. First, he claims that an astonishingly high 48 percent of American adults have "inadequate literacy skills" and only about 20 percent can independently read and understand "most patient education material and consent forms." Then too, he notes that health care information is typically ambiguous, inadequately disclosed, and altered midway. He concludes, "there is no reliable way to give consumers information adequate to clarify the [choice] among plans . . . until federal policy makers standardize benefits, proscribe risk selection, [and] enforce quality standards, and take other legislative steps to smooth the rougher edges of competition."[43]

In other words, consumers are so dumb and health care information is so ambiguous and complex that it can be understood only when choice is standardized and regulators tell health care providers how to practice medicine. The "rough edges" he proposes so casually to "smooth" represent the guts of a truly competitive market—differentiated products.

Federal Reserve chairman Alan Greenspan would no doubt be surprised by this dour assessment of the intellectual ability of the average American. For one thing, the percentage of workers with post-high school education has risen 15 percent in the past two decades.[44] And in Congressional testimony, Greenspan has attributed the surge in the U.S. economy's productivity to Americans' remarkable interest in education, noting: "The average age of undergraduates in school full time has gone up several years. Community colleges have burgeoned in size and on-the-job training has gone up very substantially. They are pressing very hard for higher levels of education and capacity and ability. [Education] has induced a significant increase in their real incomes."[45]

Further, the technocrats' critique implicitly assumes that professionally trained people are more capable of interpreting complex information than are average consumers. Yet studies show that health care practitioners, the very technocrats who pooh-pooh the abilities of others, are hardly wizards when it comes to information. For example, in a simple algebra test, only 53 percent of health care providers—doctors, nurses, and Ph.D.'s—could answer all the questions correctly.[46] And after all, if the experts who control the health care system are so wonderful, how did we get into the present mess?

Yet the professor of public health is hardly alone in his assessment of consumers' limited ability. His view is supported by many studies that demonstrate the consumers' ignorance of the ABCs of health care. A perennial favorite in the health policy press is a series of papers in which the writers cluck about the American public's ignorance of the most rudimentary aspects of health care. For example, in 1995, the experts tsk tsked that 60 percent of the public thought the health care system was changing slowly or not at all, in direct contradiction to the experts' view of the subject; in 1997, researchers noted that many could not explain the terms *HMO* and *managed care* to the experts' satisfaction;[47] and a 2001 report pointed out that "fewer than one-third of all consumers accurately reported all four health plan attributes."[48]

In the eyes of these experts, consumers are not only ignorant but also obdurate, failing to heed useful health care information. For example, consumers are legendarily indifferent to the health plan performance data contained in HEDIS (Health Plan Employer Data and Information Set), a survey by the industry's quality enforcer, NCQA (National Committee for Quality Assurance), that tracks process measures such as health plans' rates of immunizations and mammograms.[49]

To my mind, these judgments ignore the fundamental tenet of information-seeking behavior:

Consumers seek only the information that is directly pertinent to their needs.

I cannot describe exactly how cars work. Nevertheless, I am an intelligent buyer of cars because I seek the information that assesses those qualities of an automobile in which I am interested. Health care consumers are most interested in provider outcome data for medical conditions similar to their own, treated in people they consider as peers.[50] Thus it should come as no surprise that Americans cannot describe an HMO to the questioners' satisfaction or that they are uninterested in data about their health plans. Consumers clearly attribute health quality to their providers, not to their health plans.[51] And they are much more impressed by *outcome* data than by reports on *process* measures. Indeed, NCQA rankings had no correlation with consumers' assessments of care by their health plans.[52]

Is lack of use of the available information an indictment of consumers or an indictment of the poor quality of the data provided?

Two authors have concluded that the fault lies largely with the information provided. In their judgment it frequently is not sufficiently comprehensive and relies excessively on the process of care (for example, mammograms received), rather than the care outcome (for example, breast cancer mortality statistics by provider). And when outcome data are available, they are "so broadly aggregated that the results may be of only limited value to consumers."[53] Further, many users do not trust the data and cannot readily access it; for example, Pennsylvania's risk-adjusted cardiac surgery outcomes by hospital were mailed out only once.[54] Last, most consumers cannot act on the data because they lack choice and control.

A survey of small business owners and employees found that health plan information competes for their limited time with many other sources of information. The researchers concluded that these consumers must be convinced that "the time and effort involved in knowing more about health plans . . . will affect [them]," and they recommended three sensible changes to increase receptivity to health information:

- Focus on measuring the kind of medical care that "makes a difference" when the patients' health is in jeopardy and that patients cannot undertake themselves (for example, focus on outcome measures for heart surgery rather than on outcomes of taking aspirin daily).
- Focus on physicians and hospitals.
- Use the measures to drive quality-improvement programs.[55]

Grading the Providers. If Americans rely on their providers for health care quality, why are provider performance data so notable for their absence?

One report explains that the cost of collecting the data no doubt exceeds the information's benefits. The cost? "As much as $.59 to $2.17 per member per month." And the benefits? The report does not answer that question, perhaps because the costs of providing medical care dwarf those of collecting performance data, and high benefit-to-cost ratios for performance data collection can be easily achieved. For example, if performance data improve the costs of treating a person with diabetes by as little as 1 percent, in a population of 1,000 enrollees the collection costs will be repaid fiftyfold in less than one year.[56]

The same report also notes that many data cannot be reliably measured for most doctors because they treat so few of the sick. For example, "a physician would need to have more than 100 patients with diabetes . . . for a profile to have a reliability of .8 or better, while more than 90 percent of all primary care physicians at the HMO [studied] had fewer than 60 patients with diabetes."[57]

This conclusion trades off the interests of the patient for those of the provider. After all, sick people are likely better treated by physicians who see enough patients like them to register reliable outcome measures.[58] Dealing with a complex illness such as diabetes is akin to servicing a fighter plane. Should this plane be serviced at the corner garage or in a fighter plane specialty center? The providers whose small patient populations deter reliable performance measures are probably not the ones who can best serve such a challenging problem.

A more understandable provider concern is with the poor quality of the underlying data with which physicians' performance may be evaluated. For example, the U.S. General Accounting Office found severe flaws in the federal government data bank of the adverse actions taken against physicians and dentists. But as U.S. Representative Thomas Bliley (R-Va.) noted, the best way to improve the quality of these data is not to suppress them but rather to open them to the public. Paraphrasing former U.S. Supreme Court justice Brandeis, he noted that "the best disinfectant is some sunshine."[59]

One of the most important reasons for the absence of provider performance ratings lies with the providers' considerable political power. Their clout no doubt dampens others' ardor for publication of outcome data. "We don't do anything to make providers mad," explained an official about his state's ban on publishing such data.[60] Similarly, the executive director of a Cleveland business council felt that the Cleveland Clinic opted out of an areawide process of measuring hospital outcomes because "they could. They do have a third of the hospitals in Northeast Ohio." Adding further fuel to the powerful clinic's decision was the fact that it "was not always the best in every specialty." In some areas, ratings were worse than predicted.[61]

Is Information Good for Your Health? There is considerable evidence that the publication of health care performance data affects providers.[62] In the accounting literature, this phenomenon is well known as the *audit effect*:[63] firms clean up their acts in anticipation of an accounting audit. In the health care sphere virtually all the reviews of the impact of published performance data on physicians, hospitals, and insurers have concluded that they resulted in improved outcomes or processes. Further, the positive impact of the information appears to increase over time.[64]

For example, studies of the effect of New York State's and Pennsylvania's publication of risk-adjusted mortality rates for open-heart surgeries, by hospital and surgeon, concluded that they had substantial impact. In New York, they correlated with sharply reduced death rates from the procedure,[65] and a comprehensive study concluded that these favorable results were not obtained by avoiding sicker patients. To the contrary, even though the state's patient population was older than the average, its mortality rates from open-heart procedures declined much faster than the national average.[66]

The mechanism of action appears to be an increase in internal quality control procedures. An in-depth study in Pennsylvania demonstrated that its hospitals implemented more dramatic changes in their governance and clinical care than those in neighboring New Jersey, a state that lacked a system of publicly reported performance. For example, 38 percent of the Pennsylvania hospitals and none of the New Jersey ones used performance information to recruit staff thoracic doctors.[67] Similarly, in New York the data were used to discourage low-performance doctors and improve hospital procedures.[68]

Similar results were obtained in Cleveland and Minnesota. Cleveland's Health Care Quality Choice initiative published risk-adjusted mortality and length of stay outcome data, by hospital, for intensive care, medical-surgical, and obstetrical admissions, and patient satisfaction data from obstetrical and medical-surgical patients. In all cases mortality rates and lengths of stay dropped. Other health measures improved too. The rates of vaginal birth after a cesarean section were double those achieved elsewhere in Ohio, for example. Patient satisfaction ratings simultaneously improved.[69] Similarly, an analysis of the impact of Minnesota's mandatory report card for consumer satisfaction with health plans found that within four years some of the plans had restructured their quality improvement process and service quality to improve their ratings.[70]

How to Make It Happen. Every interest group that has been required to measure its outcomes has likely claimed that its work is so diffuse that its impact cannot be measured. Such claims delayed the measurement of the performance of business enterprises until the mid-1930s. The delay is surprising because accounting, the measurement tool of business performance, has been around since the middle of the fifteenth century when double-entry bookkeeping was first codified.[71] But executives' claim that accounting could not accurately measure company performance and that the cost of measurement exceeded its benefits prevented the widespread accounting for the economic performance of the firms they led.[72] President Franklin Roosevelt finally forced such measurement in 1934, when he promulgated the laws that created the U.S. Securities and Exchange Commission (SEC). The SEC requires regular compilation of financial statements and their broad dissemination by publicly traded firms. In Roosevelt's view, the SEC was "The Truth Agency."[73]

Accounting was not nearly as accurate a measure of performance in 1934 as it is now. And no doubt accounting will become much better still in the future. That is the way it is with all measuring tools: they improve with use. In 1687, Newton first measured gravity. By 2000, physicists could measure the minute energy of a *tau-nutrino* buried deep within an atom.[74] In 1953, Crick and Watson first measured the structure of DNA. By 2001, biologists could measure the structure of individual genes.[75]

So it is with health status measures. Epidemiologists can now create relatively crude measures of health status. With practice and patience they will refine those measures of outcomes and relate them more accurately to their causal agents.

The Likely Availability of Relevant Performance Data. Information is essential to a competitive market. When consumers are presented with genuinely differentiated choices, they turn to information sources to help them separate the wheat from the chaff. In a consumer-driven health care system, consumers will seek out information sources to help them choose appropriate providers and insurers. The providers' reluctance to permit measurement of their performance will crumble in the face of competitive pressures or government requirements. And entrepreneurial providers will rush in to provide these data.

After all, in a consumer-driven system, what consumers want is what consumers get.

And what present-day consumers want is information.

The Risks of Risk Adjustment. The absence of risk adjustment of the prices paid to health insurers and providers rewards those who seek out the well and punishes those who treat the sick. In a cruel irony, as I noted earlier, in today's system, health insurance and integrated health care are not for the sick. This consequence of our average cost payment system is not only morally repugnant but also economically undesirable. After all, sick people account for most of our health care costs. Improved treatment of their illness will lower costs and improve their health status. But the absence of risk adjustment deters those who excel in treating the sick.

Is risk adjustment feasible?

Some assert that it is. For example, a comprehensive review of the experiments with risk adjustment conducted by four state Medicaid and other large buying groups concluded that "[p]ayment accuracy is improved . . . health plans generally were supportive of the payment changes . . . [and] the implementation of risk-adjustment was largely invisible to . . . key stakeholders."[76] Anecdotal data, too, has shown that risk adjustment is desirable. In Minneapolis, care systems whose payment was adjusted for their enrollees' risk noted their interest in attracting the chronically ill.[77] And in Colorado and Oregon, preliminary results indicate that risk-adjusted payments "can succeed in getting money to the HMOs that most people think have the sickest enrollees."[78] One interesting study demonstrates how even less than optimal risk adjusters can substantially improve the health status of enrollees relative to the results obtained by average-cost payment.[79]

That private sector firms are attempting to predict risk more accurately also attests to its feasibility. Some early results indicate the fruits of their research. The Haelan Group in Indianapolis, Indiana, claims 70 percent accuracy, achieved with the aid of patient-completed questionnaires, in predicting high-cost health care needs. London-based Willis Group Ltd. predicts those at high risk for certain health care problems with neural networks that associate the data contained in disparate islands of insurance claims information.[80] PacificCare Behavioral Health has developed a predictive mechanism for mental health status.[81] Continual review of risk-adjustment protocols like these will improve the process.[82]

But Joseph Newhouse, a health economist, speaks for many when he asserts that the shortcomings of risk adjustment are so severe that it should be implemented only as a partial payment mechanism.

Like many other health policy analysts, he sees a third party administering the risk-adjusting weights and the payments to which they are applied. He does not conceive of risk adjustments set competitively, either by third-party firms or by the insurers or providers themselves. In his view, "Government is the natural agent to do this."[83]

Government may be a natural, but it is not a winner. The pitfalls he sees standing in the way in the government's efforts to determine risk adjustments include the costliness of obtaining reliable, stable data; the difficulty of rendering judgments about the right price for treatments; the danger of physicians' using their superior knowledge to dump enrollees for whom the risk-adjusted payments are set too low and to attract those whose payments are set too high; and the incentive to upcode diagnoses to obtain higher payments. To avoid shortchanging sick people in their care, he recommends a payment scheme that blends actual costs and risk-adjusted payments.[84]

So, is risk adjustment feasible or not?

And if it is not feasible, is payment for average costs the sole alternative to risk adjustments?

The Rise and Fall of Transfer Pricing. When I began my doctoral studies, transfer pricing was a hot issue in economics. Like risk adjustment, transfer pricing was an attempt to emulate the working of the market with prices simulated by technocrats. You may never have heard of it. That is because it is no longer a hot issue.

The reason for its rise and fall contain important lessons for the current hot health economics issue, risk adjustment: simulation of market prices is beyond our ken, and only markets themselves can determine the right prices.

In the end, technocratically determined transfer prices were abandoned largely because of the pernicious results they induced. They were supplanted with market-based pricing.

The rise. Way back in the 1970s, many U.S. firms were vertically integrated. Their managers had convinced themselves that they could produce better and cheaper goods if they owned all the components of their final products. For example, in 1973, Time, Inc., owned not only its magazine empire but also a paper mill, to produce the paper on which the magazines were printed, and a forest, to supply the trees from which the paper was made.[85] Ownership of a forest and paper mill, Time's management reasoned, could help the company avoid paying profits to independent timber and paper suppliers. In effect they were saying that Time's managers were so competent that they could earn profits in the notoriously difficult publishing business, while any idiot could raise, cut down, and grind trees and mash the resulting pulp into paper.

Yet the managers of Time, and other vertically integrated firms, were not totally blinded by hubris about their managerial skills. They knew that internal suppliers, cushioned from the rigors of the external marketplace by a corporate parent, could become fat and lazy. To ensure that their component parts remained competitive, they measured their performance with an income statement. The revenues in the income statement were earned when one part of the company sold a product to another part of the company.

The ideal price for these transfers was equal to the market price.[86] Valuing the sales among internal divisions at market prices would enable measurement of the financial performance of the component divisions of vertically integrated firms as if they were independent companies. Had Time, Inc., used this policy, for example, the timber harvested by the forest division and sold to the paper mill would have been priced at the market price of identical timber sold at the same time. If the forest division could earn profits at this market price, then it was somewhat competitive with the independent forests that required a profit to survive because they could not rely on the deep pockets of a corporate parent. If not, the resulting loss would signal a managerial problem.

There was one small problem, however. Determining the market price of any interdivisional transfer is incredibly difficult. In the case of Time, Inc., it would have involved measuring the market price for each quantity and type of timber sold by the forest to the paper mill at exactly the time of the transfer. Who knew that price?

The accountants rushed in to solve this problem. No, they did not know the market prices, but like all good technocrats they thought they could simulate them by using the standard costs of production—the average costs of producing timber and paper under optimal conditions. If the transfer prices were set equal to the average full standard costs, the internal divisions whose actual costs exceeded the standard would be clearly labeled losers, organizations whose actual costs exceeded the optimal ones.[87]

Of course, standard costs were not equal to market prices, but they were better than nothing. Or so the accountants said.

The fall. But the use of standard costs as a surrogate to determine the revenues of the firm's internal suppliers had a problem from a managerial point of view. A big problem. Standard costs treat fixed costs—those of raising the trees—and variable costs—those that change with volume, such as the costs of harvesting the timber—as if they were the same. But they differ significantly. After all, fixed costs remain fixed. But variable costs change with every transaction.

The ideal transfer-pricing system between the forest and the paper mill would motivate the internal purchaser to consider the decision about the quantity of timber to be purchased from the same perspective as Time's general managers. From their vantage point the paper mill should consider only the variable costs of buying the timber in this decision. After all, Time's fixed costs would remain fixed whether the paper mill purchased one cord of wood or ten million. But if the transfer price were set at variable costs, the seller—the forest division—could never show a profit, whereas the buyer—the paper mill—would show enormous profits with its cost of goods sold equal only to variable costs.

However, if the transfer price were set equal to standard costs, including an expense for the fixed cost of the forest, the buyer would be charged for those fixed costs that from Time's general perspective were not relevant. Time's general managers feared this charge would unnecessarily limit the amount of lumber the mill purchased from the forest.

Either of the two technocratic approaches to transfer pricing created pernicious consequences for the parent firm.

If the transfer price were set at average full standard cost, the internal buyer would unnecessarily limit the quantity purchased.

If the transfer price were set at variable cost, the internal seller would always show a loss and the internal buyer a huge profit. The motivational value of the transfer-pricing system would be lost.

Although many theorists addressed this problem, the discussion became so arcane that real-world managers lost interest in it. (I can personally testify to this lack of interest from my experiences in teaching the subject to senior managers of large corporations.) Instead, managers insisted that vertically integrated firms always buy from their internal providers at a transfer price set at average full standard cost.

The results?

Disastrous. For example, the manager of a vertically integrated company hired me to consult on the impact of its transfer-pricing policy on his business plan for a new product. The standard costs of the firm's internal provider were substantially higher than the prices charged by external competitors. The firm's requirements for transfer pricing of internal purchases at standard costs eliminated the profits of the new business he championed, even though external procurement of the components would have made the idea extremely attractive. Ironically, the firm's standard cost transfer pricing policy forced the exclusion of new business ideas that a competitor, who was not saddled with the firm's vertical integration, would enthusiastically adopt.

What was the solution?

Was ever more refined, technocratically derived transfer pricing the answer?

Not at all.

It is not feasible to simulate a market price.

Instead, firms dismantled their vertical integration. They realized that vertical integration, accompanied by transfer pricing among the components at a nonmarket price, cushioned internal suppliers from the discipline of the market.

Not surprisingly, when Time, Inc., for example, finally shed Temple-Inland, its forest and paper mill, it took a pounding on the sale. Noted one analyst:

> There's no question that Time invested more money in Temple-Inland than it produced. How much, no one knows.
>
> Arthur Temple, however, probably has a pretty good idea. That's because the Temples clearly seem to be the shareholders who fared the best in this deal. As the majority stockholder, they sold their company to Time 11 years ago for Time shares then worth about $100 million. They wind up with 13 percent of Time's common, now worth about $345 million, and about $92 million of Temple-Inland stock. And the Temple family still controls its original company, expanded, modernized and broadened. If that's a divorce, it has to be one of the nicest divorces in history.[88]

Likely Impact on Risk-Adjusted Pricing.   So, what does all this have to do with consumer-driven health care risk adjustment? As in transfer pricing, the best way for insurers to price policies that cover people of different risks of illness is with prices they quote, not with prices centrally prescribed by a government.

Consider this hypothetical example of the virtues of market-based risk pricing:

> **Baetena prices an insurance product that provides focused, integrated care for people with diabetes at $11,000 per year.**
>
> **An employer makes this option available to its enrollees. If Baetena earns profits at the $11,000 price, it will attract competitors who will reduce the price. If it loses money, it will either raise its price or exit the market. If Baetena's product is of low quality for the money, it will lose enrollees. If it is a good value, it will gain enrollees.**

In other words, when an insurer is free to set its prices for high-risk or low-risk enrollees, market forces will compel it to be efficient and effective.

Alternatively, a market for risk adjusters would enable employers to judge which risk-adjustment system best meets their needs. Mark Tierney, chairman of eBenX, is an early-stage creator of such an exchange. It is his thinking that

> Change will not occur in the system . . . unless we mitigate (note I said mitigate not eliminate) the impact of adverse selection on the carriers. Plans must be paid more for attracting the greater risk. We can do it, the technology and actuarial science are in place, now we need only to get limited groups of the carriers to accept this new form of payment from employers and employees who purchase through the exchange.
>
> We have two clients that are doing some form of risk adjustment and six carriers who have agreed to accept prospective risk-adjusted payments through our exchanges. The carriers include Anthem, Kaiser, and four other large carriers. (We are not yet in a position to demonstrate positive results. That will take another 12–18 months.)
>
> The concept here is the right one. It will cause more competition at the customer level, not the benefit manager level. It is designed to support partial or fully at-risk integrated delivery systems. It will allow for true consumer-driven health care to occur at the employer level.[89]

Market-based pricing risk adjustment avoids the technocratic risks Newhouse identified. It does not require centralized collection of data, and it does not pose the dangers of upcoding. It also reduces the dangers of excessive profits or losses. The providers who profit hugely because they are paid excessively for their patients will attract competitors. Those who underprice will raise their prices at the next opportunity.

Risk-adjusted pricing at market rates does raise two dangers, however. One is that the providers may be incapable of realistic risk-adjusted pricing because they do not understand their own cost structure. Then too, risk adjustment could invade privacy. After all, the more that is known about the health status of the enrollees and their prior use of the health care system, the higher the accuracy of the risk adjustment.

The experiences of California physicians, more of whom offered insurers a full capitated price for all their services than did the physicians in other parts of the United States, indicate the extent of the first problem. The California Medical Association reported that in 1999, 90 percent of the state's physician organizations were in financial trouble and at least thirty-four medical organizations were facing bankruptcy.[90] These experiences have been echoed elsewhere in the United States.[91] The reason? All too many physician organizations simply do not understand their cost structure. To dramatize how little cost knowledge exists, consider that the giant, long-established Northern California Kaiser did not know its costs for treating various kinds of cancer until it conducted a major study, published in 2001.[92] The CEO of one of the most successful of these physician groups explains the problem this way: "I think you have to look at some core issues which are organizational and structural."[93]

The problem of vendors that offer unrealistic prices is well known in industry. Purchasers that want stable, long-term relationships with their vendors ensure the maintenance of such relationships by carefully "qualifying" potential bidders on the basis of their quality, efficiency, and stability. Unrealistic, low-ball bidders are frequently eliminated or counseled.[94] Employers could undertake similar qualifying programs with their health care insurers and providers to avoid unstable, naive risk-adjusted pricing.

The privacy concerns raised by risk pricing of health insurance are addressed by Steve Hyde and Al Lewis in Chapters Thirteen and Fifty-Three of this book. As a practical matter, most risk adjusters restrict their variables to demographic ones, such as age and gender, to avoid invasion of privacy.

Status Quo Naysayers

Some of those who control the present, employer-centered system fear that a consumer-driven health care system may strip them of their power. They include executives of the firms that sell health insurance to large groups, the health care human resource (HR) managers of large corporations, and officials of unions and employer coalitions and their lobbying arms.

They may well believe that they add considerable value to the health care system and that this value will be lost under consumer control. Their belief in the value added by their activities is illustrated by the results of a survey of employers and providers. When asked how to make health care both cheaper and better, the HR representatives judged the tools at their disposal, "selective-contracting" and "negotiation," as more important in increasing productivity than the tools controlled by providers and consumers, summed up under the heading "improved delivery of health care." In the providers' eyes, in contrast, "negotiation" was a weak lever, and "improved delivery of health care" was given the highest ranking.[95]

On a personal level, these naysayers would not be human if they did not fear that consumer-driven health care will disrupt their professional power base.

Health Care HR Mavens. The response to my keynote speech to a large group of representatives of employer-sponsored health care illustrates the personal concerns of these professionals. In this vignette, Bruce, the fictitious managed breakfast insurance HR maven from Chapter Three, stands in for the people I actually talked to.

I first met Bruce at a briefing of congressional staffers. He was the health care human resource manager of a major U.S. corporation. He seemed affable enough. Although his talk was filled with the usual top-down, corporate managed care notions, Bruce told me that he would support a market-based health insurance system in his firm when the right time came.

I next met Bruce at the speakers' table of a national convention of his peers. Bruce was not nearly so affable this time around, as he fumbled with the laptop he had set up on the table. Bruce was scheduled to speak after me. I noticed he was typing rapidly on the laptop during my lecture. When he rose to speak, I knew what all the typing was about.

Bruce's talk was a rebuttal to mine. It was based on the haunted house model of consumer-driven health care: employers' contributions to employee health insurance would be newly subjected to income taxes, employees would be forced to shop for their own health insurance, and sick people would be left out in the cold because no insurer would want to cover them.

As an old teacher I simply could not resist correcting his points. At the question-and-answer session following his talk, I noted that in a consumer-driven health care system:

- Employers and employees would continue to contribute to the purchase of health insurance on a pretax basis.
- Employers would present their employees with a large number of differentiated health insurance options. They would do the initial shopping, not their employees.
- Risk adjustment would provide better care for the sick than they receive under the present uniform pricing system.

And as always, I concluded by saying that as a result of competition and differentiated pricing, consumer-driven health care would increase quality relative to costs.

Bruce was clearly unnerved by my response and not because of my debating skills. Bruce was unnerved because, in his insular world, he had never before heard these points rebutted.

At any rate, he turned to me, sweeping his arm to include the crowd of his peers seated before him, and said, "What are all these HR people going to do in a defined contribution health insurance system?"

Aha!

Bruce had stated the nub of his problem with consumer-driven health care—*loss of power.*

In my experience as a member of the boards of directors of many corporations, I have noted that all too many CEOs do not value their HR staff highly. I do not agree with their assessment, but it is what it is. For a time, human resource health care specialists were the exception. Because of their special status, most CEOs delegated substantial power to them, including the power to terminate health insurers' plans and providers, renegotiate prices, redesign benefits, and modify employee contributions.[96] They were even allowed to encroach on the sphere of health care providers. For example, the Leapfrog Group, a coalition of large purchasers staffed primarily by HR managers, is pressing hospitals to adopt three safety standards: computerized entry of prescriptions, the presence of a trained physician in intensive care units, and referrals to high-volume hospitals.[97]

In the corporate world few human resource officials have such powers over vendors. These are tasks more normally undertaken by line managers, not by staff personnel.

Consumer-driven health threatens this rare HR corporate power and glory.

This concern lay at the heart of Bruce's opposition to it.

My response to him was that HR officials had an important role to play in a consumer-driven health care world: they will be the ones who will select the policies, provide employees with information, and oversee the process. Bruce seemed little mollified. In a consumer-driven health care world, he would be reduced to the same level of power as the HR professionals overseeing other employee issues.

Group Health Insurers. Some group health insurers likely favor the prospect of consumer-driven health care little more than Bruce. It is not that their status quo is so wonderful. The health insurance industry experiences underwriting cycles that whipsaw the participants from boom to bust.[98] When profits are high, insurers expand. The expansion causes new entrants to compete for business by cutting prices. Lower prices reduce profits. Weak participants exit the business. The remaining participants can now afford to raise their rates because they have relatively fewer competitors. As their profits rise, the cycle begins anew.[99]

But on the plus side group health insurance is not so bad a business. As a wholesale business it has only a few big clients, unlike a retail business that must satisfy hundreds of millions of potential customers. And the group insurance business does not require minutely detailed cost accounting systems. If the customer is big enough, the insurer is pretty much assured that the health care costs of the whole group will not explode if a few of its members incur heavy expenses. So the need for exquisitely detailed cost accounting is minimized. And the sector is not dauntingly competitive because the HR customer requires only a low level of product differentiation.

The individual insurance market is quite a different business from group insurance. The latter is characterized by many small competitors selling many different products. In a multistate survey, the U.S. General Accounting Office found from seven to over one hundred such insurers per state. These insurers offered policies that varied widely in their benefits, cost-sharing provisions, payments to providers, and provider networks. For example, one plan limited its benefits to specific diseases and major medical expenses. Although insurance policies like these are unusual in the group setting, they are pervasive in the individual market. In North Dakota, for example, they accounted for more than half of the individual market enrollees.[100]

To make matters worse, not only do the firms in the individual health insurance market face ferocious competition from many competitors that sell differentiated products, but they also cannot rely on the safety of large numbers. They need superb cost-accounting as well as retail marketing skills to succeed. Perhaps for this reason, one of the country's largest insurers, United Health, purchased Golden Rule—a firm specializing in individual policies—for a sum of nearly half a billion dollars in 2003.

The consumer-driven health care world will require health insurers to sell to both corporations and, just as mutual funds do, individuals. Because there will be many competitive insurance products, each with its own distinct features, retail marketing will become a major challenge. As for the protection once provided by insuring a big group, forget about that. It is likely that the big groups will now be carved up among competitors. So knowledge of the health care costs of individuals will be a must. If the industry suffered from cycles when its few participants sold similar products to a few large clients, what will happen when it sells dissimilar products to many clients?

Not surprisingly, many of the surveys supported by those who favor the status quo demonstrate that employees want the present employer-based system to be maintained. Consider, for example, the survey results presented by the Employee Benefit Research Institute (EBRI) and its subsidiary, the Consumer Health Education Council (CHEC). (EBRI researches employer-provided benefits, and CHEC is funded by the health insurance industry and groups representing doctors and hospitals.[101]) Their *2000 Health Confidence Survey* found that although 43 percent of employees were very or extremely confident that their employers or unions had selected the "best" health insurance for them, only 33 percent expressed the same confidence in their own ability to choose the "best" health insurance for themselves.[102] Similarly, The Commonwealth Fund, a long-time advocate of universal health insurance, found that 73 percent of those with employer coverage think their employers generally do a good job of selecting quality health plans, and 50 percent think that employers should continue as a main source of health coverage in the future.[103]

The message of these surveys is clear as a bell: maintain employers as the shepherds of health insurance. Employees are frightened by the prospect of choosing for themselves.

Yet surveys by organizations that are not wedded to employer-supported health care report conflicting results. For example, the Progressive Policy Institute found that 64 percent of its respondents agreed that "individuals are best able to choose the health care coverage they want so they should have that option and not have to take just what coverage their employer provides," and only 27 percent agreed with the statement that "employers are better able to find the best health plan to offer their employees."[104]

I do not question the integrity of the pollsters, but subtle, unwitting variations in the phrasing of questions may elicit the results desired. Indeed, some of the data contained in the very surveys in which respondents appeared to advocate continuance of the status quo raises questions about the surveys' overall con-clusions. For example, The Commonwealth Fund survey showed that those insured by government programs preferred themselves as purchasers over the government. The uninsured also favored making their own purchases rather than having the government make them.[105] Similarly, the EBRI survey revealed that 73 percent of its respondents favored a consumer-based solution to Medicare's problems, one "allowing beneficiaries to choose from many private health plans, where the government contributes a fixed amount to the cost of each plan."[106]

Government-Controlled, Universal Health Care Naysayers

For many years, ideologues have urged the adoption of universal health care in the United States. I agree with them: all Americans should have access to health care. Equality is what the United States is all about.

But once more the devil is in the details.

Most of the universal health care crowd wants the government to run the resulting system, either by managing the provision of health care, as in the United Kingdom, or by determining the providers' budget, as in most of Europe and Canada. They argue that having one-payer, the government, will reduce the administrative costs of having many competing health insurers.[107]

This "detail" is where they lose me. Government-control smothers competi-tion in a blanket of uniformity, but competition to improve the quality of health care services provides the best opportunity for cost control. Consumer-driven competition for the best health promotion, the best focused health care, and the best technology will create more for less. This is the kind of competition that will ultimately control costs and raise quality.

The impact of laws that dictated minimum lengths of hospital stays for newborns and their mothers illustrates the problem of government control. The laws were passed for the best of motives—in response to complaints about drive-through deliveries in HMOs, but their effect was disastrous. Although innovations such as new drugs and devices lowered all hospital lengths of stay by nearly 8 percent in the period from 1995 to 1997, the length of childbirth stays increased by 14 percent.[108]

If one-payer economies suppress the innovations that increase productivity, significant cost control in these systems can come about only by rationing health care services.[109]

A mountain of evidence points to rationing in government-controlled universal health care systems. One result is the cruel fate of British women diagnosed with breast cancer or those stricken with heart disease. They suffer from one of the worst survival rates found in developed countries. The reason? The shortage of doctors, nurses, and beds in the British health care system and the difficulty of obtaining referrals to hospitals or specialists.[110] In the estimation of the World Health Organization, 25,000 British cancer deaths per year would not have occurred in the United States.[111]

When I lectured in Canada to the Ontario Hospital Association about *Market-Driven Health Care,* the results of a first-ever patient survey were announced. It revealed that almost half of those with a recent stay in a hospital graded their quality of care as barely passing.[112] Other Canadian polls revealed especially high dissatisfaction with waiting times for specialized surgery. And these waits were not costless. Waiting patients suffered major and irreversible losses in health status.[113]

Human tragedies also result inevitably from rationing health care. In Toronto a desperate father took a physician hostage in an effort to obtain quicker treatment for his sick child. He was shot to death by the police. In Montreal a grandmother lay in a hospital's hallway on a gurney, awaiting open-heart surgery. She had been on a waiting list for five years.[114] The decision by Quebec's premier to have surgery for his melanoma performed in the United States says it all.[115]

Although the long-suffering, stoical British are so wedded to the goal of social equality that 50 percent of them rated their medical care as excellent or very good, their evaluations of their actual health care experiences belie these overall ratings. Thirty-one percent experienced doctor visits shorter than five minutes and 34 percent visits shorter than ten minutes, only 19 percent rated the care they received at their last doctor visit as excellent, and 33 percent endured waiting times of four months or more for elective surgery. In contrast, among U.S. respondents, only 30 percent had a doctor visit shorter than ten minutes; 29 percent rated the care received at their last visit with a doctor as excellent; and only 1 percent had a wait of more than four months for an elective procedure.[116]

Sadly, the deprivations endured by the British and Canadians did not lead to equality of health status.

One English scholar concludes: "Social inequalities in health care continue to be a major (and increasing) problem."[117] Similarly, a Canadian review of cancer incidence noted that "[d]espite Canada's universal health insurance . . . the association between lower socioeconomic status and the incidence of many consumer cancers is just as strong in Ontario as it is in the United States."[118] Providers of cardiovascular care in Canada concluded that preference in accessing care is given to those who are politically or economically powerful or potentially litigious.[119]

The ideologues who favor government-controlled universal health care are so steeped in rationing as a cost controller that they predict that consumer-driven health care will create this self-same limitation in the U.S. health care market: they expect access to health care to be rationed inversely to income levels.[120] One, for example, forecasts a four-tier market under consumer-driven health care whose ease of access to providers increases with the enrollees' income: lower-income employees will encounter hard-to-access, tightly managed HMOs and upper-income ones will wallow in easily reached, luxuriously appointed doctors' offices.[121]

In this view, the universal health care ideologues entirely miss the point of consumer-driven health care. The competition inherent in consumer-driven health care increases productivity; it makes things better and cheaper. The results benefit rich and poor alike. Elsewhere in our economy, all income classes have access to the better, cheaper food, appliances, financial products, computers, and cars that competition created. A competitive, consumer-driven health care health care system will fashion similar innovations in the delivery of health care.

THE ROLE OF GOVERNMENT IN A CONSUMER-DRIVEN HEALTH CARE SYSTEM

In any consumer-driven democracy, the government fulfills three crucial roles: it oversees the solvency and integrity of the participants, subsidizes the purchase of needed goods or services for those who cannot afford them, and provides transparency in the market.

When applied to a consumer-driven health care system, these principles imply that the government must

- Prosecute fraudulent providers, enrollees, and insurers and ensure the financial solvency of insurers
- Subsidize those who cannot afford health insurance
- Require the dissemination of audited data about the performance of insurers and providers

The first two government functions seem to me to be obvious. Although some argue that markets can function without government oversight because competition will drive weak providers out of business, health insurance is too important to be left without government safeguards. And even though others might feel that consumer-driven health care will eventually make health care affordable for all, or that insurance is not really needed because charitable providers will care for the poor uninsured, to me these objections border on fantasies. Health insurance will never be as affordable as a bag of potato chips, and why should poor people scrounge for charitable care while the rest of us can choose the care we prefer? In our prosperous land we should subsidize health insurance for those who cannot afford it so they can obtain health care in the same way as the rest of us.

The third role of government, that of providing accountability, is surprisingly controversial. Although many complain about the absence of good consumer information, not all agree on the role of government in providing it. In a poll performed by a Democratic party think tank, nearly 60 percent of the respondents agreed with a statement that "health care companies and doctors should disclose how well they perform so consumers can judge where to spend their money."[122] The wired generation is even more demanding—80 percent of respondents noted that the absence of quality information was the most negative aspect of e-health plans.[123] Yet no less an observer than the Nobel laureate economist George Stigler argued that the truth will out in markets as competitors expose each others' weaknesses or market analysts dig it up.[124]

Although Stigler may be correct in general, to my mind so many fraudulent, incompetent, and inefficient suppliers flourish in the sectors of the economy that are not required to release performance data that the prospect of unleashing consumers in a health care market that lacks these performance data is downright frightening.

The New York State data cited previously in this chapter illustrate the results when government requires meaningful health care information. Using his clout, in 1989, the New York state commissioner of public health requested data by surgeon and hospital for the risk-adjusted death rates among patients who had had open-heart surgery. By 1992, the state had achieved the lowest risk-adjusted mortality rates for these surgeries in the country.[125] Physicians and hospital executives with low-performance scores typically revamped their protocols in response to these data.[126] Most studies found that the fears that surgeons would abandon sick patients to improve their performance ratings were unfounded and that the severity of illness among New York patients having coronary artery bypass graft (CABG) surgery increased.[127] Although one excellent study concluded that the ratings led to "a decline in the severity of illness" of CABG patients, even this study concluded: "Our results do not imply that report cards are harmful in general. . . . [R]eport cards could be constructive if designed in a way to minimize the incentives and opportunities for provider selection."[128]

Similar results have been obtained in other instances of required performance disclosure. When Minnesota's state government required all insurers who served state employees to be evaluated by their enrollees in a report card, some plans restructured significantly to improve their quality ratings.[129] Similarly, the Pennsylvania hospitals whose performance data were measured and disseminated by a public agency used the results to change their patient care and governance to a greater extent than neighboring New Jersey hospitals, whose performance data were not released. The important changes included board reviews of the data and reworkings of the patient care procedures.[130] And all these results were obtained in the absence of consumerism. In New York State, for example, the data themselves caused hospitals to improve and to restrict the privileges of low-performance surgeons.[131]

Absent government involvement, information that evaluates providers will not be forthcoming. Most voluntary efforts are typically duds, and employers simply are not that interested in the data and are unclear about how to interpret it. Consider the case mentioned earlier of a voluntary Cleveland coalition to collect hospital performance data. The effort was widely lauded. For example, one hospital claimed that the decrease in its rate of cesarean sections from 30 percent of all births to below 20 percent was "purely driven by the Cleveland Health Quality Choice."[132] An evaluation concluded that reductions in risk-adjusted mortality rates and lengths of stay were linked to the performance reports.[133] Nevertheless, the effort collapsed when the Cleveland Clinic left the group, allegedly because it did not like the performance ratings it received. Noted a local doctor, "What the Clinic really didn't like is that they weren't shown to be the best at everything."[134] In addition, the employer community that sponsored the effort did not actively use its results. For example, the only hospital to achieve better-than-expected ratings hoped that the results would yield many new patients as employers referred their enrollees there, but the predicted surge never materialized. Notes one employer, "We weren't that aggressive."[135]

As for the voluntary, industry-led mechanisms for accountability, they are so weak that in 2001, *Modern Healthcare,* the industry's leading journal, demanded the resignation of Dennis O'Leary, the head of JCAHO (Joint Commission on Accreditation of Healthcare Organizations), whose governance is dominated by providers. The editorial declared: "O'Leary and JCAHO have . . . repeatedly failed at initiatives designed to judge hospitals and other healthcare providers based on their performance—how well they take care of sick people. The projects always are announced with much fanfare and heady names such as 'Agenda for Change.' And they're invariably scrapped, watered down or delayed."[136] An evaluation headed by John Gifford, a professor at the University of Michigan, for example, found no correlation between JCAHO scores and outcome measures, including mortality and complications, for the hospitals studied.[137]

Organizations conducting voluntary efforts also frequently dilute their reports to consumers. In Cleveland, for example, the data revealed to consumers were not nearly as precise as those provided to payers. The hospitals agreed not to use them in advertising because, as one Cleveland Clinic official said, "They could confuse the public."[138] Finally, industry–focused efforts rarely reflect the diverse perspectives of all the participants in the system even though these can differ significantly. Consider, for example, the evaluation of Washington, D.C., HMOs that found Kaiser rated near the top by employers, in the middle by users, and near the bottom by doctors.[139]

In the absence and failure of voluntary mechanisms for the provision of performance data and in view of its importance to a consumer-driven health care system, the federal government should require the collection and dissemination of information about provider performance. The results would likely replicate those obtained by President Roosevelt when he chose to rescue the depressed U.S. capital markets by forming the Securities and Exchange Commission. Bucking powerful business opposition, inconsistent state involvement, and his own advisers' counsel that he grade the firms in the security markets, FDR instead created the SEC to compel audited disclosure, using generally accepted accounting principles (GAAP), about the performance of publicly traded firms.[140]

It is the SEC that requires disclosure, but the promulgators of GAAP have been housed in private, nonprofit, standard-setting organizations, such as the Financial Accounting Standards Board. The successful European Union model for setting standards in health, safety, environment, and consumer protection follows a similar public-private structure.[141]

Like all human endeavors, the SEC is not without faults. The accounting and governance problems of Enron—a firm that in 2002 went into the nation's largest bankruptcy up to that time—were exacerbated by laxity in SEC enforcement.[142] Nevertheless, the transparency created by the SEC has enabled the celebrated broad participation of average Americans in the securities markets and these markets' legendary efficiency. Perfect cannot be the enemy of good: Imagine the U.S. capital markets without the trust that the SEC inspires.

The DC retirement arena once again illustrates appropriate roles for governments in consumer-driven health care. There, the federal government broadened the safety net through oversight. For example, government rules to protect against excessive participation in pension plans by high-income employees helped to energize marketing efforts to lower-income ones. Similarly, the small-employer market expanded its 401(k) plans when government rules simplified plan administration. Last, firms like Morningstar could not measure investment performance absent the SEC's standard definitions for returns and yields.[143] Nevertheless, powerful special interests, especially providers and technocrats, oppose the idea of a health care version of the SEC.

Most providers like the theory of consumer-based choice and information, but some hate the reality—the requirement that they be held as accountable for their performance as everybody else. Providers understandably resist measurement of their performance and advance many claims to urge their case. Some claim that performance is intrinsically unmeasurable—a palpably ludicrous claim. After all, if the performance of medicine cannot be measured, there is no basis for teaching or practicing in the field. Others claim that only they can correctly interpret the data. In this claim they misunderstand how markets work (see the section titled "How Markets Work" in Chapter One of this volume).

Yet others argue against performance measures by noting that it is impossible to obtain reliable data about the performance of providers who see few patients with a particular medical condition.[144] But this argument seems exactly backward. The purpose of performance measurement is to protect the patient, not the physician's practice. The physicians who see many people who are struck by one disease are more likely to develop the expertise needed to care for it. In a consumer-driven health care world, the low-volume physicians who cannot generate statistically reliable outcome data for specific patient conditions will likely lose their patient load to those who generate excellent outcomes, in part because they see so many individuals with the specific problem.

A more serious objection is voiced by the technocrats who point out that outcome measures are not as accurate in 2002 as they will be in 2020.[145] First, the language for measuring performance has yet to be defined. Second, the risk adjusters that would make it possible to compare the performance of high-risk specialists to those who treat less severely ill patients are in an early state.

These are substantial issues. In the absence of solutions to them the outcome measures that are crucial to consumer-driven health care will be seriously distorted. For example, a study that compared hospitals' rates of cesarean sections both with and without adjustment for the patient characteristics that affect the likelihood of needing the procedure found that after adjustment the performance of five of the twenty-one hospitals in the study changed dramatically: among other changes, two hospitals that had been classified as outliers were reclassified as normal and some that were classified as normal were reclassified as outliers.[146]

The impact of imperfect measures extends to providers too. Physicians may be dissuaded from caring for very sick patients by a concern that their outcome measures will not correctly reflect severity of patient illness.

Measurement issues like these can be solved with time. Among others, prescient employers in Florida and payers in Washington have already used risk adjusters successfully (for further information, see Chapters Twelve, Eighteen, and Forty-One in this volume). The continually evolving measures of performance of investment management—such as GAAP and beta, the measure of risk of different investments—provide a good example of how difficult measurement problems are solved. Beta, as discussed in Chapter One, has been continually refined since it was first suggested in 1952. Similarly, the system used by Morningstar to rate the investment performance of mutual funds has evolved over time. In 2002, for example, it was changed to allow for the difficulty of generating earnings in some types of investments. It now permits mutual funds operating in poorly performing sectors, say technology, to earn high ratings if they have performed substantially better than their peers.[147] Moreover, as the refinement of these measures of financial performance continues, investors have had access to ever-better data with which to evaluate the performance of their mutual funds and stocks.

Patients who put their health on the line deserve no less.

CONSUMER-DRIVEN HEALTH CARE: YEA OR NAY?

Consumer-driven health care is challenged by those who for reasons of ideology, elitism, or self-interest do not wish the reins of health care turned over to consumers. These players have long had their turn at the bat: the technocrats and keepers of the status quo have controlled the U.S. health care system for decades, and universal health care ideologues have shaped most of the European and the Canadian health care systems. The results? In the United States, high costs, uneven access, and quality chasms. Similar results have been obtained elsewhere, except for cost control, which has been achieved in some other countries at the price of rationing health care for the sick.

Consumer-driven health care will liberate consumers to drive the results their actions have achieved elsewhere in our economy: better quality and better cost control.

Notes

1. "Xerox May Pay Workers to Buy Own Insurance." *Los Angeles Times,* Dec. 4, 1999, p. A1.

2. U.S. Bureau of Labor Statistics, "Issues in Labor Statistics: Summary 00-11." In *Consumer Expenditure Summary, 1997.* Washington, D.C.: U.S. Bureau of Labor Statistics, May 2000.

3. Dutton, G. "The Shrinking Pool of Plans." *Business & Health,* Annual 2001, pp. 14–16.

4. "Quality Concerns Ensure Consumers Will Gain Clout." *Managed Care,* Jan. 2002, p. 44.

5. Gabel, J. R., Lo Sasso, A. T., and Rice, T. "Consumer-Driven Health Plans." *Health Affairs* ("Web Exclusive"), Nov. 20, 2002, p. W405.

6. Damato, K. "Index Funds." *Wall Street Journal,* Apr. 9, 2001, pp. R4, R9.

7. Jacobius, A. "Good Times May Be Over for 401(k)s." *Pensions & Investments,* Apr. 30, 2001, p. 1.

8. "An Increase in Households Owning Mutual Funds." *New York Times,* Nov. 13, 2001, p. C6.

9. "Databook." *Pensions & Investments,* Dec. 24, 2001, p. 41; also see [www.vanguard.com].

10. Freudenheim, M. "A New Health Plan May Raise Expenses for Sickest Workers." *New York Times,* Dec. 5, 2001, p. A1; Silow-Carroll, S., and Duchow, L. *E-Health Options for Business: Evaluating the Choices.* New York: Commonwealth Fund, Mar. 2002, pp. 13–15.

11. Benko, L. B. "Coalitions Lose Mission." *Modern Healthcare,* May 14, 2001, *31,* 56–58.

12. SalomonSmithBarney. "What We Learned at Humana's Investor Day." New York: SalomonSmithBarney, Sept. 25, 2002.

13. Greenwald, J. "Self-Funding of HMOs on the Rise: Rate Hikes, Tax Savings Spur Employer Interest." *Business Insurance,* Jan. 28, 2002, p. 1.

14. Mark Tierney, chairman of eBenX, personal communication to the author, May 2002.

15. American Medical Association, *Competition in Health Insurance: A Comprehensive Study of U.S. Markets.* Chicago: American Medical Association, Jan. 2003.

16. "U.S. Healthcare." In *Hoover's Handbook of American Business.* Austin, Tex.: Hoover's Business Press, pp. 90–91.

17. Robinson, J. C. "At the Helm of an Insurance Giant." *Health Affairs,* Nov.–Dec. 1999, *18,* 89–99.

18. Martinez, B. "Aetna Tries to Improve Bedside Manner in Bid to Help Bottom Line." *Wall Street Journal,* Feb. 23, 2001, pp. A1, A9.

19. Silow-Carroll and Duchow, *E-Health Options for Business,* p. 1.

20. Barr, S. "Looking for Ways to Soften the Blow of Rising Health Insurance Costs." *Washington Post,* Dec. 12, 2002, p. B2.

21. Dennis, W. J. "Wages, Health Insurance and Pension Plans: The Relationship between Employee Compensation and Small Business Owner Income." *Small Business Economics,* Dec. 2000, *15,* 247–263.

22. "For Many Generation X'ers Grass Is Greener at Home." *New York Times,* Dec. 11, 2001, p. C2.

23. Fronstin, P. "Trends in Health Insurance Coverage: A Look at Early 2001 Data." *Health Affairs,* Jan.–Feb. 2002, *21,* p. 191, exhibits 2, 3.

24. Cowan, C. A., McDonnell, P. A., Levit, K. R., and Zezza, M. A. "Burden of Health Care Costs." *Health Care Financing Review,* Spring 2002, *23,* 131–135.

25. U.S. Census Bureau. *Statistical Abstract of the United States, 1999.* Washington, D.C.: U.S. Government Printing Office, 2000, p. 573, table 911.

26. The Commonwealth Fund, Pub. #672, Oct. 2003. [www.cmwf.org/programs/insurance/glied-largefirms-672.pdf], Oct. 2003.

27. Fronstin, "Trends in Health Insurance Coverage," pp. 188–193, exhibit 3; for hourly pay data, see U.S. Bureau of the Census, *Statistical Abstract of the United States, 1999,* pp. 436–438, table 690.

28. Dana E. McMurty, vice president, health policy and analysis, WellPoint, personal communication to the author, May 3, 2002. The $80 figure relates to employee-only contracts for subscribers aged eighteen to thirty-nine on the Basic PPO plan.

29. The Commonwealth Fund, Pub #672.

30. Trude, S., and others. "Employer-Sponsored Health Insurance: Pressing Problems, Incremental Changes." *Health Affairs,* Jan.–Feb. 2002, *21,* 66–75; Stires, D. "The Coming Crash in Health Care." *Fortune,* Oct. 14, 2002, pp. 205–212.

31. "An Engineering Icon Slips." *Wall Street Journal,* Feb. 4, 2002, p. B1.

32. "Safety in Numbers." *Business Week,* May 7, 2001, p. 127.

33. "The Road to Chapter 11 Is Littered with Misconceptions." *New York Times,* Feb. 3, 2002, business section, p. 4.

34. "The Economics of Panty Hose." *Forbes,* Aug. 23, 1999, p. 70.

35. Silow-Carroll and Duchow, *E-Health Options for Business,* p. 15.

36. Howatt, G. "New Health Plan Fares Poorly at 'U': Workers Pick Old Favorites over Newcomers." *Star Tribune,* Dec. 15, 2001, p. 1D.

37. Burda, D. "What We've Learned from DRGs." *Modern Healthcare,* Oct. 24, 1993, p. 42; Gardner, J. "Wrestling with Medicare Doc Fee Schedules." *Modern Healthcare,* Oct. 2, 1995, p. 88.

38. Available at [www.sec.gov/edgar.shtml]. EDGAR stands for *electronic data gathering, analysis, and retrieval.*

39. See, for example, safety data for cars at [www.nhtsa.gov] and for planes at [www.faa.gov].

40. Barringer, F., and Fabrikant, G. "Coming of Age at Bloomberg L.P." *New York Times,* Mar. 21, 1999, p. 1.

41. Sell, S. "Martha in Bloom: An Empire Grows from Stewart's Home." *USA Today,* July 3, 2000, p. 1D.

42. Hunt, D. L., Jaedke, R., and McKibbon, K. "User's Guide to the Medical Literature," *Journal of the American Medical Association, 283*(14), Apr. 12, 2000, 1876–1879.

43. Brown, L. D. "Public Policies to Protect Choice in Health Plans," *Medical Care Research and Review, 56* supp., Sept. 1999, 159–162.

44. "Blunt Portrait Drawn of U.S. Work Force in 2000," *New York Times*, Aug. 30, 2002, p. C4.

45. "State of the Economy," *Federal News Service*, Jan. 20, 1999.

46. Estrada, C., Barnes, V., Collins, C., and Byrd, J. C. "Health Literacy and Numeracy," *Journal of the American Medical Association, 282*(6), Aug. 11, 1999, 527.

47. Robert Wood Johnson Foundation, *Community Snapshots Consumer Survey.* Princeton, N.J.: Robert Wood Johnson Foundation, 1995; Princeton Survey Research Associates, *National Survey of American Views on Managed Care.* Princeton, N.J.: Princeton Survey Research Associates, 1997, p. 44.

48. Cunningham, P. J., Denk, C., and Sinclair, M. "Do Consumers Know How Their Health Plan Works?" *Health Affairs, 20*(2), Mar./Apr. 2001, 159.

49. Gabel, J. R., Hunt, K. A., and Horst, K. M. KPMG Peat Marwick, *When Employers Choose Health Plans.* New York: Commonwealth Fund, 1998.

50. See, for example, Hubbard, J. H., and Jewett, J. "Will Quality Report Cards Help Consumers?" *Health Affairs, 16*(3), May/June 1997, 218–228.

51. See, for example, Pacific Business Group on Health, *Report on Qualitative Research Findings: California Health Care Smart Shopper Public Education Campaign.* San Francisco: Pacific Business Group on Health, Mar. 1998.

52. Landon, B. E., and others. "Health Plan Characteristics and Consumers' Assessments of Quality." *Health Affairs*, Mar.–Apr. 2001, *20*, p. 274.

53. Bates, D. W., and Gawande, A. W. "The Impact of the Internet on Quality Measurement." *Health Affairs*, Nov.–Dec. 2000, *19*, p. 106. For an expanded discussion of this topic, see also Herzlinger, R. E., and Bokser, S. "Note on Health Care Accountability and Information in the U.S. Health Care System." Harvard Business School Case No. 302-007. Boston: Harvard Business School, 2001.

54. Bates and Gawande, "The Impact of the Internet on Quality Measurement."

55. Legnini, M. W., Rosenberg, L. E., Perry, M. J., and Robertson, N. J. "Where Does Performance Measurement Go From Here?" *Health Affairs*, May–June 2001, *19*, 173–177.

56. This figure is based on costs of $10,000 per patient and an incidence of diabetes of 7.5 percent, which produces annual diabetes costs per 1,000 enrollees of $750,000. A 1 percent reduction in these costs, $7,500, will pay for collecting performance data from twenty-five doctors at a monthly cost of $2.50 per member. Because the number of doctors covering 1,000 enrollees is typically 0.5, the payback is fiftyfold.

57. Hofer, T. P., and others. "The Unreliability of Individual Physician 'Report Cards' for Assessing the Costs and Quality of Care of a Chronic Disease." *Journal of the American Medical Association*, July 9, 1999, *281*, 2098–2105.

58. Halm, E. A., Lee, C., and Chassin, M. R. "How Is Volume Related to Quality in Health Care? A Systematic Review of the Medical Literature." In M. Hewitt, *Interpreting the Volume-Outcome Relationship in the Context of Health Care Quality.* Washington, D.C.: National Academy of Science, 2000, pp. 27–62.

59. Landers, S. J. "Physician Data Bank Records Found Inaccurate, Incomplete." *American Medical News,* Dec. 18, 2000, *43,* 1–2.

60. "Data Needs for Measuring Competition and Assessing Its Impact." HCFO [Changes in Health Care Financing and Organization] *News & Progress,* July 1999, p. 3.

61. McEnery, R., and Golov, D. "Project's Collapse Shuts Off Information on Hospital Care." *The Plain Dealer,* Aug. 23, 1999, p. 1A.

62. Because of the virtual absence of effective choice in the health insurance market, there has been little opportunity to evaluate the impact of information on consumers' health status. A study of one of the few early adopters of consumer-driven health care, BHCAG, demonstrated virtually no impact from information, perhaps because the information contained no clinical data, all the care options covered the same benefits, and enrollees could "shop with their feet" because they could easily rotate from one care group to another on a monthly basis. See the discussion of BHCAG's experience in Chapter Forty-Two.

63. Churchill, N. C., and Govindarajan, V. "Effects of Audits on the Behavior of Medical Professionals Under the Bennett Amendment." *Auditing,* Winter 1982, *1,* 69–90; Kaplan, S. E., Menon, K., and Williams, D. D. "The Effect of Audit Structure on the Audit Market." *Journal of Accounting and Public Policy,* Fall 1990, *9,* 197–201.

64. Romano, P. S., Rainwater, J. A., and Antonius, D. "Grading the Graders." *Medical Care,* Mar. 1999, *37,* 295–305.

65. Chassin, M. R., Hannen, E. L., and DuBuono, B. A. "Benefits and Hazards of Reporting Medical Outcomes Publicly." *New England Journal of Medicine,* Feb. 8, 1996, *334,* 394–398; Bentley, J. M., and Nash, D. B. "How Pennsylvania Hospitals Have Responded to Publicly Released Reports on Coronary Artery Bypass Graft Surgery." *Journal of Quality Improvement,* Jan. 1998, *24,* 40–49.

66. Petersen, E. D., and others. "The Effects of New York's Bypass Surgery Provider Profiling on Access to Care and Patient Outcomes in the Elderly. "*Cardiac Surgery,* Oct. 1998, *32,* 993–999.

67. Bentley and Nash, "How Pennsylvania Hospitals Have Responded . . .," p. 45.

68. Chassin, M. R. "Achieving and Sustaining Improved Quality: Lessons from New York State and Cardiac Surgery." *Health Affairs,* July–Aug. 2002, *21,* 40–51.

69. Sirio, C. A., and Harper, D. "Designing the Optimal Health Assessment System." *American Journal of Medical Quality,* Spring 1996, *11,* S66–S69.

70. Changes in Health Care Financing and Organization (HCFO). "Health Plan Report Cards May Influence Insurers More Than Consumers." Findings Brief. Washington, D.C.: HCFO, Apr. 2000, pp. 1–2.

71. Chatfield, M. *A History of Accounting Thought.* Huntington, N.Y.: Krieger, 1997, p. 32.

72. Carey, J. *The Rise of the Accounting Profession.* New York: American Institute of Certified Public Accountants, 1970, pp. 1–16.

73. Seligman, J. *The Transformation of Wall Street.* Boston: Houghton Mifflin, 1982, p. 41.

74. Schwarzschild, B. "The Tau Neutrino Has Finally Been Seen." *Physics Today,* Oct. 2000, *53,* 17–19.

75. Robert, L. "A History of the Human Genome Project 2001." *Science,* Feb. 16, 2001, *291,* 1195–1200.

76. Dunn, D. L. "Application of Health Risk Adjustment." *Inquiry,* Summer 1998, *35,* 145.

77. Knutson, D. "The Minneapolis Buyers Health Care Action Group." *Inquiry,* Summer 1998, 35, 176.

78. "Health-Based Payment System Offers Some Promise." HCFO [Changes in Health Care Financing and Organization] *News & Progress,* Nov. 1999, p. 10.

79. Goodman, J. C., Pauly, M., and Porter, P. K. "The Economics of Managed Competition." Working Paper, National Center for Policy Analysis, Nov. 2000.

80. Hatcher, C. S. "Predictive Modeling Can Trim the Waste and Keep Providers Fiscally Fit." *Managed Healthcare Executive,* Mar. 2001, pp. 37–38.

81. "Predicting Employee Health." *On Managed Care,* Mar. 2001, p. 3.

82. See, for example, Iezzoni, L. I., Ash, A. S., Coffman, G., and Moskovitz, M. A. "Predicting In-Hospital Mortality." *Managed Care,* Apr. 1992, *30,* 347–359; Iezzoni, L. I. "The Risks of Risk Adjustment." *Journal of the American Medical Association,* Nov. 19, 1997, *278,* 1600–1607.

83. Newhouse, J. P. "Risk Adjustment: Where Are We Now?" *Inquiry,* Summer 1998, *35,* 122–129.

84. Newhouse, "Risk Adjustment," p. 124.

85. "Time to Buy Temple Industries for $153 Million." *Wall Street Journal,* Feb. 16, 1973, p. 10.

86. Deardon, J., and Henderson, B. D. "New System for Divisional Control." *Harvard Business Review,* Sept.-Oct. 1996, *44,* 144–156

87. Deardon and Henderson, "New System for Divisional Control."

88. Blyskal, J. "A Divorce Made in Heaven." *Forbes,* May 21, 1984, pp. 80–82.

89. Mark Tierney, personal communication to the author, 2002.

90. "The State of Risk Contracting in California." *The Aventis Risk Report,* Spring 2000, pp. 4–11.

91. Gold, M. R., Hurley, R., and Lake, T. "Provider Organizations at Risk." *Health Affairs,* Mar.–Apr. 2000, *19,* 175–180.

92. Fireman, B. H., and others. "Cost of Care for Cancer in a Health Maintenance Organization." *Health Care Financing Review,* Summer 1997, *18,* 51–76.

93. "An IPA Success Story." *Modern Healthcare,* Sept. 13, 1999, p. 68.

94. Corey, E. R. *Procurement Management: Strategy, Organization and Decision-Making.* Boston: CBI, 1978, pp. 52–56.

95. Watson Wyatt Worldwide and Health Care Financial Management Association. *Delivering Value in Health Care.* Washington, D.C.: Watson Wyatt, Spring 1998.

96. Lo Sasso, A. T., and others. "Beyond Cost: Responsible Purchasing of Managed Care by Employers." *Health Affairs,* Nov.–Dec. 1999, *18,* 219.

97. Hofmann, M. A. "Health Care, Retirement Aetna's Key Businesses." *Business Insurance,* Apr. 27, 1998, *32,* 125–126.

98. See, for example, Grossman, J. M., Strunk, B. C., and Hurley, R. E. *Reversals of Fortune: The Rise and Fall of Medicare Plus Choice.* Washington, D.C.: Center for Studying Health System Change, May 2002, p. 2; Himmelstein, D. U., and Woolhandler, S. J. "A National Health Program for the United States: A Physician's Proposal." *New England Journal of Medicine,* Jan. 12, 1989, *320,* 102–108.

99. Gabel, J., and others. "The Changing World of Group Health Insurance." *Health Affairs,* Summer 1988, *7,* 48–66.

100. U.S. General Accounting Office (GAO). *Private Health Insurance.* Washington, D.C.: GAO, 1996, pp. 3, 38.

101. Employee Benefit Research Institute (EBRI). "Most Americans Dissatisfied with Health Care." News Release. Washington, D.C.: EBRI, Nov. 3, 2000.

102. Employee Benefit Research Institute (EBRI). *2000 Health Confidence Survey.* Washington, D.C.: EBRI, June 2000, p. 15.

103. Commonwealth Fund. *Listening to Workers.* New York: Commonwealth Fund, Jan. 2000, p. 8.

104. Penn, M. J. "Health Care Is Back." *Blueprint,* Spring 2000, p. 71.

105. Commonwealth Fund, *Listening to Workers,* p. 8.

106. Employee Benefit Research Institute, *2000 Health Confidence Survey.* p. 21.

107. See, for example, Woolhandler, S. J., and Himmelstein, D. U. "The Deteriorating Administrative Efficiency of U.S. Health Care." *New England Journal of Medicine,* 1991, *324,* 1253–1258.

108. "Moms Gaining Time in Maternity Wards." *New York Times,* June 15, 1999, p. F8.

109. It is difficult to compare the costs of private and government-run health care systems in various countries because of differences in accounting practices. For example, governments do not reflect the depreciation expenses of most of their assets whereas private firms do, and the employee pension expenses of many governments are accounted for separately from the health care entities.

110. "The Doctor's Dilemma." *The Economist,* Jan. 22, 2000, p. 55.

111. Lyall, S. "In Britain's Health Service, Sick Itself, Cancer Cure Is Dismal." *New York Times,* Feb. 10, 2000, p. A1.

112. Daly, R. "Hospitals Just Pass Patient Ratings." *Toronto Star,* Nov. 2, 1998, p. A1.

113. Naylor, C. D. "Health Care in Canada." *Health Affairs,* May–June 1999, *18,* 21.

114. Brooke, J. "Full Hospitals Make Canadians Wait and Look South." *New York Times,* Jan. 16, 2000, p. A3.

115. Frogue, J. "A High Price for Patients." Heritage Foundation *Backgrounder* No. 1398, Sept. 26, 2000, p. 14.

116. Donelan, K., and others. "The Cost of Health System Change." *Health Affairs,* May–June 1999, *18,* 214.

117. Marmot, M. "Acting on the Evidence to Reduce Inequalities in Health." *Health Affairs,* May–June 1999, *18,* 42.

118. MacKillop, W. J., Zhang-Salomons, J., Boyd, C. J., and Groome, P. A. "Association Between Community Income and Cancer Incidence in Canada and the United States." *Cancer,* Aug. 15, 2000, *89,* 901–912.

119. Alter, D. A., Basinski, A.S.H., and Naylor, C. D. "A Survey of Provider Experiences and Perceptions of Preferential Access to Cardiovascular Care in Ontario, Canada." *Annals of Internal Medicine,* 1998, *129,* 567–572.

120. Naylor, "Health Care in Canada," pp. 22–24.

121. Parrish, M. "When Patients Buy Their Own Health Care." *Medical Economics,* Mar. 5, 2001, p. 106.

122. Penn, "Health Care Is Back," p. 71.

123. Holmes, B. J. *HMOs' eHealth Plan Threat.* Techstrategy Report. Cambridge, Mass.: Forrester Research, Jan. 2001, figure 2.

124. Stigler, G. J. "The Economics of Information." In K. R. Leube and T. G. Moore (eds.), *The Essence of Stigler.* Stanford, Calif.: Stanford University and Hoover Institution Press, 1986, pp. 46–66.

125. Hannan, E. L., Siu, A. L. Kumar, D., and Chassin, M. R. "The Decline in Coronary Artery Bypass Graft Surgery Mortality in New York State." *Journal of the American Medical Association,* 1995, *273,* 209–213; Dziuban, S. W. "How a New York Cardiac Surgery Program Uses Outcome Data." *Annals of Thoracic Surgery,* 1994, *58,* 1871–1876.

126. Chassin, "Achieving and Sustaining Improved Quality."

127. Peterson and others. "The Effect of New York's Bypass Surgery Provider Profiling . . ."

128. Dranove, D., Kessler, D., McClellan, M., and Satterthwaite, M. "Is More Information Better? The Effects of 'Report Cards' on Health Care Providers." Working Paper w8697, National Bureau of Economic Research, Jan. 2002.

129. Changes in Health Care Financing and Organization, "Health Plan Report Cards . . ."

130. Bentley and Nash, "How Pennsylvania Hospitals Have Responded . . ."

131. Becher, E. C., and Chassin, M. R. "Improving the Quality of Health Care: Who Will Lead?" *Health Affairs,* Sept.–Oct. 2001, *20,* 164–179.

132. McEnery and Golov, "Project's Collapse Shuts Off Information . . ."

133. Sirio, C. A., and Harper, D. "Designing the Optimal Health Assessment System: The Cleveland Quality Choice Example." *American Journal of Medical Quality Care,* Spring 1996, 11, S66–S69.

134. "Operation That Rated Hospitals Was a Success, but the Patient Died." *Wall Street Journal,* Aug. 23, 1999, p. A1.

135. "Operation That Rated Hospitals Was a Success . . .," p. A1.

136. Taylor, M. "Another Provider Files Antitrust Suit." *Modern Healthcare,* Dec. 10, 2001, p. 26.

137. Lavern, E. "Good Scores Don't Equal Good Care." *Modern Healthcare,* Jan. 14, 2002, p. 7.

138. "Operation That Rated Hospitals Was a Success . . .," p. A1.

139. Watson Wyatt Worldwide. *Purchasing Value in Health Care.* Bethesda, Md.: Watson Wyatt Worldwide, 1997.

140. Seligman, *The Transformation of Wall Street,* p. 41; Herzlinger, R. E. "Finding the 'Truth' About Managed Care." *Journal of Health Politics, Policy and Law,* Oct. 1999, *24,* 1077–1093.

141. Mattli, W. "Global Private Governance for Voluntary Standards Setting: National Organizational Legacies and International Institutional Biases." Working Paper RPP-2001-06, Regulatory Policy Program Center for Business and Government, John F. Kennedy School of Government, Harvard University, May 2001.

142. Mclean, B. "Why Enron Went Bust." *Fortune,* Dec. 24, 2001, pp. 58–68.

143. Robert Pozen, former vice chairman of Fidelity Investments, personal communication to the author, Apr. 2002.

144. Hofer and others, "The Unreliability of Individual Physician 'Report Cards' . . ."

145. Newhouse, "Risk Adjustment."

146. Aron, D. C., Harper, D. L., Shepardson, L. B., and Rosenthal, G. E. "Impact of Risk-Adjusting Caesarian Delivery Rates When Reporting Hospital Performance." *Journal of the American Medical Association,* June 24, 1998, *279,* 1968–1983.

147. "Mutual-Funds Ratings Stars Are Changing." *Wall Street Journal,* Apr. 23, 2002, p. C1.

CHAPTER EIGHT

How to Make Consumer-Driven Health Care Happen

Consumer-driven health care will be fueled by employers, created by insurers and providers, overseen by governments, and funded by the public.

NEW ROLES FOR ALL

This brief chapter summarizes their new roles in making consumer-driven health care a reality.

The Fuelers of Change: Employers

To enable consumer-driven health care, employers must create a framework that empowers their employees with control, choice, and information.

Control. Create a level playing field. Give each employee the same amount of money, adjusted for risk status. Do not subsidize different plans at different rates.

Choice. Enable competition by offering insurance options that are genuinely differentiated from each other in benefits, term, provider structure and payment, and out-of-pocket maximums. Risk-adjust payments so that insurers are equally interested in insuring the sick and the well. Do require a minimum level of catastrophic insurance.

Information. Arm employees with helpful, clear information to guide their decision making.

The Engines of Change: Insurers and Providers

To create consumer-driven health care, insurers and providers must respond with consumer-friendly, higher-quality, lower-cost innovations. Insurers must craft genuinely differentiated product offerings. Providers must completely re-create the process of care through focused factories, integrated patient medical information, and personalized medical technology. Insurers must accept the providers' prices and bundles of care and not dictate them. And both must cooperate with attempts to measure their performance.

The Overseers of Change: Governments

To oversee consumer-driven health care, governments must provide sunshine—through a "truth agency" that assures excellent, relevant, timely evaluations of insurers and providers—and regulation of insurers and providers to ferret out unscrupulous, undercapitalized, anticompetitive, and fraudulent participants.

The Funders of Change: Consumers

To create a universal consumer-driven health care system, the American public must be willing to support expansion of the safety net of health insurance to those who cannot afford to buy it. After all, we are all part of history's greatest successful experiment in structuring a democratic, affluent, fulfilled society. How can we leave the poor out of it?

CONSUMER-DRIVEN HEALTH CARE GUIDELINES

These roles are revolutionary, and they will require revolutionary changes in the way we deal with our health care system.

Employers and their human resource agents must switch from micromanaging insurers and providers to empowering employees. In the words of Corbette Doyle, Aon Healthcare Alliance CEO and an early adopter of consumer-driven health care, "management must believe in the strategy and clearly communicate its support and trust."[1]

Insurers must depart from offering standardized, one-price-fits-all products that minimize their risk and start offering differentiated products. Managed care is best implemented in the costly to-implement, difficult-to-manage staff or group models in which insurers are closely integrated with their providers.

Providers should call a cease-fire in their turf battles and integrate to provide high-quality, efficient services that are focused on the patients' needs.

Governments should halt their micromanagement of the structure of insurance policies and the payment of providers and instead oversee insurers' and providers' integrity and shed sunlight on their outcomes.

Consumers must end their ostrichlike denial of the hardships faced by the poor uninsured and instead enable all to attain the benefits of the new consumer-driven health care system.

These changes will require dedication and persistence as the many powerful special interests in this sector try to shanghai the revolution for their own purposes.

One overriding principle must guide the movement: *every change must help the health care consumer.*

Note

1. Corbette Doyle, personal communication to the author, Feb. 2002.

PART TWO

VISIONS AND MODELS

The authors in Part Two flesh out the vision of consumer-driven health care and provide various early-adopter models, both in the United States and abroad. A diverse, expert group of respondents then comments on these visions and models. Additional chapters can be found at http://www.josseybass. com/go/herzlinger. They include those by James Garrison, former CEO of the Delta Dental Association, who uses the dental market to illustrate how traditional insurance can cause the inflation and inappropriate use that a consumer-driven health insurance plan avoids; Tom Beauregard, of Hewitt, and Thomas Kuhlman, of Towers Perrin, who provide us with their advice; and Mark Litow, Miliman & Robertson's renowned actuary, who outlines the guts of the cost-accounting systems that will support the competitive prices that will be required of consumer-driven health care.

Here is a likely scenario of how consumer-driven health care will be implemented by employers:

Step 1. The employer either transfers a flat sum to the employees or helps to pay for their health insurance and health care expenditures through various savings accounts.

This step enables employees to pay for health insurance with pretax income.

Step 2. The employer offer its employees a large number of health choices, as diverse as those in a 401(k) plan. The plans differ in benefits, term, provider groups, provider payments, out-of-pocket costs, and price. This step enables consumers to choose the plans that best meet their needs. Differentiation drives the competition among insurers and providers that will help the health care system improve quality and lower costs.

Step 3. New, neutral intermediaries or the insurers and providers themselves step in: they risk-adjust the payments and provide enrollees with the information and support they need to make a choice.

The risk-adjustment step captures interest in the sick and thus maintains product differentiation. Absent risk adjustment of prices, insurers are motivated to design more or less uniform policies with features that attract healthy enrollees, and providers are penalized for treating sick patients. The information and support helps enrollees to sort out the pros and cons of different policies and providers.

Step 4. The employees choose the health insurance options that best meet their needs, subject to the requirement of purchasing a catastrophic insurance policy. If their choice costs less than the amount transferred by their employer, in most cases they can save the difference in cost for other health care needs.

Consumers who allocate funds they view as theirs now have "skin in the game." They will choose the plan that offers the best value for the money and trade off expenditures for additional health insurance versus expenditures for other health care needs.

The chapters in this part of the book contain the visions and models that put flesh on this skeleton and commentaries on those visions and models.

Chapters Nine, Ten, and Eleven present various visions of consumer-driven health insurance policies. Chapters Twelve through Sixteen offer analyses of the tax status and risk-adjustment issues that must be addressed in implementing these visions. Together these eight chapters underscore the energy and competence of those who are behind this new movement. Chapters Seventeen through Twenty-Three illustrate early-adopter models of consumer-driven health insurance in the United States and internationally. These models are fascinating in their breadth and illuminating in their success. Representatives of different perspectives and interest groups respond to these visions and models in Chapters Twenty-Four through Thirty-Two.

THE VISION

Every movement requires a tipping point if it is to succeed. In the case of U.S. health insurance, our major corporations' adoption of innovative products provides that point. They are the leaders of the consumer-driven health care charge.

William ("Bill") George's discussion, in Chapter Nine, of a consumer-driven health care system that provides the right care describes how Medtronic, the extraordinary medical device company he led for many years, both exemplifies this vision and helps to advance it. Medtronic is not only an early adopter of consumer-driven health insurance but also the creator of a revolutionary class of medical devices that can help those with chronic diseases to help themselves. Brian Marcotte is vice president of benefits and compensation programs at Honeywell, a company that provided the tipping point for managed care when in 1988, as AlliedSignal, it became the first large firm to enroll all its employees in managed care with a single national vendor. Although the firm received many accolades for its courage, Marcotte now writes, in Chapter Ten: "that bold move has become a dubious honor . . . we are looking to a consumer-driven health market as the next sea change."

These chapters explaining the business rationale for consumer-driven health care are followed by one that elucidates the nature of insurance. In Chapter Eleven, John Goodman, the founder and leader of the Dallas-based National Center for Policy Analysis, takes us with him on a thought experiment to fashion the ideal health insurance policy that provides financial protection, motivates health promotion, and yet involves the users in resource allocation. (This policy is similar to the one widely used in South Africa, whose impact Shaun Matisonn describes later in Part Two.)

IMPLEMENTATION ISSUES

The next five chapters address the critical implementation issues of tax status and risk adjustment. In Chapter Twelve, Harvard Medical School professor Lisa Iezzoni guides us through three cautionary case studies of risk adjustment, and in Chapter Thirteen, Steve Hyde, a health care entrepreneur and actuary (as he inaccurately describes himself, "I didn't have the personality to be an accountant") proposes a broad-based market system that obviates the need for risk-adjustment. Then, Jeanne Brown (Chapter Fourteen), Charles Klippel (Chapter Fifteen), and Bonnie Whyte (Chapter Sixteen) discuss the tax implications of consumer-driven health savings and flexible spending accounts, from their perches in the Evergreen Foundation, Aetna, and the Council on Flexible Compensation, respectively.

U.S. AND INTERNATIONAL MODELS

The next eight chapters describe models of consumer-driven health insurance, both in the United States and abroad, that incorporate these visions and illustrate how some of the implementation issues have been successfully addressed. The U.S. models include the Federal Employees Health Benefits Program, as explained by its long-time director James Morrison (Chapter Seventeen); the

State of Washington, which successfully used risk adjustments and information for its health insurance programs, as described by Vicki Wilson, Jenny Hamilton, Mary Uyeda, Cynthia Smith, and Graydon Clouse (Chapter Eighteen); the Buyers Health Care Action Group, whose risk-adjusted payments to providers and wide choice for consumers has led to exemplary cost control and enrollee satisfaction, as articulated by Ann Robinow, a long-standing BHCAG executive (Chapter Nineteen); and the forays of WellPoint, the country's most admired health insurance firm, into consumerism, as recounted by its CEO, Leonard Schaeffer (Chapter Twenty).

The international scene provides a treasure trove of consumer-driven initiatives. In Chapter Twenty-One, Bruno Holthof, of McKinsey & Company, analyzes their impact in European countries such as Switzerland, Holland, and France, as does Paul Belien, of the Centre for the New Europe, in Chapter Twenty-Three. In Chapter Twenty-Two, Shaun Matisonn, of South Africa's Discovery Health, details the extraordinary cost reductions that that organization's consumer-driven policy achieved, apparently without diminishing health status. On the Web site, Dr. Wilfred Prewo analyzes how Germany's health care system can become consumer driven.

RESPONDENTS

What do informed outside readers make of these visions and models?

Their responses are many and varied.

In Chapter Twenty-Four, Alvaro Salas-Chaves, Costa Rica's former minister of social security, analyzes how Latin America's health care systems can become consumer driven. Professional investor Eugene Hill worries that government will gum up the works and diminish the flow of capital to this new area (Chapter Twenty-Five). Although the three physician spokespersons—Jesse Hixson, former principal economist of the American Medical Association (AMA), past AMA president Daniel Johnson, and Harvard Medical School professor Warner Slack— welcome the change (Chapters Twenty-Six, Twenty-Seven, and Twenty-Eight, respectively), Johnson cautions about the new kinds of accountability it will require of the profession. Corbette Doyle, CEO of AON Healthcare Alliance, wonders if the movement will truly control costs (Chapter Twenty-Nine), and two veteran health benefits consultants, Robert Coburn, of Mercer Human Resource Consulting (Chapter Thirty), and John Erb, of Deloitte & Touche (Chapter Thirty-One), are either not optimistic about the pace of change (Coburn) or urge the importance of a central government role for financing and oversight (Erb). Last, in Chapter Thirty-Two, John Rother, of the American Association of Retired Persons, worries about the ability of the public, especially those who are most in need and most vulnerable, to manage consumer-driven health care initiatives absent the necessary information and risk adjusters.

CHAPTER NINE

The Future of Twenty-First Century Health

William W. George

As the twenty-first century begins we are witnessing a major revolution that will shape our health care system throughout the next century. The revolution to which I am referring is not managed care, a creative new government payment plan, or the coming revolution in genetic therapy, important as it will be in offering new treatments and healing options.

The real revolution is consumer-driven health care, the *empowerment of patients* in becoming full collaborators with their health care team in managing their health. This is the long wave that will dominate twenty-first century health care.

Today, we think of the patient as the "product" of the health care system, a rather helpless being whom we treat as best we can and then release, with occasional follow-up. The insurance and managed care systems refer to these people, rather coldly, as *covered lives*. To the government's quality and mortality tables, they are but mere statistics, whose personal stories have little or no impact on their outcomes.

No longer! Across the United States patients are becoming empowered to take responsibility for their own health. Dissatisfied with a system that directs their health care through a maze of insurers, clinics, and physicians—none of whom seem to communicate with any of the others—patients and their families are attempting to take control over their health care destinies. With increasing frequency they are seeking second opinions and alternate providers. They also deal with their frustrations by going outside the health care system in search of herbal medicines, complementary therapies, improved diet and nutrition, and intense exercise plans with personal trainers.

Patients are being empowered by the availability of information about their health: information about diseases, treatment options, new therapies, integrated healing, differences in quality of physician groups and hospitals, information on the latest clinical trials, and the case histories of other patients. No longer are these data the exclusive domain of physicians. Now patients and family members can access a vast amount of health information on the Internet—some valid, some not, but all freely available.

Patients' newly found empowerment is part of the backlash against managed care. Empowered patients and their families react negatively to being controlled by the managed care system, especially when they sense the system is not acting in *their best interest.* They will expend great energy to get the health care they need. If they cannot gain access or treatments they need, they will fight with their insurers, go around their providers, or even engage their elected representatives to get it.

Rather than encouraging patients' newfound empowerment, the health care system seems to be threatened by it. Instead, the health care system should channel these energies to facilitate patients' getting *the right care.* The system should empower patients to become full collaborators in their prevention and healing processes. To make this approach work, patients must become accountable for their decisions and bear a larger portion of the cost.

THE RIGHT CARE

What is the right care? It is an integrated approach to patients' health needs for the long term. It is care that involves the most knowledgeable physicians and health care workers acting in unison to see that patients receive the care they need to be restored to full health. It is based on disease management care paths developed from broadly based statistical data on patient outcomes. It seeks to minimize the frequency of patient interactions with the health care system and draws heavily on disease prevention as well as recurrence prevention. By expanding conventional allopathic therapies with the use of complementary therapies, it offers a fully integrated approach that takes into account the needs of the whole patient.

Unfortunately, today's health care system is a long way from delivering the right care. Patients who need to see a specialist to get the proper diagnosis are often retained by their primary care clinic or denied the tests required to diagnose their disease properly. Patients suffering from chronic disease are often not followed by their specialist after receiving a procedure. Those with heart ailments, for example, wind up back in the emergency room or, worse yet, in the intensive care ward, when all they needed was to have someone follow up on the progress of their medications. Far too often patients with life-threatening diseases are not properly instructed as to the lifestyle changes they should make to prevent the recurrence of the disease or how to live with their disease. So the condition comes back or gets worse, and they have to start the process all over.

RETHINKING OUR HEALTH CARE SYSTEM

Correcting these ills and preparing our health care system for the empowered patient of the twenty-first century is no easy task. It cannot be done by "tinkering around the edges" or passing legislation that encourages more litigation. What is required is a fundamental rethinking of the nature of disease itself and of the organization of health care in order to address the diseases that are prevalent today using all the available tools, especially the power of individuals to take care of themselves.

In the United States today less than 25 percent of each health care dollar is spent on prevention and acute care. More than 75 percent of that dollar is used for the treatment and management of chronic disease. Let us separate health care into these two rather broad categories—prevention and acute care on the one hand and chronic disease on the other—and envision how our system might be organized to manage them.

Prevention and Acute Disease

In my experience the primary care system is well equipped to handle acute diseases of a wide variety, with only occasional referrals to specialists. This part of the system is relatively well managed and fairly efficient. However, the primary care system does not do nearly enough in the area of disease prevention, especially in addressing the needs of the whole person—body, mind, heart, and spirit.

Prevention should be the primary responsibility of the individual. People must take responsibility for their own health, or of course they will wind up sick. But prevention by individuals must be facilitated by the health care system. Our health care system can and must do a whole lot more to encourage people to modify their behaviors and lifestyles to prevent disease. From free flu shots and inoculations to smoking cessation classes to regular exercise programs to dietary education, much more emphasis on prevention will be the winning ticket—for the individual and for the system.

Paul Ellwood's original, 1970s concept of the *health maintenance organization* was a clinic where healthy people could go on a regular basis to have checkups of their physical condition and to review their complete lifestyles with a team of health care workers that included nurses, dietitians, exercise therapists, and even psychologists and counselors. It is a pity we have gone so far away from this concept because this is precisely what we need today: a place where people of all ages can go for a regular checkup followed by a lifestyle consultation to help them prevent disease. I do this every year without fail and have for the past thirty years. My physician gives me two full hours for these discussions, one for diagnosis and one for feedback. With today's managed care organizations pressing physicians for "productivity" by trying to limit patient visits to ten minutes per patient, this kind of time is hard to come by, but it is invaluable.

I envision a series of *wellness clinics,* run by primary care physicians, that focus on the needs of the whole patient—body, mind, heart, and spirit. They would offer a full range of complementary therapies such as acupuncture, chiropractic treatment, massage and energy work, instruction in meditation and stress reduction, and consultations with psychologists, physical therapists, dietitians, and nutritionists.

Who would pay for all this? To answer this, I believe that the *value of prevention* must be recognized by the people paying the bills—employers, governments, and consumers themselves—so they will make the necessary investments to make prevention happen through wellness clinics and similar centers. The good news is that *all* the individual resources required to deliver this kind of integrated prevention exist today, but unfortunately, the system is not organized to carry out this delivery. Instead, these resources operate independently, *without* looking at the whole person, and often they wind up competing with each other or, worse yet, giving the individual conflicting advice.

As a company dedicated to "restoring people to full life and health" and an employer of 23,000 people, Medtronic, Inc., where I was CEO from 1991 to 2001, recognizes fully the value of prevention. All Medtronic's medical coverage in the United States is through health plans, rather than insurers, and we are fully self-insured. Prevention is an integral part of everything we do, from the offerings of our providers to the plethora of "healthy lifestyle" things we do inside the company. For example, all our major facilities have fitness centers, which are filled eighteen hours a day. We will spend any amount on smoking cessation classes for employees and their families, but we do not permit smoking *anywhere* on company property. This includes the grounds and our parking lots and covers all international operations, including Japan. We sponsor regular noontime "brown-bag lunches" that feature speakers on healthy living, and our internal e-mail is filled with regular messages on stress reduction, diet, and nutrition. Once a quarter the mammogram van pulls up for free checkups, and employees are offered free flu shots every fall. Among our biggest health care concerns are the "weekend warriors" who rupture ligaments in their knees or fracture their bones playing sports. As a result of all these efforts, our health care costs have risen only 4 percent per annum over the past five years, and we are experiencing much greater productivity among our employees. *Prevention works!*

Chronic Disease Management

The management of chronic disease, as I have mentioned, is the area that already generates 75 percent of the health care costs even though it applies to a small proportion of the population. However, with the aging population resulting from greater longevity and the movement of the baby boomers into their later years, the incidence of chronic disease is certain to increase, regardless of the breakthroughs envisioned in medical therapy.

In the past, people suffering from a chronic disease often died within the first few months or years after onset, or they died suddenly of a heart attack or a stroke. Today we can diagnose these diseases much earlier so they can be treated, if not cured, and a patient can live with his disease for many years, perhaps decades. The real question here is can the patients manage themselves or will they be a high-cost burden on the health care system and on their families? In the vast majority of cases today the latter is the case: chronic diseases are an extraordinary economic burden on the system, especially toward the end of life.

Today's health care system frequently manages a chronic, incurable disease as a series of acute events. Rather than having a well-defined disease management plan that the patient follows, the specialist typically performs a procedure on the patient and returns her to her primary care physician without a rigorous plan for preventing recurrence of the disease and for ongoing follow-up. Patients who receive one of Medtronic's stents in an angioplasty procedure may go home thinking they are cured and make no changes in their lifestyle, not comprehending that they still have coronary artery disease that is highly likely to progress.

In chronic disease management I believe that improved care paths hold the potential for much better patient outcomes, less need to access the system, and dramatic cost savings. For each disease this process should be led by physicians who specialize in that disease and who treat a large number of patients annually. Of course they need a complete support team, including experienced nurse practitioners and a geographically based network of primary care doctors to support them locally. These specialists should be organized around large specialty practices and into multispecialty clinics and associated with a major tertiary hospital. The freestanding "heart hospital" may be an efficient way to get procedures done, but it begs the question of ongoing care of the disease and the treatment of complications that require the intervention of other disease specialists. It also puzzles me why so many sophisticated specialists want to do procedures at multiple hospitals rather than settling in at one principal hospital where they have the guaranteed support of a top-quality team with all the required follow-up systems in place.

The management of disease—be it cardiovascular disease, cancer, the wide array of neurological diseases, spinal or joint diseases, diabetes, or some other chronic condition—is so complex today and changing so rapidly that it must be directed by a specialty team. It is here—in the long-term treatment of chronic disease—where the greatest costs are being incurred throughout the system and, consequently, where the greatest savings can be made by improving the care plan. The specialists need to develop rigorous, evidence-based disease management plans for each category of disease they treat. These plans should draw on the longitudinal histories of their patients and clinical research studies conducted by other institutions. To realize the potential savings, all patients with a given disease should be under the direction of the same specialty team working with a defined disease management plan.

Why is this systemic change required? The management of these chronic diseases is so multifaceted that only specialists who see hundreds of patients each year with a particular disease can understand and manage that disease. To do so, they must be fully current on all the new technologies and treatment options and the status of the latest clinical trials and medical research. Seeing a large number of patients with subtle variations of a disease gives physicians an experience base to draw on in making intuitive judgments about both diagnosis and therapy. Further, the technology available for chronic disease management, whether it is implantable devices or advanced diagnostic imagery, requires a specialist to monitor and to interpret it.

What then is the role of the primary care physician in chronic disease? My belief is that when there is a preliminary indication of the possibility of a chronic disease, primary care physicians will serve as *traffic directors,* referring their patients to the best available specialist for definitive diagnosis and treatment. The primary care physician will retain the patient for normal health care interventions and do much of the follow-up in conjunction with the prescribed disease management plan, but the specialist will be the patient's principal physician in the ongoing treatment of the chronic disease.

Emerging Medical Technologies

In the years ahead the treatment of chronic disease will be dramatically affected by the new technologies and new therapies which are on the horizon. Today, the Internet *informs* patients about their disease. In the future, the new technologies will enable patients to be *connected directly* to their special physician and their health team.

For those patients with an implantable device such as a pacemaker, a defibrillator, or one of the emerging new class of implantable monitors, this *connectivity* will be enhanced many times over. Devices will transmit real-time cardiac rhythms and other stored information from a remote transmitter in the patient's home directly to the physician via the Internet. The new monitoring devices will provide blood pressure readings, stored EKGs, and body weight and will be augmented with ischemia sensors and sensors for other physiological measures.

Eventually, the physician will be able to titrate the patient's medications by a simple command delivered via the Internet.

In the future, gene therapy and new classes of biotech drugs will dramatically alter the treatment of cardiovascular disease. Human genome testing will enable us to measure the individual's propensity to incur various types of heart disease, and to begin treatment much earlier in the cycle.

Let us examine how some of the emerging medical technologies will provide greatly improved care at much lower costs:

- *New diagnostic imaging tools* will provide substantially improved diagnosis and do it much earlier in the disease cycle, but they will also require centralized monitoring and sophisticated interpretation.

- *Embedded computers* in implanted devices will give physicians the capability to monitor, diagnose, and treat patients with these devices, but effective use of this technology will also require substantial expertise. Let me illustrate: Medtronic's implantable defibrillator can discriminate between a wide array of arrhythmias and deliver the appropriate therapy on a "closed loop" basis, as well as record all the significant events taking place in the patient's heart.

- *New patient management systems* will evolve in which the Internet serves as a connection vehicle between patient and specialist. This will require sophisticated software and special security provisions to protect the patient's confidential medical information. All of the information gathered by the new implantable monitors and other devices will be read remotely by the physician through telemetry.

- The *human genome* project will provide a vast amount of diagnostic information. However, sophisticated evidence-based disease management tools will be required if this information is to be used appropriately.

- Many of the *new class of biotech drugs and gene therapies* are likely to need a site-specific drug delivery device to administer them and knowledge of both the drug or gene therapy and the device delivery technology.

- Physicians will able to dialogue with patients, often in their homes, using *videoconference tools* and having *access to real-time monitored data and historical data from patients' electronic records*. This, plus the availability of extensive data on patient outcomes, will enable health care specialists to improve the timing and effectiveness of interventions.

Putting together the best integrated therapeutic treatment plan for the individual patient in the future will require extensive knowledge in all these areas, both of the technologies and of the therapies.

AFFORDABILITY OF THE RIGHT CARE

Considering both the desire of patients to receive the best care and the cost of the new technologies, the obvious question is whether we can afford the right care. I believe that a restructured system that is based on both the involvement of empowered, economically at-risk patients and the use of these new technologies will dramatically *reduce* the long-term cost of managing patients throughout the course of a chronic disease. This favorable outcome will result from

- Creating better clinical pathways for treating chronic disease, based on documented clinical outcomes research

- Reducing the variability of care management

- Reducing the frequency of inappropriate interactions of the patient and the health care system

- Having the patients take greater responsibility for their healing, rather than relying as heavily as they do now on their physicians

- Eliminating or greatly reducing the array of middlemen who gatekeep, process claims, and attempt (often futilely) to "manage" the process

Shifting more patients to high-volume, more cost-effective specialty groups will force the elimination of low-volume, less-efficient groups, thereby reducing the total system cost. Direct connectivity between specialist and patient will reduce the duplication caused by multiple physicians interacting with the patient for the same purpose. Finally, I believe that efficient use of the new technologies will enable patients to be treated primarily from their homes, not in emergency rooms, intensive care units, extended hospital stays, or nursing homes.

Regardless of the status of individuals' health, whether patients are well or in the midst of a chronic disease, they need to have an economic stake in their health. It is not satisfactory to make health care options essentially free to the user and at the same time try to suppress users' utilization of the system by bureaucratic rules and constraints or by limiting the availability of needed services. Given the political malaise in Washington surrounding health care, I believe employers must take the lead in shifting a greater portion of the economic burden to their employees. The most promising approach at present is to convert from a *defined benefit* to a *defined contribution* plan, giving employees choices among a series of approved health plans with add-on options. To eliminate concerns over financial hardship from an extended chronic disease, catastrophic coverage should be automatically provided through an insurance-based plan. In the future we may have laws enabling real medical savings accounts (MSAs), and that will make MSAs a very viable option.

A CASE STUDY: CONGESTIVE HEART FAILURE

To understand better how the new system of treating chronic disease might work, let us look at the example of a fifty-five-year-old person recovering from angioplasty. The cardiologist at Integrated Health Center (IHC) develops a healing plan with the patient, which includes a regular exercise plan, strict low-fat diet, and stress reduction techniques such as meditation and massage therapy, as well as quarterly monitoring of his or her condition at IHC. In spite of all these efforts, five years later at age sixty the patient suffers a mild heart attack. In this regard they are following in the footsteps of their father, who suffered a similar event in his early fifties and, unfortunately, did not survive it. Thanks to randomized scientific studies showing the high risk of sudden cardiac arrest among first time myocardial infarction sufferers, the patient's cardiologist implants a dual chamber defibrillator prophylactically, to help regulate the heart and protect against sudden cardiac death.

Over the next ten years, the patient enjoys a fully active life, among other pursuits, jogging, hiking, and playing golf. At age seventy he or she is diagnosed with early congestive heart failure, which progresses to stage three by the time he or she reaches seventy-five. At this point the fifteen-year-old defibrillator is upgraded to a new generation device with cardiac resynchronization capability, more advanced diagnostic tools, the ability to titrate medications, and a remote monitoring capability with "hands free" telemetry. The latter is required because the patient has moved to Fort Myers, Florida, but wants to retain the existing IHC specialty team. In Florida, the patient establishes a relationship with a local internist but looks to the IHC cardiologist for monitoring heart failure.

In ongoing communication with the team at IHC, the implanted device transmits the patient's heart condition to a remote bedside monitor, which in turn transmits it over the Internet directly to IHC. For specific consultations the patient has a "virtual" meeting with the IHC team, via a videoconference. As a result of each consultation, the drug regimen may be altered and the pacemaker reprogrammed, all via remote electronics. Invisible to the patient is the IHC patient management system, which makes all of the treatments possible.

The result of this treatment is that the patient enjoys another five to ten years of quality living, in spite of the eventual progression of the disease. However, he or she is able to live at home, and has no unscheduled interactions with the medical system. The patient uses the medical savings account to pay an annual fee to IHC for managing the disease; this fee is only half of the traditional cost for stage III/IV heart failure patients. This is true even in the final stages of life, which are managed from the patient's home and attended by a hospice nurse. The final stage is ameliorated by the terms of the patient's *living will*, which limits high-cost interventions at the end of life.

The remarkable thing about this example is that *all* of the technologies described are feasible today! What is needed is the development of optimal disease management care paths, the tailoring of these technologies to optimize those paths, and most important, the transformation of our health care system to ensure that each patient receives the right care.

CONCLUSION

If these new therapies for managing chronic disease with the aid of emerging technologies are more effective and reduce the total cost of long-term care, what is preventing their adoption? Some would cite political realities, systemic and cultural barriers, physician resistance, and patient ignorance about how to navigate the system. No doubt all these factors are impeding the emergence of the optimal system.

I believe the key is the organization of the health care system around prevention and acute disease and the establishment of integrated disease management systems to treat chronic disease. In comparison to our current system, a reorganized system along the lines I have outlined will enable patients to receive the right care and take greater responsibility for their own healing, leading to an enhanced sense of well-being and higher quality of life throughout their lifetimes, and it would be much more cost effective.

CHAPTER TEN

How Employers Can Make Consumer-Driven Health Care a Reality

Brian J. Marcotte

In 1988, AlliedSignal, subsequently known as Honeywell, was the first company to enroll all employees in managed care with a single national vendor. Many firms followed, hoping to stay 18 to 20 percent annual increases in health care costs. Thus began the transformation of how employers purchase health care. We at AlliedSignal were optimistic that the concept of contracting with the best providers and using data to reduce treatment variability would improve quality and lower costs and that our purchasing leverage would instill competition among the health plans. AlliedSignal received many accolades for what was considered a bold move at the time.

Much of the promise of managed care, however, has not been fulfilled. Health care costs are back on the rise. Many of the problems that plagued the managed care movement in the early 1990s (such as users' difficulty in obtaining referrals, providers' dissatisfaction with their contracts, balance billing, and poor customer service) continue to exist today. And the pillars of managed care—aggressive provider contracting and utilization management—are now today's cost drivers. At Honeywell, where I am vice president for the Benefits and Compensation Program, health plan provider contracts have increased by as much as 40 percent in some markets and inpatient utilization is up 15 percent after ten years of steady decline.

Today Honeywell spends $650 million annually on health care. With 12 to 15 percent annual cost-increase trends, Honeywell's costs will nearly double in five years. We now have 98 percent of our employees in managed care plans. We believe the lifecycle of this strategy is near its end and we, like others, are look-ing to a *consumer-driven health care market* as the next stage in the evolution of health care purchasing.

There are many obstacles to consumer-driven health care given the current delivery systems. Consumerism is discouraged because providers and con-sumers are insulated from health care costs. There is a lack of information to support consumer health care decisions. Incentives do not exist for health plans or providers to treat the chronically ill. Competition at the health plan level has proven to be ineffective. And the individual market is not mature enough to sup-port an influx of 150 million consumers from the employment-based system.

But if employers helped build the managed care model, they can certainly be the catalyst for creating a consumer-driven market. Who better to drive it than corporate America? All the best examples of success and failure in serving consumers exist there. If employers play their role, the government creates no obstacles, and we embrace the Internet as an enabler for purchasing health care, a consumer-driven model could be several transformation steps away from replacing the current managed care system.

FROM MANAGED CARE TO CONSUMER-DRIVEN CARE

Employers jumped on the managed care bandwagon to build an element of cost accountability into the market. The quid pro quo for the employee who joined a managed care plan was a very rich in-network benefit (for example, low copays, no deductible, and no or little coinsurance). Employers essentially told their employees, "Sit back and relax: your primary care physician will navigate you through the health care delivery system . . . send you to a specialist if you need a specialist . . . direct you to the emergency room if it's an emergency . . . it's not your responsibility."

While employers were enjoying the benefits of the flat cost trends of the mid-1990s, they were creating a workforce of passive health care consumers who were fully insulated from costs and had no responsibility for managing care. Even consumers who wanted to play an active role were at the mercy of the system and succumbed to letting the system manage them.

After more than a decade of passivity, employers need to prepare, condition, and encourage employees to play an active consumer role. In a consumer-driven model, health care plan designs are structured to provide a financial stake for consumers. Consumers are armed with decision support resources—both high touch and Internet based—to help them make purchasing decisions.

In this consumer-driven system, consumers purchase health care like any other product or service every time they access the health care system—not just at annual enrollment. In other words, competition takes place at the *provider* level not just the *health plan* level. Providers are encouraged to compete for each encounter on price, quality, and service.

It will take time to engage the health care consumer and to prepare the market to support a consumer-driven model. Given their purchasing leverage and captive audience, employers are in the best position to simultaneously prepare and condition both the consumer and the market.

KEY STRATEGIES FOR TURNING EMPLOYEES INTO CONSUMERS

When we at Honeywell look at the health care delivery system today, we know that there is still significant variation in provider pricing and health condition management. We also know through our experience with managed care that health care decisions cannot be imposed on consumers; instead, consumers must be enabled and encouraged to drive efficiency. The opportunity in health care lies in addressing these factors through strategies employers can implement to encourage consumerism.

There are six key strategies that employers must implement or influence to encourage consumerism to take hold:

1. Give employees financial accountability by decoupling the relationship between company contributions and health care costs, that is, move to a defined contribution approach.

2. Improve clinical outcomes for high-cost conditions.

3. Build consumer involvement in care decisions at all levels.

4. Create provider contracting methodologies to give consumers a quality-based system.

5. Delegate the purchasing of health care to consumers.

6. Enable redesigned benefit options that give consumers greater control over how they spend their health care dollars.

These strategies, combined with the delivery power of the Internet, can facilitate the development of a consumer-driven health care market by the middle of this decade.

Move to Defined Contribution

Employees must begin to view health care less as an *entitlement* and more as *compensation* they can use to purchase the coverage that best meets their needs. Employers need to move away from providing the *employee* with the benefit entitlement and establish for the *consumer* a set amount that the company will contribute for health care.

Choice is essential in defined contribution approaches to health care plans, therefore a full spectrum of plan options—from indemnity to HMO—should be available. If an employee chooses a more expensive plan, like a PPO or indemnity, for convenience and flexibility, she pays the difference. If she chooses a lower-cost plan, the savings are hers.

Some employers have made this transition or are in the process of doing so. It is a key step in creating one level of consumerism and begins to break the entitlement mentality. However, defined contribution cannot be a strategy unto itself. Health care must remain *affordable* for the consumer. Therefore employers must make inroads into condition management and decision support and begin to realign incentives for consumers and providers *before* defined contribution is fully implemented. Although it is important to decouple the relationship between company contributions and health care costs, this change should evolve over time, as the other strategic elements take hold.

Improve Clinical Outcomes for High-Cost Conditions

Regardless of how employers reshape plan design to encourage consumerism, condition management (or care management) is the critical element in improving health outcomes. Conditions whose treatment displays high variation from evidence-based medicine guidelines and with the greatest potential return on investment from a financial and outcomes perspective must be identified and aggressively managed. We need to establish critical drivers of positive outcomes for each condition managed.

At Honeywell, we know that 10 percent of our population generates 70 percent of our costs. This 70 percent is spent primarily on treating chronic and severe or life-threatening acute conditions. We have had some success improving chronic conditions with disease management programs, but they lack the design incentives, decision support, and aggressive education and follow-up necessary to maximize compliance and reach the full at-risk population. Honeywell is now working with several health plans to take a new, aggressive approach to care management that incorporates new process, plan design, and decision support elements. Medical and prescription drug claims and predictive modeling will be used for high-risk identification. Incentives for compliance with treatment protocols will be incorporated into plan designs. *High-touch* decision support tools will be provided, in line with the severity of the condition. And a concierge approach to nurse outreach will be provided to encourage compliance and assist employees in navigating the system.

An example of our aggressive approach toward care management is our new diabetes disease management program. The target population will be identified via medical and prescription drug use (as in other diabetes programs). However, the target population will then be *engaged financially* in a two-step program. The first step is a health risk assessment survey that will both enable risk stratification of our diabetes population and establish a baseline of that population's compliance with five key drivers of improved outcomes. Participants will be paid $25 from the health plan upon their completion of the survey. The second step is a simple, yet aggressive process to maximize compliance around the five key drivers. These drivers include having the following tests completed annually: two hemoglobin A1c tests, one comprehensive cholesterol screening, one retinal eye exam, one foot exam, and one urine protein test. In addition to completing these tests, members of the target population must also establish a remedial action plan with their doctor if their HA1c or cholesterol levels fall outside an established norm. Participants who complete step two will be reimbursed $150 from their health plan upon annual completion. It is important that reimbursement is in no way tied to how one's body performs; it's tied only to making a relatively simple effort to manage one's health.

Build Consumer Involvement in Care Decisions at All Levels

Care management targets a specific at-risk population. But if we expect employees to play a more active role in managing their care, we need to provide decision support for care decisions. According to a multiemployer focus group study conducted by Hewitt Associates,[1] employees feel there is little or no information available regarding hospitals and doctors and there is no other market in which they have so little information with which to make decisions. In their words, there is no *Consumer Reports* available for health care.

Many companies are now providing on-line resources to support enrollment decisions. These resources include plan comparisons, rates, provider information, and decision modelers to help employees see which options best match their priorities. However, according to a 2002 survey on consumer attitudes toward health care, also conducted by Hewitt Associates,[2] only 31 percent of employers felt that providing employees with access to experts to advise on treatment options, doctors, or hospitals was a high priority, whereas 61 percent of consumers believed it was a high priority.

At Honeywell we have established a resource for our employees called LifeLine—a place where employees can go to get help on anything from child- and elder-care referrals to employee assistance programs and financial and legal assistance. It is also the point of entry for a medical decision support service provided through a company called Consumer's Medical Resource (CMR). CMR was implemented in July of 1999 and helps our employees who have been diagnosed with life-threatening and serious medical conditions such as cancer, HIV, or multiple sclerosis. It provides access to a group of leading medical researchers and physicians on staff at Harvard Medical School. CMR provides current, comprehensive, and objective information to employees about their medical conditions and their treatment options. It is customized to the individual and arms employees with real-time information to help them better participate with their physician in important decisions about their care.

For example, the three-year-old son of one employee was born with congenital heart defects, including a ventricular septum defect (VSD) and a missing aortic valve. The child's physician recommended a heart transplant "right now or he will not survive the summer." The employee called CMR to get information on heart transplantation, VSD, and options that might exist. CMR's customized response included information on all treatment options, several of which had not been discussed with the employee previously. After reviewing the new information with the doctor, the employee decided to seek another opinion. The new opinion confirmed that other, less radical procedures were available and should be attempted before the transplant. Having learned more, the employee decided not to proceed with the heart transplant and to attempt additional repair surgery. Months later, the child was healthy again and is now unlikely ever to need a transplant. As in this example, given the information, consumers can be self-confident, assertive, and engaged. Decision support services like CMR will be essential in a consumer-driven system. They make it possible for consumers to have an informed discussion with their provider and be genuinely involved in making decisions about treatment options.

This service has proven to be very powerful. At Honeywell, 428 employees who had used the service over the past thirty months participated in a survey. At a minimum, CMR has made 72 percent of survey respondents more comfortable than they initially were that the treatment recommended by their physicians was the best course for them. However, one in six survey respondents had changed a treatment to the treatment of choice, or *best practice*, revealed by CMR, eliminated or minimized side effects of treatment, and changed physicians. Additionally, one in fifteen had discontinued unnecessary or questionable treatment, and one in twenty-nine had identified an incorrect diagnosis. Eighty-seven percent rated CMR's overall service as "excellent," and 17 percent rated it as "very good." All survey respondents stated they would recommend CMR's service to other employees. Savings to Honeywell have been at least twice the cost of the service over that time period.

Still, CMR and care management reach only a small segment of Honeywell's employee population, those with chronic, severe, or life-threatening acute conditions. In order to create a consumerism mind-set among employees whenever they access the health care system, we need to build consumer involvement in care decisions at all levels—from choosing a physician to determining the right course of treatment for prostate cancer.

Supplying consumer-friendly health care data has always been a challenge, but the need for qualitative and cost tools for navigating a consumer-driven health care marketplace is now unavoidable. Several companies, such as Subimo and Dr. Quality, have begun to breach the Internet space to provide solutions.

These companies demystify health care for consumers and help them answer such questions as which hospital is best for them. Sharing this Internet marketplace are broader tools such as WellMed and Optate, whose products help employees access their health risk information, participate in disease management programs, compare benefits, and look for potential drug interactions. Most of these broader tools have also partnered with existing qualitative providers or offer homegrown solutions. The integration of on-line tools with high-touch services like CMR will be key to a successful decision support program.

Create Competitive Provider Strategies

How can employers also influence the provider community and encourage them to play in a new game? Current practices like capitation, discounted fees, managed care reporting, and contracting run counter to the effort. Again, competition needs to take place at the *provider* level not the *health plan* level. We need to engage both providers and payers at the point of service in the financial transaction. We need to provide the right incentives for providers to compete for market share and for the 10 percent of chronically ill consumers who account for 70 percent of health care cost.

This will not happen overnight. We can begin by varying copays in existing provider networks to encourage the use of cost-efficient physicians and facilities. These multitier networks introduce a level of defined contribution to provider reimbursement. Providers who charge more will need to justify their fees to the consumer—not the health plan. Many consumers, however, associate high quality with high cost, and until we can provide consumers with data to prove otherwise, these designs will be viewed by employees as nothing but another cost shift.

Delegate Purchasing to Consumers

Defined contribution, care management, and decision support tools begin the transition to a consumer-driven model. Through funding, plan design, and information we have a means of awakening the health care consumer. But behavioral change cannot be sustained if we do not change the underlying delivery system. We still need to involve the patient along with the provider in the financial transaction and eliminate the insulation factor that managed care has created. And we need to create new drivers for quality care and employee satisfaction with the health care system.

When employees pay for care directly—which is rare today—they do so as consumers, carefully considering both cost and quality. The relatively new Lasik surgery for correcting vision (which is typically not covered by an employer plan) is a perfect example: consumers are responsible for the cost, know the price going in, and pay at the point of service. In fact the cost of Lasik surgery has decreased over the past five years—which is also a rarity in health care—from approximately $4,000 per eye when it was first approved in July of 1998 to about $500 per eye today. Because Lasik surgery is discretionary, the example cannot be applied broadly. However, it does point out how price insulation makes health care very different from other markets. If Lasik surgery was a covered benefit, it would probably still cost employees about $500 per eye (their coinsurance) and employers perhaps as much as $4,000 or more.

Enable Redesigned Benefit Options

The question is, could we encourage the same kind of employee purchasing behavior, by offering employees plans that lift barriers to care and provide them with more control over how health care dollars are spent? One approach currently being tried in the marketplace is to offer as an option in the menu of choices available to employees a high-deductible *catastrophic plan* that is accompanied by a *health account,* or medical spending account-like, feature. This may seem like a retreat from employer funding of health care, but the intent is not to retreat but rather to engage employees more. The lower cost of the catastrophic plan would leave some employer dollars available to fund the health account. For example, the health account could be $500 with a deductible of $1,000. Employees would use the health account to pay for routine expenses such as office visits, prescription drugs, and so forth. What they do not spend rolls over each year and builds over time. Initially, provider networks would be maintained to retain discounts. Over time a fee schedule could be established for all other care—acute to catastrophic. Now consumers become the gatekeepers who can control how health care dollars will be spent, while still having the financial protection they need for high-cost illness or injury. Decision support services like CMR and Subimo will aid them. Employees who are frustrated with the bureaucracy of managed care will choose this option gladly, employees who value the first-dollar coverage of managed care will resist, and to maintain positive employee relations many companies will continue to offer other options alongside the new alternative.

It is our intent at Honeywell to pilot a catastrophic plan with a health account. However, these plans do have a number of issues that need to be addressed. There is concern that young, healthy employees will opt into the catastrophic plan whereas older employees in greater need of health care will stay in the traditional managed care plan. How will employers adjust for risk selection? How will the health account balance be managed? What happens to the balance when an employee leaves the company or retires? Will the health account be capped? Will there be a vesting requirement? These issues will be addressed as employers continue to experiment with catastrophic plans.

MAKING THE INTERNET AN ENABLER

The Internet can be the place in health care where cost and quality data come together to help consumers make decisions at the point of service. As Internet-based solutions such as Subimo and Optate emerge, qualitative data will allow employees to understand that there is not necessarily a direct link between cost and quality. Consumers will be able to access patient safety data based on the number of procedures a hospital has performed, the complication rate, staffing standards, and postoperative infection rates, as well as other factors important to them. These services will provide independent validation of the providers in a given market.

Honeywell will use a Web-based decision support tool in combination with a multitier hospital network. The multitier network will vary hospital-day copays from $150 for more efficient hospitals to $350 for average hospitals to $500 for less efficient hospitals. We compared hospital qualitative data for four surgical procedures (coronary artery bypass, prostatectomy, mastectomy, and gall bladder removal) to the cost of facilities in the multitier network. We found, for each condition, examples where medium- or low-cost facilities had quality rankings higher or about the same as the rankings among high-cost facilities.

The Internet offers many demonstrations of breaks with traditional buying paradigms that can be applied to health care. There are, for example, a number of Web sites where you can enter the specifications of the car you want to buy, your zip code, and your e-mail address, and the site will provide competitive quotes from several car dealers in your region. You can also obtain vehicle performance and quality information to aid in your decision. And if you buy a book or CD from amazon.com, its Web site will suggest other titles that may be of interest to you.

Despite these precursors, the task of pulling qualitative, cost, health assessment, disease management, and benefit comparison information into one useful tool is daunting. The vision is to create an e-health decision support service that will not only provide employees with comparative benefit and premium data at the health plan level but will also—with an amazon.com-like front-end portal—interact with consumers who need assistance with chronic conditions; provide reminders for care management follow-up, appointments, routine exams; and meet other health care information needs.

If we take this Internet vision to the next level, consumers who elect to participate in a catastrophic insurance and health account option could purchase health care *services* over the Web. Could the "price of admission" for a provider to participate in a network be meeting a specific level of quality? Could we do away with capitation and per diems and let providers bid for services over the Web in a *virtual PPO*?

In a virtual PPO (I'll call it "healthcarebuy.com"), the e-health vendor would contract with providers based on their quality. The lure of not having to deal with capitation and the hassles of managed care, coupled with the leverage of the employer community, would draw providers to participate. A consumer could get on line with healthcarebuy.com and enter his name, zip code, the type of service requested, and e-mail address. The e-health vendor would then relay a list of providers and price information back to the consumer, along with benefit coverage levels and quality and satisfaction data. Lasik surgery is again a good example of how this could work because it is not covered by most health plans and the method of purchasing it is similar to the way consumers purchase other goods or services on-line today.

When the service required is a covered benefit, a fee schedule would be established for services available through the virtual PPO. This could be a case rate that the plan would pay for diabetes management or prenatal care through a focused factory or center of excellence. It could be a fee schedule for an office visit, orthodontia, or a crown. Consumers would view on-line provider pricing, quality and outcomes information, and the plan's payment toward the service. They then would make a selection based on price, quality, service, and convenience. If the deductible of the catastrophic plan had not been met, the consumer would pay directly out of the health account. Credit card technology could link all three players in the transaction, and process the "claim" at the point of service. This approach creates a dynamic free-market system and gets health care back in the hands of physicians and patients.

For routine and acute care, the e-health vendor would have to establish a *base network*. But even here, why could a consumer not customize the base network? Consider how you can buy a computer on-line today through Dell or Micron. You can choose whether you want a Pentium II or Pentium III or IV processor, Sony's large monitor or standard monitor, upgraded sound board, upgraded graphics card, and so on. Each option affects the price. If you choose components that are incompatible, you are immediately redirected to other options.

Granted, a network of providers is different from the components of a computer, but for the process of selection the analogy holds. Do I want to receive my routine care from physicians affiliated with the local hospital or the teaching hospital? Do I select centers of excellence or a broad network? If I select physicians who are not affiliated with my hospital selection, I can be redirected. And my selections affect the overall cost of my plan.

CONSUMERS AS PRIMARY PURCHASERS OF HEALTH CARE

As U.S. health care evolves to a consumer-driven model, the role of the employer changes and ultimately becomes less important. Consumers become the primary purchasers of health care. Employers may still establish relationships with health plans and provide decision support services, but they are delegated a secondary purchasing role. We may reach a time when employers are no longer needed to play any purchasing role, and a new market entity emerges that will contract with health plans or providers for coverage and handle enrollments, communications, and decision support.

THE END GAME

In the ultimate vision of a consumer-driven system, employees receive dollars from their company to purchase *affordable* health care in an open market. They have the tools and resources to make informed decisions and weigh the trade-offs. The employer has transferred the risk of managing health care to the employee and provides a total compensation package that includes dollars for health care. The employer also plays a secondary purchasing role and provides employees with tools and resources that enable decision making. Providers are accountable to consumers for costs and outcomes and can charge whatever the market will bear.

One last thought illustrates the profound impact that consumer-driven health care can have. Today an employee who goes to her physician's office, waits two hours, and is dissatisfied with the physician visit itself, nevertheless pays her copay, say $10. She then calls the *employer* to complain about the *health plan*. When this same scenario happens in a consumer-driven system in which the employee has to pay the full cost of the visit, say $100, out of her health account, her complaints will be directed at those who can more readily act to correct them—the providers. And consumers would have the most powerful weapon of all in this system, they could choose never to return.

Notes

1. Hewitt Associates. *Employee Perspectives on Health Care Consumerism.* Lincolnshire, Ill.: Hewitt Associates, 2002.

2. Hewitt Associates. *Consumer Attitudes Toward Health Care Innovations: What Every Employer Should Know.* Lincolnshire, Ill.: Hewitt Associates, 2002.

CHAPTER ELEVEN

Designing Health Insurance
for the Information Age

John C. Goodman

The modern era has inherited two concepts of health insurance: the fee-for-service model and the HMO model. Even when combined with the latest techniques of managed care, neither model is appropriate or workable in the information age.

Both models assume that (1) the amount of sickness is limited and largely outside the control of the patient, (2) methods of treating illness are limited and well defined, and (3) because of patient ignorance and asymmetry of information, treatment decisions will always be filtered—made by physicians based on their own knowledge and experience or clinical practice guidelines.

However, an explosion of technological innovation and the rapid diffusion of new knowledge about the diagnosis and treatment of disease have rendered all these assumptions obsolete.

WHY TECHNOLOGICAL CHANGE AND THE DIFFUSION OF KNOWLEDGE HAVE MADE TRADITIONAL HEALTH INSURANCE MODELS OBSOLETE

Although the HMO model is often viewed as the more contemporary of the two models, it is actually the least compatible with the changes our society is undergoing. The traditional HMO model is fundamentally based on patient ignorance.

Figures and tables were not available at time of printing.

224

The basic idea is a simple one: make health care free at the point of consumption, and control costs by having physicians make rationing decisions, thus eliminating options that are judged "unnecessary," or at least not "cost effective." But this model works only as long as patients are willing to accept their doctor's opinion. And that only works as long as patients are unaware that there are other (possibly more expensive) valid options.

The technological reality is that we in the United States could spend our entire gross domestic product on health care in useful ways. In fact we could probably spend the entire GDP on diagnostic tests alone—without ever getting around to treating a real disease. The information reality is that patients are becoming as informed as their doctors—not about how to practice medicine but about how the practice of medicine can benefit them.

Combine the potential of modern medicine to benefit patients with patients' general awareness of these benefits and zero out-of-pocket payments, and the HMO model is simply courting financial disaster.

The fee-for-service model is only a slight improvement. It tries to control demand by introducing deductibles and copays. But these financial incentives are too weak. Systemwide, in 1997, third parties paid almost ninety-eight cents of every dollar spent in hospitals, eighty-eight cents of every dollar spent on physician services, and eighty-two cents of every dollar spent on health care generally. The incentives for patients were to consume hospital care until it was worth only two cents on the dollar, physician care until it was worth only twelve cents, and health care generally until it was worth only eighteen cents.[1]

To see where these incentives could easily take us, consider just a few of the ways we could spend health insurance dollars usefully if price were no object:

- The Cooper Clinic in Dallas offers an extensive annual checkup to such clients as Ross Perot and Larry King; if everyone did this, at $1,200 a pop, we would increase our nation's annual health care bill by more than 25 percent.

- There are now nine hundred tests that can be done on blood alone; if we spent only, say, $4,000 on them as a part of everyone's annual checkup, we would double the nation's annual health care spending.[2]

- Americans purchase nonprescription drugs almost twelve billion times a year; if we sought a physician's (free) advice before making such purchases, we would need twenty-five times the number of primary care physicians we currently have.[3]

Notice that, in all these cases, we have tested and diagnosed but have not actually done anything to cure an illness!

Some believe that managed care can solve these problems. They are wrong. Imagine grocery insurance that allows you to buy all the groceries you need, but as you stroll down the supermarket aisle, you are confronted with a team of bureaucrats prepared to argue over your every purchase. Would anyone want to buy such a policy?

Traditional health insurance is not designed to work much better.

Accordingly, I propose a new approach. It combines an old concept, casualty insurance, with two relatively new concepts: universal medical savings accounts (to control demand) and a proliferation of focused factories (to control supply).

DESIGNING AN IDEAL HEALTH INSURANCE PLAN

Let us begin by wiping the slate clean. Imagine you could get together with 999 other people and create an insurance plan just for all those in your group, 1,000 people. These 1,000 people are not alike. Some are old, some young. Some are male, some female. Some are in good health, some are not. Given these and other differences, how can you design a plan that all would want to join? In answering this question, forget the normal insurance industry bureaucracy. Forget state and federal regulations. Forget federal tax law. Forget everything else that would pose an artificial impediment to achieving the ideal. You are on your own. You must design the plan that will come closest to meeting your needs and those of your colleagues. What follows is a discussion of some problems you will inevitably encounter and some proposed solutions.

Terms of Entry

One of the first decisions we must make in designing a plan of this kind is what premiums should be charged to people when they join the insurance pool? No matter what benefits we decide to include in the plan, we have to collect enough premiums to cover all the costs. So, how much should each person pay? I have a suggestion that will not only solve this problem but also avoid others. In fact, failure to follow my suggestion on this issue will virtually guarantee that our group will not agree on anything else. My suggestion is this: each person should pay a premium equal to the expected health care costs he or she adds to the 1,000-person pool. If individual A will add $1,000, the right premium for A is $1,000. If B's expected costs are $5,000, B should pay $5,000. If C's expected costs are $10,000, C should pay $10,000.

What if the premium is so high for some people that they cannot afford to pay it? Then either they will be left out of the pool or others must make a charitable contribution on their behalf. Because all agreements are voluntary in this imagined scenario, coercion is not an option. Politicians usually try to "solve" the problem by keeping the premium artificially low for people with high health care costs. But if some people are undercharged, others must be overcharged.[4] People who are overcharged will want less coverage than they otherwise would, and those who are undercharged will want more. If we want people to make economically rational decisions, they must be charged a premium that makes the expected benefit of their additional coverage equal to its expected cost.

Terms of Renewal

At the end of an insurance period of, say, one year, on what terms should people be allowed to renew? Should those whose health has deteriorated be charged more? Should people whose health has improved be charged less?

Insurance is like gambling. Our decision to charge each entrant in the pool a premium equal to his or her expected costs makes the gamble a "fair" bet for all. But changing premiums based on changes in health status would be like changing the rules after throwing the dice. It would defeat the purpose of insurance—which is to share risk with others. Therefore, a reasonable rule is to raise or lower everyone's premium at renewal time, based on whether the whole group's costs have been more or less than expected. Those who got sick and generated high medical costs after joining the pool would not be penalized but would get the full value of the insurance.

Such a rule is broadly characteristic of the market for individual insurance. At the time of initial enrollment, people may be charged different premiums, based on age, sex, and perhaps health status. But once in a plan, no one can be expelled from it or charged an extra premium because his health deteriorates. Renewal is guaranteed, and if premiums are increased, they must be increased proportionately for everyone.

The small-group market now operates quite differently in most states. A firm's premiums are readjusted annually, based not on the experience of the larger group with which the firm's employees have been pooled but on the firm's employees' own experience over the previous year. In effect, every firm's employees are kicked out of the pool at the end of the year and allowed to reenter only if they pay new premiums based on the changes in their expected health costs. Subject to regulatory constraints, in the small-group market people can buy insurance only one year at a time. If this practice were applied to life insurance, everyone's premium would be reassessed annually, and rates for those diagnosed with cancer or AIDS during the previous year would be astronomical. Such a practice would virtually destroy the market for life insurance. Small wonder that small-group health insurance markets are in perpetual crisis.

The features of the individual market described previously come closest to emulating what most economists would consider a free market for health insurance, although that market is also far from perfect. In contrast, the features of the small-group market are almost totally the product of unwise public policies embodied in federal tax law and state regulation. Not surprisingly, this market has generated the most frequent complaints, particularly from small business owners. Unfortunately, most states try to deal with the problem by piling on more regulations rather than by confronting its cause.

Third-Party Insurance Versus Self-Insurance

The decision about what services to cover is closely related to the decision about how to allocate financial responsibility. For reasons that will become clear, the financial question needs to be addressed first. Federal law *excludes* employer-paid premiums from the taxable income of employees. But with some exceptions, funds employees set aside to pay medical bills directly are fully taxed (as discussed in Charles Kippel's Chapter Fifteen). Thus federal tax law encourages people to give all their health dollars to third-party payers. But if federal tax law were neutral, which services would we choose to pay for directly and which would we insure for? That is, what medical costs would we want the pool to pay, and which ones would we want to pay from our own resources?

Any time people transfer their resources to an insurance pool, there are two negative consequences (increased cost, at least for the group as a whole, and decreased autonomy) and one positive consequence (reduced risk). The problem is to ensure that the reduction in risk is worth the extra premium we must pay to obtain it. Our imaginary insurance pool faces the same problems as every other insurance scheme. Any time insurance pays a medical bill the incentives of the patient are distorted. All of us tend to overconsume when someone else is paying the bill, and this tendency, which economists call the problem of *moral hazard,* raises costs.[5] To counteract the tendency, we will want to consider some of the techniques of managed care. But these techniques will restrict our choices, reduce our autonomy, and perhaps reduce the quality of the care we get. Even if the quality is not diminished, administering the techniques will be costly.

Thus, no matter how well the plan is designed, for the group as a whole the cost of medical care will be higher than it would be if individuals simply purchased the same care on their own. Presumably, the higher costs are worthwhile if we enjoy enough reduction in risk. But at what point does the price we are paying for risk reduction become too high? Specifically, when is it worthwhile to transfer risk to a pool, and when does it make better sense to self-insure by putting funds into an account we own and control? Three general questions can help us arrive at an answer:

1. Is the medical service to be purchased prompted by a risky event, or is it the result of individual preference?

2. Is the price of transferring risk to a third party high or low?

3. Does the failure to obtain a service or the purchase of an inappropriate service have the potential to create costs for others in the pool?

The first question relates to the terms under which people obtain health care services. People differ in their attitudes toward medical care. They also differ in their aversion to risk. Take diagnostic tests for the detection of cancer. The more frequent the tests, the higher the cost. But medical science cannot tell us how frequent such exams should be.[6] That's largely a value judgment, and people's values differ. In general such exams are not prompted by a risky event. They are highly influenced by individual preferences.

As a general rule, the more expenditures depend on personal choices rather than external events, the greater will be the problem of moral hazard. This consideration suggests we should encourage individuals to purchase directly most diagnostic tests and most forms of preventive medicine.

The second question reinforces this conclusion. On one hand, transferring the risk of cancer treatment to an insurance pool is relatively low cost. For each dollar of exposure transferred, the extra premium is only a few pennies. On the other hand, transferring diagnostic testing to an insurance pool is relatively high cost. For each dollar of exposure transferred, the extra premium is a large part of a dollar. So the payoff for using insurance to cover cancer treatment is high, while the payoff for covering cancer detection is low.

The third question is whether the medical consequences of one's decision will generate costs for other members of the pool. Take immunization for childhood diseases. Studies show that these procedures pay for themselves by avoiding future health care costs that are greater than the costs of the vaccinations.[7] This implies that members of an insurance pool have an economic self-interest in seeing that all children covered by the pool are vaccinated. It may make economic sense for the pool to pay for vaccinations, thereby incurring more cost than self-pay would generate, or to require that members obtain them, thereby reducing autonomy.

Closely related to the problem created by the failure to obtain a desirable service is the problem created by the purchase of the wrong service. Suppose our plan has a $3,000 deductible and a member is diagnosed with cancer. Under this arrangement the patient would pay the first $3,000 of treatment costs and presumably would make her own decisions about how to spend that $3,000. But that $3,000 worth of decision making could have a large impact on her later treatment costs, and bad decisions early on could generate larger subsequent costs for the group. Such considerations may create a presumption in favor of paying for all treatment costs from the pool in cases where the entire treatment regime promises to be expensive.

Third-party payment for every medical service is potentially very wasteful. Such waste can be controlled only by invasive, expensive third-party oversight of individual medical care consumption. Such control necessarily interferes in the doctor-patient relationship. Some people may prefer this sacrifice of autonomy, and that may explain why there has always been a market for the traditional HMO. But many people will prefer self-pay and self-control—especially where no real reduction in financial risk is achieved by transferring control to a third-party payer. Even after taking into account each of the considerations discussed here, some health services will remain outside of unambiguous self-pay or third-party–pay categories. Ideal health plans, therefore, might have considerable discretion, and how they exercise it would depend on their members' preferences. What is important is to recognize that in the ideal insurance arrangement, some decisions will be individual and others will be collective.

Financing Mechanism for Self-Insurance: Health and Medical Savings Accounts

A common objection to individual control is that individuals will not always make wise decisions. But in our imaginary pool, everyone must voluntarily agree to the design of the plan, so we cannot entirely escape individual choice and preference. In addition, even with the most comprehensive coverage, individuals must make decisions about when to see a doctor and whether to purchase nonprescription drugs. So even if a patient wanted to turn all decisions over to someone else, that would be impossible. A more sophisticated objection is that most medical expenditures tend to be irregular and are hard for people living from paycheck to paycheck to incorporate into a budget.

One answer to this objection is the *medical savings account* (MSA).[8] Many employers make monthly deposits to accounts from which their employees can pay expenses not covered by the employer's health plan. Money not spent for medical care must remain in the account until the end of the insurance period, usually one year, after which the employee can withdraw it and use it for other purposes. MSAs make individual self-insurance workable for families who otherwise might find direct payment too burdensome. But how should such accounts be designed in conjunction with third-party insurance coverage? (*Health savings accounts* are discussed in Chapter Fifteen.)

Implications for MSA Design

Under the most common design the plan pays all costs above a deductible of, say, $3,000, and the MSA deposit is, say, $2,000. Thus the employee pays the first $2,000 of medical expenses from the MSA and the next $1,000 is paid out of pocket. Any remaining costs are paid by the plan. This structure is actually required by law under the current federal pilot program that makes MSA deposits tax free for the self-employed and employees of small businesses.[9]

However, MSAs designed in this way are not necessarily ideal. A better design is a flexible one, under which the deductible or copay varies depending on the service. A flexible MSA has a further advantage: it can fit into existing managed care plans and may partially resolve a problem these plans have with maintaining member satisfaction. For example, Alain Enthoven, a professor at Stanford University, in a well-publicized letter to then California governor Pete Wilson,[10] described a woman who was angry at her HMO doctor because he refused to give her a "medically unnecessary" sonogram. Enthoven surmised that if she had had to pay $50 out of her own pocket for the service, she would instead have thanked her doctor for saving her the expense. This and other incidents have convinced Enthoven, who had been wedded for years to the concept of first-dollar coverage, that patient out-of-pocket pay is essential to make managed care work.

There is one place in the world where flexible MSAs are a reality—South Africa.[11] Since 1993, a remarkable experiment has been under way in this southernmost African country. Due partly to liberal insurance regulations and partly to a favorable ruling from the South African equivalent of the IRS, virtually all major forms of insurance—HMOs, PPOs, and MSAs—are competing on a level playing field. Anyone with an idea on how to design a better health insurance plan has been free to try it out. And within the last few years MSA plans have soared from nowhere to capture roughly 50 percent of the market for private health insurance. Under the U.S. federal pilot program, a tax-free MSA for an American family was required to have a $3,000 deductible, which applied to all services—drugs, physician care, hospital care, and so on. South African MSAs are more flexible. The typical plan has first-dollar insurance coverage for most hospital procedures, on the theory that hospital patients don't have much opportunity to exercise choices. Conversely, a high deductible (about $1,200) applies to "discretionary expenses," including most services delivered in doctors' offices.

South Africa's more flexible approach also allows more sensible drug coverage. Although the high deductible applies to most drugs for ordinary patients, a typical plan pays from the first dollar for drugs for diabetes, asthma, and other chronic conditions. The theory here is that it's not smart to encourage patients to skimp on drugs that prevent expensive-to-treat conditions from developing.

Design of Third-Party Payment

One of the fastest-growing health insurance products in the U.S. market today is the point-of-service (POS) option. This option is popular because it answers some employee complaints about the restrictiveness of closed health care networks. Yet some analysts say that POS options can raise the cost of health insurance significantly.[12]

The approach I have been summarizing points to a partial solution to this problem. The reason out-of-network doctors might cost more, even when paid the same fees as in-network physicians, is that they are likely to order more tests and generate the use of more ancillary services. But this would be of much less concern if third-party payment were restricted largely to curative services and patients paid with their MSA funds for diagnostic services.

The problem of how to control curative costs without unduly restricting patient choice or endangering quality remains. A possible solution is a variant on an old idea: a fee schedule. From time to time the insurance industry has flirted with plans that pay doctors a set fee for various services. When patients selected doctors who charged more, they paid the difference out of pocket. However, in modern medicine that fee is only one part of a complex array of costs that a doctor can generate. So controlling the physician's fee isn't enough. But why not fix the plan's cost for an entire treatment regime? Suppose a patient is diagnosed with cancer, and the health plan normally would contract to pay a fixed fee to a medical facility to cover all costs. If the plan could be assured that this fixed fee were its maximum exposure, the plan would have no economic interest in restricting the patient's choices. It could, for example, allow the patient to go to an alternative provider and pay more, if needed, out of pocket or from an MSA. In this way the plan controls its costs, but patients can still exercise choice, and the exercise of choice would put pressure on the plan to maintain quality in its own preferred medical facility.

The decision to take the plan's money and seek treatment elsewhere would need not to be made once and for all. For chronic conditions, such as diabetes, it could be reaffirmed annually. Because traditional care for diabetes has been less than optimal,[13] many patients and doctors have long maintained that patients (with the help of a physician) can manage diabetes more efficiently than managed care can.[14] Why not let them try? The health plan might make an annual deposit to the patient's MSA and shift the entire year's financial responsibility to the patient. If there were concern that the funds might be wasted, the health plan could hold the account and monitor it. An example of the range of possibilities is again provided by the experience in South Africa. Discovery Health (one of the largest sellers of MSA plans there) gives its patients with diabetes the opportunity to enroll in a special diabetes management program. Discovery pays the program about $75 per patient per month, and the patient pays another $25 from an MSA account. Discovery is considering handling many other chronic diseases in the same way.

Casualty Insurance Model

To appreciate where this line of thinking might lead, compare casualty insurance with traditional health insurance. After an automobile accident, a claims adjuster inspects the damage, agrees on a price, and writes the car owner a check. Hail damage to a home's roof is handled in the same way under a homeowner's policy. In both cases the insured is free to make his or her own decisions about paying for damage repair. In contrast, traditional health insurance is based on the idea that insurers should pay not for conditions but for medical care. That health insurers rejected the casualty model is not surprising. After all, Blue Cross was started by hospitals for the purpose of ensuring that hospital bills would be paid. Blue Shield was started by doctors to ensure that doctor fees would be paid.[15] Had auto insurance been developed by auto repair shops, they also would have rejected the casualty model.

I am not suggesting that we give ourselves complete freedom of choice when we are patients. Paying people for a health condition and allowing them free rein to the point where they could decide to forgo health care and spend the money on pleasure may not be in the self-interest of a health insurance pool because an untreated condition today could develop into a new and more expensive-to-treat condition later on.[16] But I am suggesting that if people were largely free to make their own treatment choices and the market were free to meet their needs, health insurance would make a major step in the direction of the casualty model.

Covered Services

One of the most contentious issues in health politics today is that health insurers' services are required to cover an array of services, some of them costly. Special interests have persuaded state legislatures to require insurers to cover these services whether or not those buying the insurance want to pay for that coverage.[17] In our imaginary plan, however, these special interests get no voice. Only the 1,000 enrollees count. That said, traditional insurance has made a lot of arbitrary distinctions that an ideal plan need not make. For example, traditional insurance has paid for treatment of back problems by an M.D. but not a chiropractor. It has paid for mental health services provided by a psychiatrist but not a psychologist. The rationale was partly a misplaced attempt to save money, but it also reflected the physician interest in promoting insurance that pays for the services of medical doctors rather than the individual's interest in protection against catastrophic costs.

The casualty model of insurance helps solve this problem. Health plans could control costs and give patients greater freedom to choose among competing providers at the same time. Coupled with the idea that people should pay their full cost when entering a health plan and that medical consumption decisions not arising from a risky event should be paid by the individual from an MSA, our ideal health plan should make coverage decisions easier.

Terms of Exit

Recall that insurance contracts in the individual market are almost always guaranteed to be renewable. Once in an insurance pool people are entitled to remain there indefinitely and pay the same premiums others pay, regardless of changes in their health status. That commitment is completely one-sided, however. The insurer makes an indefinite commitment to the members, but the members are free to leave the pool at any time.

This one-way commitment creates the following problem. New insurance pools attract mainly healthy people because insurers tend to deny coverage to persons who are already sick or to attach exclusions and riders limiting these individuals' coverage (a process known as *medical underwriting*). As time passes and some enrollees get sick, the premium paid by all must be increased to cover the cost of their care. Thus mature insurance pools will almost always charge higher premiums than young pools. This gives healthy people an incentive to leave the mature pool. By switching to a young pool, healthy people can escape high premiums. But this option is not open to the sick members of the mature pool. If they try to switch, the new pool will either deny them coverage or charge them a higher premium because of their medical condition. As a result it is not unusual in the individual market to find an insurer providing the same coverage to various pools but charging vastly different premiums, depending on the age of the pool. Members of a mature pool, for example, might pay $1,000 a month or more for their coverage, whereas entrants into a young pool might pay only a few hundred dollars. Clearly, these are not the features of an ideal insurance system.

A possible solution is to make the long-term commitment apply both ways. In return for an indefinite commitment on the part of the insurer, members would commit to the pool for a period of three, four, or five years. This does not mean that people would remain stuck in a plan they wished to leave. It does mean that leaving the pool would require the consent of the pool. For example, if a healthy member left high-cost plan A to join low-cost plan B, B would compensate A for its loss. Conversely, if a sick member left A to join B, A would compensate B to take the member and pay for the higher expected cost of care. In this model, recontracting is always possible but *only the type of recontracting that leaves everybody better off.*[18]

Moreover, in the ideal system described here, people would have far less reason to switch insurers because their pool would be providing mainly financial (insurance) services rather than health care. A member would not need to switch from plan A to plan B to see a particular doctor or gain a higher quality of care.

CAN MARKETS DEVELOP IDEAL HEALTH INSURANCE PLANS?

The ideas outlined here are merely suggestive. And individuals are not expected to develop their own health plans. That's what competition and markets are supposed to do. Entrepreneurs are supposed to innovate and experiment to find the products people want to buy. But intrusive regulations aside, can we rely on the market to achieve the best result?

Patients as Buyers of Health Care

One objection to asking individuals to pay directly for most diagnostic and preventive services is that they would not get the lowest price or find the highest quality. But anecdotal evidence suggests that uninsured individuals, spending their own money, get as good a discount as do large buyers.[19] Even if this were not true, there is no reason why the health plan itself cannot negotiate discounts for its members even if the members spend their own money when they receive the services.

The issue of quality is a bit more difficult. But the solution is not first-dollar managed care for every service. Suppose that as part of its HMO network, Blue Cross set up primary care clinics for its members. Blue Cross asserts that these clinics deliver high-quality, cost-effective care. If the assertion is true, why limit the care to the HMO members? Why not allow anyone to enter the clinic and pay out of pocket for the same services? This is already happening in cities across the country—proving that fee-for-service payment and cost-effective care are not inconsistent, provided incentives are not distorted in other ways. There is no reason why a health plan should object to patients directly contracting for their health care as long as the plan's own costs do not go up.

Centers of Excellence and Focused Factories

Can there be a workable market for expensive, curative services—with patients paying the bill? In some places there already is. Managed care advocates often point to the Mayo Clinic as an example of cost-effective medicine. They ignore the fact that most of Mayo's customers are fee-for-service patients. What Harvard University professor Regina Herzlinger calls *focused factories,* health care business which provide highly efficient, specialized care, are becoming a reality.[20] They deliver lower prices, lower mortality rates, shorter stays, and higher patient satisfaction. For example, the Johns Hopkins Breast Center is a focused factory for mastectomies. The Dartmouth-Hitchcock Medical Center in Lebanon, New Hampshire, is a focused factory for heart surgery. The Pediatrix Medical Group, which manages neonatal units and provides pediatric services in twenty-one states, is another example.[21] Focused factories also are cropping up around the country to provide cancer, gynecological, and orthopedic services. One spectacular success story is that of Bernard Salick, a physician and kidney specialist who has become a millionaire by pioneering a national chain of round-the-clock cancer clinics.[22]

Patients on their own can already take advantage of these emerging markets. Indeed, some focused factories are advertising directly to patients. In a *New York Times Magazine* advertisement, for example, Memorial Sloan-Kettering Cancer

Center boasted "the best cancer care anywhere" and described how its specialists saved a life after doctors at other hospitals had given up hope.[23]

Role of Employers

Some believe that in the absence of federal tax law, employers would never have become involved in their employees' health insurance. Yet there are two reasons offered why employers might become involved even with neutral government policies. One is the economies of group buying. Signing one contract for all employees involves less overhead than having agents sell individual insurance household by household. There may be some merit to this argument, but it is a rationale exaggerated by people who focus only on the first-year cost. Under current practice, employer group plans are renegotiated *every year,* whereas individuals usually stay in their plans for several years. Taking into account all costs over several years, the difference in cost between the two approaches is much less. This presumably is why employers rarely get involved in their employees' purchase of automobile or homeowners insurance and play only a minor role in the purchase of life insurance.

A second reason for employers' involvement relates to the adverse selection problem. Medical underwriting—attempting to determine everyone's health status at the point of entry into a plan—is costly. Employer-sponsored group insurance avoids this cost by enrolling everyone—the sick as well as the healthy—at once. Further, group contracts are written in ways that discourage individuals from gaming the system by remaining out of the pool while they are healthy and then joining the pool once they get sick. In the typical arrangement the employer pays a large share of the premium, so employees do not save much by remaining uninsured. In addition, new employees have to make the decision to join the pool on a certain date. Thus the timing of the decision to insure does not coincide with the timing of illness.

Having acknowledged that there may be good reasons for employers to play a role independent of government policies designed to encourage them to do so, let us also acknowledge that the appropriate role of the employer does not have to be settled by armchair theorists. We can let the market decide. Increasingly, employers are moving away from a defined benefit approach and toward a defined contribution approach. This means that employers make a commitment of a certain dollar amount to each employee, and employees then make their own insurance choices. Remember, this is the approach taken by the federal government for its employees, by most state and local governments for their employees, and by some large private employers. Potentially, this approach can minimize the role of the employer in a way that allows employees to reap the economies of group purchase and avoid the costs of medical underwriting yet also acquire personal, portable individual coverage.

CONCLUSION: THE BENEFITS OF IDEAL HEALTH INSURANCE

Three features of ideal health insurance would make it especially superior to the health insurance arrangements that prevail today.

Ideal Health Insurance Is Patient Centered

A large portion of our health care dollars would be placed in accounts that we would individually own and control. Patients would pay for the vast majority of medical services from these accounts, and the doctors treating them would be free to act as agents for their patients, rather than as agents for third-party payers. Because patients would be spending their own money when they enter the medical marketplace, physicians would be encouraged to become financial advisers as well as health advisers. Doctors would compete not only on the basis of quality but on the basis of value for money.

Ideal health insurance also would be patient centered in the treatment of expensive conditions. Rather than have a third party pay every medical bill, insurers would make regular deposits to the MSAs of patients with chronic conditions, leaving them free to choose among competing focused factories for ongoing treatment. Rather than have a third party dictate terms and conditions for the delivery of expensive acute care, patients would be able to draw on a fixed sum of money and get their health needs met at a center of excellence or a focused factory of their own choosing.

Ideal Health Insurance Allows Insurers to Specialize in the Business of Insurance

One of the consequences of the managed care revolution is that insurers have been turned into providers of care. That is, the entity that pays our medical bills is the same entity that delivers our medical care. This development has had three negative consequences.

First, when the business of insurance and the business of health care are merged, health plans have perverse incentives to deny care. The rash of news stories reporting on the tragic consequences of underprovision of care are testimony to what can go wrong.

Second, when the choice of insurer is also effectively a choice of provider networks, consumers are forced to make decisions that are humanly impossible. Ideally, one should not have to choose a cardiologist until one has a heart problem. One should not have to choose an oncologist until one gets cancer. But in today's market, when you choose your insurer you are at the same time choosing your heart specialist and your cancer specialist, whether you are aware of it or not.

Third, the managed care revolution has delegated to those on the buyers' side of the market (insurers) the responsibility of forcing those on the sellers' side of the market (doctors, hospital administrators, and the like) to deliver care efficiently. In no other market that I know of do we depend on buyers to tell sellers how to efficiently produce their product. Undoubtedly there are good reasons why other markets are not organized this way.

Ideal health insurance, in contrast, allows insurers to specialize in what they do best: the management of risk. The supply side of the market would be encouraged to organize into focused factories and adopt other efficient techniques in order to produce high quality for low cost. The market would still be free to combine insurance and health care delivery where the combination makes sense. It may turn out that for such specialized services as cancer care, efficiency warrants specialized insurance products. Ideal health insurance would allow those market developments by providing a mechanism for people to leave one insurance pool and join another (without extra cost) when their health condition changes.

Ideal Health Insurance Is Improved by the Free Flow of Information

Under the current system consumer information is a threat to the stability and peace of mind of typical HMO personnel. The more patients learn, the more they are likely to demand. Under ideal health insurance, in contrast, accurate consumer information is a positive. The reason is that the insurer and the insured are on the same team, with a similar interest and objective—acquiring good value in a competitive market.

Needless to say, the changes outlined here will require appropriate changes in public policy. Of these, three are particularly important.[24]

First, federal tax law must create a level playing field for third-party insurance and individual self-insurance through medical savings accounts. Under current law, only employer payments to third parties are excluded from the employee's taxable income. This is a generous subsidy that can cut the aftertax cost of health insurance in half. Individual preference and market competition, not the peculiarities of the tax law, should determine the appropriate division.

Second, federal tax law must create a level playing field for employer purchase and individual purchase of health insurance. Although employers can purchase employee health insurance with before-tax dollars, people who purchase their own insurance get virtually no tax relief and must pay with aftertax dollars. An exception to this generalization is the self-employed, who get partial tax relief. Beginning in 2003, it will be 100% deductible for the self-employed. Employers may have an important role to play in helping people obtain health insurance, but this role should be determined by the marketplace—not by tax law.

A third important change needs to be implemented at the state level. Many employers would like to move to a defined contribution approach to employee health insurance. Instead of herding all their employees into a single health plan, these employers would like to allow their employees to make their own choices. As a result employees could enter a health insurance pool and stay there—taking their insurance coverage with them as they travel from job to job. Personal and portable health insurance is an idea whose time has come. Yet virtually every state has made this approach (technically known as *list billing*) either illegal or prohibitively impractical.

These changes will not solve our most important health insurance problems. Instead, they will create a legal environment in which individuals, their employers, and their insurers—pursuing their own interests—will create the needed institutions.

Notes

1. Levit, K. R., and others. "National Health Expenditures in 1997: More Slow Growth." *Health Affairs,* Nov.–Dec. 1998, *17,* 99–110; Health Care Financing Administration. *Highlights of National Health Expenditures, 1997.* [www.hcfa.gov/stats/nhe-oact/tables/tablist.htm], Sept. 2003.

2. Goodman, J. C., and Musgrave, G. L. *Patient Power: Solving America's Health Care Crisis.* Washington, D.C.: Cato Institute, 1992, p. 79.

3. Rottenberg, S. "Unintended Consequences: The Probable Effects of Mandated Medical Insurance." *Regulation,* Summer 1990, *13,* 27–28.

4. For the perverse incentives created when competing health plans are forced to charge premiums that do not reflect enrollees' expected costs, see Goodman, J. C., Pauly, M. V., and Porter, P. "The Economics of Managed Competition." Unpublished manuscript, available from National Center for Policy Analysis, 12655 N. Central Expressway, Suite 720, Dallas, TX 75243.

5. Manning, W. G., and Marquis, M. S. "Health Insurance: The Tradeoff Between Risk Pooling and Moral Hazard." *Journal of Health Economics,* Oct. 1, 1996, *15,* 609–639.

6. Tengs, T. O., and others. "Five-Hundred Life-Saving Interventions and Their Cost-Effectiveness." *Risk Analysis,* 1995, *15*(3), 369–390; Eddy, D. M. (ed.). *Common Screening Tests.* Philadelphia: American College of Physicians, 1991.

7. Tengs, "Five-Hundred Life-Saving Interventions . . .," p. 379.

8. Bond, M. T. "The Financial Impact of Medical Savings Account Plans." *Business Horizons,* Jan. 2001, pp. 77–83; see also Goodman, J. C. "Medical Savings

Accounts: The Private Sector Already Has Them." Brief Analysis No. 105. Dallas, Tex.: National Center for Policy Analysis, Apr. 20, 1994.

9. See Matthews, M. "Medical Savings Account Legislation: The Good, the Bad and the Ugly." Brief Analysis No. 211. Dallas, Tex.: National Center for Policy Analysis, Aug. 19, 1996.

10. Letter from Alain Enthoven to Governor Pete Wilson and others, Jan. 6, 1998. [http://chpps.berkeley.edu/publications/MCRF_Report_Vol_2.pdf]

11. Matisonn, S. "Medical Savings Accounts in South Africa." Policy Report No. 234. Dallas, Tex.: National Center for Policy Analysis, June 2000.

12. A mandatory point-of-service option when combined with a requirement to reimburse at the same rates in and out of network can raise the cost of health insurance by as much as 11.3 percent, according to the estimates of Milliman and Robertson for the National Center for Policy Analysis. See Matthews, M. "Can We Afford Consumer Protection? An Analysis of the PARCA Bill." Brief Analysis No. 249. Dallas, Tex.: National Center for Policy Analysis, Nov. 24, 1997.

13. Herzlinger, R. E. *Market-Driven Health Care: Who Wins, Who Loses in the Transformation of America's Largest Service Industry.* Reading, Mass.: Addison-Wesley, 1997, p. 173.

14. For a survey of the efficacy of self-monitoring see Faas, A., Schellevis, F. G., and Van Eijk, J. T. "The Efficacy of Self-Monitoring of Blood Glucose in NIDDM Subjects: A Criteria-Based Literature Review." *Diabetes Care,* 1997, *20*(9), 1482–1486.

15. See Goodman and Musgrave, *Patient Power,* chap. 5.

16. Although for the terminally ill, this is an idea worth considering.

17. See Jensen, G. A., and Morrisey, M. A. "Mandated Benefit Laws and Employer-Sponsored Health Insurance." Washington, D.C.: Health Insurance Association of America, Jan. 1999.

18. What is envisioned here is a market for individual patients. For those who doubt that such a market could develop, recall that the same objection was once raised against a reinsurance market for residential housing.

19. The reason is that sellers have an incentive to charge marginal cost when no third party is involved.

20. Herzlinger, *Market-Driven Health Care.*

21. Meyer, H. "Are You Ready for the Competition?" *Hospitals and Health Networks,* Apr. 5, 1998, *72,* 25–30.

22. Bianco, A. "Bernie Salick's Business in Cancer." *Business Week,* June 22, 1998, pp. 76–77.

23. "I Wasn't Ready to Die. Thank God Somebody Wasn't Ready to Let Me." *New York Times Magazine,* May 3, 1998, p. 60.

24. For a fuller discussion, see Goodman, J. C., and Matthews, M. "Reforming the U.S. Health Care System." Policy Backgrounder No. 149. Dallas, Tex.: National Center for Policy Analysis, Apr. 26, 1999; Pauly, M. V., and Goodman, J. C. "Incremental Steps Toward Health System Reform." *Health Affairs,* Spring 1995, pp. 125–139; Goodman and Musgrave, *Patient Power,* chap. 20.

CHAPTER TWELVE

Risk Adjustment

An Overview and Three Case Studies

Lisa I. Iezzoni

On average, sicker people cost more to treat and do less well than their healthier counterparts. From a health policy perspective this virtual truism would not matter if people were randomly assigned to health care providers and insurance plans. But they are not. Instead, finding a source of care is affected by many factors, ranging from specific health concerns to financial considerations to preferences and expectations for health care services.

Not surprisingly, therefore, the mix of persons treated by different providers and plans varies. These differences have consequences. Most important for quality measurement, persons with complex illnesses, multiple coexisting diseases, or other significant risk factors will generally develop more complications and have worse outcomes, even with excellent care, than will healthier individuals. Similarly, providers and health insurers with sicker patients will experience higher costs.

Also not surprisingly, patients' outcomes and costs of care vary, sometimes widely, across doctors, hospitals, and health plans. Many diverse patient attributes affect risks for different outcomes, as suggested by the following list:

Potential Risk Factors

- Age
- Sex
- Race and ethnicity

- Acute physiological status or clinical stability
- Principal diagnosis (case mix)
- Severity of principal diagnosis
- Extent and severity of coexisting diseases (comorbidities)
- Physical functional status
- Psychological, cognitive, and psychosocial functioning
- Cultural and socioeconomic attributes and behaviors
- Health status and quality of life
- Attitudes, expectations, and preferences for outcomes

In general, risk adjustment aims to account for differences in these clinical and other characteristics that people bring to their health care encounters.[1] The specific purpose of risk adjustment and the relevant risk factors vary, however, depending on the context—that is, whether one is assessing quality or determining payment levels.

RISK OF WHAT?

The phrase *risk adjustment* is meaningless without first answering the question, risk of what? Replies fall broadly into two camps: potential quality indicators (that is, *outcomes of care,* such as deaths, iatrogenic complications, physical functioning, satisfaction with services) and measures of resource consumption (for example, costs of care). For clarity, time frames are also required—risk of what *over how long?* For example, is one interested in deaths within thirty days or within ninety days of hospital admission? Does one want to know the costs for a single hospitalization or for a year of care?

For quality measurement the goal of risk adjustment is to control for intrinsic, patient-related factors when comparing outcomes across providers or health plans, thus leaving residual differences in outcomes to suggest relative quality.[2] The underlying assumption is that outcomes result from a complex mix of factors:

Patient Outcomes = Effectiveness of Treatments + Patient Risk Factors Affecting Responses to Treatment + Quality of Care + Random Chance

Controlling for risk begins to isolate quality differences. Risk adjustment levels the playing field, or to change the metaphor, it facilitates comparisons of apples with apples. Therefore, for example, New York State's annual *report card* on hospital- and surgeon-specific death rates for coronary artery bypass graft

(CABG) surgery explicitly adjusts for such risk factors as patients' heart function (left ventricular ejection fraction), extent of coronary artery disease (> 90 percent narrowing of the left main coronary artery), coexisting illnesses (for example, diabetes mellitus), and whether the patient has had a prior CABG.[3]

For determining payment levels or evaluating costs, risk adjustment similarly accounts for patient factors affecting use of health services.[4] The classic risk adjuster for payment is diagnosis related groups (DRGs), over 500 categories grouping diagnoses or procedures that are reasonably clinically homogeneous and exhibit similar hospital costs. In 1983, Medicare's prospective payment system began paying hospitals a bundled payment determined by the DRG, rather than itemized fees for each individual inpatient service.[5] A shorthand measure of a hospital's risk in terms of the costliness of its patient population is the case mix index (CMI), the average relative payment weight of its patients' DRGs.

Perceptions of whether one patient is sicker than another often differ across clinical and cost perspectives. For example, consider these two patients:

Two Patients with Lung Cancer

Mr. A: Small, isolated pulmonary nodule ("spot") found on routine chest x ray. No symptoms or comorbid illnesses; former smoker. Needle biopsy of lung determines that nodule is cancer (adenocarcinoma). Blood tests find no evidence of liver involvement. Computed tomography of lungs and upper abdomen finds no local spread of tumor. Mediastinoscopy with lymph node sampling finds no metastases. Lung segment containing tumor surgically removed. Good chance of surgical cure.

Mr. B: Lung cancer diagnosed several years previously. Cancer now metastatic to liver and bones. Desires "comfort measures only" (that is, no testing or active therapeutic interventions); "do not resuscitate" order signed by physician. Asks to go home with hospice support. Placed on intravenous morphine drip to control pain.

Mr. A's technologically intensive workup and operation for lung cancer are costly, but the tumor is small and easily removed; Mr. A has a good chance of surgical cure. In contrast, with widely metastatic disease, Mr. B requests not to be resuscitated, desiring "comfort measures only." Therefore even routine blood tests are eliminated, and Mr. B is kept comfortable in the least intensive setting possible. Mr. A generates high costs but with low likelihood of imminent death, whereas Mr. B incurs relatively lower costs but is likely to die soon.

Thus risk factors that predict one outcome (for example, imminent death) may not predict another outcome (for example, costs) in the same way. For example, when refining DRGs to improve their sensitivity to severity of illness, researchers found that medical inpatients dying within two days of admission generated relatively low costs.[6] In addition, risk adjustment methods for one quality or cost measure may not work for another. For instance, New York's risk adjustment method for CABG mortality is irrelevant for examining obstetrical complications; DRGs are suitable for acute-care hospital payments but inappropriate for reimbursing rehabilitation hospitals or setting capitation levels. Despite pressing health policy demands for risk adjustment, few methods have gained widespread acceptance.

NEED FOR DATA

Inadequate information about patients' risk factors is the single largest impediment to risk adjustment. Data determine the clinical credibility, validity, reliability, and accuracy of risk adjustment. Data thus dictate the scope and strength of inferences that can be drawn from risk-adjusted outcomes—that is, whether results are believable. In addition, for widespread quality measurement or setting payment levels for individuals, the data must be readily available, computer readable, and relatively inexpensive to obtain.

Today three major data sources exist:

- *Administrative data:* large, computerized data files generally compiled in administering health care services and containing such information as claims for hospitalizations or encounter records for office visits
- *Medical record information:* data extracted manually, usually retrospectively, from paper or automated medical records
- *Patient-derived data:* information collected directly from patients through interviews or questionnaires

Boundaries among these three sources are blurring considerably. Patients can now enter data about their health and personal risk factors at computer terminals in doctors' offices or over the Internet in their homes; clinical data, formerly confined to paper records, is increasingly flowing electronically; routine administrative transmissions for each health care encounter will contain more clinical information. Although completely paperless medical records remain unlikely, the volume of health care data available in electronic form is growing significantly. Nevertheless, today the three major data sources remain largely distinct, and each has pros and cons.[7]

Administrative Databases

Administrative data files contain information used to pay and adjudicate claims or meet other administrative requirements. Beyond patients' age, sex, and sometimes race or ethnicity, administrative files include diagnoses coded using the World Health Organization's *International Classification of Diseases, Ninth Revision, Clinical Modification* (ICD-9-CM) and procedures coded in various ways (for example, ICD-9-CM and the American Medical Association's *Current Procedural Terminology*). Administrative data are readily available, inexpensive to acquire, computer readable, and they typically encompass either entire populations within regions or large, well-defined segments of populations (for example, persons covered by specific insurers).

Virtually by definition, administrative data contain little of the clinical information especially essential for quality measurement. Nonetheless, because of their ready availability, they have frequently been used for quality measurement. For example, beginning in the mid-1980s Medicare started using its voluminous claims files to examine hospital mortality rates for its beneficiaries. Through Freedom of Information Act requests, the press gained access to these figures, and their release soon became an annual event.

Over time, Medicare's risk adjustment methods have improved. For instance, an advantage of Medicare data is the ability to link information longitudinally at the patient level. Medicare's later risk adjustment methods used information on patients' prior hospitalization experiences, as well as such risk factors as age, sex, and major chronic comorbid illness.[8] However, questions lingered about what the data really meant, and although initial data releases generated avid press attention, later publications sparked little interest. The public seemingly ignored this information when choosing hospitals.[9] In June 1993, newly appointed Medicare administrator Bruce Vladeck discontinued publication of the hospital mortality reports, blaming inadequate risk adjustment for unfairly penalizing inner-city public facilities, which year after year were flagged as egregious outliers.[10] When asked if he believed the data were valid for other institutions, Vladeck responded, "My answer is quite literally that we don't know."[11]

Beyond reservations about the clinical content of data, questions also inevitably arise about whether financial motivations compromise the accuracy of administrative data. For example, soon after implementation of DRG-based payment, the possibility of *DRG creep*—"a deliberate and systematic shift in a hospital's reported case mix in order to improve reimbursement"[12]—raised suspicions about the accuracy of hospital-reported diagnosis codes. New words entered the diagnosis-coding vocabulary, such as *optimization* and *maximization*. Some hospitals moved medical record departments from general administration to financial divisions.

Medical Records

In contrast, medical records indisputably offer rich information, including not only text notes by clinicians but also the laboratory, radiology, and diagnostic test reports that provide the foundations for clinical decision making. Thus these data carry immediate clinical credibility. However, well-known differences in practice patterns across providers could affect perceptions of risk. In addition, certain types of information, such as functional status, are poorly documented in medical records.[13] If a clinical attribute is not measured or documented, it cannot contribute to patients' severity ratings.

An oncologist from Pennsylvania, where all hospitals have been required to report MedisGroups severity information, recounted a story epitomizing this problem.[14] MedisGroups, a commercial product, had rated severity using extensive key clinical findings abstracted from medical records.[15] Shortly before releasing this information to local news media, state officials warned the oncologist's hospital that its MedisGroups severity-adjusted mortality rates for cancer patients were much higher than expected. Numerous deaths among patients with the lowest severity scores (0 or 1) raised particular concerns. When the oncologist investigated, he found that these deaths had occurred among patients like Mr. B (described earlier), who desired "comfort measures only." Even routine blood drawing for serum chemistry and blood count testing was suspended. As a result no test values were available to indicate these patients' true severity.

A related issue is whether or not results from specific tests or sophisticated technologies are designated risk factors. Using such findings could potentially bias risk estimates against hospitals with lesser technological capabilities or restrained test-ordering behaviors. Finally, just as DRG-based payment precipitated ICD-9-CM code creep, publication of risk-adjusted report cards could shift medical record documentation. Green and Wintfeld analyzed the prevalence of reported risk factors around public releases of New York's CABG mortality data.[16] They found that the rates of CABG risk factors—chronic obstructive pulmonary disease, unstable angina, and low cardiac ejection fraction—reported by providers increased sharply in the first quarter of 1990, immediately following publication of the first mortality report. New York State officials instituted chart audits to monitor this practice.[17]

Patient Reports

Patients' views are increasingly valued. Not only are patient-reported observations used as outcome measures (for example, self-reported health status) but patient-generated information also conveys important risk factors. Sometimes the complexities of instituting clinically credible risk adjustment prove so daunting that obtaining information directly from patients seems much simpler. For example, in 1995, the Massachusetts Health Quality Partnership (MHQP) debated which quality measures to adopt for its new initiative comparing hospital performance, immediately dismissing administrative data-based approaches as insufficient. Initial plans to compare mortality rates following selected hospital admissions (for example, for heart attack) collapsed because of the conceptual and logistical complexities of risk adjustment. MHQP decided to start by comparing patients' experiences and satisfaction with care, carrying out risk adjusting by using self-reported overall health status. Other efforts have examined the value of self-reported health status for adjusting capitation levels.[18]

Obtaining information directly from patients, however, inevitably generates a question: how good are patients' reports? Are patient-generated data the only authentic data about patients' perceptions, functioning, health status, and quality of life? Several studies have compared patients' reports to outside "gold standard" measures of more "objective" indicators (for example, hypertension, diabetes, smoking history), with mixed results.[19] Gathering this information raises numerous logistical concerns as well. Some patients are physically or cognitively unable to respond. Cross-cultural differences in attitudes toward health, symptoms, and disease are crucial considerations in applying or translating surveys for use across cultural or linguistic subpopulations. Although mailed questionnaires are indisputably cheaper than interviews, functional illiteracy complicates matters, potentially biasing results.[20]

THREE CASE STUDIES

Numerous initiatives nationwide have instituted risk adjustment, for either quality measurement or setting capitated payment levels. Three examples exemplify the complexities and pitfalls of these activities, especially difficulties arising from inadequate data sources:

- The California Hospital Outcomes Project arose amid consternation over the cost of data for risk adjustment, but highlights the downside of relying on administrative data.

- The Cleveland Health Quality Choice (CHQC) program, a voluntary coalition of businesses, hospitals, and physicians, originally was willing to pay for clinically credible risk adjustment but that willingness foundered when CHQC's most prestigious member refused to play, arguing that its patients were sicker.

- The 1997 Balanced Budget Act required Medicare to adjust capitation payments for health status, but owing to inadequate data, Medicare's strategy has an ironic twist: to increase payments, capitated plans—renowned for trying to keep their members out of hospitals—must now hospitalize those members.

California

In 1989, representatives of Pennsylvania-based Hershey Foods enthusiastically recommended the MedisGroups initiative to California's business community. As mentioned previously, for several years, Pennsylvania hospitals had abstracted MedisGroups severity information from medical records, which state officials then used to generate report cards containing risk-adjusted mortality and morbidity rates by facility. Hershey Foods officials used these reports in negotiating with local hospitals; they credited this information with saving Hershey millions of dollars while improving quality of care for their employees. Excited by these testimonials, in March 1990 California business leaders asked the state legislature to pass a bill that would require state officials to either select a method for evaluating hospital quality by a specified date or adopt Pennsylvania's approach.

The California Association of Hospitals and Health Systems disagreed vigorously. Its representatives argued that the implications of implementing MedisGroups risk adjustment were poorly understood, and they projected over $61 million in annual costs for data gathering and administrative expenses. California's legislature adjourned before completing debate over this bill, but the 1991 proposal did not mention Pennsylvania's methodology. The mandate that was eventually passed reflected two concerns: first, that collecting additional data directly from medical records was prohibitively expensive and inadequately justified, and second, that no existing risk-adjustment method sold by vendors was sufficiently clinically and statistically rigorous. Thus Assembly Bill 524, enacted in 1991, required California state officials to create homegrown risk-adjusted outcome measures, using the state's existing administrative database (that is, computerized hospital discharge abstracts from acute-care facilities).

Investigators from the University of California led initial development of the risk-adjustment models, assisted by state coding experts, epidemiologists, and local physicians.[21] California's data benefited from containing twenty-five diagnosis and twenty-five procedure coding slots, compared to the five diagnosis and three procedure slots then typical of many other state databases. The first California Hospital Outcomes Project report, published in December 1993,[22] showed hospitals' death rates for acute myocardial infarction (AMI) and rates of complications and unusually long hospitalizations following back surgery (cervical and lumbar disk excisions). Risk adjustment included demographic characteristics and ICD-9-CM codes representing chronic illnesses and complications of the principal diagnosis. Because of the limitations of coded diagnoses (they give no indication whether secondary diagnoses were present prior to admission), the report presented two models—a conservative model including only conditions that should be preexisting and a comprehensive model containing all potential risk factors.

California physicians, especially, raised questions about the accuracy and completeness of the data, particularly the coding of postoperative complications for diskectomy cases.[23] Because of such questions and concerns about inappropriately harming hospitals with reasonable outcomes, the first report did not identify hospitals with higher than expected rates of poor outcomes. Instead, by comparing their actual outcomes with predicted, risk-adjusted outcomes, hospitals were sorted into two groups: "significantly better than expected" and "not significantly better than expected." The report used statistically conservative cutoffs to make these assignments.

Some of California's most prestigious hospitals fared poorly. One reason was that these hospitals had aggressively coded surgical complications to boost their

DRG-based payments[24]—complications sometimes direct patients to the better-paid of paired DRGs. Recurrent concerns about data quality prompted the state to pursue a novel and very public examination of data accuracy. California officials reabstracted medical records of 974 patients with AMI to determine the accuracy of coded diagnoses, especially conditions used in risk adjustment. They sampled cases in three hospital strata—risk-adjusted AMI mortality better than expected, neither better nor worse, and worse than expected.[25] They found wide variations in coding accuracy across hospitals. Rates of uncoded risk factors ranged from 45 to 87 percent across facilities: 65 percent of discharge abstracts were missing at least one clinical risk factor, and 31 percent were missing two. Hospitals in the three mortality categories demonstrated similar rates of missing risk factors.

More troubling were findings of "unsupported risk factors"—coded conditions without adequate confirmatory evidence in the medical record. Almost 32 percent of discharge abstracts contained at least one unsupported risk factor. Low-mortality category hospitals overcoded much more than did intermediate- or high-mortality hospitals (37 percent versus 29 percent). Overcoding rates ranged from 10 percent at one high-mortality category hospital to 74 percent at a low-mortality facility. Variation in coding accuracy explained part of the differences between hospitals with high and low mortality performance. By overcoding, hospitals made their patients look sicker, so lower than expected mortality rates were not surprising. Overcoding would make predicted mortality rates artificially high, lowering the ratio of observed rates to predicted rates.

The second California Hospital Outcomes Project report was released in May 1996, and contained information on risk-adjusted in-hospital death rates within thirty days of admission for AMI.[26] The report excluded deaths after thirty days of in-hospital care because these deaths might reflect social problems or unrelated conditions. It classed hospitals into three categories, including significantly better than expected and worse than expected. The report no longer used conditions identified as poorly or questionably coded in the risk-adjustment model. California's effort to validate its data source is unique.

Cleveland

In 1989, Cleveland business leaders gave local health care providers an ultimatum. Health care costs had escalated incessantly, with no corresponding evidence about quality. "Either you quantify quality," business leaders in effect asserted, "or we shall do it ourselves." The Cleveland Health Quality Choice (CHQC) program resulted, the product of a voluntary coalition including Cleveland Tomorrow (an association of the chief executive officers of fifty major, local businesses), the Greater Cleveland Hospital Association, the Health Action Council (an association of health care purchasers), the Academy of Medicine, and the Council of Smaller Enterprises. The coalition members' initial challenge was to find fair and reliable measures that both business leaders and providers could support and find useful.

After much discussion they focused on three areas: observed versus expected intensive care unit (ICU) death rates; in-hospital deaths and prolonged hospitalizations in the areas of general medical, surgical, and obstetrical care; and patient satisfaction. The clinicians and hospitals insisted on clinical credibility for the patient outcome measures, and they were willing to pay for it—the use of administrative data was immediately dismissed. To examine ICU outcomes, CHQC contracted with APACHE Medical Systems, vendor of the Acute Physiology and Chronic Health Evaluation (APACHE III) risk adjustment methodology. This method relies on vital signs, routine ICU test results, and specified diagnoses to rate patients' risks of in-hospital death.[27] APACHE was a well-accepted standard in the ICU field. Questions arose, however, about appropriate risk adjustment for the medical, surgical, and obstetrical outcomes. With world-renowned institutions such as the Cleveland Clinic among their ranks, clinicians reacted critically to most options. Although CHQC representatives first considered existing severity measures, including MedisGroups, they finally decided to develop their own.

Working with Chicago-based physician consultant Michael Pine, M.D., medical and business advisory groups developed medical record review–based severity measures for each condition to be studied. Cleveland officials believed that this local input, especially from the medical community, was critical to ensuring acceptance of CHQC's findings as clinically credible. Furthermore, they insisted on consensus on various decisions, prolonging the development process and increasing its expense. The resultant risk adjustment method, CHOICE (Cleveland Hospital Outcomes Indicators of Care Evaluations), relied on dozens of condition-specific clinical variables abstracted from medical records.

Initial CHQC data were released privately to hospitals. Anecdotal evidence suggested that this helped some hospitals identify problem areas and improve patient care procedures. The first public CHQC report, *The Cleveland-Area Hospital Quality Measurement and Patient Satisfaction Report*, was released in April 1993. The one hundred–page report contained 261 measurements from twenty-nine Cleveland hospitals. By January 1995, the fourth Cleveland hospital outcomes report was able to display three-year trends. Mortality for selected medical diagnoses at the twenty-nine participating hospitals had fallen from 7.85 patients per 100 in 1991 to 7.04 patients in 1993, but as the report's authors acknowledged, many factors could explain that drop (for example, changes in discharge practices).

By 1996, however, simmering disagreements about the risk adjustment methods finally boiled over, with public assertions by the Cleveland Clinic that the methods were hopelessly flawed. The clinic also argued that the $2 million annual price tag for gathering the data was too high. Since the outset Cleveland

Clinic officials had protested that the clinic's patient population had special characteristics ignored by the CHOICE measures. For example, a Cleveland Clinic Foundation cardiologist argued that "[at] one point, the Cleveland Clinic received poor ratings in heart failure, even though we have very sick patients who receive left ventricular assist devices and heart transplants, and most of the other hospitals did not even determine the patients' ejection fraction. With the garbage that goes into the model for risk adjustment, how can outcomes be compared in a meaningful fashion?"[28] The Cleveland Clinic moved to suspend CHQC until it could be substantially revised. However, several important representatives of other major academic institutions backed CHQC. In addition, the *Plain Dealer,* Cleveland's premier newspaper, strongly backed CHQC in influential editorials. By fall the Cleveland Clinic had backed down and remained, tentatively, in the program.

Meanwhile, also in 1996, the Health Action Council of Northeast Ohio, comprising 140 large businesses, announced that CHQC had published enough longitudinal information on hospital performance to guide contracting decisions. The council proposed establishing a limited purchasing program that would contract directly with "centers of excellence," such as heart surgery or joint replacements programs, at selected hospitals. The council sent invitations to apply for direct contracting to only a handful of hospitals participating in CHQC, stipulating that to continue to qualify for the contracts, hospitals must remain in the CHQC program.[29] The businesses intended that purchasing decisions be guided not only by price but also by quality.

But this effort never took root, and the Cleveland Clinic's protestations persisted. Finally, on February 26, 1999, the CHQC announced that it would disband in July because nine Cleveland Clinic Health System hospitals (a third of the participating institutions) refused to continue submitting their data voluntarily. In writing its epitaph, the CHQC claimed credit for checking the uncontrolled cost escalation that had previously characterized Cleveland's marketplace.[30] As further justification for its withdrawal, the Cleveland Clinic noted, somewhat ironically, that the CHQC's expensive data were not being used.

Medicare's Health Status Adjustment of Capitated Payments

The 1997 Balanced Budget Act (P.L. 105-33) not only balanced the federal budget for the first time in decades but also mandated major changes in Medicare. One goal was to expand health plan choices for Medicare beneficiaries in order to control aggregate program costs through competition and risk sharing. The resulting Medicare + Choice provisions broaden health plan options, with a special emphasis on capitated managed care plans. However, questions arose about whether all beneficiaries would share equally in these choices. Would capitated plans willingly enroll potentially expensive persons—those in poor health or with disabilities?

Medicare has encouraged enrollment in capitated health plans since the early 1970s, with mixed success.[31] In 1998, about 22 percent of Medicare beneficiaries in major urban centers had capitated plans, compared to only 0.6 percent of rural residents.[32] More troubling, capitated plans appeared to enroll members who were healthier and less costly than average Medicare beneficiaries.[33] In the six months prior to their enrollment, new members of capitated plans have had 35 percent lower costs than Medicare's fee-for-service average.[34] Some plans specifically marketed to healthy persons[35] profited handsomely: Medicare overpaid capitated plans by 5 to 20 percent because of healthier members.[36]

To lessen financial incentives to seek healthy enrollees and to pay more fairly for sick and disabled people, the Balanced Budget Act required Medicare to link capitation payments to health status by January 1, 2000—that is, to risk adjust reimbursement. Although accounting for health status in setting capitation levels is laudable, quantifying risk is difficult. In determining its risk adjustment method, inadequate data wedged the Health Care Financing Administration (HCFA), renamed the Centers for Medicare and Medicaid Services (CMS) in 2001, the federal agency administering Medicare, between "a rock and a hard place."[37]

For many years HCFA had adjusted capitated Medicare payments using the adjusted average per capita cost (AAPCC) formula, accounting for residence county and for age, sex, Medicaid status, and institutional and employment status.[38] The AAPCC explained only 1 percent of health care cost variations[39] and ignored the significantly better health of capitated plan members.[40] Nevertheless, despite its inadequacies, the AAPCC used routinely available administrative information.

In contrast, risk adjustment by health status requires clinical information. Under fee-for-service plans, hospitals, physicians, and other providers submit payment claims to HCFA, reporting diagnoses and procedures. However, HCFA did not require capitated plans to submit similar *encounter* records for hospitalizations or outpatient services. Some capitated plans minimized administrative burdens on participating physicians by not requiring any reports on individual services. The Balanced Budget Act mandated new reporting requirements. As of January 1998, health plans were required to report information on all hospital discharges. (CMS anticipated requiring information on all visits and services, regardless of setting.

Thus inpatient information was the only comprehensive clinical data imminently foreseeable. Under fee-for-service payment, hospital claims including diagnoses are essential to generate Medicare DRG payments; therefore, to obtain inpatient data, health plans needed only tap into existing hospital reporting systems. Extracting data from other health care delivery settings, such as individual physicians' offices and outpatient clinics, would require fundamental and costly changes in electronic information systems for both plans and providers. Health plans also pleaded burdens caused by readying computers for Y2K compliance. Recognizing these impediments, HCFA indicated that outpatient visit reports would not be required until sometime after October 1, 1999.[41] The renamed CMS's final plan required insurers to report only a limited set of diagnoses.

The data-processing constraints of capitated health plans may limit the clinical content of even the hospitalization records. For example, some plans capture only one inpatient diagnosis code rather than multiple diagnoses. Therefore, HCFA proposed risk adjusting based on a single inpatient diagnosis, using the principal in-patient diagnostic cost groups (PIP-DCGs) method.[42]

HCFA's PIP-DCG method involves eighty-six diagnostic groups defined by ICD-9-CM diagnosis codes—such as acute myocardial infarction, bacterial pneumonia, and breast cancer—that represent clinically significant disease, often require hospitalization, and predict higher future medical costs. Using fee-for-service data from hospitalizations of Medicare beneficiaries during 1995, each diagnostic group was assigned to one of ten PIP-DCGs, with all the groups in each PIP-DCG having roughly comparable predicted costs.[43] One to seventeen diagnostic groups went into each PIP-DCG; thus most PIP-DCGs are clinically heterogeneous. For example, one PIP-DCG encompasses nine diagnostic groups that include liver cirrhosis, congestive heart failure, and lung cancer; despite this clinical heterogeneity all nine groups generate similar future costs.

The PIP-DCG method uses an additive approach to set capitated payment levels. First, each age and sex category generates its own payment amount. For example, capitated plans would receive annual base payments of $2,439 for women aged sixty-five to sixty-nine years and $5,592 for women aged eighty-five to eighty-nine years. For hospitalized persons, principal diagnoses are first assigned to diagnostic groups, then to PIP-DCGs. Persons with multiple hospitalizations are assigned to the single highest PIP-DCG generated by their principal diagnoses. Each PIP-DCG adds a specific dollar amount to the annual payment based on age and sex. For example, the PIP-DCG described in the prior paragraph adds $12,883 to the annual base payment; a PIP-DCG that contains a single diagnostic group (metastatic cancer) adds $21,881.

PIP-DCGs predictions come closer to actual costs than do predictions based on the AAPCC formula and would therefore pay health plans more fairly for members hospitalized for these conditions.[44] Although the AAPCC explains 1 percent of variation in future costs, the PIP-DCGs explain 5.5 percent.[45] However, using all claims, including outpatient records, and an approach similar to that of the DCGs performs better, explaining almost 9 percent of variations in costs.

Although clinical risk adjustment could make capitated Medicare payments more equitable, Medicare's current plans were built on several ironies.[46] At the outset, relative payment levels among diagnostic groups derive from fee-for-service experience—the only comprehensive Medicare data currently available.

Also, methods based on inpatient diagnoses explicitly require admissions to boost payment levels. As HCFA acknowledged, this incentive contradicts capitation's goal of preventing costly hospitalizations while maintaining good outcomes.[47] In addition, to deter plans from frivolous hospital admissions, HCFA proposed not considering information from hospitalizations lasting only a day. Given these various considerations, Medicare's approach could penalize plans appropriately providing high-quality care in outpatient settings.

Relying on principal inpatient diagnoses for risk adjustment was supposed to be short-lived. Adding outpatient diagnoses will better capture the burden of chronic illness and debility, improving fairness of capitated payments. Health plans and their affiliated physicians have not, however, moved expeditiously toward reporting all encounter data. The costs of managing computerized information systems within health plans, doctors' offices, and clinics are one issue, and beyond that, other impediments to generating good data persist. Busy physicians have limited time to code each patient's multiple conditions. Fee-for-service evidence suggests that outpatient diagnosis codes are frequently inaccurate and incomplete.[48] Implementing risk adjustment based on all diagnoses offers opportunities for code creep, and audits will be required to ensure coding accuracy.

Even with better methods, using risk adjustment to set capitation payments remains an unproven strategy for encouraging enrollment and excellent care of potentially costly persons. Risk-adjusting capitated payments has been tried in only a few programs nationwide, such as initiatives involving relatively small or targeted populations in California,[49] Colorado,[50] Washington State,[51] and Minneapolis.[52] It has been eschewed by private employers, for various reasons.[53] Experience thus far suggests that risk-adjusting capitation payments is technically feasible but is an "evolutionary process," requiring clear objectives and recognition of the real operational challenges to generating data and ensuring their quality.[54] Some health plans drop out, as did several in California for a variety of reasons.[55] Others find that risk adjustment increases payments, reflecting their sicker members.[56]

Medicare's foray into diagnosis-based risk adjustment has thus far been tentative, involving a small fraction of total payments. The full impact of these changes is still unfolding, but accumulating anecdotes suggest growing problems with access to care. As of January 2001, Medicare capitated plans had dropped over 933,000 elderly and disabled beneficiaries, leaving beneficiaries scrambling to find new health plans.[57] Among people dropped from these Medicare plans, 43 percent now worry about paying their health care bills.[58] Politicians agree that Medicare is in trouble, with health care costs now rapidly rising in both public and private sectors,[59] but remain unable to articulate the problems clearly or to craft solutions. Juxtaposed against high costs are persistent inequities in access to care, racial and other disparities in health, concerns about health care quality, and questions about what we achieve by spending over $1.3 trillion annually for health services.[60]

WHY RISK ADJUST?

Given these difficulties with risk adjustment, the initial question returns: why should we risk adjust? The answer is simple. Without risk adjustment, resulting information could be inaccurate or misleading. Consumers, policymakers, and other health care stakeholders will not have valid information for decision making. The best-known example of misleading results involved Medicare's first public release of hospital-level mortality figures, in March 1986.[61] One hundred and forty-two hospitals had significantly higher death rates among Medicare patients than the government had predicted. At the facility with the most aberrant results, 88 percent of Medicare patients died compared to the 22 percent predicted. But Medicare's risk adjustment was faulty. The outlier institution was a hospice caring for terminally ill patients.

Another goal of risk adjustment is to motivate improvement of care and to encourage providers and plans to accept sick patients. Without risk adjustment, providers and plans argue that they are being treated unfairly: "My patients are sicker, that's why my results are worse." Providers could avoid high-risk patients who are more likely to do poorly and thus "discredit" them. Failure to risk-adjust hampers attempts to engage providers in a meaningful dialogue about improving performance. Among health plans, inadequate payment rates may impede access to insurance among the most vulnerable in our population.

WHEN IS RISK ADJUSTMENT ENOUGH?

No risk adjuster will be perfect, so efforts must concentrate on identifying those that are "good enough." Statistical measures of model performance (for example, percentage of variation explained) alone cannot answer the question of the adequacy of a risk adjustment method. Such statistical measures reveal little about whether systematic errors in predictions occur for selected subgroups of patients or whether important risk factors are present and appropriate. From a practical perspective the question about adequacy of risk adjustment is perhaps best answered through the behavior of the target audience: risk adjustment is adequate when those most affected act as if they believe it.

Designing a clinically reasonable but logistically feasible risk-adjustment strategy requires trade-offs. Adjusting for all patient characteristics is neither necessary nor possible. Most important, risk-adjustment methods must assess risk within groups of patients without bias, and unmeasured risk factors must be unlikely to alter substantially the risk-adjusted findings. However, in a highly charged health policy environment, criticisms of risk adjustment are almost inevitable and are often more political than methodological.

Notes

1. Iezzoni, L. I. (ed.). *Risk Adjustment for Measuring Healthcare Outcomes.* (2nd ed.) Chicago: Health Administration Press, 1997.

2. Iezzoni, L. I. "The Risks of Risk Adjustment." *Journal of the American Medical Association,* 1997, *278,* 1600–1607; Greenfield, S., and others. "Profiling Care Provided by Different Groups of Physicians: Effects of Patient Case-Mix (Bias) and Physician-Level Clustering on Quality Assessment Results." *Annals of Internal Medicine,* 2002, *136,* 111–121; Eisenberg, J. M. "Measuring Quality: Are We Ready to Compare the Quality of Care Among Physician Groups?" *Annals of Internal Medicine,* 2002, *136*(2), 153–154.

3. Hannan, E. L., and others. "Adult Open Heart Surgery in New York State: An Analysis of Risk Factors and Hospital Mortality Rates." *Journal of the American Medical Association,* 1990, *264,* 2768–2774.

4. Newhouse, J. P. "Risk Adjustment: Where Are We Now?" *Inquiry,* 1998, *35*(2), 122–131; Ash, A. S., and others. "Using Diagnoses to Describe Populations and Predict Costs." *Health Care Financing Review,* 2000, *21*(3), 7–28; Kronick, R., Gilmer, T., Dreyfus, T., and Lee, L. "Improving Health-Based Payment for Medicaid Beneficiaries: CDPS." *Health Care Financial Review,* 2000, *21*(3), 29–63; Rice, N., and Smith, P. C. "Capitation and Risk Adjustment in Health Care Financing: An International Progress Report." *Milbank Quarterly,* 2001, *79*(1), 81–113.

5. Vladeck, B. C. "Medicare Hospital Payment by Diagnosis-Related Groups." *Annals of Internal Medicine,* 1984, *100,* 576–591.

6. Freeman, J. L., and others. "Diagnosis-Related Group Refinement with Diagnosis- and Procedure-Specific Comorbidities and Complications." *Medical Care,* 1995, *33,* 806–827.

7. Iezzoni, *Risk Adjustment for Measuring Healthcare Outcomes.*

8. Sullivan, L. W., and Wilensky, G. R. *Medicare Hospital Mortality Information, 1987, 1988, 1989.* Washington, D.C.: U.S. Department of Health and Human Services, Health Care Financing Administration, 1991.

9. Vladeck, B. C., Goodwin, E. J., Myers, L. P., and Sinisi, M. "Consumers and Hospital Use the HCFA 'Death List.'" *Health Affairs,* 1988, *7*(1), 122–125; Dubois, R. W. "Hospital Mortality as an Indicator of Quality." In N. Goldfield and D. B. Nash (eds.), *Providing Quality Care: The Challenge to Clinicians.* Philadelphia: American College of Physicians, 1989.

10. U.S. General Accounting Office, Health, Education, and Human Services Division. *Employers and Individual Consumers Want Additional Information on Quality.* GAO/HEHS-95-201. Washington, D.C.: U.S. General Accounting Office, Sept. 1995.

11. Podolsky, D., and Beddingfield, K. T. "America's Best Hospitals." *U.S. News & World Report*, 1993, *115*(2), p. 66.

12. Simborg, D. W. "DRG Creep: A New Hospital-Acquired Disease." *New England Journal of Medicine*, 1981, *304*, 1602–1604.

13. Bogardus, S. T., and others. "What Does the Medical Record Reveal About Functional Status? A Comparison of Medical Record and Interview Data." *Journal of General Internal Medicine*, 2001, *16*(11), 728–736.

14. Iezzoni, *Risk Adjustment for Measuring Healthcare Outcomes.*

15. Iezzoni, L. I., and Moskowitz, M. A. "A Clinical Assessment of MedisGroups." *Journal of the American Medical Association*, 1988, *260*, 3159–3163; Steen, P. M., and others. "Predicted Probabilities of Hospital Death as a Measure of Admission Severity of Illness." *Inquiry*, 1993, *30*, 128–141.

16. Green, J., and Wintfeld, N. "Report Cards on Cardiac Surgeons: Assessing New York State's Approach." *New England Journal of Medicine*, 1995, *332*, 1229–1232.

17. Chassin, M. R., Hannan, E. L., and DeBuono, B. A. "Benefits and Hazards of Reporting Medical Outcomes Publicly." *New England Journal of Medicine*, 1996, *334*, 394–398.

18. Gruenberg, L., Kaganova, E., and Hornbrook, M. C. "Improving the AAPCC (Adjusted Average Per Capita Cost) with Health-Status Measures from the MCBS (Medicare Current Beneficiary Survey)." *Health Care Financing Review*, 1996, *17*(3), 59–75; Hornbrook, M. C., and Goodman, M. J. "Chronic Disease, Functional Health Status, and Demographics: A Multidimensional Approach to Risk Adjustment." *Health Services Research*, 1996, *31*, 283–307; Fowles, J. B., and others. "Taking Health Status into Account When Setting Capitation Rates: A Comparison of Risk-Adjustment Methods." *Journal of the American Medical Association*, 1996, *276*, 1316–1321; Pope, G. C., Adamache, K. W., Khandker, R. K., and Walsh, E. G. "Evaluating Alternative Risk Adjusters for Medicare." *Health Care Financing Review*, 1998, *20*(2), 109–129.

19. Bowlin, S. J., and others. "Reliability and Changes in Validity of Self-Reported Cardiovascular Disease Risk Factors Using Dual Response: The Behavioral Risk Factor Survey." *Journal of Clinical Epidemiology*, 1996, *49*(5), 511–517; Kravitz, R. L., Greenfield, S., and Rogers, W. H. "Patient Mix and Utilization of Resources: In Reply to the Editor." *Journal of the American Medical Association*, 1993, *269*, 44; Greenfield, S., and others. "Outcomes of Patients with Hypertension and Non-Insulin-Dependent Diabetes Mellitus Treated by Different Systems and Specialties: Results from the Medical Outcomes Study." *Journal of the American Medical Association*, 1995, *274*, 1436–1444; Katz, J. N., and others. "Can Comorbidity Be Measured by Questionnaire Rather Than Medical Record Review?" *Medical Care*, 1996, *34*(1), 73–84.

20. Weiss, B. D., and Coyne, C. "Communicating with Patients Who Cannot Read." *New England Journal of Medicine*, 1997, *337*, 272–274; Sullivan, L. M., and others. "A Comparison of Various Methods of Collecting Self-Reported Health Outcomes Data Among Low-Income and Minority Patients." *Medical Care*, 1995, *33*(4),

AS183–AS193; Kefalides, P. T. "Illiteracy: The Silent Barrier to Health Care." *Annals of Internal Medicine,* 1999, *130,* 333–336.

21. Romano, P. S., and others. "The California Hospital Outcomes Project: Using Administrative Data to Compare Hospital Performance." *Joint Commission Journal of Quality Improvement,* 1995, *21,* 668–682.

22. Wilson, P., Smoley, S. R., and Werdegar, D. *Annual Report of the California Hospital Outcomes Project.* Sacramento: Office of Statewide Health Planning and Development, 1993.

23. Romano and others, "The California Hospital Outcomes Project."

24. Jost, T. S. "Health System Reform: Forward or Backward with Quality Oversight?" *Journal of the American Medical Association,* 1994, *271,* 1508–1511.

25. Wilson, P., Smoley, S. R., and Werdegar, D. *Second Report of the California Hospital Outcomes Project: Acute Myocardial Infarction,* Vol. 1: *Study Overview and Results Summary.* Sacramento: Office of Statewide Health Planning and Development, 1996; Romano, P. S., Luft, H. S., Rainwater, J. A., and Zach, A. P. *Report on Heart Attack, 1991–1993,* Vol. 2: *Technical Guide.* Sacramento: California Office of Statewide Health Planning and Development, Dec. 1997.

26. Wilson and others, *Second Report of the California Hospital Outcomes Project.*

27. Knaus, W. A., and others. "The APACHE III Prognostic System: Risk Prediction of Hospital Mortality for Critically Ill Hospitalized Adults." *Chest,* 1991, *100,* 1619–1636.

28. Vogel, R. A., and Topol, E. J. "Practice Guidelines and Physician Scorecards: Grading the Graders." *Cleveland Clinic Journal of Medicine,* 1996, *63*(2), 124–128.

29. Mazzolini, J. "Area Businesses to Give Hospital Contracts Based on Performance." *The Plain Dealer,* May 17, 1996, p. 1A.

30. "Pacesetting Quality Measurement Project Closing in Cleveland." *Medicine & Health,* 1999, *53*(10), 1.

31. Greenwald, L. M., Esposito, A., Ingber, M. J., and Levy, J. M. "Risk Adjustment for the Medicare Program: Lessons Learned from Research and Demonstrations." *Inquiry,* 1998, *35*(2), 193–209; Sing, M., Brown, R., and Hill, S. C. "The Consequences of Paying Medicare Managed Care Plans Their Costs." *Inquiry,* 1998, *35*(2), 210–222.

32. Medicare Payment Advisory Commission. *Health Care Spending and the Medicare Program: A Data Book.* Washington, D.C.: July 1998, p. 35.

33. Riley, G., Tudor, C., Chiang, Y. P., and Ingber, M. "Health Status of Medicare Enrollees in HMOs and Fee-for-Service in 1994." *Health Care Financing Review,* 1996, *17,* 65–76; Morgan, R. O., Virnig, B. A., DeVito, C. A., and Persily, N. A. "The Medicare-HMO Revolving Door: The Healthy Go In and the Sick Go Out." *New England Journal of Medicine,* 1997, *337,* 169–175.

34. Medicare Payment Advisory Commission, *Health Care Spending and the Medicare Program.*

35. Neuman, P., and others. "Marketing HMOs to Medicare Beneficiaries." *Health Affairs*, 1998, *17*(4), 132–139.

36. Greenwald and others, "Risk Adjustment for the Medicare Program."

37. Greenwald and others, "Risk Adjustment for the Medicare Program"; U.S. Department of Health and Human Services, Health Care Financing Administration. "Medicare Program: Request for Public Comments on Implementation of Risk Adjusted Payment for the Medicare + Choice Program and Announcement of Public Meeting." *Federal Register*, Sept. 8, 1998, *63*, 47506–47513.

38. Greenwald and others, "Risk Adjustment for the Medicare Program"; U.S. Department of Health and Human Services, Health Care Financing Administration. "Medicare Program: Establishment of the Medicare + Choice Program, Final Rule." *Federal Register*, June 26, 1998, *63*, 35004–35007.

39. Medicare Payment Advisory Commission. *Report to the Congress: Medicare Payment Policy*, Vol. 1: *Recommendations*. Washington, D.C.: Medicare Payment Advisory Commission, Mar. 1998.

40. Riley and others, "Health Status of Medicare Enrollees . . ."

41. U.S. Department of Health and Human Services, "Medicare Program: Request for Public Comments on Implementation of Risk Adjusted Payment . . ."

42. U.S. Department of Health and Human Services, "Medicare Program: Request for Public Comments on Implementation of Risk Adjusted Payment . . ."; Ellis, R. P., and others. "Diagnosis-Based Risk Adjustment for Medicare Capitation Payments." *Health Care Financing Review*, 1996, *17*, 101–128; Pope, G. C., and others. "Principal Inpatient Diagnostic Cost Group Model for Medicare Risk Adjustment." *Health Care Financing Review*, 2000, *21*(3), 93–118.

43. U.S. Department of Health and Human Services, "Medicare Program: Request for Public Comments on Implementation of Risk Adjusted Payment . . ."

44. Pope and others, "Principal Inpatient Diagnostic Cost Group Model . . ."

45. Greenwald and others, "Risk Adjustment for the Medicare Program."

46. Iezzoni, L. I., Ayanian, J. Z., Bates, D. W., and Burstin, H. "Paying More Fairly for Medicare Capitated Care." *New England Journal of Medicine*, 1998, *339*, 1933–1938; Pope and others, "Principal Inpatient Diagnostic Cost Group Model . . ."

47. Hellinger, F. J. "The Effect of Managed Care on Quality: A Review of Recent Evidence." *Archives of Internal Medicine*, 1998, *158*, 833–841; Iglehart, J. K. "Bringing Forth Medicare + Choice: HCFA's Robert A. Berenson." In J. K. Iglehart (ed.), *Medicare and Managed Care*. Millwood, Va.: Project HOPE, 1999, pp. 30–40.

48. Fowles, J. B., and others. "Agreement Between Physicians' Office Records and Medicare Part B Claims Data." *Health Care Financing Review*, 1995, *16*(4), 189–199.

49. Bertko, J., and Hunt, S. "The Health Insurance Plan of California." *Inquiry*, 1998, *35*(2), 148–153.

50. Tollen, L., and Rothman, M. "Case Study: Colorado Medicaid HMO Risk Adjustment." *Inquiry*, 1998, *35*(2), 154–170.

51. Wilson, V. M., and others. "Case Study: The Washington State Health Care Authority." *Inquiry,* 1998, *35*(2), 178–192.

52. Knutson, D. "Case Study: The Minneapolis Buyers Health Care Action Group." *Inquiry,* 1998, *35*(2), 171–177.

53. Keenan, P. S., Buntin, M.J.B., McGuire, T. G., and Newhouse, J. P. "The Prevalence of Risk Adjusting in Health Plan Purchasing." *Inquiry,* 2001, *38,* 245–259; Glazer, J., and McGuire, T. G. "Private Employers Don't Need Formal Risk Adjustment." *Inquiry,* 2001, *38*(3), 260–269.

54. Dunn, D. L. "Applications of Health Risk Adjustment: What Can Be Learned from the Experience to Date?" *Inquiry,* 1998, *35*(2), 132–147; Rogal, D. L., and Gauthier, A. K. "Are Health-Based Payments a Feasible Tool for Addressing Risk Segmentation?" *Inquiry,* 1998, *35*(2), 115–121.

55. Bertko and Hunt, "The Health Insurance Plan of California."

56. Tollen and Rothman, "Case Study."

57. Thomas, J. "H.M.O.'s to Drop Many Elderly and Disabled People." *New York Times,* Dec. 31, 2000, p. 14A.

58. Laschober, M. A., and others. "Medicare HMO Withdrawals: What Happens to Beneficiaries." *Health Affairs,* 1999, *18*(6), 150–157.

59. Heffler, S., and others. "Health Spending Projections for 2001–2011: The Latest Outlook." *Health Affairs,* 2002, *21*(2), 207–218.

60. World Health Organization. *The World Health Report 2000: Health Systems: Improving Performance.* Geneva: World Health Organization, 2000; Institute of Medicine, Committee on Quality of Health Care in America. *Crossing the Quality Chasm: A New Health System for the 21st Century.* Washington, D.C.: National Academy Press, 2001; Institute of Medicine, Committee on the Consequences of Uninsurance. *Coverage Matters: Insurance and Health Care.* Washington, D.C.: National Academy Press, 2001; Mechanic, D. "Disadvantage, Inequality, and Social Policy." *Health Affairs,* 2002, *21*(2), 48–59.

61. Brinkley, J. "U.S. Releasing Lists of Hospitals with Abnormal Mortality." *New York Times,* Mar. 12, 1986, p. 1.

CHAPTER THIRTEEN

Consumer-Driven Health Care

Dialogues with Socrates

Stephen S. Hyde

Cast

Socrates

Regina "Regi" Herzlinger

Steve Hyde

SOCRATES: Why is it that consumers are able to intelligently purchase such complex goods as financial products, cars, and computers but not health care services?

REGI: They have never been allowed to.

SOCRATES: Why is that?

REGI: There are two reasons. First, the health care system has long been structured under the implicit assumption that only doctors, governments, and employers—not consumers—are able to decide such matters. Second, federal tax policy has powerfully penalized direct consumer purchase of health care benefits, thus defaulting the decision to employers.

SOCRATES: Is that good?

REGI: No.

SOCRATES: Why is that?

REGI: Because it substitutes a very inefficient structure for the market-based mechanisms that would otherwise allow many individual buyers to independently deal with many sellers and thus maximize the buyers' individual and collective benefit.

SOCRATES: Can this be remedied?

REGI: Oh, yes. What is needed, and indeed what is now beginning to evolve, is a system that

1. Emphasizes and supports self-care, particularly among those with chronic conditions.
2. Offers focused services, or *focused factories,* which eliminate the undesirable variability now prevalent in health care services.
3. Furnishes horizontally integrated providers, which improves access in rural and low-income areas.
4. Provides sufficient information to consumers so that they can purchase their own health services and manage their own health care.
5. Encourages financing and payment mechanisms that encourage and support wise consumer choice.
6. Provides government regulation and tax policy that is minimal but sufficient to encourage all of the above.

SOCRATES: This sounds pretty good. Is it?

REGI: Yes, it is. But I'm also a tad biased. Why not ask somebody else?

SOCRATES: Good idea. Whom do you suggest?

REGI: Ask Steve.

SOCRATES: OK. Steve, is this as wonderful as it sounds?

STEVE: Yes, it is.

SOCRATES: How so?

STEVE: This program gets to the heart of the problem in health care. That problem is essentially a dysfunctional separation of authority from responsibility from accountability. In a healthy economic system you find all three residing in virtually every institution and individual. But in health care, providers have traditionally held the authority over what health care consumers get. Third-party payers have had the responsibility to pay for it. And consumers are stuck with the ultimate accountability, in the form of their lives and their health. In recent years, HMOs have tried to assume more of the authority, but the consumer still bears ultimate accountability. And the consumer still has little say in what health services to buy and how much to pay for them. It is not a good system.

It's as though you were allowed to eat only at a single restaurant, that restaurant could decide what you could eat, and your parents had to pay for it. You would probably be fed a lot of expensive, nutritionally questionable food, at least until your parents called up the restaurant and demanded restraint in quality, quantity, and price. You would not have much say in the matter, and no one would really need to listen anyway. Come to think of it, it would be like a college dorm cafeteria. Fortunately, the real world lets you decide what restaurant you eat at, what food you will eat, and how much you're willing to pay for it. The rest of the country's economy works this way too—except for health care.

SOCRATES: Yes, Regi mentioned that. How do you see her prescription for a consumer-driven health care system remedying these ills?

STEVE: First, this consumer-driven health care system is comprehensive. Most proposals, particularly legislative ones, are piecemeal approaches, and seriously vulnerable to unintended consequences. Second, this concept focuses on fitting an economically aberrant industry into a well-established economic model that has a long history of functioning in an efficient, effective, and humane manner. Third, it puts authority, responsibility, and accountability into better economic balance, with consumers being the big winners, along with those insurers and providers who are responsive enough to provide true consumer value.

SOCRATES: It's pretty clear that you are enamored of every single detail of Regi's schema, right?

STEVE: Well . . .

SOCRATES: Is that your Jack Benny impersonation or do you have reservations?

STEVE: There is one part that troubles me.

SOCRATES: Why didn't you say so?

STEVE: Because it's technical and would likely bore you.

SOCRATES: Nonsense. Tell me about it.

STEVE: Well, in an earlier career, I was an HMO actuary.

SOCRATES: [Yawn.] How fascinating.

STEVE: Yes, it's true, I lacked the personality to be an accountant. But it's the actuary in me that is troubled by Regi's proposal to support risk-adjusted premium payments to third-party payers so that the sick and their providers are not discriminated against. It's too complicated and also unnecessary.

SOCRATES: Please, do go on. But I have to leave for a while—my car needs an oil change. Just speak into this microphone and be assured that I will give your recorded comments the full attention they deserve upon my return.

STEVE: HMOs and insurers essentially set their premiums based on the Pareto principle, more commonly referred to as the 80/20 rule. That is, they figure that roughly 80 percent of their members will be healthy and 20 percent will be sick. Thus the premiums of the healthy help cover the costs of the sick. It is very important to keep this ratio in balance. If you don't get enough healthy consumers to offset the cost of treating the sick, you go broke.

Traditionally, there have been two ways for insurers to deal with this risk. One is to do health screening on individuals seeking to buy health insurance. The healthy are let into the plan at normal prices, and the sick may (1) pay more, (2) pay the same but be subjected to preexisting-condition limitations, or (3) be excluded altogether. Regi has suggested that a modified form of this approach be used for all health plan enrollments and that it be enforced by the federal government. This is the part of her program that I question.

The second method has been to offer health benefits only to employer groups and their families but without any health screening. This has long been the most common method for achieving an acceptable mix of healthy and sick members for the insurer. It has worked reasonably well because (1) the employer usually pays most of the premium, so the healthy employees have no financial reason not to enroll; (2) employed consumers tend to be healthier than unemployed consumers; (3) people enrolled as groups are statistically more likely to yield an acceptable cross section of health risk to the insurer than are people enrolled individually; and (4) premium pricing can be greatly simplified, allowing all members of the group to be charged essentially the same rate, weighted only for objective factors like age, gender, and geographical location.

Add to this the fact that employers can deduct 100 percent of health insurance premiums for income tax purposes (individuals cannot), and you can see why most insured people are enrolled through their employer rather than individually. Medicare and Medicaid are special cases, but the same principles generally apply.

Unfortunately, there are serious problems with group purchases. First, you, the consumer, have no incentive to save money on the health care you consume because employer-paid care is essentially an entitlement, under which anything you pay bears little or no relationship to the actual costs of care that you receive. You neither know, nor have any reason to care, how much anything costs. That's the essential reason health care costs are rising so rapidly. Second, you lose any freedom of choice beyond the health plans, benefits, and providers offered by your employer. Third, if you lose your job, you either lose your coverage or have to pay its full cost in order to continue it. Fourth, if you're not an employee of an organization that offers a health care benefit, your only hope for health insurance is via individual coverage (requiring a health screen), which may cost more than you can afford, if it's available at all.

Much better would be a system where individuals could choose whatever health plan they wanted and could afford, with employer assistance available for paying premiums but without any employer decision on choice of plans, benefits, or providers. However, this system would have to be arranged in a way that yields sufficient revenue to provide care for the sick—remember the Pareto principle. There are at least two ways to do this. One way is to charge everyone the same premium rate but do so in a way that ensures adequate enrollment of healthy members (meeting the 80/20 rule). In essence that means making it advantageous for the healthy to join while they are healthy rather than waiting until they become sick. The other way is simply to charge according to the likely cost of treating a given individual (that is, a medical condition–adjusted pricing arrangement), as determined by a prospective health assessment. I believe the former is much preferable to the latter. Regi tends toward the latter view.

I would argue that there are serious barriers to effectively mandating a standard system of risk adjustment at the individual level. First, it would be impractical to apply it to insurance other than large-group insurance, because charging individuals or small groups for their coverage based on health status would make that coverage unaffordable to anyone once he become seriously ill. Second, mandating federal regulation and oversight would require a bureaucracy that would likely be large, politically vulnerable, and I believe, ultimately unworkable. Third, the requirement for employers to pay higher premiums for their sick employees would create a strong incentive, especially for smaller employers, to get rid of such high-cost workers, regardless of any protective rules. Fourth, the opportunity for dysfunctional political favor seeking would be irresistible, with those who perceived personal disadvantage pushing for preferential treatment under the rules.

A simpler, more effective method of providing consumer choice would be a defined contribution system based on modified community rating. Under such a system, each individual consumer would receive a voucher provided, as appropriate, by an employer or by the government (to replace Medicare, FEHB, Medicaid, and the military dependent system) or purchased by the individual herself. These vouchers would be denominated in dollars, in whatever amounts the issuer selects. (I realize that the term *voucher* is laden with political baggage from its use in another context. However, it is still preferable to repeatedly saying something like "payment under a defined contribution system.")

All health plan premiums would be calculated under a modified community rating system, adjusted for such objective factors as age, gender, and geographical location, but not for individual health condition. This means, for example, that any fifty-two-year-old male living in Dubuque who buys Plan Green from Bob's Insurance Company in January 2004 would pay the same premium as any other fifty-two-year-old male from that community signing up at the same time for the same coverage from the same insurer, regardless of medical condition. All other rating methods, such as experience rating and medical condition–adjusted rating, would be forbidden, putting everyone on a level playing field. This is essential.

Each person with a voucher would, during an annual open enrollment period, be eligible to pick any insurance plan on the market. If the plan costs less than the voucher's stated value, any remainder could go into a tax-free individual medical savings account (MSA) to pay for health services not covered by insurance, or the person could decide to spend the extra money on a more comprehensive plan. If the plan chosen costs more, the consumer could make up the difference from her own funds or choose to purchase less expensive coverage.

There would be no requirement for consumers to purchase such benefits, but there would be two strong rule-based incentives to do so. The first rule would be that vouchers could be redeemed only for insurance and MSA-style spending account contributions. Thus everybody with a voucher from an employer or the government would almost certainly sign up to buy insurance because she couldn't derive the voucher's value any other way. This would not, however, ensure that self-employed or other individuals would sign up. Without a second rule, they would have a strong incentive to save money and wait until they got sick to sign up for insurance.

The second rule (and this is also how to avoid making participation mandatory) would be that the self-employed can buy their own vouchers but must either enroll at the outset of the national voucher system or be locked out for a two- or three-year period before becoming eligible again. That is, anyone who did not sign up initially would have no available coverage beyond her own financial resources until the next available window of enrollment two or three years hence. Thus a healthy, self-employed person who might not otherwise sign up (and prefer to save her money and wait for the appearance of a health problem) would think long and hard about having to go for a period of years without coverage because a single illness could bring bankruptcy. Such a rule, well publicized, offers a completely voluntary method to ensure that healthy individuals will participate in sufficient numbers to allow the 80/20 rule to work.

Overall this voucher system offers significant advantages. First, it gives consumers much greater choice than they currently have in the selection of health plans, benefits, and providers to suit their own needs and means.

Second, it enhances patient privacy, because employers and government voucher providers would be completely out of the patient medical information loop.

Third, coverage is not dependent on employment but is portable across employers—or lack thereof.

Fourth, the adjusted community rating system of pricing is relatively simple and is well established.

Fifth, there are strong financial incentives for the consumer to be a cost-conscious purchaser of health services.

Sixth, the enrollment process is blind to the health condition of the consumer, thus minimizing incentives and opportunities for inappropriate discrimination against the sick.

Seventh, although not entirely solving the problem of the large number of currently uninsured consumers, it dramatically simplifies the solution by encouraging affordable coverage.

Eighth, it gets employers and government out of the business of defining what benefits must be offered, leaving that up to the market.

Ninth, it gets government out of the business of regulating prices. One employer (or government agency) might be able to afford only a $1,500 annual voucher, whereas another could spend $6,000. The consumer receiving the voucher could then use it to purchase an insurance and MSA package within those limits, and might add additional funds of his or her own for a better package.

Tenth, health insurance would become more like life insurance. During one's youth the adjusted community-rated premiums for health insurance would be relatively low, as would be the vouchers. If the individual prudently chooses a high-deductible insurance plan (that is, a low-premium plan), the MSA contribution portions would be relatively large. More important, these contributions are early and would compound tax-free over many years to provide a substantial nest egg to cover the higher premiums and higher costs of later life, including long-term care.

Ultimately, such a system would inject traditional market economics into a seriously dysfunctional health care system, with providers and insurers competing vigorously to provide consumers with continually better service and higher value.

And there's one final piece. Under my proposal there is nothing wrong with insurer payments to medical providers being based on an individual's medical condition. Only the premiums paid to the insurers themselves need be calculated on the adjusted community-rating basis. Payments to providers may be on any basis that the insurers and the providers can mutually agree on.

SOCRATES: I'm back.

STEVE: How's your car?

SOCRATES: I got there just in time. I think it's going to make it.

STEVE: I'm thrilled. Want to hear the recording?

SOCRATES: You bet. I'll get to it right after I mow the lawn. But before you go, why don't you give me a quick summary?

STEVE: Consumer-driven health care is the only way we are going to dramatically improve the health care system in this country. It will require tweaking in some technical areas, but the big picture (with most of the details) is solid. What do you think?

Socrates: I [yawn] need a drink.

CHAPTER FOURTEEN

Employee Tax Payments and Consumer-Driven Health Care

Jeanne A. Brown

In a defined contribution (DC) plan, an employer allocates to each employee a set dollar amount for the purchase of health care services—that is, for the purchase of the health care policy or for an allocation into a health care account or for both. The allocation can be used for the premium only, for the employer-owned health care account only, or for a percentage of each. DC allows employees to fine-tune coverage to their individual needs. This contrasts with the present typical defined benefits plan wherein the employer does all the legwork, employees' options are limited, and satisfaction is often limited.

Of course there are income tax considerations when an employer changes from a defined benefit to a defined contribution plan. I review the major considerations here.

The first question the employer will need to ask is, Are defined contributions tax deductible—like defined benefits? The answer is yes.

The answer to the next important question—What is the impact of the transition from defined benefits to defined contribution on the income tax situation of the employee?—is less clear.

APPLICATION OF THE TAX LAW TO DC PLANS

Section 106 of Title 26 of the U.S. Code governs the application of federal and state income tax to a defined contribution health care plan:

Sec. 106. Contributions by employer to accident and health plans.

(a) General rule

Except as otherwise provided in this section, gross income of an employee does not include employer-provided coverage under an accident or health plan.[1]

Although the plain language of the statute is broad, fortunately federal regulation 1.106-1 makes it clear that a defined contribution is both viable and excludable from taxable income:

Sec. 1.106-1. Contributions by employer to accident and health plans.

The gross income of an employee does not include contributions which his employer makes to an accident or health plan for compensation (through insurance or otherwise) to the employee for personal injuries or sickness incurred by him, his spouse, or his dependents, as defined in section 152. The employer may contribute to an accident or health plan either by paying the premium (or a portion of the premium) on a policy of accident or health insurance covering one or more of his employees, or by contributing to a separate trust or fund (including a fund referred to in section 105(e)) which provides accident or health benefits directly or through insurance to one or more of his employees. However, if such insurance policy, trust, or fund provides other benefits in addition to accident or health benefits, section 106 applies only to the portion of the employer's contribution which is allocable to accident or health benefits. (See paragraph (d) Sec. 1.104-1 and Secs. 1.105-1 through 1.105-5, inclusive, for regulations relating to exclusion from an employee's gross income of amounts received through accident or health insurance and through accident or health plans.)[2]

IMPLEMENTATION OF THE LAW

The method of implementation of a DC program affects the tax status. Several revenue rulings and U.S. Tax Court cases address the issue.

A revenue ruling[3] released in 1961 concluded that reimbursements by an employer to his employees for the employer's share of the premiums for hospital and medical insurance provided or purchased by his employees may be considered as contributions by the employer to accident or health plans for his employees. A designation of the reimbursements by the employer would result in the exclusion of such payments from the gross income of the employees under section 106 of the Internal Revenue Code of 1954. (The current code includes section 106.)

The application of section 106 and the exclusion of taxable income to the employees were distinguished by the administration of the reimbursement. In this case an employer had a group plan in which some of his employees participated. The employer also reimbursed employees who did not participate in the group plan for individual insurance expenses. The ruling turned on the following points:

To facilitate payment of his share of the premiums paid directly by the employees to the insurers, the employer used the following methods:

(1) reimburses each employee directly once or twice a year for the employer's share of the insurance upon *proof of prior payment of the premiums by the employee;* or

(2) issues to each employee a check payable to the particular employee's insurance company, *the employee being obligated to turn over the check to the insurance company;* or

(3) issues a check as in method (2) except the check is made payable *jointly to the insurance company and the employee* [emphasis added].[4]

The Internal Revenue Service (IRS) concluded that each of these methods constituted employer payments of accident or health insurance premiums for employees because all met the necessary proof requirements. Both methods 2 and 3 included proof via checks from the employer made directly or jointly to the carrier and method 1 required proof of prior payment of premiums. Accordingly, the IRS concluded the amounts paid were excludable from the gross income of the employees under section 106 of the Internal Revenue Code.

In contrast, a previous revenue ruling[5] addressed the allotment of a defined contribution as a part of wages in the context of a negotiated agreement between an employer and an employee union. The conclusion reached by the IRS confirms that certain payments made to employees pursuant to a union contract constitute "wages" for federal employment tax purposes.

In the case on which the ruling was made, an employers' association negotiated an agreement between the association on behalf of its members and the employees' union, obligating the member employers to pay a stipulated weekly sum to each employee covered by the agreement for the purchase of individual hospitalization and surgical insurance coverage. The parties specifically agreed that the sum paid was to be used for the "express purpose" of purchasing the hospitalization and surgical insurance benefits for covered employees. The union made direct arrangements with a hospital service for the stated purpose, and payments made under the contract were used exclusively for the contracted purpose.

Under the U.S. Code, "wages" consist of all remuneration for services performed by an employee for his employer, including the cash value of all remuneration paid *in any medium other than cash,* with certain immaterial exceptions.[6] The IRS concluded that the payments in questions were required under the terms of a labor agreement governing employee relations of the employers involved, the payments were directly related to the services performed by the employees, and the payments were made directly to each employee. "Thus," according to the ruling, "they constitute a basic part of the compensation of each employee involved. Accordingly, it was held that such payments which are made by the employers directly to the employee constitute 'wages' for 'employment' for purposes of the Federal employment taxes and are includible in the gross income of the employees under section 61 of the 1954 Code." The fact that the union assumed the responsibility for the disposition of such payments by the employees was deemed immaterial.

ADMINISTRATIVE IMPLICATIONS

The ruling against the union muddies the 106 waters for employers of "union member" employees, who have submitted to employer-provided "mandated" health care benefits determined by a collective bargaining agreement. (The tax court can, and probably will, rule that by definition, wages and remuneration dictated by collective bargaining—regardless of form: for example, benefits, health, retirement, and so forth—are all included in the collectively bargained "wage package.")

However, exceptions to the ruling can occur for nonunion employers, particularly small employers (less than one hundred employees), or for union employees whose health care packages are tailored to them and not tied to the collective bargaining agreement. (How to accomplish this is another question.)

Thus whether a DC plan can be excluded under section 106 seems to depend on the existence of an "open" health care plan, that is, one that is not a mandatory employer-provided (collective) benefit, as part of wages or salary. The way benefits packages are structured and presented to employees may well determine the application of 106.[7]

The revenue rulings addressed here in the text and the notes are the only rulings that relate directly to defined contributions. (Most of the tax court rulings have been modeled on Revenue Ruling 61-146.)

Although the case law is limited, it is probable that some direction can be drawn from pension fund litigation, particularly that involving 401(k) plans. A 401(k) plan is somewhat analogous to a defined contribution health care plan in its administration, implementation, and application.

OTHER RULINGS RELEVANT TO DC PLANS

In 1989, the U.S. Court of Appeals in the Sixth Circuit discussed the possible implications and restrictions of defined contributions health care plans. In this case, *Adkins v. United States*,[8] lump-sum payments to employees (taxpayers) made in settlement of lawsuits against a former employer concerning the employer's proposed termination of contributions to a hospital-medical benefits plan did not fall within provisions of section 106, which excludes contributions by employer to accident or health plans from gross income. The statute did not provide exemption for payments made by the employer directly to employees.

The petitioners in this case were the employees, both current and former, of a corporation that proposed in 1984 to terminate its contributions to a health benefits program for eligible pensioners and surviving spouses. A temporary settlement to the employees' suit implemented a temporary modified contributory health insurance program. The employer offered employees who did not want to wait for the outcome of the negotiations or the litigation in the case the choice of a lump sum payment or continuing monthly case payments, which would be in full settlement of any claim against the corporation. The lump sum payments ranged from $6,000 to $20,000 and were dependent on each recipient's age and marital status. The decision to accept the lump sum payments was entirely voluntary. The pensioners choosing the lump sum payments had to fill out an election and release form and return both to the corporation. The election form advised the pensioners that there could be tax consequences subject to either election. The pensioners who chose the election were not required to use the lump sum or monthly cash payments for the purchase of medical insurance. Several pensioners, including petitioners in this case, made the lump sum payments election and sued to exclude it from taxable income under section 106 of the Internal Revenue Code.

The conclusion reached by the tax court in this case was predictable. What is more telling for the purposes of a defined contribution plan, however, is both the reasoning and the language used by the court:

> The pensioners who made the election were not required to use the lump sum or monthly cash payments for the purchase of medical insurance. Some pensioners . . . who elected lump sum payments did not use the payments for the purpose of medical insurance. . . .
>
> Section 106 clearly applies to contributions made by the employer to hospital, medical and accident benefit insurance programs, trusts, or funds. *Section 106 does not contemplate, or infer, direct payments to the employee.* . . .
>
> It is undisputed that in this case the corporation paid the lump-sum payments in question directly to taxpayers without any use restrictions. The payments are accessions to wealth which must, therefore, be included in income the year of receipt, unless the taxpayers can show that Congress has unequivocally provided an exemption for the payments. See, e.g., *United States v. Wells Fargo Bank,* 485 U.S. 351, [citations omitted] (1988) ("exemptions from taxation are not to be implied; they must be unambiguously proved"). . . .
>
> The exclusion from income provided in section 106, by its plain terms, applies only to an employer's "contributions" to "accident or health plans." There is nothing in the language of the statute that provides an exemption for payments made by an employer directly to employees. As the Tax Court held in *Laverty v. Commissioner,* 61 T.C. 160, 165 (1973), *aff'd,* 523 F.2d 479 (9th Cir. 1975). . . .

Section 106 has no application to payments an employer makes directly to his employee. . . . It deals only with the treatment of *contributions* by an employer to an accident or health plan for the benefit of his employees, either in the form of contributions to a separate fund or trust or by the payment of premiums on a policy of accident or health insurance. . . .

Taxpayers assert that the lump-sum payments were *"earmarked specifically for hospital and medical care."*. . . This argument fails because it ignores the fact that the statute also requires that the funds *be part of a plan.* . . .

Finally, it is worth noting that Congress amended section 106 by section 1151(j)(2) of the Tax Reform Act of 1986 (Public Law 99-514, 100 Stat. 2085). Section 106(a) now provides that "[g]ross income of an employee does not include employer-provided coverage under an accident or health plan."[9] [emphasis added]

In *Cernik* v. *Commissioner,*[10] a former municipal employee sued to have his disability payments excluded from taxable income. The tax court ruled against Cernik. Disability payments are not exclusions from income under section 106. The outcome in *Cernik,* as it was in *Adkins,* was predictable. However, once again the language is informative. The court stated:

A former municipal employee could not exclude from gross income either the short-term or the long-term disability benefits that he received under employer-sponsored disability plans because the benefits were either paid directly by the employer or were attributable to employer contributions that were not includible in the employee's income. Pursuant to Code Secs. 104(a)(3) and 105(a), premiums paid by the taxpayer to a prior disability plan outside the relevant three-year look-back period were not taken into account for purposes of determining whether the benefits at issue were "attributable to contributions by the employer.". . .

The taxpayer's alternative argument that his disability payments were excludable under Code Sec. 105(c) as amounts received through accident or health insurance for personal injuries or sickness was rejected because the benefits were not computed with reference to the nature of his injury. Instead, the record established that the benefits were calculated with reference to the taxpayer's salary and his years of service and did not vary depending on the injury or illness suffered.

SUMMARY

The plain language of section 106 of the U.S. Code, the revenue rulings, and the tax court rulings discussed here suggest that a defined contribution health plan is a viable alternative to current defined benefits plans. The big questions arise in the administration of and transition to a DC approach.

The rulings make it clear that a trust or voucher system is necessary—wherein both proof of purchase and system accountability are in place. Merely *earmarking* funds for employee use is not enough.[11] The employer must maintain a separate trust account that uses either a voucher program or a joint payee program.

Any program adopted by the employer should include a mechanism of proof of health insurance purchase by the employee to avoid employer contributions from being subject to taxation as wages to the employee. In a voucher program, employees would submit vouchers to the trust administrator to pay the employer's contribution to the carrier for the employee-selected plan. Payment for employee plans that exceeded the employer's contribution limit would have to be supplemented by the employee.

Alternatively, employers could set up a system that allowed employees to submit premium notices to the administrator of the trust or a paymaster, who would in turn cut checks made payable jointly to the employee and the carrier.

It is certain that a defined contribution health care plan is a viable alternative to the current defined benefits health care plans. Section 106 of Title 26 of the U.S. Code makes it clear that a defined contribution by an employer to an employee health care plan would be excludable from the employee's taxable income. Thus the first hurdle in a defined contributions plan is crossed. The other areas that need to be more fully examined are the administration, implementation, and application of a defined contribution plan, as well as the possible application of ERISA, COBRA, and other applicable federal and state labor laws and regulations.

But from a tax perspective, the good news remains that a defined contribution model is an avenue for possible reform.

The latest revenue ruling directly affecting DC plans was issued June 26, 2002, by the IRS and the U.S. Treasury Department regarding the tax consequences of HRAs[12] (health reimbursement arrangements), which are in the defined contribution (DC) health plan family. To the extent that an HRA is an employer-provided accident or health plan, coverage and reimbursements for medical care expenses of an employee and the employee's spouse and dependents are generally excludable from the employee's gross income under sections 106 and 105.[13] The revenue ruling and notice contain some much-needed guidance as well as some good news. First, HRAs that are funded solely by the employer (and not by salary reductions) can permit carryovers of unused amounts from year to year (*that is, the use-it-or-lose-it rule does not apply*).[14] Second, HRAs are not subject to the onerous rules[15] that apply to health FSAs (flexible spending arrangements).[16]

Several other points of note regarding HRAs include the following:[17] (1) HRAs can reimburse only substantiated medical expenses, as defined in U.S. Code section 213(d); (2) HRAs may reimburse employees for the purchase of health insurance (beware of potential HIPAA as well as other issues); (3) for employers with both an HRA and a salary reduction–funded health FSA, the HRA may specify that coverage under the HRA is available only after expenses exceeding the dollar amount of the health FSA have been paid (that is, the health FSA pays first and the HRA pays second); (4) HRAs may provide for continued access to unused HRA amounts by former employees (including retirees), but cash-outs are not permitted; and (5) HRAs are subject to COBRA'S continuation requirements.

Notes

1. *Internal Revenue Code. U.S. Code,* Title 26, §106 (2000).

2. *Internal Revenue. Code of Federal Regulations, Title 26,* § 1.106-1.

3. Revenue Ruling 61-146. 1961-2 *Cumulative Bulletin,* 25.

4. Revenue Ruling 61-146.

5. Revenue Ruling 57-33. 1957-1 *Cumulative Bulletin,* 303.

6. *Internal Revenue Code,* §§3121, 3306, 3401.

7. The importance of the implementation rules was underscored by a recent revenue ruling (Revenue Ruling 2002-3) in which the IRS held that the exclusions from gross income under Internal Revenue Code sections 106(a) and 105(b) are not applicable to an employer's reimbursements to employees for health care premiums paid via salary reductions. In the case addressed by the ruling, Employer M provides health care coverage for its employees through a group health insurance policy that qualifies for the tax exclusion under section 106(a). Employer M has a payroll arrangement whereby employees' salaries are reduced, and M applies the salary reduction amounts to the payment of the health insurance premiums for the employees. In addition, M makes "reimbursement" payments to the employees for the health insurance premiums in amounts that cause employees' after-tax pay to be the same as it would have been had there been no salary reduction and no "reimbursement" payments.

Applying its application of Revenue Ruling 61-146, addressed earlier, the IRS concluded, in Revenue Ruling 2002-3 (Dec. 22, 2001):

> [S]ection 106 allows an employee to exclude employer reimbursements for health insurance premiums, but only if those premiums are actually paid by the employer. When M applies the amount of employees' salary reduction to pay health insurance premiums, the premium payments are paid by M, not the employees.
>
> Although the section 106 exclusions apply to the health insurance premiums paid by M, there is no employee-paid premium for M to "reimburse," and therefore the reimbursement payments that M makes to employees are not excluded from gross income under section 105 because they do not reimburse employees for expenses incurred for medical care. Accordingly, the reimbursement payments are not excluded from income tax withholding. In addition, because the reimbursement payments are not reimbursements of expenses incurred for medical care, they are not excluded from FICA taxes or FUTA taxes.

In essence the IRS has eliminated what it considers to be a double-dipping of sorts. Employers had created health plans wherein employees pay premiums through pretax contributions deducted from their wages. Thereafter the employer reimburses the employees for some or all of the premiums on a pretax basis, thus reducing employee and employer contributions for FICA and FUTA taxes and lowering the employee's reported gross income. This revenue ruling holds that such a health care plan is not supported by the tax code because it does not comport with the limitations expressed in sections 106(a) and 105(b). The revenue ruling did note, however, that employer-provided health and welfare benefit coverage remains tax qualified. Employers may reimburse employees on a pretax basis for individual accident and health insurance premiums paid by the employee to the insurer if the employer has a benefit plan that permits such reimbursements and the reimbursement is of premiums actually paid by the employee. The DC plan discussed above is an example of a health plan that comports with the IRS ruling.

8. *Adkins v. United States*, 882 F.2d 1078 (6th Cir. 1989).

9. *Adkins v. United States*, 1079, 1080, 1081.

10. *Cernik v. Commissioner*, 78 T.C.M. (CCH) 471 (1999).

11. Whether or not employers would be allowed to pool their collective resources into MEWAs (multiple employer welfare associations) or other cooperative trust vehicles is at present unknown.

12. Treasury Notice 2002-45 defines an HRA as

> [A]n arrangement that: (1) is paid for solely by the employer and not provided pursuant to salary reduction election or otherwise under § 125 cafeteria plan; (2) reimburses the employee for medical care expenses (as defined by §213(d) of the Internal Revenue Code) incurred by the employee and the employee's spouse and dependents (as defined in §152); and (3) provides reimbursements up to a maximum dollar amount for a coverage period and any unused portion of the maximum dollars amount at the end of a coverage period is carried forward to increase the maximum reimbursement amount in subsequent coverage periods.

13. *Internal Revenue Code*, §105, 106.

14. Revenue Ruling 2002-41, June 26, 2002.

15. Q/A-7 rules in proposed Treasury Regulation §1.125-2.

16. IRS Notice 2002-45. *Internal Revenue Bulletin*, June 27, 2002.

17. IRS Notice 2002-45.

CHAPTER FIFTEEN

The Implications of Tax Rulings on "Savings Accounts"

Charles H. Klippel

When the history of consumer-directed health plans is written, one of the more intriguing chapters will relate to their treatment under federal tax law. The concept of a health benefits account had two key precedents under the tax code: flexible spending accounts (FSAs) and medical savings accounts (MSAs)—sometimes known as Archer MSAs after Representative Bill Archer (R-TX), who was instrumental in their creation. For early champions of the consumer-directed model, however, neither of these authorities was particularly helpful. FSAs, which allow employees to defer a portion of their salary into a pretax spending account, were subject to a strict annual use-it-or-lose-it requirement that precluded any accumulation of funds from year to year. MSAs permitted accumulation but were available only to small employer groups. (Most of the early adopters of consumer-directed plans were large, national employers.) Worse, the authorizing legislation for MSAs limited their number to no more than 750,000 nationwide, restricted other coverage to relatively unattractive high-deductible plans, and contained a cutoff provision that froze the program to new entrants at the end of 2003.

Tax advisers contemplating the early consumer-directed plans found themselves in uncharted waters. With understandable caution, many felt obliged to point out that FSAs and MSAs were both creatures of specific enabling legislation, something that the *account* portion of the consumer-directed plans lacked. By long-standing tradition, group health coverage was defined in annual terms; the notion of an accumulating, multiyear benefit structured as an account was

279

a novelty. But by focusing on the distinction between *employee* funding of FSAs and *employer* funding of consumer-directed benefits, proponents of the new plans saw (or at least hoped they saw!) sufficient authority for this new idea in the basic employee health benefits sections of the code. The U.S. Treasury Department agreed, and—anxious to lead rather than follow this emerging trend—rearranged its 2001–2002 departmental priorities to develop supporting guidance for these plans within the context of the existing tax law. The result was a new acronym, the HRA (for health reimbursement arrangement), and a remarkably robust, coherent, and detailed framework for the implementation and operation of HRA-based plans.

The Treasury's HRA guidance clearly reflected at least three core principles that emerged from the department's internal deliberations: durability, flexibility, and consumer protection. A number of early commentators had suggested that by virtue of the way an *employee* is defined in relevant sections of the code, it should be possible to carry the accumulated benefits into retirement. The Treasury confirmed this view and went a step further by permitting other postemployment carryovers if elected by the employer. Employers could also define the scope of coverage for HRAs, allowing broad FSA-style use of the funds, mirroring the limitations of the plan's more traditional companion benefits, or something in between (for example, an employer that does not otherwise offer dental coverage may permit employees to use their HRA accounts for dental services).

Perhaps most challenging was the Treasury's goal of embracing the emerging consumer-directed model—which combines the flexibility of a benefit account with more conventional coverage for serious illnesses—without opening too wide a door for less consumer-friendly defined contribution schemes. Even this was accomplished by carefully crafting the guidance around a revenue ruling *safe harbor* predicated on a hybrid plan design. Not bad for an initiative based entirely on existing law!

MIXING AND MATCHING ACCOUNTS

In developing its guidance on HRAs, the Treasury knew that many employers would offer these plans in conjunction with FSAs. A modest debate had already developed among early proponents of the plans as to the proper payment order for an expense covered by both an FSA and the as-yet-unnamed HRA. Some advocated that the HRA pay first, preserving the employee's FSA funds for services not covered by the employer's plan. Others suggested the FSA should be used first, protecting the more durable HRA dollars. Still others suggested that the employee should be allowed to choose on a claim-by-claim basis, a consumer-centered if administratively daunting solution.

The Treasury embraced a relatively pragmatic middle ground, permitting FSAs to be offered with HRA plans and allowing the employer to establish in advance of each plan year the order of payment between the two accounts. Significantly, this ordering rule applies only when a claim is covered by both accounts. Most of the first-generation HRAs provide first-dollar coverage, followed by a deductible. It is not difficult to imagine a second generation in which the deductible must be met before the HRA is available. When offered with an FSA these plans could represent something of a hybrid, allowing the FSA to pay first up to a fixed liability (the deductible), beyond which remaining FSA funds would be reserved for noncovered expenses during the year.

Because of the annual use-it-or-lose-it requirements of FSAs, many consumers today use these accounts only to fund predictable, discretionary health expenditures—for example, orthodontia—not covered by their health plans. Others estimate "likely" expenses for deductibles and copayments as well as noncovered services; for these consumers a hybrid HRA plan with a fixed deductible might work quite well.

Employers may, of course, define coverage under their HRA plans to include services traditionally covered by an FSA, such as orthodontia or laser refraction surgery. The HRA guidance for permitted coverage virtually mirrors the FSA rules, although in one key area the HRA rules are more generous: if permitted by the employer these accounts can be used to pay for qualified long-term care premiums.

Have employers chosen to use this flexibility? The early indications are that some have, whereas others retained common coverage definitions for both the HRA and the plan's other benefits. It appears that the flexibility may be used primarily by employers not currently offering a standard coverage such as pharmacy or dental benefits. They could allow these services to be covered by the HRA without altering their underlying plans.

ARCHER MEDICAL SAVINGS ACCOUNTS

Perhaps not surprisingly, the Treasury guidance did not address the interaction of HRAs and MSAs. MSAs continued to be fairly rare, constrained by perceptions that administration was complex and that the authorizing legislation was in effect an experiment. Significantly, HRAs were conceived as first dollar coverage accounts, which if provided by an employer would preclude the employee from maintainng the supplemental Archer MSA.

The idea of a first-dollar discretionary spending account, however, did have appeal for some small employers, and health insurers, led by Aetna, began to incorporate HRA-like accumulating benefit "funds" into fully insured plans suitable for this market segment. While the accounts are not portable beyond the coverage period, these plans do provide much of the flexibility, cost transparency, serious illness protection and benefit accumulation features of sophisticated HRA-based plans offered by larger employers. Notably, the Federal Employees Health Benefits Program has elected to include this fully insured model among the plan offerings available to Federal employees beginning in 2004.

THE NEW ACRONYM IN TOWN: HSAS

The remarkable market interest in consumer-directed health plans, including new opportunities to accumulate health benefit dollars, did not escape the attention of Congress. As part of the 2003 Medicare reform initiative various tax-favored health savings alternatives were proposed, including a limited roll-over of FSA dollars and relaxation of some of the Archer MSA restrictions. A series of new acronyms also appeared in the debate, including HSAs (Health Savings Accounts), a supplemental fund for high-deductible plans broadly following the MSA model, HSSAs (Health Savings Security Accounts), an even more flexible savings vehicle, and RMBAs (Retirement Medical Benefit Accounts), an allied notion focused specifically on retirement health savings that were championed by, among others, the 401(k) management community.

HSAs and HSSAs were incorporated into early versions of the House Medicare reform bill, although HSSAs in particular seemed unlikely to survive as the bill was scored. The fate of the HSA provision was debated in the final reconciliation of the House and Senate bills and ultimately survived as Title XII of the *Medicare Prescription Drug, Improvement and Modernization Act of 2003*.

Like Archer MSAs, HSA balances can be carried forward from year to year, rolled over from one account to another and, subject to a tax penalty, can even be withdrawn in cash. Also like MSAs, HSAs can only be funded by individuals covered under a high-deductible medical plan, but HSAs are not subject to a sunset nor are they restricted to the small employer market. An HSA may be funded by the eligible individual, his or her employer, a relative, or any combination of these sources.

HSAs seem destined to replace Archer MSAs. They are also likely to replace many FSAs, although (at least for the time being) only for individuals who are covered under qualified high-deductible plans. The extent to which these consumers can or will maintain both an HSA and some form of FSA remains to be seen based on future regulation and possible additional legislative changes.

THE FUTURE OF HRAS

In addition to Rep. Archer, HSAs clearly owe a debt to the creative thinking of the Treasury Department embodied in its HRA guidance. There are significant differences between the two concepts, however, suggesting that HRAs are likely to continue to play a role in the design of employee health benefit plans for the indefinite future.

One key distinction is that HRAs can be self-funded. Self-funded employers tend to be larger companies, many of which provide more than basic high-deductible coverage for their employees. These companies may elect to adopt high-deductible plans and supplement that coverage through contributions to an HSA, but the HRA model provides substantially greater flexibility in both plan design and funding. The paradigm of HRAs as first-dollar benefit funds may also change, permitting an employer to structure a portion of its benefits as an accumulating "fund" without disqualifying employees from maintaining a supplemental HSA.

Perhaps most significantly, additional funding may be contributed to an HRA after the retirement of the employee and without the requirement that the account be coupled with a high-deductible plan. The ultimate legacy of the HRA may be its application to post-retirement benefits as employers, driven by FASB 106 and other considerations, continue to move away from defined benefit retirement health plans.

TAX POLICY, CONSUMERISM, AND CONSUMER PROTECTION

Tax policy has always been a critical lever for the federal government to encourage consumer savings. In the emerging field of health savings the stimulus provided by the HRA rulings and HSA legislation is likely to be particularly compelling, since the funds are not just tax-deferred but truly tax-exempt if used for health services. At the same time both the Treasury and Congress have sought to balance a complex set of consumer issues—encouraging more flexible benefit designs, greater cost awareness, and opportunities for savings while preserving the traditional protection of defined benefit coverage for significant illnesses and injuries—while living within the increasingly stringent fiscal realities facing the government. Congress had the advantage of being able to rewrite the law, and the HSA rules are as a result fairly prescriptive. The Treasury Department needed to find new answers within old law and did a remarkably good job. The two solutions overlap, but ultimately may work in concert to shape the emerging era of consumer-driven health benefits.

CHAPTER SIXTEEN

You Just Can't Pay Tom, Juan, and Ashley the Old Way Anymore

Bonnie B. Whyte

Abstracts from the Headlines

CalPers expects 25% health premium increases

Factories move to Canada and Mexico

The face of U.S. business is changing daily, becoming more diverse, more global. The company town, the corporate pension after twenty-five years with the same firm, as well as the classic nuclear family, are artifacts from another age.

The same is true in health care. The family doctor dispensing wisdom and penicillin is equally long gone.

The new model has every Tom, Juan, and Ashley working at a variety of employers over their lifetimes, in different configurations, just as their families and lifestyles also evolve. They are also consumers of new drugs and new therapies and use new diagnostic equipment and highly trained specialists. They will live longer and consume more health care, and it will cost a lot.

What can employers do to attract and retain the best workers? How can they stay competitive in a continually reconfigured environment? How can they prosper and achieve appropriate bottom-line results? Fortune 500 firms have long recognized these challenges. They began changing their compensation and benefits models in the late 1970s to meet the needs of the evolving workforce. At that time, employers had a static and paternalistic model: a pension after ten years of service, standard life insurance that assumed a male head of household and a nonworking spouse, and family health insurance from Blue Cross that was both expensive and unappreciated.[1] Employees wanted different things: more money and faster retirement—with portability if they left for another job. Regulatory and accounting requirements for recognition of the net present costs of defined benefit pensions in corporate financial statements caused additional problems by forcing disclosure of uncertain, large negative numbers. Employers responded. Today nearly all major corporations have 401(k) plans. Defined benefit pensions are declining in number, as mergers, acquisitions, layoffs, and early retirements take their toll.

DEFINED CONTRIBUTION RETIREMENT SAVINGS: LESSONS FROM 401(K)

The growth of 401(k) plans since their introduction has mirrored the changes in employee demographics and the dynamics of the boom-and-bust business cycles. The 401(k) plan, a section of the tax code, is widely interpreted to allow deferred compensation through savings, profit sharing, stock bonuses, or pension plans purchased with pretax money. Employees may take certain compensation as cash or defer the compensation into a plan. Most 401(k) plans accept salary reduction contributions and, due to discrimination regulations, most employers match employee contributions, thus doubling their funds, up to a certain level.

Section 401(k) plans are the only deferred compensation that can be linked directly with section 125 cafeteria plans, creating a three-way trade-off among cash, deferred compensation for retirement, and welfare benefits, which include health, accident, and disability coverage. Their success has fueled the stock market, through plan purchase of company stocks and mutual funds. Employees receiving monthly or quarterly statements of their increased retirement savings see and appreciate the growth. The relative portability of these individual accounts has proved its value for both employee and employer alike as jobs and workers move around. The decline of the old-fashioned defined benefit plan, with its unchanging but permanent benefits, has resulted in fewer workers with guaranteed retirement benefits but more workers with retirement savings accounts.

The same trends are happening in health benefits. Dual-income families had needs different from those of single-income families and costs were rising at exorbitant rates; health maintenance organizations and managed care plans promised better care for stable costs. Thus the stage was set for the birth of full defined contribution plans for health care as well as for retirement plans.

CAFETERIA OR FLEXIBLE BENEFIT PLANS

With refinements in the tax code, *cafeteria,* or *flexible benefits,* plans emerged in the 1980s that allowed employers to offer a variety of retirement and health options to their employees. Employees loved having choices. Employers loved it too.[2]

How does it work? Flexible benefits, or more briefly, *flex,* refers to programs governed by section 125 of the Internal Revenue Code. These plans are cafeteria-style benefit arrangements. Generally, the employer must have a written plan that offers the employee a choice between cash and nontaxable *qualified* benefits, without discrimination in favor of highly paid employees. In return both the employer and participants receive certain tax advantages (tax deductibility for the employer and pretax money for benefits for the employee), employees may have the freedom to choose cash in place of unwanted or unneeded benefits, and the employer can attach a known cost rather than an uncertain estimate to the benefit expenses in the firm's public financial statements.[3]

Section 125 allows an exception to the concept of *constructive receipt,* so an employee can choose from a group of benefits and receive them without paying social security or income tax on those benefits. Qualified benefits include group term life insurance, disability benefits, accidental death and dismemberment benefits, dependent care assistance, and the big-ticket item of accident and health benefits.[4]

Large employers have moved to a full-choice model of benefits, offering everything from retirement to health, from buying and selling vacation days to fitness programs. In a sense, benefits are a vital element of the total compensation model employers wanted.[5] Employees see what they are buying, and employers have a more complete handle on their compensation structure.

FLEXIBLE SPENDING ACCOUNTS

Where, then, is the movement among employees in their health coverage? How are they coping with managed care, copays, and the booming area of alternative therapies? After all the ebbs and flows, employers are seeing employees use flexible spending accounts in creative ways to supplement health plans.[6]

A flexible spending account (FSA) is a reimbursement account for either child or elder dependent care assistance or, for purposes of this discussion, health expenses. An employee may have two reimbursement accounts, one for health and one for dependent care expenses. To fund these accounts, employees agree to have their salaries reduced by a uniform amount over a year. Employees can then draw funds from these employer-administered accounts to pay medical expenses not covered by health insurance.[7] Health FSAs are generally used to pay for copays and deductibles. Employees can do extremely well by planning for health expenses that are frequently not fully covered by health insurance, such as dental, eye care, and mental health expenses. Employees who anticipate elective procedures, or who use out-of-network physicians, are finding FSAs a way to buy out of their managed care plan. They can get the benefit of plan discounts for most of their medical needs but use their FSA funds for special needs or care.[8]

Eligible medical expenses are regulated by the definitions of section 213 of the Internal Revenue Code. In some, for example, cosmetic improvements, general wellness therapies, and nonprescription or over-the-counter drugs, herbs, and vitamins could not be reimbursed,[9] but alternative therapies for medical conditions often could.

FSA Problems: Use It or Lose It

In 1999, an estimated thirty-six million workers had cafeteria plans and sixteen million were offered flexible spending accounts. Among the latter, approximately 22 percent actually participated in an FSA, with a median contribution of $568 annually. This low FSA participation rate of fewer than one in four has been fairly constant, despite an increase in the number of employers offering flex.[10] This is surprising. Survey after survey has shown that employees value their health benefits second only to paid vacation. The annual Workplace Pulse Survey conducted by the Employers Council on Flexible Compensation (ECFC) has shown that employees want a choice in their benefit package, especially in health coverage.[11] In 1998, most employees (70.2 percent) were covered by a private insurance plan offered through employment.[12] Employers with diverse employee populations see a wide variety of usage of the different plans, proving that one-size-fits-all health coverage is inappropriate.

What is holding employees back from using a spending account?

Fear.

If an employee does not spend all the money in his account, it is generally returned to the plan for administrative expenses. The phrase "use it or lose it" appropriately describes this IRS policy. Under IRS regulations, employees must sign up for a twelve-month plan year and not make any changes. It is easy to understand why an employee would hate to "lose" money from his paycheck. However, smart employees also realize that their tax savings can add up significantly. At a minimum the employee is saving social security (FICA) taxes, as well as federal and most state taxes. Thus an employee in a 15 percent bracket who sets aside $1,000 annually is saving at least 22.65 percent (15 percent plus 7.65 percent FICA) for an annual minimum savings of $226. For those in higher tax brackets, the savings are even greater.[13] The employee would still be significantly ahead of the game even if he "left" $50 in the FSA account and "lost" it at the end of the year. This is still a difficult concept for employers to communicate to their employees and for employees to accept.

The use-it-or-lose-it aspects of FSAs also create some perverse behavior at the end of the year. Employees who find they have not spent all their FSA funds go to their dentist for an extra cleaning or their optician for extra eyeglasses. There is no incentive to save this money; the very design of an FSA encourages wasteful spending.[14]

The current design of FSAs and cafeteria plans has other flaws. Only employees may participate in cafeteria plans. This leaves the self-employed out in the cold for similar benefits. Small businesses may not want the administrative expense.[15] Many small businesses contract out payroll and benefit administration. Flex administration, particularly for FSAs, is more expensive than basic payroll and is more akin to health benefit administration. For businesses with fewer than one hundred employees, the required tests for nondiscrimination may create serious limitations for higher-paid employees and owner-employees. Those "key employees," may not receive more than 25 percent of the total benefits provided to all employees under the plan. It takes only a few well-paid or many low-paid workers to throw a small business's plan out of compliance and require all key employees to receive their benefits on a taxable basis.

Medical Savings Accounts

In 1996, Congress attempted to equalize the opportunities for access to health coverage by enacting legislation authorizing medical savings accounts (MSAs). The idea is to allow individuals and those in small businesses the option to buy high-deductible insurance and put up to $5,500 in a trust account for reimbursement of medical expenses. The attractive feature of the plan is that the funds can be saved from year to year if not spent, rather than lost as is the case with a cafeteria plan's flexible spending account.[16]

Unfortunately, state regulations and design limitations were great impediments to MSAs. Congress was deliberating extensions as of September 20, 2003. Despite the problems, nearly one out of four MSAs has been bought by a person previously uninsured.[17] With wider availability, MSAs could be a good start on resolving the vast problem of encouraging and promoting health care access for the nearly forty million uninsured Americans.[18]

The Medicare Prescription Drug law, passed in late 2003, included new "new Savings Accounts" or HSAs. These are a "new, improved" Medical Savings Accounts that are available to all individuals and offered by all employers on a tax-favored basis. The HSA itself is tied to a mandatory high-deductible health insurance plan and any unused funds in the account roll over indefinitely in an individual's account. As products emerge, individuals and small- and medium-sized employers should be moving in the HSA direction. Larger employers with more compensation and benefit options will have more difficulty integrating HSAs into their comprehensive plans.

Legislative Efforts

The debate over MSAs has reopened the issue of FSAs and the use-it-or-lose-it provision. President Bush campaigned to permit an annual $500 rollover of FSA funds. Measures have been introduced to allow $500 or up to $2,000 to be rolled over annually within an FSA or into an MSA or even a 401(k). This would have the desirable effect of preventing the annual loss of an employee's unspent FSA funds, avoiding an end of year rush to incur medical expenses, and encouraging employees to save money for the day when they retire or have extraordinary medical expenses.[19]

The House-passed version of a Prescription Drug Bill included the $500 rollover provision, but the flexible spending account rollover did not make the final cut in the Medicare bill. It remains an achievable legislative goal in future health care reform, however.[20]

FSA reform efforts remain hostage to the congressional health care debate. However, the forecast is brighter given current administration support. Reform remains popular to workers who continue to consider funds "their money" until that money is given to tax collectors, as opposed to those who consider funds not taxed "revenue foregone" or a tax "expenditure impacting the budget."[21] The debate over health reform and how to allow consumers to buy their own health care will continue as long as revenue estimates drive medical reform decisions. Market-driven choices must be permitted to flourish. The current managed care debate will have far-reaching implications in the health and compensation fields. Populist feelings run strong over the right to good health care. Balancing our social needs and the market forces of the health business will be a critical challenge for this country as it faces continued change in the twenty-first century.

Notes

1. Gifford, D. L., and Seltz, C. A. *Fundamentals of Flexible Compensation.* New York: Wiley, 1988.

2. Manin, M. B., Sciandra, F. G., and Frayling, L. *Flexible Benefits Answer Book.* (2nd ed.) New York: Panel, 1998.

3. Johnson, R. E. *Flexible Benefits: A How-To Guide.* (4th ed.) Brookfield, Wisc.: International Foundation of Employee Benefits Plans, 1992.

4. Employers Council on Flexible Compensation. *Guidelines for Administrative Support for Cafeteria Plans.* Washington, D.C.: Employers Council on Flexible Compensation, 1995.

5. Hewitt Associates. *Survey Findings: Hot Topics in Designing and Providing Benefit Choices.* Lincolnshire, Ill.: Hewitt Associates, 1997.

6. *ECFC Flex Reporter* (Employers Council on Flexible Compensation), Sept. 1998; *ECFC Flex Reporter,* Mar. 1999; *ECFC Flex Reporter,* Sept. 1999.

7. Gifford and Seltz, *Fundamentals of Flexible Compensation.*

8. Manin, M. B., Sciandra, F. G., and Frayling, L. *Flexible Benefits Answer Book: 1999 Supplement.* New York: Panel Publishers, 1999.

9. Internal Revenue Service. *Medical Expenses.* Publication 502. Washington, D.C.: U.S. Government Printing Office, 2001.

10. U.S. Department of Labor, Bureau of Labor Statistics. *Employee Benefits in Private Industry, 1999.* National Compensation Survey. Washington, D.C.: U.S. Department of Labor, 2001; *Employee Benefits in State and Local Governments, 1998.* National Compensation Survey. Washington, D.C.: U.S. Department of Labor, 2000.

11. These surveys are published each June by the Employers Council on Flexible Compensation, Washington, D.C.

12. U.S. Census Bureau. *Current Population Survey.* Washington, D.C.: U.S. Census Bureau, Mar. 1999.

13. Manin and others. *Flexible Benefits Answer Book.*

14. Employee Benefit Research Institute (EBRI). "Flexible Benefits, Choice, and Work Force Diversity." Issue Brief. Washington, D.C.: EBRI, July 1993.

15. Segal Company. "Flexible Benefits for the Small Organization: Why Flex Plans Are Not Just for Large Corporations." New York: Segal Company, Aug. 1993.

16. Manin and others, *Flexible Benefits Answer Book, 1999 Supplement.*

17. Internal Revenue Service. Announcement 99–95. Internal Revenue Bulletin 1999-42, Oct. 18, 1999.

18. U.S. Census Bureau. "Health Insurance Coverage: 2000" Press Release. Sept. 21, 2001.

19. Moffit, R. E., and Beach, W. W. "Rollover Flexible Spending Accounts: More Health Choices for Americans." Heritage Foundation *Backgrounder* 1159, 1998.

20. Employers Council on Flexible Compensation. "Contentious Prescription Drug Conference to Continue into September." *Bulletin.* Washington, D.C.: Employers Council on Flexible Compensation, Aug. 1, 2003.

21. U.S. General Accounting Office. *Tax Policy: Effects of Changing the Tax Treatment of Fringe Benefits.* Report to the Joint Committee on Taxation, U.S. Congress. Washington, D.C.: U.S. General Accounting Office, 1992.

CHAPTER SEVENTEEN

The Federal Employees Health Benefits Program

James W. Morrison Jr.

In 2000, the Federal Employees Health Benefits Program (FEHB) provided health care coverage for nearly ten million employees, retirees, and their dependents. From its beginning in 1960,[1] it has been the world's largest employer-sponsored, voluntary health insurance program. The FEHB is notable as a consumer choice, price-competitive model with participating private sector carriers bearing substantial risk.

EVIDENCE OF NEED

When the FEHB was enacted into law, the U.S. federal government was perceived to lag behind large, private sector employers and some large states and cities in providing health care coverage to its employees. Before the law's enactment, only about 70 percent of the government's employees had any form of health insurance protection.[2] Individuals obtained coverage through private policies or group plans offered by unions and various agency associations. Few employees had major medical coverage. Many had no coverage at all, owing to either preexisting conditions or prohibitive cost.

The FEHB allowed most employees to upgrade their coverage substantially. Of the approximately four million eligible employees and retirees, all but about 15 percent elected to do so. (A number of those who declined to participate may well have had spousal coverage elsewhere.)

A BRIEF DESCRIPTION

Like all public sector programs established by statute, the FEHB's basic structure reflects a number of political horse trades and legislative compromises. The law provides for two government-wide plans (which Congress intended to be the major source of coverage), employee organization plans (included to accommodate the various unions and associations that were already providing coverage to federal employees), and *comprehensive medical plans* (a category coined by the FEHB act to accommodate the then emerging group practice and individual practice prepayment plans). Even though several amendments to the law have updated elements of the program, such as the government's contribution to premiums, antifraud protections, and a number of administrative issues, in 2000 the FEHB remains configured largely as it was when established forty years ago.

The FEHB is administered by the U.S. Office of Personnel Management (OPM), the federal government's central personnel policy agency. Congressional oversight is performed not by health policy committees, but by the Senate and House committees responsible for overseeing general government management. The entry of government-wide plans and employee organization plans into the FEHB is controlled by statute. The indemnity benefit plan slot, vacant since Aetna withdrew from the FEHB in 1989, could have been filled by another insurer via a noncompetitive contract with OPM, but any additional government-wide plan or employee organization plan can be admitted only by an amendment to the law. In 2000, there was one government-wide plan and twelve employee organization plans. Health Maintenance Organizations (HMOs) are admitted to the program upon application to, and approval by, the OPM on an annual basis. In 1999, there were nearly three hundred HMOs in the program.

The government's contribution to premium is set by law at 72 percent of the weighted average of the premiums of all plans, but the contribution to a given plan cannot exceed 75 percent of that plan's premium. Separate premiums have been established for the two enrollment categories: self only and self and family. Premium payments by enrollees are withheld from salaries (or annuities for retirees) and, together with the government contribution made by each employing agency (and by OPM for retirees), deposited in the Health Benefits Fund. Disbursements are made to carriers via letter of credit draws. The desired level of plan reserves is set by regulation and held by the government in accounts earmarked for each plan. Annually, each enrollee can switch plans or decline coverage during an "open season." Generally, only about 5 percent of all enrollees elect to change plans in any year.

EVIDENCE OF EFFICACY

The FEHB has been studied repeatedly.[3] Yet, specific, objective measures of cost effectiveness are difficult to come by. Most studies have attempted to compare FEHB benefit values with those of plans offered by large private employers; others have compared elements of the program, such as FEHB administrative expenses, with similar elements of large public programs; and some have simply tried to compare the rate of premium increases over time. Although all have provided interesting and generally useful information, the many unique features of the FEHB tend to frustrate attempts at apples-to-apples comparisons.

For example, some comparisons concluded that federal employees pay slightly more of their health care costs in premiums, deductibles, and coinsurance than enrollees in the private sector. But few private sector plans offer retirees a benefit and premium package identical to that offered active workers, and few private plans have the range of choices afforded FEHB participants. Some features, such as immediate coverage from the date of employment, that have been part of the FEHB since its inception were virtually unheard of in the private sector prior to the enactment of the Health Insurance Portability and Accountability Act. With regard to controlling costs, most data have shown the FEHB outperforming Medicare, and some show a similar performance against private sector plans. But again, the analysis has been hampered by the absence of standard, authoritative published data on private insurance costs over time.

One measure of the FEHB's efficacy is the degree of consumer satisfaction the program achieves. Customer surveys are conducted annually (by the program and by many participating plans also) and the results are published in the official open season enrollment guide. Categories such as the choice of doctors available in a plan, the extent of coverage, access to medical care, and the timeliness of claims payments are among the elements measured. Generally, most plans in the FEHB have achieved favorable scores and enrollees have expressed a high degree of satisfaction with their plans.

OTHER APPROACHES

There have been no significant competitor approaches to providing health benefits coverage to federal employees and retirees. Unlike the government's life insurance program, in which offerings by private companies and even one by an organization of federal employees compete, in health care coverage there are no alternative health insurance programs for permanent, full-time employees and retirees. For a brief period, some of the government's financial agencies, for example, the Federal Reserve Board and the Federal Home Loan Bank Board, offered their own plans, but they have since returned to coverage under the FEHB.

SOCIETAL IMPACT

From its beginning the FEHB has had a significant impact on the government's ability to attract and retain qualified employees. The availability of comprehensive coverage without regard to health status has been a compelling feature for many people entering government service. And the FEHB has also affected the health benefit systems of other public employers, as several states have copied the federal program. And unlike Medicare, which has imposed, by legislative or administrative fiat, below-market rates of reimbursement on hospitals and doctors, the FEHB has remained a market-based system of private sector competition. Finally, because of its size, perceived performance, and enduring stability, the FEHB is cited frequently as a model for reforming other large health care systems, especially Medicare.

CRITICISMS

Among astute observers, the FEHB is sometimes referred to as an "accidental success." This characterization is largely true. Initially, the government set out to provide commercially available, fee-for-service insurance coverage through a government-wide plan, but political imperatives forced an accommodation for the service benefit and cash indemnity types of plans, for the existing union and association plans already engaged in providing coverage, and for the then very few group and individual practice plans. Thus the notion of competing plans was the result of political necessity, not health care policy. Subsequent external factors, such as the Health Maintenance Organization and Resources Development Act of 1973 (Public Law 93-222), which encouraged the development and expansion of HMOs generally, also facilitated rapid program growth.

Some health policy analysts believe that the accidental beginning and the haphazard way the FEHB has grown have created severe structural defects in the program. They criticize the multiplicity of choices, the apparent adverse selection and risk segmentation, and the manner in which competition actually occurs in the FEHB.

For example, one study characterized the vast array of benefit choices as "the most striking feature of FEHB which causes it to stand out as a bizarre aberration among other large employers' health benefit plans."[4] This view holds that federal employees and retirees find it too daunting to make an informed choice among the large number of available plans. Other analysts assert that this same array of choices allows better-informed individuals to switch from plan to plan in ways that may be personally beneficial but harmful to the program as a whole. To these critics, younger and healthier enrollees opt for lower-priced, suboptimal coverage, whereas older and sicker enrollees stay in familiar plans, thereby driving up premiums in these plans. (This phenomenon might be described more precisely as adverse retention.) In the view of these critics, limiting the range of choices would enlarge, and improve, the FEHB's risk pool. Finally, the criticism that competition is inadequate at the consumer level is premised on the belief that meaningful enrollee choice cannot simply evolve from individual preferences but must be prescribed by the employer or plan sponsor. An element of this criticism is the statutory basis on which plans are admitted to the FEHB. These critics believe that plans must be competitively selected by the employer to avoid plan complacency and inadequate service.

A RESPONSE

These criticisms are based on values other than consumer empowerment. In fact, employer-prescribed benefit choices and plan selection is the antithesis of consumer empowerment. It is not that these criticisms are without some merit. But they have more validity if one believes that average individuals are not sophisticated enough to make appropriate choices for themselves and their families, or if one believes that only the government is capable of doing the "right" thing, or if one values standardization and administrative tidiness over the rough and tumble of the marketplace.

So the real question is what is a reasonable price to pay for personal freedom, individual choice, and customer satisfaction? What is the societal value of a satisfied consumer? If that customer's plan choice is different from the considered choice of a health care "expert," is the value of her satisfaction greater than the value she would get by following the expert's choice? Is it better for a bureaucrat to decide the appropriate benefit package for enrollees, or should health plans in the marketplace design products in response to expressed consumer preferences?

If the ability of consumers to choose among competing products is a hallmark of a healthy marketplace, the FEHB is a success. If choice is associated with increased consumer satisfaction, the FEHB is a sterling example. In assessing the efficacy of the FEHB, it might be useful to consider that this program provides coverage for the U.S. president and vice president, Supreme Court justices, and members of Congress as well as rank-and-file civil servants, and also covers their families. They are all consumers. Clearly, if they were not satisfied with this particular consumer-driven model, it would be changed.

RECOMMENDATIONS

Today, it would be extremely difficult to replicate the FEHB exactly in structure and form, even for the federal government it serves. It would certainly be difficult to do in the private sector. Public disaffection with managed care, the paucity of health plans with a number of carriers that compete to insure the same group of enrollees, and the belief on the part of some that professional benefit managers, or group purchasers, are better equipped than individual consumers to discern differences in value and exercise informed choices, have combined to produce an entirely different setting from what existed in 1960.

But the FEHB offers many lessons for today's examination of the efficacy of consumer-driven health care. It has demonstrated that a limited government role, coupled with an appropriate role for the private sector, is a model worth emulating. It has demonstrated that an array of consumer choices forces competing health plans to strive constantly to bring attractive products to market and to place a high value on customer service, especially in a program where individual underwriting is prohibited. It has demonstrated that adverse selection and risk segmentation are manageable, even though some enrollees make choices that health policy "experts" consider unwise. And the FEHB has demonstrated that the ability to choose from a menu of health plans is correlated with high levels of consumer satisfaction.

Notes

1. The FEHB was created by the Federal Employees' Health Benefits Act of 1959 (Public Law 86-382) enacted September 28, 1959. The program became operational on July 1, 1960.

2. Detwiler, M. L. *History of the Federal Employees Health Benefits Program, Inception to 1970.* Washington, D.C.: U.S. Civil Service Commission, Bureau of Retirement, Insurance, and Occupational Health, 1971.

3. See, for example, the following studies: U.S. House of Representatives, Committee on Post Office and Civil Service. *Review of the Federal Employees Health Benefits Program.* Committee Print 97-8. Washington, D.C.: Committee on Post Office and Civil Service, 1982; U.S. General Accounting Office. *Health Insurance: Comparison of Coverage for Federal and Private Sector Employees.* HRD-87-32 BR. Washington, D.C.: U.S. General Accounting Office, 1986; U.S. Office of Personnel Management. *Study of the Federal Employees Health Benefits Program.* Washington, D.C.: U.S.

Office of Personnel Management, 1988; Congressional Research Service. *The Federal Employees Health Benefits Program: Possible Strategies for Reform.* U.S. House of Representatives, Committee on Post Office and Civil Service, Committee Print 101-5. Washington, D.C.: Congressional Research Service, 1989; Creedon, J., Allison, T., Mellman, R., and Sherman, W. *Report on Federal Employees Health Benefits Program.* U.S. House of Representatives, Committee on Post Office and Civil Service, Committee Print 102-6. Washington, D.C.: Committee on Post Office and Civil Service, 1992.

4. Creedon and others, *Report on Federal Employees Health Benefits Program*, p. 75.

CHAPTER EIGHTEEN

Health-Based Premium Payments and Consumer Assessment Information

Vicki M. Wilson, Jenny M. Hamilton,
Mary K. Uyeda, Cynthia A. Smith,
with Graydon M. Clouse

The Washington State Health Care Authority (HCA) was created in 1988 to help ensure that the state could continue to provide comprehensive health care coverage to its employees.[1] Among several approaches adopted by the HCA to accomplish this directive are the two described in this paper:

- *Health based premium payments.* Premium payments to health plans are adjusted for the underlying risk of the populations enrolled in each plan.

- *Consumer assessment of health plans.* Consumer reports are provided to enrollees based on their fellow employees' assessments of health plan experiences.

Motivating these two approaches is the HCA's commitment to eliminating barriers to enrollees' exercising the full range of choices available to them. The

This chapter was initially written by the first four authors in 1999. It was updated by Grady Clouse in 2002. The Washington State Health Care Authority (HCA) gratefully acknowledges colleagues at the University of Washington, William M. Mercer, Inc., Kaiser Permanente Center for Health Research, and Healthcare Business Services International, Inc., for their invaluable development and implementation work leading to health-based premium payments. This work was funded by a grant from the Robert Wood Johnson Foundation to the University of Washington and the Washington State Health Care Authority. The HCA also is indebted to the Harvard Medical School team, a part of the CAHPS™ consortium, for selecting the HCA as a 1997 CAHPS demonstration site and to the Picker Institute for its work and guidance in implementing CAHPS for Washington State public employees.

comments presented in this chapter are from the perspective of a large purchaser whose influence on the health care market is due as much to size as to government status. However, as a government agency, HCA's role includes the obligation to (1) be public in decisions, actions, rationales, and methods so that others can benefit and (2) model decisions and approaches that go beyond HCA's self-interest.

The HCA context is that of competitive bidding by capitated managed care plans and a self-insured preferred provider organization (PPO), all administered within a managed competition framework to a commercial population. In 1999, sixteen plans were offered to public employees; choices ranged from two to twelve depending on county of residence. In 2000 and 2001, eleven plans were offered.

APPROACH 1: HEALTH-BASED PREMIUM PAYMENTS

This section discusses how to risk-adjust payment.

Evidence of Need

There is ample discussion in the literature regarding the need to fairly compensate health plans and providers for the predictable illness burden of their enrollees.[2] For HCA the move beyond age and gender for adjusting plan premiums was motivated by consistently unequal distribution of risk among HCA health plans. In the early 1990s, at the urging of participating plans, the HCA began to look closely at risk distribution. From 1991 through 1997, the spread of risk among plans ranged annually from 16 percent to over 30 percent. For example, in 1991 the risk mix for nine plans available to employees ranged from .92 to 1.08. In 1997, the range for twenty available plans was .98 to 1.32. There was increasing concern that if capitated premiums were not more closely aligned to each plan's risk mix, employees' options for coverage could be severely curtailed. At worst, plans could use subtle marketing or provider-contracting practices to steer higher-need individuals elsewhere, and at best, plans could become reluctant to advertise their expertise in treating special need individuals.

In addition, the future viability of the state's self-insured PPO (offered statewide) was in question. It was becoming populated with higher-risk enrollees as healthier enrollees migrated to capitated managed care plans. It was critical to HCA's commitment to consumer choice that this PPO remain a viable option.

Approach Description

Two models for assessing relative risk among health plans are used.[3] The first model is based solely on enrollee demographics; the second includes enrollee demographics plus a measure of enrollee health status based on diagnostic cost groups (DCGs).[4] The demographic variables include enrollee age, gender, member status (subscriber, spouse, or dependent), family tier (employee only, employee and spouse, employee and children, or full family), retiree status, and COBRA status. In the future, HCA planned to adopt an internally developed diagnostic model.

Each model gives an expected monthly cost per enrollee, that is, an assessment of each enrollee's expected illness burden or risk. The expected cost is the product of two predictions: (1) the probability that an enrollee will incur some medical cost and (2) the enrollee's monthly cost, assuming that some cost is incurred. The individual assessment information is aggregated to the plan level and used to adjust health plan bid rates. Health plans bid on the average HCA population; their bids are then adjusted up or down depending on the relative (to the population average) risk mix of enrollees served by the plan. Money is moved among plans so that HCA pays in total no more based on the risk-adjusted premiums than it would based on the original bid rates. All plans, including the HCA's PPO, are included in the process.

An example underscores the value of using an assessment model that includes a diagnostic measure of health status. HCA's demographic model predicts a monthly expense of $92 for a forty-year-old male employee. The health status model predicts a monthly expense ranging from $34 to $2,311 for a forty-year-old male employee, with health status varying from healthiest to sickest, respectively.

Between 1998 and 2000, the HCA phased in health-based risk adjustment. In 1998 and 1999, the demographic model was the base. Additional adjustments for health status were made to the base—up to +2 percent in 1998 and ±5 percent in 1999, using the health status model. Beginning in 2000, the full health status model became the base; the demographic model is now used only for new public employees for whom no diagnostic experience is available.

The decision to phase in the full health status model was driven largely by data concerns. Plans were afforded the time to learn the importance of submitting accurate and complete diagnostic data and to learn the impact of this more complex methodology. In recognition that one plan's poor diagnostic data can affect the entire system and to protect plans from a catastrophic data lapse, the HCA retains the right to cap adjustments so they are no more than ±15 percent of the population average.

Evidence of Efficacy

Since inception HCA health plans have continued to vary in their risk profiles, risk adjustment has been moving money among plans, the quality of data has been improving, and plans and providers have been supportive. The following evidence is from HCA's first four years of implementation.

The range of adjustments made to health plan bid rates was –16.8 percent to +13.7 percent in 1999 and –14.6 percent to –10.6 percent in 2001. This means that in 2001 the plan with the healthiest population (relative to the average) had its bid rate decreased by 14.6 percent and the plan with the least healthy population had its bid rate increased by 10.6 percent.

The amount of premium dollars shifted among plans is substantial. In 1999, HCA's monthly premium payments to plans totaled approximately $35.9 million. About $2.3 million per month, or 6.4 percent of premium dollars, was shifted among plans. The largest donor plan lost over $300,000 per month, and the largest receiver plan gained over $1.0 million per month. The shifted dollars represent almost 97 percent of the dollars that would have been moved under the full health status model. In 2001, HCA monthly premiums were $47.8 million, with approximately 6 percent shifted among plans. The largest donor plan lost over $546,000 per month, and the largest receiver plan gained over $1,197,000 per month.

Data quality continues to improve, and this improvement is a factor driving a reduced range of premium adjustments. Plans are more proactive in reviewing quality reports. Error rates reflecting discrepancies between plan-supplied diagnostic data and HCA-supplied enrollment data are decreasing. Future improvements will come mainly from better diagnosis coding by providers and improved tracking of eligible enrollees by the plans. In the meantime, the HCA and the plans have more information than ever before to help them understand the care being delivered to enrollees.

The reactions of health plans and providers have also been positive. Plans are encouraging HCA to refine the model. Of particular concern is the changing role of drug usage and its impact on overall practice patterns. Likewise, provider groups are encouraging HCA to facilitate use of risk adjustment downstream. As one representative of physicians wrote, "From our perspective, failure to pass on to providers the effects of risk factor adjustment negates the very purpose for which HCA took this very responsible step—namely, to assure that resources are available to care for an individual's health care needs."[5] Both issues represent next steps to take for the HCA.

Attributes

Differences among purchasers in risk adjustment mechanisms are numerous and primarily driven by (1) the context in which the purchaser operates, (2) the population for whom coverage is being purchased (for example, the commercial, Medicaid disabled, individual, or small employer market), (3) the quality of the data available, (4) the administrative resources required, and (5) whether or not there is the political will to push beyond current limitations. More critical than the specific approach is the fact that adjustment occurs at all and uses a measure of enrollee health status that goes beyond simple demographics.

The positive attributes of HCA's approach include

- An emphasis on data that plans should collect and analyze as standard practice for managing care

- An effective model that recognizes health care spending patterns (for example, zero expenditures for many individuals in a given year)

- Decisions that focus on addressing predictable risk, leaving insurance risk to the health plans

- A diagnostic classification approach that is clinically meaningful, consistent with underwriters' health expenditure experience, and publicly available, and that uses both inpatient and ambulatory data

- Safeguards to ensure privacy of enrollees' medical information

- For HCA, an expense-neutral premium distribution mechanism

APPROACH 2: CONSUMER ASSESSMENT OF HEALTH PLANS

This section describes consumer assessment of the health plans.

Evidence of Need

The need of consumers to be more informed and therefore self-directed in their choice of health coverage and their care decisions, and the methods to provide them with tools to accomplish this, are under lively discussion. For HCA the decision to implement consumer reports came primarily from two directions: (1) the reintroduction in 1996 of employee premium contributions, and (2) HCA's desire to purchase based on quality as well as price.

Until 1996 (with a brief exception in the early 1970s), the State of Washington paid the entire plan premiums of its workforce. In 1996, employee contributions to plan premiums were reinstated. Employees who select health plans with premiums above a defined benchmark pay the difference. For example, in 1999, contributions ranged from $0 to $13 per month for an individual employee and from $10 to $45 per month for a full family, depending on choice of plan. The impact of direct cost to employees has been unmistakable. Between 1998 and 1999, 14 percent of members switched health plans. Of that 14 percent almost half moved into one plan where the employee's contribution dropped from $22 to $0 for an individual and from $69 to $10 for a full family. HCA saw this as an indication that members needed additional information so that their coverage decisions could be made both on price and quality. By 2001, the percentage of members who switched plans from the prior year had dropped to just over 10 percent.

The need was equally evident if HCA were to realize its goal of purchasing for value. Quality from the perspective of the consumer could be added to measures of plan clinical quality, solvency, service area, network adequacy, and price. Although not yet fully realized, the HCA's goal is to objectively enter quality into its contracting decisions.

Approach Description

Beginning in 1997 and continuing in 1999 and 2001, the HCA made consumer reports part of its purchasing program. The reports are based on surveys that assess enrollees' experiences with health plans. The model used is from the federally funded Consumer Assessment of Health Plans study (CAHPS™).[6]

The HCA adopted most of the CAHPS 2.0 revisions for its 1999 implementation, which entailed changes to the tools, protocols, and report templates originally introduced as CAHPS 1.0.[7] The 1999 survey asked consumers for information on plan and length of coverage; access to care, including primary and specialist care; provider relationship; utilization; communication with providers and staff; and plan administration. It sought overall ratings of plan, care, and providers and asked about the respondents' health status, demographics, and need for assistance in completing the survey. It also included a set of supplemental CAHPS items asking about chronic conditions, plan complaint resolution, and knowledge of out-of-pocket costs.[8]

The CAHPS questionnaire was adopted by the National Committee for Quality Assurance (NCQA) and thus became the market standard. For 2001, HCA asked plans to survey their members and remit those data to HCA. The results HCA received thus represented a commercial population broader than the HCA-sponsored population, but plan scores did not differ significantly from prior HCA-only scores.

A summary of the evolution of HCA's efforts between 1997 and 2001, many the result of consumer and health plan feedback, is presented in Table 18.1.

Starting in fall 1997, HCA provided consumer reports primarily for enrollees' use in annual open enrollment periods. As of fall 2001, all consumer reports were delivered on-line, and all enrollment changes were required to be entered on-line using a decision support tool that assisted enrollees in selecting their coverage. No printed information was sent to enrollees unless specifically requested. Beyond its primary use by HCA enrollees, there are additional uses of the consumer information. First, we provide health plans with detailed reports of their own consumer feedback, including comparisons to top performers and top priority areas for quality improvement.[9] And second, through the efforts to collect this information, the HCA is building a base of experience to use consumer assessments of plans in its future purchasing decisions.

Table 18.1 Major Changes in HCA Consumer Reporting, 1997–2002.

Category	1997–1998	1999–2000	2001–2002
Population	Public employees and dependents	Public employees, retirees, and dependents	Broad commercial population served by HCA-contracted plans
Protocols	CAHPS 1.0	CAHPS 2.0	NCQA format administered by plans
Administration	Federal project demonstration site	Competitive bid contractor	Plan
Consumer report	Older long version	Newer short version	On-line version
Experiences of people with chronic conditions	Little emphasis	More emphasis	Same as 1999–2000
Experiences of children	Some emphasis	No emphasis	No emphasis
Experiences with plan complaints	No emphasis	Some emphasis	Some emphasis
Required length of time in plan	6 months	12 months	12 months

Evidence of Efficacy

The national CAHPS team conducted a complete evaluation of the initial implementation. Ongoing feedback from evaluation surveys, enrollee focus groups, and plan interviews has reaffirmed HCA's decision to continue. The electronic enrollment tool was a great success, with nearly 17,000 hits and an estimated 10,000 users. These enrollees spent eleven minutes on average using the tool, and 80 percent found it useful and usable. Feedback from prior years indicated that compared to other sources of information, the report was identified as providing the most useful plan information. Plans' acceptance and use of the plan-specific reports for quality improvement are encouraging. Consumers can not only hold plans accountable by "voting with their feet," they can also provide detailed feedback on needed service and quality improvements. In 1999, plans requested access to even more detailed survey results. In 2000 and 2001, HCA increasingly used the results to request quality improvement strategies during contract negotiation, in an effort to keep plans focused on the customer feedback data.

The HCA's intentions for future efforts include (1) partnering with other purchasers to pilot a report using the Foundation for Accountability framework—a consumer-friendly blending of CAHPS data with clinical process and outcomes data, (2) evaluating the feasibility of assessing providers' experiences with health plans, and (3) exploring use of CAHPS at the delivery system level as well as the plan level, given the considerable overlap in provider networks among HCA plans.

Attributes

Adoption of CAHPS makes HCA part of the movement to promote a gold standard for measuring and reporting the performance of plans and delivery systems from the consumers' perspective. Other approaches are either merging with CAHPS (for example, the NCQA Member Satisfaction Survey) or are going by the wayside (for example, homegrown surveys developed by individual purchasers or plans).

The advantages for the HCA of using CAHPS and now NCQA's survey parallel the advantages of having a single national standard and include benchmarking; partnering; and credibility, reliability, and validity. First, a single standard promotes comparisons within and across states or markets, allowing identification of blue-ribbon performers and assessment of lesser-rated plans or systems against these performers. It provides a base of data from which research can identify characteristics of plans and delivery systems most likely to meet consumer needs, thus enhancing the role of consumers in defining the evolving health care system. Second, a single set of tools that can be used by public and private purchasers, health plans, consumers, regulators, accreditors, and advocacy groups affords great opportunity for partnering. Imagine the benefits of a public-private partnership that spreads costs and reduces consumer survey fatigue by collecting and reporting annually on all plans or delivery systems statewide, independent of any specific population, employer, or purchasing group. Finally, the CAHPS-NCQA instrument is continually improved by the best researchers and practitioners in the field, driven by sound scientific principles and user input. The credibility, reliability, and validity of information produced from the tools and protocols are invaluable. Their ready availability encourages the production of consumer information by those who might otherwise be discouraged by lack of resources or expertise.

BARRIERS TO DIFFUSION AND RECOMMENDATIONS

The following comments are not specific to the HCA's approaches but instead address diffusion of these efforts in general.

Commitment

Strong leadership and conviction to stay the course are important. Internal advocates whose commitment is flexible but unwavering are critical. Without that commitment there may not be the political will to withstand and overcome challenges to the need, priority, efficacy, and cost associated with these efforts.

The potential *barrier* is lack of communicated conviction; the *answer* is committed, vocal leadership.

Expectations

Understanding what can and cannot be achieved by these approaches is important to sustaining them over time. The causal link between intervention and behavior or policy goal is not always direct and clean. Setting expectations about desired outcomes and which of these outcomes can be reasonably measured is useful. It is especially important to understand that trying to achieve perfection in one step is limiting.

The potential *barrier* is misplaced expectations; the *answer* is clarity of policy goals and definitions of success.

Health Plans as Stakeholders

For health plans, these initiatives are likely to affect the dollar bottom line—enrollees may come or go depending on survey results, and substantial dollars can move based on relative risk. Plans need to be active advisers and reviewers as approaches are developed, rolled out, and refined.

The potential *barrier* is stakeholder resistance; the *answer,* at least partially, is securing active involvement.

Consumers as Stakeholders

This barrier arises primarily in relation to consumer assessment and reporting. The assumption that consumers must have better information to be more active in health coverage and care decisions may well be true. However, the understanding of what information is needed and how much is needed is elusive. Consumers are overwhelmed with information; they also are overwhelmed with efforts to gather it. Respondents' sense of burden and their cynicism about the applicability of the information are growing.

The potential *barrier* is consumer overload on many levels; the *answers* lie in continued research, public education about "what's in it for me," and partnerships among purchasers to achieve economies and reduce consumer burden.

Technical Complexity

Consumer assessment and risk adjustment are technically complex, involve many policy and implementation decisions, and are still evolving—inspiring uncertainty in even the most dedicated purchaser: Am I doing the right thing? What will be the unintended consequences?

The potential *barrier* is paralysis; the *answer* is "just do it" and, if necessary, buy the expertise to do it.

IMPACTS ON SOCIETY AND LINKS TO CONSUMER-DRIVEN HEALTH CARE

It is not clear how the U.S. health care system will evolve over the next five to ten years. However, it is reasonable to assume that consumers will play a large role in shaping it.[10] Whether it becomes consumer driven or simply consumer focused, the approaches described in this chapter will likely be relevant. Listed here are the policy goals used at HCA to frame its approaches (some goals apply to both approaches, some to only one). We at HCA believe our realization of these goals will facilitate important changes in the market, helping us to remove consumer access and decision-making barriers.

- Promote competition and market efficiency
- Enhance HCA and health plan ability to understand the care and service needs of our population
- Provide a level playing field for consumers and health plans, in which prices reflect quality and efficiency, not risk selection
- Encourage a focus on care management rather than risk management by providing reasonable payment for predictable risk
- Expand the range of tools to use in making value-based decisions
- Inform and educate consumers about information important to their coverage decisions
- Encourage plan accountability through informed consumerism
- Advance the state of knowledge about plan performance measurement, consumer information needs, and health-based risk adjustment

Notes

1. The Washington State Health Care Authority (HCA) is a cabinet-level government agency that purchases health insurance coverage for roughly 439,000 covered lives (nearly 8 percent of the insured state population). These people are enrolled in either the Public Employees Benefits Board (PEBB) program or the Basic Health Plan (BHP) program. The PEBB program covers two groups: public employees and non-Medicare retirees, combined into one risk pool, and Medicare retirees, a separate risk pool. Both pools include spouses and dependents. The BHP program is for low-income working poor and provides reduced premiums for enrollees with incomes at or below 200 percent of federal poverty. Through the Primary Health Care Services (PHCS) program, the HCA also provides grants to community and migrant health care clinics that serve under- and uninsured individuals.

The initiatives described in this chapter apply to the PEBB program. Health-based premium adjustments are made on behalf of the employee and non-Medicare group (about 314,000 individuals). The consumer reporting initiative includes the Medicare retiree group as well.

The HCA coordinates purchasing for PEBB and BHP with the state's Medicaid program, administered by the Department of Social and Health Services' Medical Assistance Administration. Together the programs cover about 1,339,000 individuals (roughly 23 percent of the insured state population). For additional information see the HCA Web site [www.hca.wa.gov].

2. See, for example, Gauthier, A. K., Lamphere, J. A., and Barrand, N. L. "Risk Selection in the Health Care Market: A Workshop Overview." *Inquiry*, 1995, *32*, 14–22; Giacomini, M., Luft, H. S., and Robinson, J. C. "Risk Adjusting Community Rated Health Plan Premiums: A Survey of Risk Assessment Literature and Policy Implications." *Annual Review of Public Health*, 1995, *16*, 401–430; Puchalski, P. J. (ed.). "New Applications for Risk Adjustment." *Inquiry*, 35(2, Entire issue), 1998.

3. This approach description is drawn from Wilson, V. M., Smith, C. A., Hamilton, J. M., and others. "Case Study: The Washington State Health Care Authority." *Inquiry*, 1998, *35*(2), 178–192. See also [http://boat.washington.edu/risk-adjust].

4. Ellis, R. P., Pope, G. C., and Iezzoni, L. I. "Diagnosis-Based Risk Adjustment for Medicare Capitation Payments." *Health Care Financing Review*, 1996, *17*(3), 101–128. See also [www.dxcg.com].

5. Marc E. Provence, director, Office of Health Plan Services, University of Washington Physicians, personal communication to Gary L. Christenson, administrator, Washington State Health Care Authority, Apr. 12, 1999.

6. Weinberger, M. (ed.). "Consumer Assessment of Health Plans Study (CAHPS™)." *Medical Care*, 1999, *37*(3, Supplement).

7. The federal Agency for Health Care Policy and Research (AHCPR) provided prerelease versions of CAHPS 2.0 tools and protocols. Information can be obtained from the AHCPR clearinghouse at 800-358-9295. See also [www.ahcpr.gov].

8. The CAHPS family of surveys includes a set of core surveys (adult, child, adult Medicaid managed care, child Medicaid managed care, Medicare managed care) and sets of supplemental questions for adults and children.

9. The 1997–1998 plan-specific reports included information on the following: background of the survey methodology, instructions for using the results, and summary charts and tables that (1) compared a plan's score to the statewide average and the best scoring plan on each item, (2) identified a plan's problem areas related to low consumer satisfaction, and (3) provided question responses cross-tabulated with respondents' health status, age, gender, race, time in health plan, and high-user status (defined as three or more visits to the plan within six months).

10. See, for example, Coile, R. C. "Anticipating the Millennium: Healthcare Environment Will Be Driven by Consumerism, Cyberhealth, and Co-Opetition." In R. C. Coile Jr., *Millennium Management*. Chicago: Health Administration Press, 1998, chap. 12.

CHAPTER NINETEEN

The Buyers Health Care Action Group

Creating Incentives to Seek the Sick

Ann L. Robinow

T alk about perverse incentives. Today, health plans and providers commit economic suicide when they attract more than their share of sick patients, and improve their bottom line by skimming the better risks. The health insurance industry is organized around this economic reality. Plans with sicker than average enrollees are noncompetitive and unprofitable. And as providers increasingly accept financial risk, they too are driven by this reality. Those with sicker than average patients outspend their capitation dollars or ruin their provider performance profiles, risking bankruptcy or termination from health plan provider panels.

Many of the business practices of health plans, and much of the provider and public discontent with plans, can be traced to this perverse economic incentive. Benefit design and underwriting practices whose purpose is to exclude costly enrollees, and barriers to care through gatekeeping and limited networks, are common, pernicious attempts to deal with adverse selection.

The author would like to acknowledge Barbara O. Johnson, M.P.H., senior consultant, Reden and Anders, Ltd., for her invaluable assistance in the preparation of this chapter and the implementation of the risk-adjustment program described.

BHCAG: CARE SYSTEMS COMPETE FOR PATIENTS

The Buyers Health Care Action Group (BHCAG), a purchasing coalition, organized and owned by forty-seven self-funded employers in and around the Minneapolis-St. Paul area, created a new consumer-driven health care system to reverse this ugly reality.

Responding to a BHCAG request issued late in 1995, Twin Cities providers organized themselves into fourteen provider groups, called *care systems*, distinct from one another at the primary physician level. (An additional ten care systems participate outside the metropolitan area.) Care systems must meet BHCAG standards, including having the ability to meet the full continuum of patient care needs. Essentially every provider in the service area is available through one care system or another. Annually, each care system sets a per capita claim target, or price per member, that assumes standard benefits and an average population. Each employer establishes a defined contribution at no more than the cost of the lowest-cost care system, so that employees pay more for care systems that set higher claim targets. Benefits are identical across all care systems, and all care systems are offered. Employees and their family members may each choose a different care system. They are provided with extensive information on each care system and its physicians, including consumer-derived information on quality and satisfaction, and care system cost (as demonstrated in Table 19.1). During the plan year, dissatisfied enrollees can switch to another system as long as it costs the same or less than their current system.

THE RESULTS

In BHCAG, care systems are accountable to consumers rather than to employers or plans. In its third year, BHCAG data about enrollment patterns clearly showed consumer migration toward lower-cost, better-performing care systems. If all care systems performed at the most efficient level or all enrollees moved to lower-cost care systems, combined employer and employee savings would have approximated 20 percent of total health care costs. Downward price pressure in the setting of claim targets occurred among what were formerly high-cost care systems. These systems include those where the majority of the BHCAG population was enrolled in the past. Illness burden information enabled BHCAG to better understand whether cost increases are caused by changes in the health status of the population or other factors, such as price or utilization patterns. Since 1997, BHCAG has seen increases in per-member per-month costs, but review of the illness mix of the covered population over time demonstrated that this increase has been largely due to an influx of sicker enrollees.

Table 19.1. How Care Systems Compare: Twin Cities Metro Area.

Adult's Care

	How People Rated Their Clinic	How People Rated Their Doctor or Nurse	How Well Doctors Communicate	Getting Referrals and Care	Getting Care Without Long Waits	Courtesy, Respect, and Helpfulness of Office Staff
Cost Group I $						
★Children's Physician Hospital Organization	*This care system provides only children's care.*					
★St. Croix Valley Healthcare						
Wright/Sherburne County Physicians Hospital Organization		*No results — insufficient numbers.*				
Cost Group II $$						
★Access Quality Care System						
Allina Care System						
Aspen						
Fairview Physician Associates						
Family HealthServices Minnesota, P.A.						
★HealthEast Care System						
Hennepin Faculty Associates						
Minnesota HealthCare Network						
North Physicians Health Organization						
★Park Nicollet/Methodist/ HealthSystem Minnesota						
Cost Group III $$$						
HealthPartners Regional Affiliated						
HealthPartners Medical Group						
University of Minnesota Physicians Care System	*No results — care system is new.*					

Children's Care

	How Parents Rated Their Children's Clinic	How Parents Rated Their Children's Doctor or Nurse	How Well Doctors Communicate	Getting Referrals and Care	Getting Care Without Long Waits	Courtesy, Respect, and Helpfulness of Office Staff
Cost Group I $						
★Children's Physician Hospital Organization						
★St. Croix Valley Healthcare						
Wright/Sherburne County Physicians Hospital Organization		*No results — insufficient numbers.*				
Cost Group II $$						
★Access Quality Care System						
Allina Care System						
Aspen						
Fairview Physician Associates						
Family HealthServices Minnesota, P.A.						
★HealthEast Care System		*No results — insufficient numbers.*				
Hennepin Faculty Associates						
Minnesota HealthCare Network						
North Physicians Health Organization						
★Park Nicollet/Methodist/ HealthSystem Minnesota						
Cost Group III $$$						
HealthPartners Regional Affiliated						
HealthPartners Medical Group						
University of Minnesota Physicians Care System	*No results — care system is new.*					

The symbols on this summary chart show the results of statistical tests that compared the score for each Care System to the average score for all all Care Systems in the Twin Cities metro area in this survey. They show which care systems scored better or worse than the survey average for each topic, but they don't give the actual scores.

■■■ **better** than the average score for all Care Systems in the Twin Cities metro area in this survey.
■■ **about the same as** the average score for all Care Systems in the Twin Cities metro area in this survey.
■ **worst** than the average score for all Care Systems in the Twin Cities metro area in this survey.

The symbols tell you which Care Systems scored better or worse than the survey average for each topic, but they don't give you the actual scores.
★Quality Award Winner

Note: The symbols show the results of statistical tests that compared the score for each care system to the average score for all care systems in the Twin Cities metro area in this survey. They show which care systems scored better or worse than the survey average for each topic, but they don't give the actual scores.

Preliminary analysis indicates that new hires by BHCAG employers are approximately 20 percent sicker than new hires in prior years, and enrollees who have migrated into the BHCAG program from other plans have been sicker than existing enrollees. (This may be a result of very low rates of unemployment in the community, and calls for further analysis.) Many more individuals move in and out of this program during the course of the year than "snapshot" looks at total enrollment would indicate. (Evaluations of plans and providers in every market are missing important information and are likely to draw erroneous conclusions when they evaluate changes in cost and utilization without understanding corresponding changes in the covered population.) When BHCAG includes this increase in illness burden in its population in its calculations, the four-year actual and projected rate of cost increase through 2000 is running 4 to 5 percent less than benchmark increases for health plans and other large purchasers in this market. Excluding increases resulting from this change in illness burden, our four-year trend is projected to run approximately 5 percent per year.

PROVIDER REIMBURSEMENT AND RISK ADJUSTMENT

As enrollees receive care from their designated care system, providers submit claims to a common administrator. Claims are paid on a fee-for-service basis from the account of the enrollee's employer. The fee level paid is determined by a quarterly comparison of the actual financial performance of each care system to the claim target that was set by that system. As part of this comparison, the illness burden of each care system's enrollee population is measured. Care systems attracting sicker patients are expected to incur more cost; healthier patients should cost less, and claim targets are adjusted accordingly. Each quarter, care systems whose costs were less than their risk-adjusted claim target are rewarded. Their fees are raised to a higher fee schedule for the subsequent quarter. Conversely, care systems whose costs exceeded their risk-adjusted target are punished. They are paid at a lower fee schedule (see Table 19.2). Thus care systems that deliver care efficiently, after consideration of patients' needs, are paid more for each service.

Table 19.2. Sample Calculation of Quarterly Fee Schedule Changes.

Care System	Claim Target	% of Average Illness Burden	Risk-Adjusted Claim Target	Actual Claims	% Fee Change for Next Quarter
A	$100.00	88%	$88.00	$95.00	−8%
B	100.00	100	100.00	95.00	5
C	95.00	105	99.75	100.00	0
D	95.00	120	114.00	110.00	4

VARIATION IN ILLNESS BURDEN

Fair and accurate calculation of the illness burden for each care system is critical to creating the right incentives in this payment model. BHCAG uses a diagnosis-based method that involves *adjusted clinical groups* (ACGs), a method developed at Johns Hopkins University.[1] The illness burden is based on the diagnoses of each member. Each member is assigned to one of 105 ACG groups with similar expected resource requirements. Each care system's mix of enrollees is compared to BHCAG's overall distribution to determine that system's illness burden. (In determining illness burden, the impact of catastrophic claims, defined as 90 per cent of the cost over $30,000 for inpatient services or over $10,000 for professional or drug costs per enrollee per twelve months, is excluded.) Each care system's population is evaluated retrospectively using the diagnosis data submitted with claims for the same time period for which costs are being evaluated.

BHCAG data show that incentives to avoid risk are overwhelming in the absence of risk adjustment. Variation in illness burden among care systems is large and not explained by age and sex mix. The range of the illness burden among metro area care systems 1998 was from 12 percent healthier than average (a windfall under a non-risk-adjusted model) to 15 percent sicker than average, after excluding catastrophic claims (see Figure 19.1).

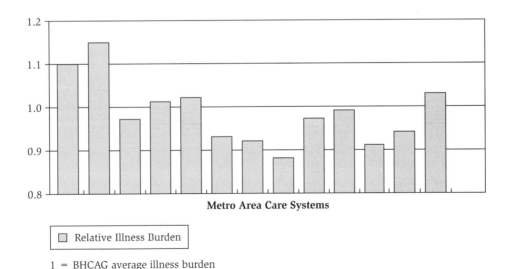

Metro Area Care Systems

☐ Relative Illness Burden

1 = BHCAG average illness burden

Values exclude 90% of catastrophic claims over $30K inpatient, $10K professional or Rx

Figure 19.1. Illness Burden Variation Among Metro Area Enrollee Populations.

BETTER INCENTIVES FOR ACCESS AND CARE

The BHCAG purchasing and reimbursement model improves incentives by removing providers' risk in relation to the illness burden of their patient populations while optimizing reimbursement levels for judicious resource use. More revenue comes with sicker patients. In addition, because care often results in lower costs (such as reduced admissions for well-managed asthma and diabetes) and because providers are rewarded for this, they are motivated to place additional emphasis on care processes and outcomes.

With this system, providers are not punished for costs in excess of their target due to their enrollees' illness burden. In addition, they do not retrospectively repay costs in excess of their target, but future fee levels are reduced. This reduces the incentive to skimp on care and the requirement for establishing solvency funds. They also need not consolidate to achieve very large patient populations across which risk can be spread. Because they do not need to be geographically dispersed or to serve every type of patient, care systems can choose to be smaller or to focus on their strengths. (Several BHCAG care systems have focused on a particular geographical area, and one care system serves only children.) With the employer as the insurer, if a provider system fails, employees are never left without coverage.

THE REAL PROMISE OF MANAGED CARE

As is typical of most patient populations, more than 80 percent of BHCAG's claims are incurred by 21 percent of the population. Changes in care processes to improve outcomes and resource use for this segment of the population offer the biggest potential returns. Achieving these improvements requires systemwide changes in care processes, or truly *managed* care. Without broad implementation of risk-adjusted payment, plans and providers who excel in the management of these patients cannot prosper because they will attract sicker patients but not the necessary additional dollars. Risk adjustment by a subset of purchasers or payers is insufficient to change overall market incentives. With appropriate risk adjustment throughout the market, the best plans and providers should seek to provide excellent care to the sickest patients.

BARRIERS TO IMPLEMENTATION

Individual plans or providers cannot drive illness burden payment adjustments because budget neutrality in risk adjustment always creates financial winners and losers. Large purchasers, such as state and federal governments, purchasing coalitions, or legislators must require and oversee the process. Although risk-adjustment efforts now are performed by states across health plans for their Medicaid populations, these efforts do not consider illness burden variation among risk-taking providers.

The challenges in implementing risk adjustment are considerable. The technical expertise required to design and implement risk-adjustment approaches is not widely available, and risk-adjustment implementation is so novel that there is little experience to draw on. The several accepted technologies have only recently moved from academia into actual practice. Each technology can be used in multiple defensible ways, but differences in applications create confusion and credibility problems. Not surprisingly, those who have implemented risk-adjusted payments continue to fine-tune their programs as more is learned.

Some have questioned the adequacy of risk-assessment technologies for explaining differences in the cost of care. Studies of diagnosis-based technologies show these technologies have superior explanatory power when compared to the traditional risk adjusters, age and sex variation, especially when populations rather than individuals are evaluated.[2] Nevertheless, no risk adjuster can be expected to explain all cost differences, because other differences exist, such as unit price and practice patterns.[3] (Indeed in the unlikely case that all cost difference could be explained by illness burden variation, the role of managed care could be limited to price negotiation.)

Primary inpatient diagnosis-based risk adjustment is phased in for Medicare plans. Consequently, the industry is paying close attention to the technology and data requirements for risk adjustment and is starting to consider the change in economic incentives it will create. For example, Medicare plans that have achieved profitability by avoiding risk will need to design new strategies for managing cost when risk adjustment is fully implemented. Medicare's risk adjusters widely recognized as inadequate but realistic given the dearth of available ambulatory data. (Any provider now billing a Medicare fiscal intermediary must provide procedure and diagnosis codes on claims. Despite massive data systems tracking cash transactions, not all plans have developed the capacity to capture and analyze these procedure and diagnosis data. One wonders about the ability of plans to manage care without such data.)

In contrast, since its inception in 1993, BHCAG has required providers seeking payment to submit claims, and these claims must include procedure and diagnosis codes, both inpatient and ambulatory. This rich database is central to BHCAG's ability to risk-adjust with strong provider support. Unlike capitation arrangements, where there is no incentive to submit claims, linkage of payment to data submission results in BHCAG's having the data needed to support risk adjustment.

RISK ADJUSTMENT AND A CONSUMER-DRIVEN HEALTH CARE SYSTEM

Informed consumers should demand risk adjustment to correct the prevailing incentives against the sick. Risk adjustment is an essential step to improving the health care marketplace and providing real patient protection. A market that rewards providers and plans who attract the sick and deliver excellent care will create the right incentives to fundamentally improve how care is managed.

BHCAG and others have demonstrated that risk adjustment is possible. Political will is necessary to move the rest of the market.

Notes

1. Weiner, J. P., Starfield, B. H., Steinwachs, D. M., and Mumford, L. M. "Development and Application of a Population-Oriented Measure of Ambulatory Care Case-Mix." *Medical Care,* 1991, *29*(5), 452–472.

2. Fowles, J. B., and others. "Taking Health Status into Account When Setting Capitation Rates: A Comparison of Risk Adjustment Methods." *Journal of the American Medical Association,* Oct. 23–30, 1996, *276,* 1316–1321.

3. Dartmouth Medical School, The Center for the Evaluative Clinical Sciences. *The Dartmouth Atlas of Health Care.* (J. Wennberg and others, eds.) Chicago: America Hospital Publishing, 1998, p. 3.

CHAPTER TWENTY

An Insurance CEO's Perspective on Consumer-Driven Health Care

Leonard D. Schaeffer

Twenty-five years ago no one talked about the need for consumer-driven health care. We thought that we had it. Most Americans were enrolled in policies with indemnity coverage that gave them unlimited choice of physicians and ready access to specialty care. Medical inflation was not a concern, and for the most part, only the "kooks" in California and "socialists" in Minnesota were experimenting with health maintenance organizations (HMOs). Aside from the occasional egregious malpractice case, Americans equated choice of provider with quality care, and the consumer reigned supreme.

However, the environment has changed—radically. Exacerbated by the growth of third-party payers, including government, and the proliferation of new technologies and pharmaceutical advances, consumption of health care goods and services increased. Medical inflation surged. Health care coverage became increasingly less affordable for individuals and third-party payers. HMOs and managed care, once considered alternative systems of care, became mainstream as employers aggressively pushed for lower rates of premium increase.

Those of us in the health industry understood the need for cost control and predicted the growth in managed care. But we did not fully anticipate the impact of this paradigm shift on individual consumer perceptions, where high expectations and limited resources would collide. As the old approach to consumer-driven health care, framed by unfettered access and excess consumption, became unaffordable, new choice-reducing features such as provider networks, physician gatekeepers, and an emphasis on coordination of appropriate care forced Americans to make health plan choices with economic and access consequences. Simply put, many did not like it.

In this country's market economy a new definition of consumer-driven health care, consistent with a managed care framework, is needed. Business strategies—like those at WellPoint Health Network, where I am CEO—that offer a broad range of consumer-focused products are helping to shape that definition.

THE HEALTH SECURITY MODEL

Today, premiums for health insurance, driven by underlying medical costs, are generally rising at more than twice the overall inflation rate. We in this country have the best medical system in the world, yet it is increasingly unaffordable. The challenge for health insurers is to mitigate the increased cost of insurance while recognizing the consumer's need for choice.

WellPoint has responded to this challenge by adopting a new model that redefines the role of traditional insurance. Our model sets forth a *health security company* that is committed to providing health security by offering a choice of quality, branded health and related financial services to meet the changing expectations of individuals, families, and their sponsors throughout a lifelong relationship. *Security* is not just about *insuring* consumers through an array of products that reflects their preferences but about *assuring* consumers that the organization financing their care is fiscally sound, will provide affordable products over time, and will help them make choices as they navigate the health care system. Health security companies focus on three related areas—innovative health plan design, quality improvement through collaboration with physicians and hospitals, and programs that help members use the health care system effectively. In this chapter the emphasis is on the ways an understanding of today's "new" consumer—who has more access to health care information, more disposable income, and more experience with computers—is shaping the health plans of tomorrow. (Figure 20.1 summarizes the differences between the health security model and earlier health care plan models.)

CONSUMER-FOCUSED PRODUCTS

In our country's employer-based health care system, there are two primary customers, the employer-payer and the employee. However, each has different needs and expectations. Employers prefer closed-panel HMOs, under the assumption that these plans maximize cost controls by limiting access. Employees, in contrast, prefer coverage plans with provider choice and have been shielded from the actual costs of care because their employers generally pay a

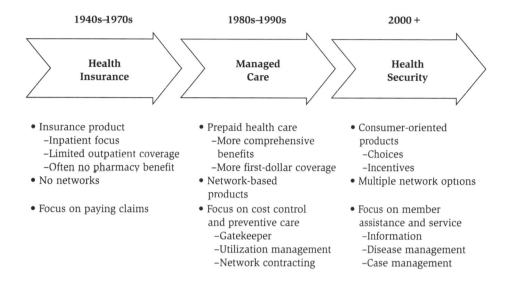

Figure 20.1. Three Models: Health Insurance, Managed Care, and Health Security.
Source: Wellpoint Health Network.

significant portion of the premium. The challenge for insurers is to design health care products that meet the needs of both employers and employees.

It is not sufficient to keep costs down. The demand for flexibility and choice is too great to be ignored. However, health insurance is not merely another consumer good or service. It is distinct from other consumer items because it has a relationship to a person's physical well-being. Consumers cannot exchange their physical health the way they might return a faulty hair dryer. Consequently, it is imperative that consumers be given as much control over decisions affecting their health as possible, from decisions about cost sharing to the choice of provider. In a voluntary environment this approach will not only help to satisfy the needs of current members but also help to attract new members, thereby reducing the ranks of the uninsured.

WellPoint has always focused on offering choice through various types of open-access PPOs, traditional HMOs, and hybrid products that combine the best features of both. Currently, a minority (about 28 percent) of our members are enrolled in an HMO product, and the rest are in open-access, network-based products. They benefit not only from the contractual relationship we have with health care professionals—that is, they get a better price—but also from their ability to control many aspects of their own health care. They choose their own doctors and hospitals, and they make these decisions based on what they believe is best for themselves and their families.

Consumer desire for choice and control has driven our product development efforts. We spend significant time and resources identifying the issues that motivate consumers and influence their health care purchasing decisions. We amplify our experience in selling a variety of products to individuals with extensive market-based research. As a result, we have been able to formulate a comprehensive portrait of key product features that motivate health care purchasers.

We have identified consumers with three distinct price purchase preferences: low, medium, and high. A low-price purchaser is likely to have limited discretionary income and may also be currently uninsured. A medium-price purchaser may want more extensive health coverage but still remains very price sensitive and faces a variety of competitive coverage options. Members of this group look for maximum dollar value in their benefits. The high-price buyer is willing and able to pay for more comprehensive coverage. In our focus groups we also discovered that most people's perception of the cost of coverage is far greater than the actual price. When they are informed of the real cost, their interest in purchasing grows. When they are also given the opportunity to choose their own provider and the level of financial protection that is right for them, their incentive to purchase coverage is maximized.

Given these factors, we introduced a new version of our PlanScape PPO program in California that reduced monthly premiums for nearly half a million members while maintaining choice and flexibility. This product was developed specifically in response to the increasing number of Californians dropping or losing their individual health coverage in the face of rising premiums. The new PlanScape offers a range of options, enabling members to make choices based on their individual financial and health care needs. They can choose a plan with more cost sharing at a lower premium, or they can pay a higher premium for coverage requiring lower out-of-pocket charges for care. Each option provides 100 percent cost coverage for eligible services received from participating physicians, hospitals, and other clinicians up to $5 million, after the initial out-of-pocket threshold is met. The amount of the threshold is selected by the member, as reflected in the premium level. Costs incurred below the threshold are financed by a wide choice of cost-sharing arrangements, such as deductibles and copays.

Consumers today are better informed about health care in general and thus are becoming even savvier about how and where their health care dollars are spent. In 1999, more than 43 percent of Americans used the Internet to search for health care information. Physicians often talk about patients who come to their offices with reams of paper they have downloaded about their particular illness or disease. This growing interest in personal health care has created a more analytical, sophisticated, and demanding consumer. Insurers must understand that this interest is not based solely on cost but also on a strong desire to take personal control over decisions relating to the health care services received, who provides them, and the appropriate level of financial security.

The consumer revolution means that consumers are going to be active participants in their health care by seeking information, expecting treatment options, and participating in the decision-making process with their health professionals. By adopting a health security approach, insurers can give consumers the control they want while meeting the needs of diverse payers and members and helping to reduce the number of uninsured.

CHAPTER TWENTY-ONE

An Alternative to Managed Care

A European Perspective on Informed Choice

Bruno L. Holthof

Increased health care spending has been of worldwide concern for at least two decades. In response, major health care payers (governments and insurance companies) started putting controls on the patient-physician interaction: *managed care* was born. Most managed care initiatives reduce the choices available to patients by restricting patients' use of health care services and imposing guidelines on physicians. These limits have created dissatisfaction among patients as well as among physicians.

This chapter describes how in Europe, as well as in the United States, increased choice for patients, if they are supplied with the right information, can lead to a more productive health care system. *Informed choice* could become an alternative to managed care.

IS MANAGED CARE REACHING ITS LIMITS?

In the 1990s, managed care was embraced in the United States and Europe. Between 1990 and 1995, the segment of insured people in the United States enrolled in a managed care plan grew to over 50 percent of the total. During this period, hospital admissions dropped by 6 percent and patient days per capita decreased by 16 percent from their 1990 level. Encouraged by these apparent successes in the United States, European governments introduced managed care into their health care systems. They transformed administrative institutions into managed care organizations with financial incentives to manage medical costs.

In the United Kingdom health care budgets were allocated to regional health authorities that bought health care services for their patients. These authorities encouraged many innovations: for example, they supported the development of GP (general practitioner) Fundholding Practices, the equivalent of capitated physician groups in the United States. In Germany, the government introduced competition between the *Krankenkassen* ("sick funds"). Before the reforms the *Krankenkassen* charged a premium to their captive membership to cover health care costs (expressed as a percentage of salary to ensure solidarity). After the reforms members could freely select their *Krankenkassen*, which led to higher enrollments at those that charged lower premiums. To charge lower premiums, *Krankenkassen* had to start managing medical costs.

Growing Patient and Physician Dissatisfaction

Unfortunately, most managed care initiatives in the United States and Europe require some form of restriction in provider choice for the patient. The Netherlands, for example, requires an obligatory enrollment with a general practitioner who acts as a gatekeeper. Swiss insurance companies charge lower premiums for enrollees in a plan that restricts provider choice. Patients, however, do not like a restriction of choice. A study conducted within a large health maintenance organization in northern California compared the satisfaction level of patients who could choose their doctors to that of patients who were assigned to specific doctors. Among 10,205 respondents, the patients who chose their doctors were 16 to 20 percent more likely than those assigned to specific doctors to rate their satisfaction level as "excellent" or "very good".[1]

Dissatisfaction with lack of choice explains the shift of enrollment from restrictive plans to nonrestrictive plans observed in the United States. In 1992, only 5 percent of all insured employees were covered by nonrestrictive plans. By 1996, this number had grown to about 20 percent. Some insurers, such as the Oxford Health Plan, have more than 80 percent of their members in nonrestrictive plans.[2]

Managed care has also not been popular in Europe. Switzerland, for example, was one of the European countries that, in 1966, introduced managed care most aggressively. Swiss consumers who enrolled in a managed care plan could obtain substantial reductions in their premiums, on the order of 10 to 20 percent. Nevertheless, in a 1999 report, only 6 percent of the population had selected a managed care solution.[3]

Marginal Improvements in Productivity

To make things worse, payers began to realize that physician behavior has not changed with the change in plan approach. Savings claimed by managed care organizations can often be attributed to an organization's (1) better risk selection of insured patients, (2) selection of physicians who already practice in cost-effective ways, or (3) receipt of discounts for services rendered in return for higher patient volumes. None of these three factors will improve the overall productivity of the health care sector (when productivity is defined as outcomes achieved divided by inputs required). For example, patients registered with the Wiedikon group in Switzerland used significantly fewer resources than a control group with the same risk profile: 36 percent fewer admissions, 16 percent shorter average length of stay in hospital, and 60 percent lower drug costs. Although these statistics imply significant savings, the differences were most likely explained by Wiedikon's selection of physicians with cost-effective practice behavior from the start.[4]

SIGNS OF AN EMERGING MODEL: INFORMED CHOICE

With increasing patient and physician dissatisfaction and cost shifting rather than cost savings, is managed care not reaching its limits? There are signs of an emerging model in which the patient plays a more important role in the struggle for more productive health care. It appears that when consumers are given appropriate information and an incentive, they make rational trade-offs among different health care offerings. The rapid evolution in information technology and information supply supports this emerging consumerism.

Increased Availability of Data

Advances in information technology and growing consumer demand will overcome the barriers that have traditionally prohibited the widespread provision of comparative information. Lack of data has been and still is a barrier to transparent and fair outcome comparisons among health care providers. For example, tertiary care hospitals, which treat sicker patients overall than other hospitals, are more likely to encounter poor outcomes or complications. A fair comparison of their performance would incorporate the severity of illness of their patients. Yet today's medical registration systems—often lacking, for example, diagnostic coding for care given in outpatient settings—are not yet sufficiently complete to allow for comprehensive risk adjustment. Reliable outcome comparisons all too often require expensive, ad hoc scientific studies that collect the required data from the medical records.

A second barrier is the reliability of the available data. Most data registration systems are used for reimbursement purposes. As illustrated by *DRG creep* (the practice in U.S. hospitals of using more complex DRG codes to obtain higher Medicare reimbursement), data registration systems are usually optimized to obtain high reimbursement. As a consequence, they may not always reflect underlying economic and clinical conditions.

Going forward, advances in information technology will likely allow collection of the required data on a broader scale. Breakthroughs in voice recognition software and new user interfaces should reduce the technical barriers to quick data entry. With increased connectivity and advances in relational databases and statistical techniques, the transmission and analyses of these data will also become easier. From a technical viewpoint the creation of large databases will ease the extraction of comparative performance information.

These advances in information technology will of course not suffice to improve the quality of comparative performance data. Physicians will have to be motivated to register correct medical information. In a managed care environment this motivation does not currently exist, as is shown by the Sésam Vitale initiative in France. A patient card, created by the French government and Social Security, was supposed to track all medical information (diagnoses, interventions) for each patient. However, by 1999, several years after launching the initiative, thirty million cards had been produced and distributed but fewer than eight hundred doctors were using the system. The major reason for this failure appears to be the doctors' reluctance to reveal patients' medical information. In addition, patient associations have been concerned that patients do not have direct access to their personal information and have wondered if the only purpose for this information is to identify patients who are outliers in medical consumption.[5]

As in this example, in a managed care environment patients and physicians do not see any benefit in proposed improvements in information systems. On the contrary they perceive them as cost-containment and control tools. In an informed choice environment this trend would likely be reversed. Increasingly, assertive consumers will demand transparent information output from their providers.

As illustrated by the following examples the pressure for good comparative information seems to be rising. In 1997 in the Netherlands, *Elsevier,* a weekly magazine, published rankings for major Dutch hospitals, examining medical capability, patient service, and reputation.[6] In France a hospital guide book ranked the country's hospitals—an initiative comparable to the famous *Guide Michelin* with its reviews of restaurants. The book was edited by three doctors in collaboration with the journal *Sciences et Avenir.*[7] The rankings displayed adjusted death rates and other indicators by specialty and by region. Judging by the extensive national media coverage that followed the book's publication, the French population is eager to learn such outcomes. The explosion of visits to medical Web sites also demonstrates that patients are indeed becoming increasingly educated and informed.

Given Information, Patients Make Good Trade-Offs

Governments and employers traditionally have been responsible for buying health care on behalf of their citizens and employees, respectively. They assumed this responsibility because they felt consumers would not be able to buy health care efficiently given the large asymmetry in the information held by consumers and providers and given the vulnerability of sick people.

However, if reliable comparative performance data on providers become available, this information asymmetry will decrease. In such cases, and when given incentives to do so, patients can make good trade-offs in buying health care services, as demonstrated by a number of ongoing experiments.

In 1999, the Netherlands planned to expand an experiment with the PGB (*persoonsgebonden budget*), a system in which individuals receive a personal budget of funds that they can spend freely to buy home care or care for the mentally handicapped. They can spend their budget to buy services from professional providers and pay them a fee for each service provided, or they can pay family members or friends who are willing to take care of them. In 1998, 7,500 patients participated—5,400 bought home care services and 2,100 bought support for the mentally handicapped. The total budget spent by these patients in 1998 was Dfl220 million (about US$111 million). PGB encouraged consumers to take the initiative, make choices on how care should be delivered, become price conscious, and start to evaluate the outcomes of care provision. For assistance in buying care, consumers could seek the advice of care brokers. For mentally handicapped care, for example, the Social Pedagogic Services (SPDs) included care brokerage in its service offering.[8]

France provides another example of consumers making health care buying decisions. In France, individuals typically have had two payers, the Social Security (government) and a complementary private insurance (*mutuelle*). For a birth, for example, the mother was reimbursed a minimum amount by Social Security. Private insurance would cover the remainder, often allocating a fixed sum for a delivery (ranging from F3,000 to F5,000 depending on the insurer). The average exchange rate in 2001 for French francs to U.S. dollars was .13667. Most parents shopped around for the best quality in a lower-cost provider because they knew that they could keep whatever money was left over from this fixed payment.

Similarly, in 1998, CNP, one of the major payer organizations in France, started an experiment with 50,000 of its members. It created a call center that collects and updates the prices of routine treatments in dental and optical specialties. When a member calls, CNP provides the patient with price comparison and alternative provider choice information free of charge. Since its inception in 1998, the call center has answered more than 30,000 calls and provided 3,000 price quotes. The cost of an average tooth filling for example has been reduced by 20 percent. This service has been successful because for dental or optical treatments neither the Social Security nor the *mutuelle* will typically reimburse 100 percent of the cost. Patients have to pay the difference out of their own pocket and therefore have an incentive to shop around.[9] These examples illustrate that when patients have the right information combined with an incentive to use it, they shop to select a provider for health care services.

LONG-TERM VISION: HEALTH CARE SYSTEMS BASED ON INDIVIDUAL BUDGETS

Because of cultural and ideological differences, differences among national health care financing systems are likely to persist. Economic pressures, however, will demand higher productivity levels in any health care system. Consumer-oriented organization of health care as described in this chapter could provide a better solution than managed care. Allocation of health care budgets to consumers will create health care markets focused on improving performance, even when individual countries still decide to fund their health care systems in different ways.

Despite Differences in Funding . . .

Discussions about the funding of the health care expenditures are usually very political because they imply choices about access and equity. In the past, Europe has opted mainly for public systems with universal coverage and for solidarity by collecting funds via taxes or social security contributions. The United States has opted for a mixed private and public system with different funding mechanisms (employee benefit programs and tax-funded government programs, respectively). Significant differences in the ways countries decide to fund their health care systems will likely remain, reflecting different viewpoints on taxation and income redistribution and on the role of government in financing health care.

. . . Consumer Budgets Could Be the Basis for Managing Expenditures

Nevertheless, regardless of the funding system, governments could base the expenditures side of their health care systems on the free but informed choice of health care consumers. For the long term they could calculate a fair health care budget that would enable each citizen to obtain minimum health care coverage. This budget would take into account each person's risk profile. Older and sicker people would be entitled to more money than younger and healthier individuals. With that budget, consumers could shop around for health care, though they would have to buy at least minimum health care coverage, with the minimum package defined by the government.

Certain parts or principles of such a system are already being applied in some countries. In Switzerland, for example, the premiums of payer organizations have been adjusted by the government based on the total risk profile of each organization's pool of patients. A 1999 report noted that Sanitas, for example, which had an unfavorable rate of high-risk patients, received 23 percent of its funds from the government, whereas Swica, which had a higher proportion of low-risk patients, obtained only 1 percent of its funds from the government.[10] A similar risk adjustment approach has been used for the regional health authorities in the United Kingdom. The poor, ill, and old North West region received 21 percent more funds per capita than the rich, young, and prosperous Anglia and Oxford regions.[11] The importance of good risk-adjustment formulas is illustrated by the German case. The *Krankenkassen* in Germany are risk-adjusted only on the basis of age and gender. A *Krankenkassen* with lower-risk patients within each age and sex group could offer a more attractive premium and hence receives an unfair competitive advantage.

Although risk-adjusted budgets are difficult to calculate, experience with this method of resource allocation exists in several European countries and could be refined over time as more accurate and complete electronic medical records become available.

CONCLUSION

Economic imperatives require increases in health care productivity. This implies encouraging better outcomes with the same resources or similar outcomes with fewer resources. Informed choice could be the driving force for more entrepreneurship and innovation in both the United States and Europe. Entrepreneurs could tap into all available technologies to create broad health care offerings for consumers. These consumers could then call on health care brokers to find matches for their individual preferences within this range of offerings. Advances in information technology will create the required transparency in the performance of health care providers. At the same time, these advances will allow the calculation of fair consumer budgets that will create the market.

Notes

1. Schmittdiel, J., Seby, J. V., Grumbach, K., and Quesenberry, C. P., Jr. "Choice of Physician and Patient Satisfaction in a Health Maintenance Organization." *Journal of the American Medical Association*, Nov. 19, 1997, *278*, pp. 1596-1599.

2. Kleinke, J. D. "Power to the Patient." *Modern Healthcare*, Feb. 23, 1998, p. 66.

3. "Die Mündiger bürger sollen selber wählen." *Basler Zeitung*, Apr. 13, 1999, pp. 338–339.

4. McKinsey & Company. Internal research.

5. Bui, D., and Mitrofanoff, K. "Santé: Le grand gaspillage" (Health: The great waste). *Challenges*, Apr. 1999.

6. Hen, P. de. "De beste ziekenhuizen" (The best hospitals). *Elsevier*, Sept. 5, 1998, pp. 115–130.

7. Houdart, P., Vincent, J., and Malye, F. "Le guide des hopitaux" (The guide to hospitals). Le Pre aux Clers: *Sciences et Aventir,* 1998.

8. Driest, P., and Weekers, S. "Het persoonsgebonden budget: Breekijzer of tijdelijke regeling?" Utrecht: Nederlands Instituut voor Zorg en Welzijn, 1998.

9. Bonnard, J. "Santé: De nouvelles pistes pour diminuer les dépenses" (Health: New approaches to reducing expenses). *Le Figaro,* Apr. 6, 1999.

10. "Risk compensation in Swiss health insurance." *Handelszeitung,* May 5, 1999.

11. United Kingdom. HM Treasury. *Supply Estimates for England, Wales and Scotland.* London: HM Treasury.

CHAPTER TWENTY-TWO

Medical Savings Accounts and Health Care Financing in South Africa

Shaun Matisonn

South Africa has made tremendous progress in the past few years in creating a nonracial democracy. Throughout this period all facets of the country have been forced to respond to rapid change and restructuring. The health care sector has proved no exception. South Africa has a population of approximately 43.5 million people and a GDP of $100 billion. Average annual income levels are disproportionately split between the various race groups, with the average white family earning substantially more than what the average black family earns.[1] This income inequality continues in the health care sector, where of the total health care expenditure of $8 billion (8 percent of GDP), 45 percent is allocated to the public sector to provide health care to 83 percent of the population. The remaining 17 percent of the population consumes, through the private sector, 55 percent of the funds spent on health care.[2]

This imbalance in spending has led to state-of-the-art health care provision for those individuals who can afford private insurance and lower and declining standards for those in the public sector. The continued pressure for high-quality health care in the private sector has led to rampant inflation in insurance contributions. Over the last fifteen years, contributions as a percentage of payroll have grown from an average of 2 percent to almost 17 percent.[3]

These high levels of medical inflation have forced employers and consumers to look for alternative solutions in the delivery of private health insurance.

MSA-BASED PRODUCTS

Until recently, traditional private health insurance has always been provided on a fee-for-service, indemnity basis, with little intervention from the funder and carte blanche for the consumer. To bring more discipline to these arrangements, a number of insurance companies, including Discovery Health, where I am head of risk management, have entered the market with alternative products.

The core of the Discovery Health product design is a medical savings account (MSA), a tax-deductible health care account that allows consumers to allocate funds for their health care spending. If these funds are not spent, the consumer saves them. Previously any unused health plan benefits were lost in future years, and so rational consumers made sure that benefits were used in the current year. The MSA encourages a radical departure from the traditional use-it-or-lose-it mentality of local consumers, a mentality exemplified in the history of low consumer savings in South Africa.

A crucial point is that the MSA does not cover all health care expenses. In its design a distinction was made between discretionary expenses, which are not insured, and nondiscretionary expenses, which are insured. Discretionary expenses were defined costs for events such as day-to-day primary care visits, spectacles, dental visits, and so forth. Nondiscretionary expenses were defined as costs for hospitalization for such problems as trauma or surgery and medication for such chronic conditions as diabetes. This distinction creates an environment where the individual is fully insured for more costly, random events and is in control of low-cost, manageable expenses. Included in the coverage for discretionary, or largely outpatient, expenditure is an annual deductible. Once the individual's cumulative discretionary expenses have exceeded the deductible, the person is covered for health care expenses above that amount. This form of coverage assumes that a need for a large amount of discretionary health care starts to become nondiscretionary and that the individual should be insured against such an eventuality.

The distinction between discretionary and nondiscretionary expenditure allows flexibility in the coverage of different treatments. A classic example is Viagra, Pfizer's erectile dysfunction pill. Viagra raises two important questions for health insurers: first, Should this pill be covered? and, second, If it is covered how much coverage should be given? The importance of these questions is enhanced by the high cost associated with Viagra: roughly half of all men aged forty to seventy experience erectile dysfunction and the cost of a pill is approximately $5 to $10 per use. Traditional insurance arrangements struggle to answer coverage questions like these, but the MSA deals with this problem neatly. In Discovery Health's opinion, Viagra is used for lifestyle enhancement as opposed to life sustainment and therefore is clearly a discretionary expenditure. It is thus covered by the MSA's discretionary funds. The MSA therefore gives consumers the freedom to choose what is most suitable for them in terms of coverage and usage, without affecting the total costs to other consumers.

The average health plan contribution is approximately $175 per month, of which 35 percent, or $61.25, is paid into the MSA. This provides an annual MSA amount of $735. The average deductible is $950. The entire contribution is treated the same from a tax perspective. Two-thirds of the contribution is tax deductible, in an environment with marginal tax rates equal to 42 percent. Different companies adopt different approaches to the investment of unused savings balances. Discovery Health pays a rate of interest roughly equal to the CPI on savings balances below $950 and then offers far higher returns on higher balances. Currently individuals can withdraw the savings balances only through contribution holidays or on withdrawal from the health plan. They can also transfer them to another carrier when MSAs are part of the new carrier's benefit design.

The use of many traditional managed care techniques, such as utilization management and provider profiling, is confined to the management of nondiscretionary expenditure. The application of these techniques often differs from that in the United States, primarily because of the shortage of medical practitioners, particularly specialists, in the South African market. South Africa has an average of approximately 1 doctor to every 2,500 patients, compared to 1 doctor to every 250 patients in the United States, and the ratio of primary care practitioners to specialists in South Africa is approximately 75:25 compared to 60:40 in the United States.[4] This relative undersupply prevents funders from contracting at discounts with limited segments of the medical community.

THE IMPACT OF MSAS ON THE SOUTH AFRICAN MARKET

The South African market has adopted MSAs enthusiastically. Discovery Health, the first company to introduce them in 1993, has grown from a base of zero covered lives to in excess of one million at the beginning of 2002. This coverage represents approximately 15.5 percent of the total private market. A recent independent survey found that 76 percent of South African companies either already use or plan to move to MSA-based product designs.[5] To determine the impact of MSAs on health care spending, an analysis was conducted using data from three different health insurance companies, two of which use MSA plans and a third that uses a non-MSA arrangement that covers discretionary expenses with a 20 percent copayment (Table 22.1 shows the detail of the data set used).[6] To ensure that we were comparing like with like, the investigation considered different age bands as well as large groups of individuals who had been exposed to the same type of underwriting regimes. The family sizes were not significantly different in the different data sets.

Table 22.1. Data Used in MSA Spending Analysis.

Age Band	Number of Families			
	Non-MSA		MSA	
20–35	2,028	28%	26,400	48%
36–50	2,447	34	22,416	41
51–65	1,683	23	5,212	10
66 +	1,071	15	503	1
Total	7,229	100	54,531	100

The starting point of the investigation was a comparison of the relative levels of discretionary spending. The results of this comparison (Table 22.2) showed dramatic savings. Under an MSA plan, spending was reduced by almost half.

We also considered the impact of these savings on the overall benefits delivered to all members under an MSA plan, given the different coverage arrangements. Figure 22.1 shows the percentage of claims covered by the plan for different levels of nondiscretionary health care spending after ensuring that the individuals were paying the same contribution under the two different plans. From the graph it is clear that consumers who are not claiming are better off under an MSA plan than under traditional insurance plans. As the MSA is depleted, consumers incur higher out-of-pocket costs. The group of moderate claimers is better off under a more traditional plan, because they incur lower out-of-pocket costs. However, the high claimers are better off under an MSA plan than under a traditional plan because the significant savings in discretionary spending allows the plan to offer superior coverage levels for catastrophic events.

Because the moderate spenders are worse off under an MSA plan, it seems likely that these moderate spenders will either become low spenders, due to more prudent use of medical services, or are on the way to becoming seriously ill and will become high spenders. The overall effect on the system, considering the value by which each of the populations is better off and the populations'

Table 22.2. Average Discretionary Cost per Family per Year (US$).

Age Band	Non-MSA	MSA	% Reduction
20–35	$1,007	$561	56%
36–50	1,529	784	51
51–65	1,717	882	51
66 +	2,278	1,060	47

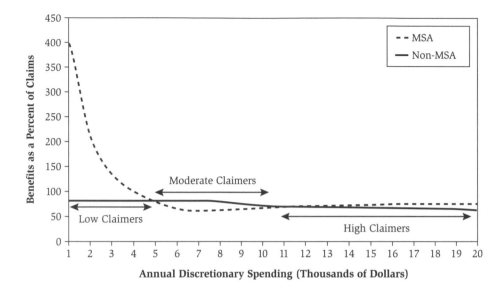

Figure 22.1. Comparison of Benefits Received in Relation to Claims Incurred.

relative weights, clearly shows improvements of as much as $167 per person under an MSA arrangement. If these gains are applied to all the privately insured individuals, they amount to over $1.2 billion.

This analysis has important implications for health insurance market risk pools. Some criticize MSAs for disproportionately attracting the young and healthy and therefore potentially destabilizing risk pools. But Figure 22.1 illustrates that even though MSAs are certainly attractive to the young and healthy, they are not unattractive to the old and sick. The findings shown here have been replicated over all ages used in the analysis.

Another criticism of MSAs is that they motivate people to turn discretionary spending into nondiscretionary spending, for example, by seeking admission to a hospital for routine care. Although plan design certainly creates this perverse incentive, carriers can implement management controls such as preauthorization to prevent this behavior. As Table 22.3 shows, these controls have been effective in controlling nondiscretionary spending in the MSA plans.

The final criticism traditionally leveled at MSAs is that they create incentives for individuals to forgo care. Although this is a difficult question to answer without a proper longitudinal analysis over a period of years, our investigation did not show a greater incidence of catastrophic claims under an MSA plan than under a non-MSA plan over one year.

This detailed analysis of actual MSA experience in the South African market shows that MSAs are an efficient means of financing health care. These benefits

Table 22.3. Average Nondiscretionary Cost per Family per Year (US$).

Age Band	Non-MSA	MSA
20–35	$ 393	$316
36–50	557	358
51–65	732	495
66 ⏐	1,369	997

Note. These costs cover primarily inpatient and chronic medication expenses.

have been translated into annual premium increases to the consumer far lower than the average increase. Whereas MSA plans have increased premiums at an average of 12 to 13 percent over the last five years, the industry average has been approximately 17.5 percent. The MSA impact is even more favorable because the inflation increase passed on to the consumer involves not only the annual premium increase but also the actual savings account balance at the end of the year. For example, consider an individual who contributes $200 per month to purchase health insurance, of which $80 goes into an MSA, for an annual MSA contribution of $960 a year. Assume further that the annual premium increase is 10 percent. If the individual spends only half of that MSA contribution ($480), he or she can apply the MSA balance of $480 toward purchasing the same benefits in the new year as in the previous year. So, in the new year the individual pays $220 ($200 + (10% × $200)) a month, less the $40 a month that can come from the savings account ($480 ÷ 12), or $180 ($220 − $40). In other words, the person who paid $200 a month last year and saved half of his or her MSA will pay only $180 after a premium increase of 10 percent to purchase the same benefits. In this way MSAs not only can reduce premium increases through more efficient use of health care resources but also can provide lower increases and often discounts to the individuals who save money.

WELLNESS AND LOYALTY PROGRAMS

In addition to this MSA plan design, Discovery Health provides an optional accompanying lifestyle and wellness program. The program costs an additional 5 percent of the total monthly premium. (Seventy-four percent of all plan members belong to the program.)

The program is designed to enhance the effectiveness of the MSA and benefit plan for the consumer. The first key element is a focus on wellness. Individual consumers earn points through taking advantage of a variety of preventive health care services such as mammograms, pap smears, and cholesterol screening. (All of these services are paid for from the MSA.) In addition, points can be earned through visits to the gym or by a passing score on a fitness test. Points allow individuals to enhance their status. As they move from blue to gold status, they become entitled to a whole range of lifestyle enhancements, the second key element of the program, such as access to a range of exclusive gyms and exotic holidays. The impact of the program has been very encouraging, through an increased emphasis on wellness and through improvement in the value provided to healthy consumers.

THE FUTURE OF MSAS

Even though MSAs have proved very successful in the South African market, further challenges exist.

The first and foremost is to ensure that empowered consumers are provided with more and better information that will enable them to navigate successfully through the health care system. We believe in leveraging technology to provide individuals with this information. With the rapid advances in the Internet and other technologies and the increasing adoption of these technologies by South Africans, particularly those who purchase private health insurance, the provision of such information to consumers begins to be achievable.

A second important challenge is to make MSA transactions seamless. Within Discovery Health we have experimented with various on-line payment mechanisms. Successful implementation has proven harder than one might think it to be. One on-line arrangement, for example, allowed the provider to check an individual's MSA balance on-line and, if appropriate, debit the individual's account. However, this seamless cash transaction had the unfortunate effect of dampening the consumers' perception that they were spending their own money and increased claims experience. I believe that technology along with partial cash payments by the consumer will be key to overcoming this particular challenge.

The final challenge in the South African MSA market is a regulatory one. Although to date, the regulatory market around MSAs has been fairly loose, the government is attempting to tighten up regulations. The government's interest underscores the maturity of the MSA market as well as the improvement in its operation, but some downside may come from an excessively restrictive regulatory environment. Presently, the government seeks to cap the maximum amount of the total contribution that can be paid into an MSA, to reduce the scope for tax avoidance.

In conclusion, significant success to date has been achieved with MSAs. We believe MSAs will continue to remain an important component in the quest for a successful solution to the problem of health care financing.

Notes

1. Sidiropoulos, E. *South Africa Survey 1996/97.* Johannesburg: South African Institute of Race Relations, 1997.

2. Health Systems Trust. *South African Health Review.* Durban, South Africa, 1998, 1997, 1996.

3. Old Mutual Actuaries and Consultants. *The 1997 Health Benefits Survey.* Cape Town: Old Mutual Actuaries and Consultants, 1997.

4. Health Systems Trust. *South African Health Review.*

5. Matisonn, S., and Kallner, H. "An Analysis of MSAs in the South African Market." Unpublished discussion document prepared for a government task force investigating MSAs, 1999.

6. Matisonn, S., and Kallner, H. "An Analysis of MSAs in the South African Market."

CHAPTER TWENTY-THREE

European Health Care

The Cost of Solidarity and the Promise of Risk-Adjusted Consumer-Driven Health Care

Paul Belien

American policymakers often look to Western Europe for an alternative to the health care system in the United States. Across the Atlantic, they hope to find the recipe for a health care system that is less costly than the American system and that provides universal access to affordable health care. European policymakers hardly ever look to the United States for an alternative to their health care systems. Many Europeans tend to consider the American health care system as inadequate because of what they perceive to be its gross violation of the equity principle.

Most of the present European health care systems, however, are as inadequate as the American system. The European countries provide more equity in health care, but they do so increasingly by shifting the price tag for health care to the next generation, by rationing care to the old, and by suppressing useful innovations. Indeed, the whole European social security system is not a solution but a time bomb.

THE COST OF SOLIDARITY

Let's look more closely at the process and cost of providing basic health care for all.

A Grandfather's Ordeal

My most direct experience with the issue of health care was the death of my grandfather a couple of years ago. My grandfather was very old—ninety-one—when he died. In his family longevity was not uncommon. One of his brothers died at the age of ninety-six, another at ninety-five. His father was ninety-four when he died. My great grandmother died at the age of ninety-nine, two months before her one hundredth birthday. The family record was set by a niece who reached one hundred and three. All had been relatively healthy up to the time of their deaths.

My grandfather had never been ill. He had never needed medical treatment. Upon reaching his nineties, however, he began to have a problem that is quite common in older men: a prostate problem. His children persuaded him to go to a hospital for surgery. It took some effort to get this ninety-one-year-old man to a hospital for the first time in his life, but he went. Like all Belgians, throughout his professional life my grandfather had paid wage-related contributions to cover health insurance. As he had never needed much health care, he had been a net contributor to the Belgian health care system. Now was the very first time he was going to claim something back.

My grandfather had his operation in May. In November he was dead. The prostate operation had gone well, but the hospital administered an antibiotic drug that caused complete deafness. Though there were other, but costlier, treatments possible, the hospital gave this drug to the old man. Hospital staff knew about the possible side effect, but it did not strike them as an unreasonable and unjust thing to do. Why should it? A man who has already had ninety healthy years of his life surely has no right to complain about deafness when some people get more seriously ill or die at far younger ages.

When my grandfather left the hospital, he was completely deaf. But his prostate problem had been cured. According to the clinic the prostate operation had been highly successful. As far as the Belgian health care statistics were concerned, my grandfather's treatment raised the quality average. It had also been cheap. Statistics show that Belgium has a high quality of health care that is relatively cheap, available to all the country's inhabitants, and virtually free of charge for the patients. It is the kind of health care that Americans, looking at comparative statistics, would envy. My grandfather, however, did not look at statistics. The fact that as a patient he did not have to pay for a treatment that caused him to go deaf did not console him. When he left the hospital, his spirit was broken. The old man thrived on having his children, grandchildren, great-grandchildren, friends, and neighbors communicating with him. Now it was all over. He loved to watch—and listen to—television every evening. The operation deprived him of this pleasure. I still see him sitting in his chair, lonely, unable to communicate, and becoming increasingly suspicious and sour. Very soon he lost his will to live. Six months after the successful prostate operation was inflicted on him, he was dead.

My grandfather's story proves not only that statistics can be misleading, but also that although free health care for everyone sounds good, sometimes it might be better not to have any service than a bad service, even if this bad service costs nothing. In other words: aiming at equity by giving everybody in a country the same rights to health care is hardly relevant. In the health care debate we should focus on health, not on health care. My grandfather would have been better off without his prostate operation. He could probably have lived with his prostate problem for a few more years. He could not, however, live with the deafness that was inflicted on him because doctors and hospitals were cutting the cost of the "free" service they delivered by reducing the quality of their service.

The Time Bomb

I have put the word "free" in quotation marks, because, of course, even in Belgium health care is not free. It costs society a fortune to provide "free" care. It is true that sick patients do not have to pay the full bill at the moment when they need medical treatment. But these same patients during their own healthy days have been paying for other people's treatment. Health care in Belgium, as in almost all the other European countries, is paid for on a pay-as-you-go basis. The healthy, usually young people of today pay for the needs of the sick, usually older people of today. In turn they rely on the future generations to pay for their needs when they are sick and old.

However, demographics are changing. The percentage of young people is steadily declining because the birthrate has been falling since the 1960s and the life expectancy of the elderly is increasing. As a result the health care system now faces serious problems. The older the population, the more health care it needs. This life cycle implies that as the number of elderly people increases, total health care costs are also likely to increase. At the same time, however, it becomes ever more difficult to find the resources to support the system, because the number of young, active people who must finance it is also dwindling. Each of these younger individuals will have to carry a bigger share of the existing burden, even as the total burden itself is constantly growing.

There are only two ways to keep this "free" system intact. Either drastically increase the financial burden on those at the paying end of the system—the young and the healthy of today—or drastically limit the quality and the availability of health care for those at the receiving end—the sick and the elderly. For the past two decades, governments in Western Europe have been increasing the financial burden on the young. As this burden has become intolerable, they are now shifting their policies toward cutting back quality. Certain medical treatments or drugs are no longer available to persons above a certain age or to persons who are considered to be too sick, or they are not made available at all. Studies of kidney dialysis, for example, show that more than a fifth of dialysis centers in Europe and almost half in England have refused to treat patients over sixty-five years of age.[1] Gradually, health care in Europe is becoming a horror story. And this is only the beginning.

My grandfather's deafness was the side effect of an antibiotic that was given to him because of budgetary constraints. More expensive drugs and treatments, with fewer side effects, are set aside for younger patients. Political authorities, claiming to be the guardians of solidarity in society, deem it less desirable for a young person to be deaf than for an old one. Hence my grandfather, after having paid heavy wage-related contributions as a young man to fulfill his solidarity with the elderly, now had to pay the price of deafness to fulfill his duty of solidarity with the young. If governments continue this policy, soon euthanasia might be the price the solidarity principle the welfare state imposes on the very old and the very sick, those people whose health care is costing society the most.[2] Some doctors have already warned about "economic euthanasia" and "government decrees which allow ministers to eliminate certain categories of people, while at the same time resolving the pension problem."[3]

In Europe old people increasingly receive less care than young people do. In the United States, ironically, the situation is the reverse. There the elderly are entitled to universal health coverage via the government-run Medicare program, and young people are not (with the exception of the very poor, who are entitled to participate in the government-run Medicaid program). In the United States the bulk of government health care expenditure goes to those over sixty-five years old, whereas in six other nations (Japan, Germany, France, Italy, the United Kingdom, and Canada) most of the government money is spent on those under sixty-five. By the year 2000, public health expenditure on those over sixty-five amounted to 3.6 percent of the American gross domestic product (GDP), compared to 2.8 percent spent on those under sixty-five. The respective figures in France, in contrast, are 2 percent for those above sixty-five and 4.9 percent for those under that age.[4] But by 2030, the Organization for Economic Cooperation and Development (OECD) estimates that not only the United States but also Japan, the United Kingdom, and Canada will spend a higher percentage of public money on those above sixty-five than on those under that age.[5] Unless, of course, governments decide to restrict access to health care and quality of care for the elderly and the very sick even further.

An Accumulation of Debts

In many Western European countries, governments are facing precarious budgetary situations. During the past twenty years, Western European nations have seen their government spending climb by an average of 0.6 to 0.7 GDP percentage points annually. Since 1970, government spending in Western Europe has risen from 36.5 percent of GDP to almost 51 percent. If the present Western European government spending process continues, in twenty years government spending will account for nearly 65 percent of GDP.[6]

The United States has also seen a rise in government spending during the past twenty years, but only from 31.5 percent to nearly 36 percent of GDP.[7] The U.S. ratio of government spending to GDP is lower because in Europe social security spending constitutes a much larger expense item. This is not true for health care, however. The percentage of government spending on health care is as high in the United States as in the average Western European country—about 6 percent of GDP.[8] Moreover, on top of government spending, Americans spend an additional 7.5 percent on health care out of their own pockets.[9] The American government provides health care only for the very poor and the elderly, leaving the middle classes almost completely to their own devices. The European governments provide universal health insurance for everyone, but they virtually monopolize the sector with the argument that it is the government's duty to guarantee equal health care for everyone. They make it very hard or almost impossible for private citizens to acquire additional health care over and above what the government provides.

Everywhere in the Western world, health care expenditure has been growing rapidly during the past decades.[10] This has caused considerable problems in the European welfare states, where health care is almost exclusively the government's responsibility. Indeed, health care is the fastest-growing segment of government spending. By 1999, Belgium government spending for health care rose a staggering 114.1 percent in ten years.[11] According to a 1993 survey by Andersen Consulting in ten Western European countries, medical costs rose by an average of 4.1 percent in real terms each year between 1970 and 1990, whereas real economic growth over the same period rose only 2.7 percent each year.[12] Government income has not risen as dramatically as its expenditure. The result is that all over Europe governments have accumulated enormous debts. In 1999, the U.S. government debt of 60 percent of GDP is in this context of small importance when compared to Sweden's 10 percent, Italy's 118 percent, Belgium's 114 percent, and even Canada's 85 percent. A public debt of 100 percent of GDP means that for a state to pay all its debts every citizen would have to work for one year giving all his or her earnings to the state. Indeed, as debt has to be reimbursed sooner or later, a rise in government debt indicates that the cost of present government expenditure is being transferred to the future.[13]

This is a moral as well as a political problem. A future generation that had no say in past political decisions is, nevertheless, forced to foot the bill for those decisions. This is a violation of the fundamental democratic principle "no taxation without representation." Hence it is no surprise that all over Western Europe the traditional parties that devised the current welfare systems are rapidly losing their electoral appeal, especially among the young. The growth of so-called extremist parties in Europe is based not only on their antiimmigration policies. The two most successful of these parties, the Freedom Party (FPOE) in Austria and the Flemish Bloc (VB) in Belgium, stress the need for welfare reform as the present systems are becoming financially unsustainable. Alexandra Colen, member of the Belgian Parliament for Antwerp, put it this way: "Most parents would be ashamed to leave their children an inheritance of debts. But this is exactly what governments have been doing in the past two decades. The current generation of Belgian taxpayers is already handing over more in solidarity payments to the former generation than to the present one. In the future this discrepancy will only grow. This situation calls for a new Boston Tea Party."[14]

DIFFERENT SYSTEMS: ARE THEY REALLY DIFFERENT?

It is the financing side of the European health care systems that is causing the European countries' problems. When we look at European health care systems from this angle, we notice that Europe has basically two types of systems.[15]

First, there is the so-called single-payer health care system. In this system health care is paid for and organized by the government, either at a national or a regional level, often with money from income taxes. Britain established this system immediately after the Second World War. It is also used in the Scandinavian and Mediterranean countries. Outside Europe, nations like Canada, Australia, and New Zealand have a similar system. A single-payer system guarantees access to health care for everyone. All citizens are covered and belong to the largest possible pool, namely the nation or province as a whole. The main problem with this system is that the health care budget is predominantly paid with tax money. Contributions are not related to (individual or collective) health risks. If the budget does not cover the costs of the health care needs, waiting lists appear. Health care is rationed, and the quality deteriorates as the budgets become more restricted.

The second type of European health care financing system is the social insurance–based system. This is a multiple-payer system. Health costs are not paid by the government but by various sickness funds. In theory these are private, independent organizations. This is the system of continental Western Europe. It is found in countries like Germany, Austria, France, Belgium, the Netherlands, and Luxembourg and also in a few countries outside Europe, such as Japan and Korea, which had close links to Germany during the first half of the century. The system was formally established by the German chancellor Otto von Bismarck, who made membership in a sickness fund compulsory for all citizens in 1883. But the roots of the sickness funds go back to the voluntary associations, or "friendly societies," that emerged in the early nineteenth century among workers to pool various individual risks.[16] Britain was a pioneer here, with numerous friendly societies in the late eighteenth century,[17] but it nationalized its whole health care sector after the Second World War.

A social insurance–based system also provides universal coverage because membership in a sickness fund is compulsory. In theory members are free to choose their fund, but in some countries they are obliged to join the fund of their profession. Members pay a premium to the fund that constitutes a certain percentage of their wages. Again this is theory. Often the members do not know the amount of the premium nor do they personally pay anything to the fund. The fund receives a sum from an official government organization in accordance with the number of its members. The amount of the premium is usually set by the government as a percentage of the wages. The premium operates like a payroll tax, paid by the employer to an official government organization. The government collects the money and distributes it among the funds. The fact that many of the Western European health care systems are paid for by wage-related contributions has also resulted in higher wage costs in Europe than in the United States. The average German worker costs his employer $26.9 an hour (of which 46 percent accounts for welfare benefits), whereas the average U.S. worker costs only $15.89 an hour (of which only 28 percent accounts for welfare benefits).[18]

Every country has its own type of funds, reflecting the different ways in which this system grew in different nations. Belgium has "ideological" sickness funds, which are closely affiliated with the different political parties. There are funds for socialists, for liberals, for Christian Democrats, and so on. Actually, it makes no difference which fund you belong to; the premium is the same for every fund and is set by the government. The coverage is the same too. France has professional sickness funds. Germany has regional funds, professional funds, and company funds. Unlike Belgium, Germany has premiums that vary within a certain range. The same is true for the Netherlands, but these ranges are not very extensive in either country. In Germany, for example, premiums range from 8 percent to 16 percent of a worker's gross salary. The national average is 13 percent. This means that healthy and young Germans handed over 13 percent of their contemporary earnings to provide for the medical care of the sick and the elderly. Given current trends, the number of active, working Germans, whose wages support the system, will fall to 84 percent of its present number in the first quarter of the twenty-first century, and the number of old people will increase to 188 percent of its present figure. And with each percentage point increase in the number of elderly in a population, the number of people needing health care rises even more dramatically. Already 20 percent of the German population is over sixty, and 33 percent of all hospital patients are over that age.

All over Europe, social insurance–based systems have run enormous deficits that the governments during the past decades have balanced with general taxation. As a consequence the theoretical distinction between health care systems financed completely from general taxation and sickness fund systems financed with a percentage of the members' wages is becoming obsolete. European health care systems are increasingly alike in their dependency on money provided by the government and their high level of political interference and state control. Even the U.S. health care system, which theoretically belongs to a third group (the private insurance–based system), is to a large extent a government-run system.[19] Indeed, almost 45 percent of health care expenditure in the United States is tax financed, as Medicaid, Medicare, and other government health care programs devour 5.9 percent of the U.S. GDP—which is 45 percent of the total amount of medical expenditure in the United States.

From the point of view of cost control the way in which the European countries have organized their systems does not seem to make much difference. No matter how they have organized their health care, they have all seen their costs rise over the past decades.[20] It made absolutely no difference whether a country had a single-payer or a sickness fund system.[21] Changing the system from a government-run, single-payer system into a social insurance–based sickness fund system, or vice versa, in the hope of lowering costs, does not make much sense.[22]

Single-payer and sickness fund systems both exhibit the same deficiencies. They both have a built-in incentive for overconsumption because they contain very few incentives for the health care consumer to spend rationally in a responsive way.[23] Hence governments, in order to limit consumption, have had no other choice but to set health care budgets. They did so traditionally in single-payer systems, but nowadays they do so in sickness fund systems too.[24] Waiting lists for certain medical services occur in Canada and Britain, which have single-payer systems, but also in the Netherlands, which has a sickness fund system.[25] Everywhere governments are rationing health care. Pressures on health expenditures have led European countries where prescription drugs were traditionally free, like Germany, to introduce price-regulating legislation. They have led countries where the choice of doctors was traditionally free, like Belgium, to consider restricting this freedom.[26] Governments talk a lot about introducing market mechanisms into the system, but even though they use the word *market* quite often, they aim for a system of managed competition, controlled and regulated from above, by the government itself.[27] Hospitals, doctors, and health care insurers are pressured by the authorities, sometimes with the threat of heavy penalties, to lower the cost of treatment. European governments are interfering more than ever in the business of the health care providers.[28] This interference started with price control in the pharmaceutical sector, but as price control did not work, it has moved on to control at the point when the doctor writes the prescription. Government agencies are starting to compare each health care provider's behavior with average behavior and are sanctioning providers whose prescription patterns differ from that average. In the end what patients get is mediocrity.[29]

In this quest for mediocrity, governments learn from each other. Approaches applied in one country are often adopted in others. The goal is always the same—to cut costs by restricting consumption. The question that no one asks, is, Does consumption have to be cut?

In markets with a free supply of services and spontaneous competition, prices decrease because of the natural expansion and differentiation of the services offered. Consumers have a real say. Because they demand, choose, and pay for a service, that service had better be good and reasonably priced. Consumers have rights—they can insist on quality—and they have obligations—to be cost conscious and limit their consumption or pay the bill themselves. In managed competition, however, consumers have no say. The "competition" they create cuts costs by lowering the quality provided or by attracting healthy patients and discouraging the sick. The patient has no real options. Cost control often means the curtailment of health care services. We can see this tendency all over Europe. The result is that Europe's health care systems are gradually beginning to resemble each other in the low level of quality they provide and in their high level of government interference.

The Quest for Mediocrity

Apart from the graying of the population, another important factor is causing health care costs to expand continuously—the fact that medical technology is constantly improving. New methods and drugs are usually very expensive at the time of their introduction. After this initial phase the prices go down. In matters of life and death, as health care sometimes is, people prefer the best treatment available, which often is the newest and most expensive.

One of the most common ways in which government-funded (and hence government-controlled) health care systems try to limit costs is by rationing, or even completely blocking, access to new and costly medical technology. New pharmaceutical drugs are often targeted. A common policy is to decree the substitution of generic products for branded drugs. Generics are copycat drugs that can be freely produced once pharmaceutical companies' patents run out. Sometimes these products are less efficient than the newer drugs and have their own side effects.[30] Another method is reference pricing. Drugs with similar therapeutic effects are grouped, and the price of the least expensive drug in the group is the price at which all the other drugs have to be sold if they want to qualify for reimbursement under social security.[31] Some governments have drawn up "negative lists" of drugs, which doctors cannot prescribe or which patients must pay for completely out of their own pocket. Drugs are put on the negative list not because they are harmful products but because they are high-quality goods that politicians and bureaucrats consider too expensive.

Limiting the state's costs, not enhancing the people's well-being, has become the primary concern of the countries in Europe. In Sweden one condition for pharmaceutical companies seeking permission to market a drug is that "the price is reasonable." After Germany introduced extremely drastic measures to curb pharmaceutical expenditure in 1993, the sales of the seven largest research-intensive drug manufacturers immediately fell by 16.5 percent, and the sales of the four largest generics makers rose by 36 percent.[32] This is a severe handicap for the research-intensive manufacturers who must reinvest profit for the development of new and better products. Less drastic cost-curbing measures in the decade before 1993 had already resulted in German pharmaceutical companies seeing their worldwide share of drug patents drop to 8 percent in 1986–1990 from 16 percent in the period from 1981 to 1985.[33]

By stifling medical innovation, state-run health care systems, like those in Western Europe, not only kill their own countries' pharmaceutical industries but also take a free ride at the expense of countries with largely private health care systems, like the United States, where the government does not cap innovation. European governments wait until the "unreasonable" prices for new drugs in the United States drop to a "reasonable" level and then they allow doctors to prescribe these drugs. As a consequence, European patients gain access to new drugs a few years later than U.S. patients. If the United States were to adopt a government-regulated health care system similar to that of most European countries, pharmaceutical innovation would come virtually to a standstill. This would harm not only U.S. but ultimately also European patients. Indeed, where would the Europeans find new drugs if the United States adopts the European health care policies? And the Europeans are not the only ones getting a free ride at the expense of the Americans. Canada's health expenditure is lower than that in the United States, but one-third of Canadian physicians admit that they have referred patients to U.S. physicians and hospitals because of the lack of availability of certain medical services in Canada and the length of time patients sometimes have to wait before receiving medical care.[34] Where would these patients go if the United States adopts the Canadian health care system?

The Private Sector: Risk-Adjusted Individual Health Insurers

The only people who can still receive quality medical care in Europe today are the privately insured. However, in many countries, it is illegal to leave the government or sickness fund system and purchase private health insurance. In countries like Britain, where individuals have the option of seeking private medical assistance and paying the full bill themselves or buying additional health insurance on top of what they already pay for the national health insurance, the number of people buying additional private insurance has risen significantly over the past years.[35] But this option, where it exists,[36] is open only to the afflu-ent citizens who can afford to pay for health care twice: once via taxes or mandatory social insurance premiums and once via private insurance or direct fees to doctors.

Only three European countries allow (some) people to acquire private health insurance without still having to pay premiums or taxes to cover health risks under the official system. These countries provide "free" health care not in the sense of the "free" services provided by the so-called solidarity based systems but in the sense that people are free to decide how to finance their health care. These countries are Switzerland—the only country in Europe with a health care system based totally on private insurance—and also to a certain extent Germany and the Netherlands. The latter two countries have sickness fund systems, but in Germany, people earning more than a certain income are allowed to opt out of the sickness fund in Germany, and in the Netherlands individuals with cer-tain health risks are required to leave the standard fund and enter a different system. (For more on the German system, see Dr. Wilfred Prewo's article, "Con-sumer-Driven Health Care in Germany: A Proposal" on www.josseybass.com/go/herzlinger.)

Private insurance health care systems are often criticized because some very high risk individual citizens cannot afford to pay premiums calculated on indi-vidual risk. This is exactly the problem in the United States. Switzerland, Ger-many, and the Netherlands, however, have each reduced this inequity in their own way. The following sections look at the Swiss and Dutch experiences as examples.

Switzerland. The Swiss give government subsidies to groups with higher health risks, so that everyone, even a high-risk individual, can obtain insurance. The amount of these government subsidies differs from canton (region) to canton, as Switzerland allows cantonal governments to decide in this matter. The over-all objective appears to be to support those most in need, such as families with children and those with low incomes. On average, approximately 5 percent of the income of the insurance funds comes from cantonal sources. In addition, the federal government provides premium subsidies too, but these are based on age and sex. These federal subsidies amount to, on average, 10 percent of health care costs for males, 35 percent for females, and 30 percent for children.[37] Because of the Swiss government's budgetary problems, these subsidies have gone down lately, and many Swiss insurance companies are now experiment-ing with American-style HMO schemes.

Switzerland is the only country in Europe with a health care system more akin to private than to social insurance. Swiss insurance payments are not linked to income but are instead set on a per capita basis, with weightings for age of entry into a fund, regional cost differences, and sex. The Health Insurance Law defines the catalogue of benefits to which all Swiss insurance members are entitled; however, individual insurance funds can offer additional benefits over and above this basic package.

To prevent the situation in which some insurance companies keep their premiums low by running hardly any risks while other insurers must ask for exorbitant premiums because they get the high-risk patients, Switzerland has introduced a risk-adjustment system. All insurers in the market must pay a portion of the premiums or contributions they collect into a central fund. The relative financial risk of each insurer is then calculated, and insurers with a larger proportion of less healthy, high-risk members receive from the fund an amount that compensates them for the higher financial risks involved in insuring their members. In effect, insurers with healthier members subsidize those with less healthy members. All the health insurers operating in a canton are subject to the same risk-adjustment mechanism. Risk adjustment is based on age and sex only. Calculations are based on actual costs, but only for care that falls under the basic benefits package. Although the system reduces differences in premiums within cantons, significant differences still exist since the risk adjustment is calculated only for care covered by the basic benefits package.

The Swiss health care system is self-managing. Health insurers set their own health premiums, subject to the risk-adjustment system. Premiums differ from insurer to insurer, but so do the services to the patient. The Swiss insurance funds have considerable freedom in the benefits packages they offer, as long as they include the basic list of services in the Health Insurance Law. Because this law specifies services in a relatively vague way, there is a considerable range of options for consumers. Insurers usually offer an array of benefit packages for their customers that can be supplemented with various programs specifically designed for children, housewives, professionals, farmers, and other such groups. In Switzerland it is the responsibility of the people themselves to purchase health insurance. Every Swiss citizen has to pay a premium. Those on low incomes receive a subsidy from the government.

Self-management tends to lead to novel and innovative contracts between health insurers and providers. Many Swiss insurance companies are experimenting with U.S.-style health maintenance organization (HMO) schemes. HMOs buy health services for their members, and by buying pharmaceuticals or medical services in large quantities, they can limit the price for each individual product. HMOs in Switzerland are medical practices that are owned by groups of insurance funds, offer primary care, and have informal arrangements with hospitals.[38] Members who join HMOs are offered lower premiums than are people in the traditional programs. Some insurers have introduced bonuses. If patients do not use any health services in a given period or spend less than a set amount, they are paid back part of the insurance premium. This encourages patients to use the system in a cost-conscious way.[39] However, the need for such a bonus does not seem to be great in Switzerland because out-of-pocket expenses are very high.

Copayments are the linchpin of the Swiss health care system. They apply to primary as well as hospital care, and cover about one-third of the annual health care expenses. Their purpose is to reduce consumption of health care services. The levels are set by the government, and in most cases the government does not allow citizens to insure against them. In the late 1990s, patients paid all their costs for ambulatory care up to the level of a deductible that was around 150 Swiss francs per year (US$125), and 10 percent of costs above this level. There was also an annual maximum level for copayments. For adults it was set at Fr500 (US$417). Insurance funds are free to offer their customers higher annual deductibles in return for lower premiums. For hospital care, patients paid the room and board costs for the duration of their stay in a hospital. It is possible to insure against payments for the room and board costs of hospital care (but never for primary care). There was also a copayment of Fr10 per day for hospital treatment costs. Citizens are not allowed to insure themselves against this type of hospital copayment.

Because one-third of Swiss health care is financed through direct patient copayments and because it is illegal to insure oneself against most of these copayments, Swiss citizens have to rely to a large extent on their private savings in order to prepare for future health risks. As a result the Swiss health care system relies on capitalization. Because they are forced to pay a significant part of the health care costs themselves, patients start capitalizing by setting aside money for future needs, and because they have to start making rational choices, which they cannot do without becoming informed about health care issues, they are forced into patient empowerment.

In terms of health care outcomes Switzerland ranks among the top countries,[40] with its position better than that of other European countries on almost all health indicators.[41] However, the Swiss system is not without problems. The Swiss devoted $2,499 per capita to health care in 1996, which was the second highest amount found by the OECD (after the United States) and the third highest if measured as a percentage of GDP.[42] Health care costs have been rising rapidly since the early 1990s, exceeding the level of premium increases.[43] According to the Swiss authorities, development of supply (expanded facilities, growing specialization, and greater use of technology) is the fundamental factor in this increase. The impact of the aging population and the escalation of social insurance benefits are not very significant.[44] The rise in health care costs due to an expansion of health care supply puts the government under pressure to increase its subsidies to people with health risks.[45]

The Netherlands. In the Netherlands, one-third of the population is privately insured, and the number is rising. The Dutch, like the Germans, can also opt out of the system, but the income threshold is lower than in Germany. The Dutch make private insurance affordable to everyone by covering the high risks—those who need so-called catastrophic health care—under a different nationwide scheme. There is a compulsory government-regulated single-payer system for the expensive health risks and a sickness fund system for the other risks. For costly risks the citizen is placed in the largest possible risk pool, namely the whole nation. When they are noncatastrophic risks, however, citizens can leave the sickness fund system if they earn above a certain income. In that case they can buy private insurance, whose premiums are affordable because the very high risks are not covered here.

LABORATORIES FOR REFORM

The few privately insured health care systems of Europe—in force for Switzerland, 10 percent of the German population, and 35 percent of the Dutch population—seem better equipped for the future than the government regulated systems. They are interesting laboratories for health care reform. They are consumer driven and they are trying out a variety of interesting ideas, such as medical savings accounts (MSAs),[46] health care vouchers, and bonuses. Private systems leave room for experimentation. If people want to join an HMO system that restricts them to certain HMO-approved doctors they can do so, but they are also free to join an insurance scheme that leaves the choice of doctor to them.[47] Or they can use the money they saved in their MSA to pay the doctor of their choice. In these systems, patients have choices; the single-payer and sickness fund systems rob them of choice. The same holds for providers—the hospitals, the doctors, and the pharmaceutical companies.[48]

It is true, however, that the European private insurance–based systems also have their problems. At present they too, like the government or sickness fund systems, are predominantly financed on a pay-as-you-go basis. If one wants to remedy health care systems, the only solution is to abandon the pay-as-you-go system of financing. Instead of funding all the health care needs of the old (and more often sick) of today with the contributions of the young (and more often healthy) of today, while the latter rely for the financing of their own future needs on the smaller number of young (and more often healthy) people of tomorrow, people should be building up reserves for the future liabilities of their own generation.

Only a system of health care financing with capitalization schemes is immune to these demographic pressures. Even the private health care insurers in Europe have hardly any financial reserves. In a capitalization system the future needs of an age group would have to be almost fully funded when that generation reaches the age where it needs health care most. For example, the fact that the German private health insurance system is not financed on a capitalization basis—and as a consequence lacks financial reserves—has two important consequences. First, there is no portability of reserves. Once a client has joined a private insurance company, he or she cannot leave the insurance company without losing the right to pay no more than the premium for the age group they belonged to when they first took private insurance. If you join your insurance company when you are twenty-five, you will still be paying the premiums of a twenty-five-year-old when you are forty-five. But if at forty-five you decide to join another private insurance company because you have come to the conclusion that its service is better, the benefits of twenty years of membership will be lost. You can join the other company only by starting all over again; you will be regarded as a new client and will have to pay the premium of a forty-five-year-old. If choosing a new insurer implies that you penalize yourself, you are hardly left with a choice. You are as trapped within your private insurance company as others are trapped within their National Health Service or their sickness fund.

Second, because the German private insurers lack financial reserves, the same demographic evolution in society that also raises the average age of their members forces them either to increase premiums dramatically for their younger members or to gradually ration health care, because they spend more money than they receive. They too, like the government, will soon start rationing health care, deciding what care their members can get and how much that care may cost. For the patient who needs treatment but cannot get it because of budget limits, it is hardly relevant whether these budget limits are imposed by a government, sickness fund, HMO, or insurance company. Therefore, privatization without capitalization is hardly a remedy for the current health care crisis.

THE CAUSE OF THE PROBLEM

We know that health care costs are rising everywhere, no matter what system nations use. Costs rise everywhere in Europe and North America for the same two reasons: aging populations and the huge costs of developing new cures and treatments. In a system based on capitalization, both problems can be neutralized. The aging of the population is not a problem because the health care the elderly receive is paid for with money they themselves set aside many years ago. The money an individual pays is not spent on the sick of today but is invested to generate new capital. One way to invest it is in the development of new cures and treatments, that is, in pharmaceutical and medical innovation.

Indeed, the capital set aside under a capitalization scheme is not buried by insurance companies or hidden in a stocking. It is put in a bank account, and the bank invests it in growth sectors of the economy. Health care could be such a growth sector.

In the Western world the major area of economic growth in the past decades has been the service sectors, whereas the manufacturing sectors have been under heavy pressure. Manufacturing sectors are vulnerable to competition from foreign and especially developing countries. The same phenomenon is true with respect to certain services,[49] but there are also services that are by definition location bound because certain jobs are by definition proximity jobs. If you are in a car accident, the ambulance will take you to a hospital in the neighborhood. When you feel sick, you go to see a doctor in your hometown.

In the health care sector, foreign competition is of only marginal importance. Modern technology such as telemedicine will not alter this materially. Your travel agent or banker can live at the other end of the world, because you can communicate effectively with these individuals electronically. Your children can get schooling from foreign teachers via television, but when they have a terrible toothache, you take them to a dentist somewhere in town. Whenever a patient has to undergo a medical examination or is in need of medical treatment, the provider of the medical treatment has to be close by. As a consequence, every expansion of the health care market is a benefit to the national labor market. For governments coping with high unemployment figures, growing health care needs should be most welcome.[50] What is more, the health care market cannot be saturated. Death is the ultimate end and pain the ultimate agony. People will always want to avoid death and pain as much as possible. Typically, the richer people get, the more they are able and willing to spend on their health.[51] One simply cannot be too healthy. This makes health care into one of the most promising growth sectors of the economy. In a capitalist economy, promising growth sectors attract money.

Why then, given its enormous growth potential, is capital not flowing to the health care sector? It is because in a variety of ways governments are preventing it from doing so. Nowhere in Europe are governments willing to give up control over health care. However, as they do not want to give up control, they have to finance the system, which they cannot do adequately because of their enormous budget problems and their lack of capital. The health care sector is in need of capital, but governments, unable to provide it, are cutting costs instead of allowing the markets to provide the necessary capital. Governments cannot provide the solution to the health care crisis the nations of Western Europe and North America are facing today. Governments are not a solution to the problem but the cause of it.

When politicians look at health care, they often make the mistake of not being humble enough. They simply do not have enough information to enable them to organize and control the whole system. They aim for cost control and hence focus so much on costs that they forget what health care is all about, namely health. When we discuss health care reform, we should bear in mind that we must focus on health rather than on health care per se. This is a point that has often been made by the Swiss health economist Peter Zweifel, a professor at the University of Zurich. If equity is needed, he says, it should be defined in terms of health, rather than health care.[52] It is important to make this point: a country may have excellent health care accessible to everyone and yet its people may be less healthy than those of a neighboring country with less accessibility to health care.

Health policy is of course a determinant of health, but access to health care seems to be less important than some people think. In 1948, Britain became the first country to provide every citizen with the same access to health care. One would expect the poor in Britain to be as healthy as others, but such is not the case. It appears that in Britain, even after fifty years of equal access to health care under the National Health Service, health is still very dependent on social class.[53] Often differences in national traditions and consumers' habits and cultures can explain such divergences. Apart from access to health care, there are many other determinants of health: genetic factors (explaining the good health my grandfather enjoyed up to a very old age), exogenous factors (such as climate and the level of environmental pollution), socioeconomic factors, and lifestyle factors. The importance of all these has been examined in a Dutch study[54] that shows, for example, that although Germany has far better health services than Greece, Greeks tend to be healthier than Germans, perhaps because of the Greek diet, which features plenty of fruit and vegetables, limited animal fat, and moderate alcohol consumption.

When we use international comparisons as a tool for health policy, all health determinants should be taken into consideration. This is a difficult exercise. The Dutch study concludes quite bluntly that at present, national health data cannot be compared at the international level because of the abundance of factors influencing health. Nevertheless, we notice that political decisions about health care that are implemented in one country often mirror the decisions of other countries without taking all the data, such as cultural differences, into account. It is no wonder that the results are not always what politicians expect them to be. Even at the national level, politicians are not as knowledgeable as policymakers need to be about health and health care. We may well wonder whether policymakers will ever be capable of taking all the determinants of health into consideration. Will they be able to centralize all the relevant information? And do they know enough to assess the decisions they make?

If we examine attempts at health care reform in Europe over this past decade, we can see that many reform measures have had unintended consequences that required improvisation and more regulation. There have been attempts in many countries to introduce certain market mechanisms into health care, but in general the role of the market has actually been diminishing. There is a tendency toward more regulation instead of less. Controls on doctors have grown tremendously. Soon their prescription patterns are going to be scrutinized. Doctors who prescribe more pharmaceuticals than the average will risk sanctions. The same is true of hospitals. Governments talk about introducing more competition into health care systems, but the competition they propose is always managed competition, regulated from above.[55]

As the finances available for maintaining health care decrease and the consumption of health care increases, the public seems more and more interested in equity—and in access to health care—than in health itself. This is likely due to a certain panic reaction now that it has become clear that the present systems are on the brink of collapse. But if we want to fix our state health care systems, the only way is to abandon our present pay-as-you-go financing policies and adopt a capitalization system. We should be opting for a decentralized system in which patients are empowered and free to choose the health care package they think will best serve their needs.[56] This requires a strongly deregulated system with many health care options. For catastrophic illnesses, for example, risks could be pooled on a national basis through mandatory insurance, and those who are too poor to pay their premiums should be able to get government subsidies. Generally speaking, however, patients should be made into responsible consumers who are capable of making their own choices.

Notes

1. Goodman, J. C., and Musgrave, G. L. *Twenty Myths About National Health Insurance.* Dallas, Tex.: National Center for Policy Analysis, 1991.

2. The Belgian minister of health, Marcel Colla, opened the euthanasia debate in Belgium in the autumn of 1995 with his public confession that he had asked doctors to provide euthanasia for his sick mother (Sheldon, T., "Belgium Brews Row over Euthanasia," *BMJ,* Dec. 9, 1995, pp. 1525–1526).

3. Malfliet, T. "Artsen en patiënten proletariaat" (Doctors and Patients Proletariat). *VAS-berichten,* May 1996.

4. Organization for Economic Cooperation and Development (OECD). *Aging Populations, Pension Systems and Government Budgets: How Do They Affect Saving?* Paris: OECD, 1995.

5. Organization for Economic Cooperation and Development (OECD). *Aging Populations . . .*

6. Real spending on social security is expected to increase threefold by the year 2015 as the percentage of West Europeans over the age of sixty almost doubles between 1990 and 2030. See, for example, "Why EU Pensions May Face the Axe." *Wall Street Journal Europe,* Nov. 14, 1994.

7. Rubenstein, E. S. *The Right Data.* New York: National Review Press, 1994, chap. 4 ("Comparative Spending of Governments").

8. The lowest Western European figure is 5.3 percent (Denmark), the highest is 6.7 percent (France), and in the United States the government spends 5.9 percent of GDP on health care. See Organization for Economic Cooperation and Development (OECD). *The Reform of Health Care: A Comparative Analysis of Seven OECD Countries.* Paris: OECD, 1992.

9. Per capita health care spending in the United States is the highest in the world. It was $4,358 in 1999 versus $2,463 for Canada and $2,853 for Germany. Other nations trail behind. See, for example, Reinhardt, U. E., Hussey, P. S., and Anderson, G. F. "Cross-National Comparison of Health Systems Using OECD Data, 1999," *Health Affairs,* May/June 2002 21(3), pp. 169–181.

10. In most countries the prices of health services have increased more rapidly than other prices in the economy. See, for example, MacFarlan, M., and Oxley, H. "Reforming Health Care." *The OECD Observer,* Feb.–Mar. 1995, pp. 23–26.

11. Van Overtveldt, J. "Spilzieke huisvader" (Over-spending Family Man). *Trends,* July 18, 1994.

12. Andersen Consulting. "Health Care Survey in Belgium, Denmark, France, Germany, Italy, the Netherlands, Norway, Spain, Sweden, and the United Kingdom." Discussed in Van Overtveldt, J. "Doctors in Management." *Trends,* June 19, 1993.

13. In Italy the total cost of public health care absorbs over 40 percent of total revenue from direct taxation and is equal to 65 percent of the public sector deficit. See, for example, Martino, A. "The 100 Trillion Lire Health Care Mess." *Wall Street Journal Europe,* Oct. 28, 1993.

14. Colen, A. "The Moral Crisis of Welfarism." *Right Now!* Apr.-June 1996, p. 9.

15. National Economic Research Associates (NERA). *Financing Health Care with Particular Reference to Medicines.* London and White Plains, N.J.: NERA, 1993. This is a multivolume report on health care systems in Western nations; volume one, *Summary and Overview,* is devoted entirely to a tour of the different health care systems.

16. "When it was first introduced statutory health insurance was modeled on existing self help ('solidarity') groups based on professions. . . . Today, solidarity means something quite different. It reflects the ideal that the entire population should have equal access to the complete range of health care services irrespective of ability to pay" (von Stillfried, D., and Arnold, M. "What's Happening to Health Care in Germany?" *British Medical Journal,* Apr. 17, 1993, p. 1017).

17. Reekie, W. D. *Government in Healthcare: Lessons from the UK.* Hayward, Calif.: Smith Center for Private Enterprise Studies, 1995, chap. 4 ("Private Health Care, Evolution and Erosion").

18. "Europe's Recession Prompts New Look at Welfare Costs: Benefits Reduce New Hiring." *New York Times,* Aug. 9, 1993.

19. "Social security [in the United States] is not what most people assume it to be. It is neither a pension plan nor a genuine trust fund. It is, rather, a redistribution system: the federal government taxes the young and gives to the old, plain and simple" ("Anti-Social Security." *The Economist*, Jan. 21, 1995, p. A30).

20. The annual average rise in real terms in Europe between 1970 and 1990 was 4.1 percent. See the discussion of the Andersen Consulting health care survey in Van Overtveldt, "Doctors in Management."

21. On the North American continent the rise was higher than in Europe (for various cultural reasons, such as litigation practices which are virtually unknown in Europe), and Canada, with its single-payer system, faced exactly the same annual rise in health care costs between 1970 and 1990 (5.2 percent) as the United States (5.3 percent). See the discussion of the Andersen Consulting health care survey in Van Overtveldt, "Doctors in Management."

22. Changing a largely private system like the one in the United States into a single-payer system like Canada's in the hope of lowering costs will not make a difference either. According to some analysts, U.S. health costs actually fall below Canada's if one takes into consideration that Canada has a younger population.

23. The main problem is that in a health care system like Germany's, money never changes hands between health care provider and patient. Nowhere is there a sense of accountability or an incentive to economize. See, for example, Bering-Jensen, H. "The German Health Care Squeeze." *Wall Street Journal Europe*, Nov. 8, 1993.

24. Budgets aim to control spending to comply with targets, but the real social costs under this strategy are likely to be high. See, for example, Danzon, P. M., "The Hidden Costs of Budget-Restrained Health Insurance Systems." In R. B. Helms, (ed.), *American Health Policy: Critical Issues for Reform*. Washington, D.C.: AEI Press, 1993; Danzon, P. M. *Global Budgets Versus Competitive Cost-Control Strategies*. Washington, D.C.: AEI Press, 1994; Looney, W. *Drug Budgets: The Hidden Costs of Control: Impact of European Drug Payment Reform on Access, Quality and Innovation*. Zellik, Belgium: CNE, 1995.

25. For example, Dutch newspapers publish monthly lists of waiting periods for specific surgical operations in hospitals in the different regions of the country. The Dutch Federation of Patients and Consumers Organizations (NP/CF) intends to provide the public with a Web site of waiting lists. According to the NP/CF: "The length of hospital waiting lists for treatment and rehabilitation has become a severe problem in the Netherlands. In 1998 people often needed to wait between two and six weeks for a first medical consultation, and for a surgical intervention, this even may take several months, depending on the type of operation and medical facility." [www.hoise.com/vmw/articles/LV-VM-07-98-28.html], May 28, 1998.

26. In June 1991, the Belgian minister of social affairs, Philippe Busquin (currently a commissioner of the European Union), put forward a proposal to introduce in

Belgium a system similar to the one existing in the Netherlands. People would have to choose a general practitioner who would then become their *vaste huisarts* ("fixed family doctor") and keep their "patient file." Patients would be obliged always to see this doctor first. Busquin intended to put an end to the phenomenon of "medical shopping around" (according to Belgian newspapers, June 13, 1991). However, the opposition to the proposal was strong and Busquin's plan was buried. In 1995, the proposal was revived by the Belgian government ("Dehaene wil een vaste huisarts" (Dehaene Wants a Family Doctor). *De Standaard,* Apr. 24, 1995) but ran into strong opposition again. In 1998, a consensus was reached whereby people over sixty are free to opt for a *vaste huisarts.* If they do so, they receive higher reimbursements ("Vaste huisarts goedkoper voor 60-plusser" (Family Doctor Is Cheaper for People over Sixty). *De Standaard,* Dec. 17, 1998).

27. Some analysts call the present evolution, rather euphemistically, one toward a "quasi-market, whereby health and social care finance remains in the hands of the state, but some kind of managed competition is introduced into the system of care provision" (Le Grand, J. "The Evaluation of Health Care System Reforms." In Ferrera, M. *The Evaluation of Social Policies: Experiences and Perspectives.* Pavia, Italy: Faculty of Political Science of the University of Pavia, 1993, p. 54).

28. The United States is also familiar with the concept of managed care, but rather than the government, private organizations are doing the managing here. See, for example, Clancy, C. M., and Brody, H. "Managed Care: Jekyll or Hyde?" *Journal of the American Medical Association,* Jan. 25, 1995, pp. 338–339. However, a government-regulated managed competition system was introduced at the state level in Tennessee in 1994, as discussed in Lemov, P. "An Acute Case of Health Care Reform." *Governing,* May 1994, pp. 44–48. Wasley, T. "TennCare: Health Care Reform: Dream of Disappointment." Heritage Foundation *State Backgrounder,* Feb. 28, 1995.

29. As one observer sees it: "The phrase managed care is as thin as a verbal fig leaf. Look it up in your glossary of contemporary survival and you'll find its true definition: restricted care" (Passaro, V. "On the Examining Table: A Patient's Wary Encounter with Managed Health Care." *Harper's,* May 1994, p. 63).

30. "Recipe Trouble: Production Problems at Generic-Drug Firm Lead to Serious Claims." *Wall Street Journal Europe,* Feb. 3, 1995.

31. An in-depth study of a reference pricing system and its consequences is Maassen, B. M. *Reimbursement of Medicinal Products: Law, Administrative Practice and Economics of the German Reference Price System.* Zellik, Belgium: CNE, 1996.

32. "Industry Profile: Pharmaceuticals." German Brief, Frankfurter Allgemeine Zeitung Information Services, Nov. 5, 1993.

33. Melloan, G. "Why Europeans Are Being Shorted on Miracle Drugs." *Wall Street Journal Europe,* Apr. 19, 1994.

34. Blendon, R., and others. "Physician's Perspectives on Caring for Patients in the United States, Canada and West Germany." *New England Journal of Medicine,* Apr. 8, 1993, pp. 1011–1016.

35. For instance, in Spain one in ten insured have purchased a second (private) insurance policy to secure coverage. See, for example, Arrumada, B. "Spain's Health Care System Needs Surgery." *Wall Street Journal Europe.* Aug. 2, 1994. In Italy, according to some estimates, over 50 percent of those entitled to "free" public health routinely resort to private provision. See, for example, Martino, "The 100 Trillion Lire Health Care Mess."

36. Sometimes individuals are legally allowed to buy additional private health care, but private health care providers are not allowed to sell them their services. The best-equipped hospital in Glasgow, Scotland, is a private hospital run by the U.S. company Health Care International. The hospital is mostly empty, and its doctors have nothing to do because although it does get some British patients, it is restricted from admitting large numbers because it is not allowed to compete with local health services in the Glasgow area. See, for example, "Empty Beds: U.S. Overconfidence Leaves This Hospital in Critical Condition." *Wall Street Journal Europe,* Dec. 20, 1994.

37. National Economic Research Associates (NERA). *The Health Care System in Switzerland.* London and White Plains, N.J.: NERA, 1994.

38. Moore, S. "Swiss Insurers Compete to Provide Health Care in More Open Market." *Wall Street Journal,* July 26, 1995. According to this article, Swiss HMOs resemble U.S. HMOs. The largest HMO network is "Swisscare—a management company formed by three leading insurers—which provides health insurance for 2.8 million people." The other big HMO is "Swica, formed by the merger of four health insurers in Nov. 1992. . . . Swica is the national pioneer in crossing the divide between insurer and health-care provider. Swica's budding national web of primary-care centers is modeled on powerful national networks assembled by American giants such as Kaiser Permanente and United Health Care Corp. Other Swiss rivals are following suit, and insurers-turned-providers now hope to adopt the full managed-care menu—including wresting volume discounts from pharmaceutical giants on drug purchases and even dispensing medicines more cheaply by mail."

39. Zweifel, P. *Bonus Options in Health Insurance.* Norwell, Mass.: Kluwer, 1994.

40. National Economic Research Associates. *The Health Care System in Switzerland.*

41. World Health Organization (WHO), Regional Office for Europe. *Country Information Switzerland.* Copenhagen: WHO, Regional Office for Europe, Dec. 1, 1997.

42. According to the Organization for Economic Cooperation and Development (OECD), in 1996 the United States devoted 14.0 percent of GDP to health, Germany 10.5 percent, and Switzerland 10.2 percent, followed by France with 9.7 percent, and Canada with 9.6 percent. The Netherlands and Sweden reached 8.6 percent, Belgium 7.8 percent, and the United Kingdom 6.9 percent (*Health Data 98.* Paris: OECD, 1998).

43. "Health Care Costs Rise." Swiss Week in Review. *Neue Zürcher Zeitung,* Mar. 22–28, 1999.

44. Switzerland. Federal Statistical Office. *Anstieg der Gesundheitskosten* (Increase in Health Care Costs), June 4, 1998.

45. These government subsidies account for about one-third of Swiss annual health care spending. According to the Organization for Economic Cooperation and Development, *Health Data 98*, in 1994 in the United States, only 44.6 percent of total expenditure on health came from public sources, whereas the Swiss figure was 72.1 percent. This was well below Belgium's 87.9 percent and Sweden's 84.6 percent, but not far from France's 74.0 percent and the 77.5 percent in the Netherlands and Germany. As I pointed out earlier the Netherlands and Germany have partially privatized health care systems, whereas the quality of public health care in France is considered so poor that most French who can afford to do so buy additional health care on the market.

46. In the United States some experiments with MSAs have led to substantial cost saving. See, for example, Tweed, V. "Medical Savings Accounts: Are They a Viable Option?" *Business & Health,* Oct. 1994.

47. U.S. employers' health care costs fell 1.1 percent in 1994 as enrollment in managed care plans rose to 58 percent of employees from 46 percent in 1993. But 15 percent of employees joined HMOs that allowed them to use doctors outside the plan, up from 7 percent in 1993. See, for example, "Employer Costs for Health Care Fall 1.1% in U.S." *Wall Street Journal Europe,* Feb. 15, 1995.

48. As private systems are more flexible than the heavily regulated public systems, they seem able to remedy their own flaws. See, for example, "While Congress Remains Silent, Health Care Transforms Itself." *New York Times,* Dec. 18, 1994.

49. For example, for an analysis of the Belgian service sectors that are moving to countries with low labor costs, see "Het hazepad van de dienstensektor." *De Morgen,* Feb. 3, 1996.

50. According to the U.S. Bureau of Labor Statistics ("A world without jobs?" *The Economist,* Feb. 11, 1995), the number of home health workers in the United States is predicted to grow by 140 percent between 1992 and 2005.

51. When a country's economy grows, its spending on health care grows even faster, as can be seen in Asia. See, for example, "Healthcare Spending Set to Race Ahead in Asia." *Financial Times,* Apr. 27, 1995.

52. Zweifel, P. *Health Care Reforms and the Role of the Pharmaceutical Industry: Proceedings of a European Workshop.* Basel, Switzerland: Pharmaceutical Partners for Better Healthcare, 1995.

53. Indeed, in many single-payer countries equity does not exist. Studies show that the Inuits and Crees in Canada and the Maoris in New Zealand receive less health care and have worse health outcomes than other citizens of those countries. See, for example, Goodman and Musgrave, *Twenty Myths About National Health Insurance.*

54. Schaapveld, K., Chorus, A.M.J., and Perenboom, R.J.M. "The European Health Potential: What Can We Learn from Each Other?" *Health Policy,* 1995, *33,* pp. 205–217.

55. This is also the conclusion of Jeremy W. Hurst in his study of health care in Belgium, France, Germany, Ireland, the Netherlands, Spain, and the United Kingdom. As Hurst sees it, all seven countries have adopted global budgets for public expenditure on health care and firm policies for making such budgets stick. It seems that central governments feel that only they can balance the marginal benefits with the marginal costs of extra public spending on health care. ("Reforming Health Care in Seven European Nations." *Health Affairs,* Fall 1991, pp. 7–21.)

56. As one analyst sees it: "Real reform of the [French] health care system seems absolutely necessary, not so much because of the high costs—as so many people wrongly believe (health is priceless)—but because it is absurd for a modern and rich nation not to have the best system possible" (Vergara, F. "An Opportunity for Real Health Care Reform." *Wall Street Journal Europe,* Dec. 19, 1995).

CHAPTER TWENTY-FOUR

Consumer-Driven Health Care

An International View

Alvaro Salas-Chaves

Consumer-driven health care can be considered the latest strategy to improve the performance of health care systems. It is politically attractive because it embodies the basis for a modern health care system that transfers increasing responsibility to the individual. In the twenty-first century politicians will support these ideas of change and self-confidence because people want to make their own decisions and take their own risks and responsibilities. It is credible because other sectors of the economy have already made great strides in improving consumer focus, with tangible benefits for the consumer. The whole economy is changing in this direction. Commerce and industry in general provide excellent examples.[1] If it works in the automobile market or in the computer market, why not in the health care market?

Consumer-driven health care is the expected outcome of decades of investment in human capital. It is the result of great efforts made by generations of hard-working teachers in schools and universities to produce educated people who are capable of making the best possible decisions. As education levels rise and information is more accessible to individuals, consumers become ever more conscious of the importance of quality health care; this new awareness, and the demands it will place on health systems worldwide, will ensure the feasibility of its implementation.

Finally, consumer-driven health care strategy is possible because it challenges intelligent managers and entrepreneurs who will strive for greater convenience at affordable prices and better quality of services and satisfaction. Until now the concept of a market for health care has been little used. Traditionally, the health care market has been overregulated by the state, with limited information about real prices, costs of interventions, and real returns. Consumer-driven health care can be the catalyst that changes this long-standing practice.

THE INTERNATIONAL CONTEXT

During the last two decades governments the world over have initiated health care reforms that aim to improve the value given for the money spent on health care.[2] Developed, underdeveloped, and poor countries alike have established task forces, steering committees, and health commissions[3] to reshape the health care system because no one is satisfied with the kind of service provided and with its costs. From Britain to Singapore and from the United States to Chile and Costa Rica, everyone agrees that there is a need for change. Countries; governments; international agencies such as the Pan American Health Organization and World Health Organization (PAHO/WHO), the World Bank, and the Inter-American Development Bank; and industrialized countries' development agencies, among others, strongly support those reforms, especially in underdeveloped and poor countries.[4]

In 1993, the World Bank dedicated its sixteenth World Development Report, *Investing in Health,* to the interaction that exists among human health, health policymaking, and economic development. As Lewis T. Preston, its then-president, stated: first, governments have to improve the economic endeavor to allow families themselves to improve their health status; second, public expenditure on health has to be reoriented toward more cost-effective programs to contribute better to the health of the poor; and third, governments must facilitate diversity and competitiveness in the financing and provision of care.[5]

It is clear that the existing systems do not work. It is also clear that even though the top-down reforms have tended to improve accessibility of services, equity, and resource allocations, health services continue to fail to meet the expectations and desires of their customers. During the millennium we are now embarking on, health care systems will take a big step forward. It is time for a bottom-up approach to organizing the health care system, time to put the customer in the center of the organization.

THE NEW MILLENNIUM, THE CONSUMER ERA

The new millennium announces a new era, the consumer era. It is informative to browse the Internet and see the vast amounts of information and services focused on the consumer. Every day the amount of information available to the consumer increases, encouraging one clear strategy: do it yourself, make your own decisions. People want to become responsible for their own destiny. People want to do the things they want, whenever they want, because they have the purchasing power and the information that empowers them to make better decisions. They want to buy goods and the services they think they need, exercising what is known as *purchasing power.* People already do so in many different ways, when they buy a car or when they buy a new house, for example, and for purchases such as these, excellent sources of information are available to help them make the best decision. Health care services are next; why should they not be?

THE ROLE OF GOVERNMENT

Governments have a fundamental role to play in increasing the feasibility of consumer-driven health care. In many areas one of the main reasons consumers can make their own decisions safely is that the product they are buying is guaranteed. That means that products have passed testing in order to be approved, released, and put on the market. No matter which make of computer you buy, all of them are surely good enough. The differences in price will relate to the capacity of the hard disk or the computer's speed; the more capacity and accessories you buy, the more you pay. But all the computers will do what a computer has to do, faster or slower, in 3D or not, with multimedia or not.

The health care market has to offer more transparent products that include basic and fundamental standards. The standardization of products and information available to consumers will have to make use of international benchmarks and best practices. In this regard governments will have to guarantee the scope, the content, and to some extent, the quality of the basic products offered to the consumers. For instance, all plans would have to comply with a mandatory set of recommendations and activities that come from committees of experts. Again, regardless of the cost of the plan, the government would have to ensure that all of them, the basic plan and the most comprehensive one, include preventive and health promotion activities as well as the curative and rehabilitation services traditionally associated with health care services. In addition, greater emphasis needs to be placed on defining the roles of government and the consumer in the provision of catastrophic services. The differences in price among plans will relate to plan comprehensiveness and options. Underlying all the plans would be the need to consider consumer preferences in order to offer an acceptable level of services.

OBSTACLES TO OVERCOME

There are major obstacles to overcome in the implementation of broad-based, consumer-driven health care. The first one is legislative approval of a new body of laws that will allow employers to transfer contributions intended to pay for health care to employees and, most important, that will elaborate a transparent definition of the process of transferring those contributions to the employees. It is fundamental to have a body of laws that regulates the transformation of the health care market. There are many advantages to this major transformation, but it is important to keep in mind that there will be winners and losers, and all of them need clear rules of the game embedded in the new framework.

Chile is an example of a Latin American country that has made it possible for employers to transfer social security contributions to employees as a salary increase. Afterward, new employees started at a higher wage and workers were responsible for purchasing their own health insurance. In months, hundreds of private insurers started new business by offering different types of plans. Today Chile's valuable experience provides important lessons regarding the implementation of a system based predominantly in individual choice. Again, there are winners and losers. In the Chilean case, major opposition was easily overcome because the president, at that time, did not need congressional approval to make this systemic change.

I have no doubt that providing adequate and comprehensible information is the second large obstacle for the broad-based implementation of consumer-driven health care. As Hibbard and Jewett explain, "Although consumers are very interested in having access to quality-of-care information about health plans, physicians, and hospitals, many of them do not understand some of the indicators appearing in health care report cards."[6] Information is the key to the successful organization of health care as consumer driven.

LET CONSUMERS EXERCISE PURCHASING POWER

There is no general solution for everyone—employers, consumers, and providers. Instead, there are different solutions for everyone. Small businesses require their own solution and large ones require their own solution, no doubt about that; the same is true for providers and insurers. What it is clear is that empowered consumers will overcome today's problems. Consumer-driven health care is the general framework in which empowered consumers will shop around, according to their expectations, convenience, and purchasing power.

Consumer-driven health care can establish a system tailored to the needs and preferences of the family, and most important, it can send a clear and vital message: "If you want to be healthy and to have a healthy family, it is time to acquire good habits, to give up smoking and drinking, and to take up a healthy style of living including good nutrition and physical exercise. When you do this, you will be rewarded with an affordable premium." Consumer-driven health care can be the key that unlocks the potential of health care systems worldwide to achieve the health status goals set forth by PAHO/WHO. Changing the health care paradigm to increase the role of the consumers has the potential to align incentives at both the personal and system levels and to drive health systems to better performance. (Figure 24.1 summarizes the key arguments and recommendations of this chapter.)

Notes

1. Herzlinger, R. E. *Market-Driven Health Care: Who Wins, Who Loses in the Transformation of American's Largest Service Industry.* Reading, Mass.: Addison-Wesley, 1997,

2. Jaramillo, I., Cleofe Molina, C., and Salas, A. *Las reformas sociales en accion: Salud* (Social reforms in action: Health). Santiago, Chile: Comision Economica para America Latina y el Caribe (CEPAL), 1996.

3. Pan American Health Organization. *Health Conditions in the Americas.* PAHO Scientific Publication No. 549. Washington, D.C.: Pan American Health Organization, 1994.

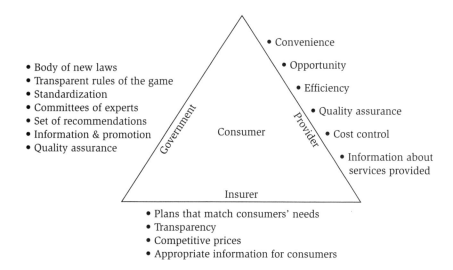

Figure 24.1. Consumer-Driven Health Care Triangle.

4. Salas-Chaves, A. *La CCSS, Presente y Futuro* (The Costa Rican Department of Social Security, Present and Future). San Jose, Costa Rica: CCSS, 1998.

5. World Bank. *World Development Report 1993: Investing in Health.* New York: Oxford University Press, 1993.

6. Hibbard, J. H., and Jewett, J. "Consumers Need Help in Understanding Health Care Report Cards." *Research Activities* (Agency for Health Care Policy and Research), No. 194, June 1996.

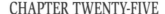

CHAPTER TWENTY-FIVE

Challenges of Consumer-Driven Health Care

Eugene D. Hill III

As a financial fiduciary and venture capitalist, my goals are to produce top-quartile, risk-adjusted returns on investment for my investors. My colleagues and I accomplish this by backing superior management teams with differentiated business strategies in large and rapidly growing markets characterized by disequilibrium.

From the investor perspective we evaluate investments with regard to market, management, method, money, and milestones. Health care easily passes the market size test and most of its segments pass the growth rate test. Owing to the dominance of nonprofit entities and government entitlement programs, entrepreneurial management teams have been scarce. There are many ways to invest in the consumer-driven health care system, each with varying market size, growth rate, operating margin, and capital intensity characteristics and further differentiated by function and method and source of payment. For example, one can choose between product or service companies and between wholesale (business to business) or retail (business to consumer) models. One can choose to be an infomediary or a traditional provider of care, either facility based or ambulatory, or a payer or care manager. In the past it has been possible to generate venture returns in such diverse entities as hospitals, skilled nursing facilities, ambulatory surgery centers, home health agencies, and managed care organizations and in such areas as physician practice management, medical devices, pharmaceuticals,

368

and health care information technology. In the late 1990s, the health care Internet companies enjoyed spectacular valuations, whereas the effects of the 1997 federal balanced budget amendments have crippled many of the service providers.

To the degree that the consumer-driven health care system reduces the failed government price controls and empowers a better-informed consumer to make direct purchases of health care goods and services, such opportunities will represent investment potential superior to that of the current highly regulated quasi-market in which consumers and providers are insulated from many of the direct economic consequences of their behavior. We will support companies that operate in a market environment and that will succeed or fail based on their ability meet consumer demand.

HEALTH MANAGEMENT PERSPECTIVE

Fragmented delivery and regulation, inefficient provision of care, perverse financial incentives, and highly variable quality have characterized the health care system in the United States. Most service providers, hospitals, and managed care organizations enjoy nonprofit tax-exempt status, and certain purchasers (employees) enjoy tax subsidization of their benefit plan purchases. Government entitlement programs (Medicare and Medicaid) are the dominant financiers of care. Disproportionate distribution costs are borne by individuals and small employers.

In response to cost-containment pressures exerted by the government and managed care, consolidation is occurring throughout the health care industry. Tax-exempt organizations are converting to for-profit status to access equity capital markets. The industry's historical underinvestment in information technology stands in stark contrast to the productivity gains and consumer service improvements achieved in other consumer service industries. Purchasing coalitions such as the Buyers Health Care Action Group (BHCAG) are attempting to standardize benefits, provide improved consumer information, and encourage evidence-based medicine. The high rates of health cost inflation that characterized the 1980s have been held largely in check in the 1990s, with prescription drugs being the notable exception.

The recent past has witnessed the bankruptcy of both large nonprofit and for-profit health care organizations due to flawed business models or execution; excessive debt leverage in a fundamentally low-margin business has proven unsupportable. Demoralization and dissatisfaction have led to calls for physician unionization and anti–managed care legislation.

CONSUMER PERSPECTIVE

The problems with wholesale employer-based distribution of health benefits are well known; excepting possibly dental insurance, health insurance is a combination of tax-subsidized, prepaid health care and catastrophic insurance protection. Moral hazard, adverse selection, benefit incomparability, and the "free-rider" problem are associated with the current system. Consumers face knowledge disparities and information deficits that render comparison shopping difficult; payment systems encourage supply-induced or -reduced demand. Except for elective procedures such as cosmetic surgery, consumers rarely know the price of goods or services in advance. In aggregate, we in the United States spend more of our resources on health care than other developed countries do, yet many of the goods and services we purchase are either not beneficial or are indeed harmful. Excessive amounts of resources are consumed by administrative activities with no added value.

SUMMARY

The challenge to the health care delivery systems will be to establish accountable, comprehensive, and competitive systems of care within local markets. The challenge to the regulators will be to remove structural barriers and let the market function, while preserving medical education, medical research, access to care in rural areas, and coverage of those with chronic conditions. The challenge to the consumers will be to take charge of their health, recognize that many health conditions are lifestyle mediated, and make better-informed purchases. The challenge to the investors will be to support enterprises that bring consumer-responsive, beneficial goods and services to the market.

By necessity, the process to achieve such changes will be evolutionary and will require substantive legislative action and initiative. Nevertheless, like the defined contribution pension plans that replaced the defined benefit pension plans, consumer-driven health care will prevail.

It is my firm conviction that the only hope we have of avoiding the kind of failure found in the socialized health benefit programs of Canada and Western Europe is to foster consumer-driven health care. It will not be easy; many entrenched economic and political constituencies will be threatened. The freedom to trust market forces and empower consumer choice will result in winners and losers, good and bad providers, and wise and unwise choices.

CHAPTER TWENTY-SIX

Making the Transition to Consumer-Driven Health Care

Jesse S. Hixson

It is hard to imagine consumer-driven health care emerging vigorously within the context and confines of our traditional employer-based health benefit system. One reason for this is that the structure of demand presented by the employer-based system cannot elicit an efficient supply response in most markets. Another is that consumers cannot express their demand to all willing suppliers in the market. In response to consumer-driven demand, providers must become patient oriented, not only packaging and marketing condition-specific sets of services but also combining these packages with a broader range of services designed to maximize convenience for patients by meeting all of their health care needs. Serving patients with chronic conditions provides the greatest opportunity for organizing a service response of this type. Forty-six percent of the people in the noninstitutionalized population have one or more chronic conditions, but they account for 76 percent of medical care expenditure. Persons with chronic conditions account for 69 percent of hospital admissions and 80 percent of hospital days; they account for 96 percent of home care visits, 83 percent of drug prescriptions, and 66 percent of physician visits.

An illustrative chronic disease market segment is diabetes. The direct cost of treating the ten million Americans with diabetes is about 5 percent of national health expenditures, but diabetes patients account for more than 15 percent of total national health expenditures. Providers targeting this segment would ideally organize services around treatment of diabetes but offer the whole spectrum of services required by these patients.

Even though this concept may sound like an HMO, it is not. Contemporary HMOs are organized around an insurance product, whereas patient-oriented provider organizations would want to market to a population owning a variety of insurance products varying widely in coverage and cost-sharing requirements. In the current employer-driven system, distinct pools of employees make up market segments. Providers who do not have access to particular employee pools are denied the opportunity to compete for patients from those pools. Each employee pool is a heterogeneous group of patients, and that forces the service response to be heterogeneous and diffuse.

In a consumer-driven system, providers must be able to compete to attract patients across all insurance pools and be able to target well-defined populations within them. This would afford the development and marketing of highly focused product lines that can be offered more efficiently, effectively, and competitively. The employer-based system of pooling risk seems to place significant barriers in the way of those who want to market their products to individuals rather than employers. In a consumer-driven system, patients must also be able to express their demands to willing suppliers. Restriction of individual access to available suppliers through managed care limits patients' ability to express their demands in the market.

Through managed care, employers have sought to reduce the amount of health care services provided to employees by placing restrictions on providers and covered services, yet they have preserved the basic incentives for employees to overconsume services. Employers have also limited the choices that employees have when choosing a plan—steering them to managed care programs through premium price differentials or offering only managed care plans. Obviously, employers are not going to be able to back away from managing their employees' consumption of health care as long as they preserve the incentives for employees to overconsume. It is difficult to conclude that consumer-driven health care can flourish as long as employers remain in the picture.

Many policymakers and consumers worry about the availability of information for patients in an era of consumer-driven health care. It is understandable that the current employer-based system does not generate consumer-oriented information, because consumers have limited choices and options and there is little payoff for producing information. If consumers come to have a spectrum of options in a consumer-driven health system, however, there will be a substantial payoff forthcoming for producers of information. For example, the Federal Employees Health Benefit Program provides extensive choice to consumers, and information is readily available to them from private sources.

CHAPTER TWENTY-SEVEN

The New Consumer-Driven Health Care System

Daniel H. Johnson

The last fifteen years of the twentieth century were a nightmare for many patients and for those who have provided their health care. In particular the patient-physician relationship has been devastated. The problems have derived from an effort by employers and government to harness runaway costs. However, both employers and government have failed to recognize the underlying basis for the rapid escalation of costs, the insulation of the person consuming the services, which is to say the patient, from the cost of those services. Just as that disconnect has been the cause of virtually all the problems that followed, the creation of a consumer-driven health care system will correct these deficiencies, increase the quality of care, and lower its cost. As traumatic as the last fifteen years of the twentieth century were, the events of those years have provoked an enormous amount of focused thinking and experimentation with our health care system, resulting in the potential for a vastly improved system that will serve as a model for all the other developed countries in the world. Out of all these lemons, we are on the verge of producing some very delicious lemonade.

Because of the folly of third-party micromanagement, some very divisive activities have taken place. The government has used preemptive and forceful tactics against medical schools, hospitals, and physicians, creating an entire new *compliance* industry. Heavy-handed insurance companies have provoked an outcry for regulations and liability exposure for insurers from physicians, people who normally dislike regulation and the tort system. Government and insurance companies and, in some cases employers, have relied on price controls to attempt to contain cost, producing the inevitable insulation of the patient from the cost. Predictably, although some brief respite from double-digit cost escalation was accomplished, insurance premiums are heading back up, and employers are threatened with the specter of liability for medical decision making.

The emerging consumer-driven system fixes all of this. Perhaps the most significant distortion of our old system was its attempt to create a market with reduced choice, a blatantly dysfunctional approach. Expanding the choices of financing mechanisms and delivery models available to patients will create a true market. Giving individuals the opportunity and the responsibility to choose and own their own insurance, with the periodic right to change if dissatisfied, will cause system accountability to flow to the patient, where it should be. It will also solve the portability problem. Moving from a defined benefit to a defined contribution system will enable the employer to continue to provide a health care benefit but will give the employer complete predictability over the cost of that benefit and will shield the employer from any liability for medical decision making.

Several innovations will be necessary if we are to implement and facilitate the new consumer-driven health care system. An advantage of the painful experiences we have just been through is the creative thinking that has gone into how to construct a better system. Examples include the idea of using *focused factories* to target expertise to difficult or chronic problems, such as the management of diabetes, asthma, cancer, long-term neurological disease, and injuries such as burns. Considerable thought has been given to how best to structure the tax system so as to permit individuals to buy insurance instead of having to obtain their insurance through their employer. Implementing the notion of a *refundable tax credit* to assist currently uninsured individuals to buy insurance will be very helpful in eliminating the cost shift that occurs in our current flawed system. Continued thinking and experimentation will be necessary to determine which, if any, is the best way to finance care for individuals with complicated problems. Should we use risk pools or risk-adjusted premiums or focused factories or direct subsidies or some combination of these? Innovative thinking is necessary in order to pool individuals together to take advantage of the rule of large numbers in spreading risk without imposing new layers of micromanagement. The unfettered *health savings account* needs to be a choice open to all individuals. The notion of creating voluntary *choice cooperatives,* as opposed to purchasing cooperatives, seems an attractive way to use market forces to increase quality and lower cost. To make a consumer-driven health care system work, we need to take maximum advantage of the *information technology* available to us now so that physicians and their health care teammates can create the most efficient processes for dealing with certain conditions and can gather and use information about what works best in a particular situation. Physicians will do the right thing when given the right information. Similarly, patients will make the right decisions when given the correct information and the incentives to do so.

In thirty years of private practice of medicine I have seen some amazing distortions. Early in my career, insurance companies would not pay for imaging procedures unless the individual was admitted to the hospital. The tests cost more in that setting. Those admissions created an artificial demand for hospital beds, leading to the oversupply we have currently. No one ever thought about the loss of productivity from incarcerating an ambulatory patient for twenty-four hours to have a thirty-minute test. Enormous utilization problems resulted from first-dollar coverage. The concept of usual, customary, and reasonable was particularly inflationary, not because it was a fee-for-service system but because it fostered a cost-plus mentality. Faced with cost escalation deriving from the insulation of employees from the cost of care, employers turned to a new mechanism to control cost that was also first-dollar coverage, namely, prepaid care. At the same time, that mechanism limited choice, and the rest, as they say, is history.

All of this, over time, has provoked a series of questions in my mind. Is it better to link the patient to the cost or to insulate the patient from the cost? If you are going to link the patient, is it better to reward the patient for using the system in a cost-effective way or to punish the patient for not doing so? Is it better to motivate or to regulate? Is it better to entice or coerce?

As we move rapidly into a new consumer-driven health care system, there will inevitably be adjustments to be made. We are going to make mistakes. When we do so, we will have to recognize them and correct them. On balance, I expect physicians to be pleased to be accountable to their patients instead of to employers or to insurance inspectors or to government investigators. Physicians will have more accountability, not less, but the accountability will be to the people to whom we have made our professional commitment. Just as no other good or service is perfect, neither will medicine be perfect. It is, after all, an inexact science. However, in an era of exploding opportunity to do more and better things for patients than we have ever been able to do before, the opportunity to do these things in a system of higher quality and lower cost is exciting indeed. From my perspective, health system reform in the 1990s has been the opportunity of a lifetime. We have, in fact, created a new consumer-driven health care system, which will put the patient in the driver's seat. What a wonderful way to begin the new millennium!

CHAPTER TWENTY-EIGHT

The Patient's Right to Decide

Warner V. Slack

During the 1960s, while at the University of Wisconsin, I developed a philosophy that I called *patient power,* in keeping with the parlance of the times.[1] In a break with the traditional paternalism of Western medicine, I argued that patients who want to should be encouraged to make their own medical decisions and helped to do so.[2] It seemed to me that communication between patients and doctors should not be used to persuade patients to do what physicians want them to do; rather, it should be used to outline the possible plans of action so that patients can make clinical decisions for themselves on the basis of their own values. As Shaw once wrote, "Do not do unto others as you would that they should do unto you. Their tastes may not be the same."[3] Controversial for its time, patient power has become more and more accepted by physicians as well as patients. Today patients are still too often deprived of their right to decide, but the people who pay the bills are the ones who deprive them.

Before the Second World War the fee-for-service system was the predominant means of payment for medical care in this country. The doctor billed and the patient paid, often on the spot. Most doctors developed their own fee systems, which depended on the patient's ability to pay. Payment was not always monetary. Commodities that the patient could afford—the proverbial sack of potatoes, for example—were sometimes accepted in lieu of cash. If a patient couldn't pay at all, the doctor would write off the bill, a form of socialized medicine, if you will. And the patient's privacy was protected within the doctor-patient relationship.[4]

376

During the 1940s and 1950s, the concept of a third-party payer—a payer outside the doctor-patient relationship—was controversial, particularly within the medical profession. The American Medical Association (AMA), as a union dutifully representing its physician members, was concerned that third-party payers would impose restrictions on fees. Group insurance programs such as the Kaiser Permanente Plan in California and the Health Insurance Plan in New York came under heavy criticism from the AMA, even to the point of organized boycotts.

In time, however, with rapidly rising medical costs and an increased demand for insurance coverage, medical insurance plans became available, both for individuals and for groups. And the number of private plans grew at a seemingly exponential rate. What were once a few tax-exempt programs, such as Blue Cross and Blue Shield, became a vast array of nonprofit and for-profit corporations. Even the federal government, despite opposition from the AMA and other economic conservatives, became accepted as a principal player with the inception of Medicare in 1965. Universal coverage is now in demand, and third-party payers are ready to market their wares.

The new kid on the block, and in some instances already the bully, was the managed care company. Some for-profit, some tax-exempt, managed care companies now wield great power over health care delivery. Marketing its medical payment plan primarily to the employer who provides coverage for its employees—the fourth-party payer, so to speak—the managed care company can determine which clinicians are participants and what services are reimbursable. The managed care company wants to know what it's paying for. And furthermore, by controlling the purse strings, it is also managing the patient's care, at least indirectly. This is particularly evident in behavioral health care, where the treatment prescribed, even the number of therapy sessions, can be dictated by the third-party payer.[5]

Proponents of consumer-driven health care, and I am a physician and professor of medicine who is one of them, seek to reverse the current trend and transfer more control to the consumer (the patient or prospective patient). With consumer-driven health care it is the consumer who chooses the health plan, rather than the employer, union, or government who supplies the funds. Armed with information to make enlightened decisions, the consumer is empowered to select the group of clinicians and medical facilities most likely to suit his or her needs. Of course, after the consumer has chosen a plan, the payer responsible for financing it is still in a position of control, because the payer can do its best to deny payment for medical services deemed warranted by the patient and physician. However, a health savings account could serve to yield control to the consumer.[6] Supplied by the employer, or by the state or federal government for those who are unemployed or whose employers have no health plan, the health savings account could be used at the consumer's discretion for routine medical expenses.

The use of a health savings account, though subject to thoughtful criticism on both medical and financial grounds,[7] offers several advantages, which I believe would outweigh the disadvantages. Such an account would give control to the patient, whose right to decide would remain sacrosanct within the limits of the account. The third-party payer would become an insurer against medical catastrophe, for which all prospective patients need financial protection. Consumer-driven health care and, in particular, the medical savings account, would also help protect the patient's privacy. For purposes of reimbursement, hospitals and clinics are now required to send confidential information, linked to charges, to various third- and fourth-party payers—strangers to the patient who are beyond the control of the hospital and doctor as well.[8] When care is financed from a health savings account, only those participating in the patient's care would need to know what is being done.

Consumers would be motivated to use the health savings account judiciously; the account would be an equity worth protecting. Patients and prospective patients would have a financial incentive to obtain good medical care, provided with efficiency as well as skill, for themselves and their families. And here the computer can help.[9] It has long been my premise that the largest yet least well utilized health care resource, worldwide, is the patient or prospective patient and that the interactive computer can be used beneficially to enlighten patients and empower them in the health care process, thereby improving the quality of care while reducing the cost. When the forces of supply and demand dictate it, patients do very well in managing medical problems. If, for example, the biochemistry of insulin were such that a child with juvenile diabetes needed only one insulin injection per year, it is likely that an academic endocrinologist in a teaching hospital would give the injection, and at considerable expense. But the need is typically twice a day, and it is the parent or older child who gives the injection at home, with admirable skill. And there are a number of other medical problems, such as headache, sore throat, hypertension, and urinary tract infection, that patients could manage themselves if provided with the clinical information necessary to do so.

Now, with more and more PCs available and worldwide communication made possible over the Internet, computer-assisted medical care in the home is becoming a reality. Web sites offer a wide range of health-related information. Although the information is usually presented in a noninteractive, didactic manner, interactive programs are becoming available to address the patient's individual needs. We are working to develop such programs in our laboratory. The idea is not to replace the doctor. The idea is to fill a void. Patients make medical decisions for themselves all the time; sometimes the most difficult one is whether to go to the doctor. The goal is to have the interactive computer help patients make health care decisions in an enlightened, knowledgeable manner.

Once consumer-driven health care is in place, physicians will welcome their liberation from the parsimonious personnel working for third- and fourth-party payers. And they will be free of much of the offensive, ill-advised, financially driven intrusion of bureaucracy into their relationship with their patients. Employers should also welcome consumer-driven health care, which will free them from the administrative and litigious responsibilities associated with reimbursement. Third-party payers may object at first because consumer-driven health care will entail fundamental corporate changes. Yet they too will be relieved of many administrative and litigious responsibilities that now accompany reimbursement for routine care. But most important, the patient and prospective patient will be the principal beneficiaries.

Notes

1. Slack, W. V. "Patient Power: A Patient-Oriented Value System." In J. A. Jacques (ed.), *Computer Diagnosis and Diagnostic Methods: Proceedings of the Second Conference on the Diagnostic Process Held at the University of Michigan.* Springfield, Ill.: Thomas, 1972, pp. 3–7.

2. Slack, W. V. "The Patient's Right to Decide." *Lancet,* 1977, *2,* 240.

3. Shaw, G. B. *Man and Superman: A Comedy and a Philosophy.* Baltimore, Md.: Penguin, 1952.

4. Slack, W. V. "The Issue of Privacy." *MD Computing,* 1997, *14,* 8–10.

5. Slack, W. V. *Cybermedicine: How Computing Empowers Doctors and Patients for Better Health Care.* San Francisco: Jossey-Bass, 2001.

6. Grahm, P. "Why We Need Medical Savings Accounts." *New England Journal of Medicine,* 1994, *330,* 1752–1753.

7. Zabinski, E., Selden, T. M., Moeller, J. F., and Banthin, J. S. "Medical Savings Accounts: Microsimulation Results from a Model with Adverse Selection." *Journal of Health Economics,* 1999, *18,* 195–218; Rind, D. "Medical Savings Account." *New England Journal of Medicine,* 1994, *331,* 1158.

8. Slack, W. V. "Private Information in the Hands of Strangers." *MD Computing,* 1997, *14,* 83–86.

9. Slack, *Cybermedicine;* Slack, W. V. "Brave New Interviewer." *Harvard Medical School Alumni Bulletin,* 1966, *69*(4), 44–49; Slack, W. V. "Patient-Computer Dialogue and the Patient's Right to Decide." In P. F. Brennan, S. J. Schneider, and E. Tornquist (eds.), *Computers in Health Care: Information Networks for Community Health.* New York: Springer-Verlag, 1997, pp. 55–69.

CHAPTER TWENTY-NINE

Comments on Consumer-Driven Health Care

Corbette S. Doyle

A shift from our current methods of delivering and paying for health care to consumer-driven health care has many implications for the government, insurers, and providers and can also be expected to affect medical technology, cost, and productivity.

THE ROLE OF GOVERNMENT

The government will need to consider how health care information will be regulated. The two key issues will be patients' privacy and the reliability of data that consumers use to make critical decisions. The Internet will likely become the major source of information that consumers rely on for health care decisions. The Net will replace the information gathering and synthesizing process that currently takes place in the human resource department of a large employer. Stories that false health care information is being disseminated via the Net are rampant already. In a consumer-driven health care model, it will be essential that consumers can be assured of the validity of the data they use for decisions. The government will not be able to ignore this.

Similarly, the demand for health care data on individuals will grow exponentially as providers, insurers, and the like seek this information for underwriting decisions and for marketing purposes. The need for these data is currently less of an issue because so many insurers' decisions are made for

380

groups of patients. As these data become more accessible and in greater demand, however, the need for consumer privacy protection will increase.

THE ROLE OF INSURERS AND PROVIDERS

Significant changes will be required of the insurance industry because many of the players are now organized to respond to the needs of large corporate buyers. The current focus on managed cost will need to shift to a true managed *care* focus because consumers will now be able to vote with their feet. Insurers, if they are smart, will reorganize their information systems so that they can provide quality of care information to consumers. Another significant change for many insurers will be the need to change their underwriting, claims tracking, and marketing processes to focus on the individual rather than the group. These changes are attractive to the extent that insurers will be forced to become more responsive to the needs of the individuals receiving the care rather than to the needs of those currently paying for the care. There will be major losers and winners during this transition process because the industry is fairly well bifurcated now between those focused on large groups and those focused on individuals and small employers. Many of the big players today do not have the structure in place to respond to individuals. The losses suffered by the firms who do not adapt well will create dislocations in the economy.

As for providers, they have proven they are not reluctant to reorganize; the real problem is that no one has, as yet, figured out an organizational model that meets the needs of all constituents. The historical, loosely organized model failed miserably to restrain cost increases. The efforts of the physician practice management firms to organize physicians failed to meet the cultural and philosophical needs of physicians. Capitation, although it puts some of the financial risk on the providers' shoulders, where it needs to be to control costs, alienates some consumer advocates.

By reestablishing the connection between consumers and their chosen providers, a consumer-driven model may provide enough stability to allow providers to select long-term organizational models with a higher likelihood of survival. Self-directed care will assume much greater significance in this model, and consumers will be interested in integrated providers who offer one-stop shopping. Nevertheless, with better information available, they will continue to demand freedom of choice. There is a risk that organized providers will try to limit choice to the providers, labs, and so forth that are part of their own organization. This would just replace the HMO restrictions we have today with provider-enforced restrictions. Thus many consumers will likely choose specialists over integrated provider groups.

THE ROLE OF MEDICAL TECHNOLOGY

Will the shift toward replacing services with technology be enhanced in a consumer-driven model? A consumer-driven model will not end the battle between cost, new technology, and imperfect information. However, to the extent that the decision is left in the hands of consumers, and not hindered by payer restraints and exclusions, then a shift toward proven technology will result more quickly than it would have otherwise.

COST AND PRODUCTIVITY IMPLICATIONS

One likely outcome is that the demarcation between the health care haves and have-nots will increase. Those who can afford to supplement their employer-paid health care budget with their own dollars will have the greatest range of options; those who cannot will have the most restrictions. If providers are not forced to rein in costs in a consumer-driven model, fixed employer budgets will eventually pay a smaller and smaller percentage of the overall cost of employee health care. This could be a dangerous precedent. If the employer no longer has responsibility for restraining costs, who will step in to fill this critical role?

Employers are just beginning to realize the value of focusing on employee productivity and absence management rather than on the budget line items for health care and workers' compensation. This is a valuable role for the economy as a whole because it implies a shift in focus away from treating symptoms cheaply and toward keeping people well. The current efforts to look at the employee's entire well-being, on an integrated basis, will be disrupted if there is a shift to individual decision making about nonoccupational health care needs and corporate decision making about occupational needs. Employers will have to reevaluate how to influence productivity in a consumer-driven model.

THE ATTRACTIVENESS OF CONSUMER-DRIVEN HEALTH CARE

A consumer-driven model is conceptually appealing and will make sense for many employers. One of the major benefits of this model would be increased employee satisfaction, at least in the short term while the employer-paid budget is adequate to cover a percentage of the total costs comparable to the past. Employer-employee relations should improve when the employer removes itself from the cost and access battle. In addition, if self-directed care becomes more prevalent, employers would benefit from a healthier workforce. In all likelihood, however, those who take care of themselves now would also do so in a consumer-driven model. Those who do not take care of themselves now will not do so in any other system unless they are given incentives or mandates.

A major risk is that as described above, the new employer focus on absence management and productivity will lose momentum. Another risk is that the largest employers will lose the relative advantage they now have over smaller employers that comes from their significant health care purchasing power. This too could cause economic dislocation. The biggest risk, however, is that health care costs will again start to skyrocket once employers feel they are responsible only for establishing and maintaining a fixed contribution rather than for paying for their employees' health care needs.

The biggest risks may well accrue to the early adopters that choose to offer a consumer-driven strategy side-by-side with a traditional HMO option rather than as a full replacement for previous plans. Assuming each employee will select the least-cost alternative based on his or her health care consumption patterns, and given such diametrically opposed plans, then each would, by definition, choose the most expensive option for the employer. Alternatively, an employer can achieve the best of all worlds by offering only health care plans that co-opt the employee in the cost-benefit trade-off.

CHAPTER THIRTY

The Evolution of Consumer-Driven Health Care

Robert W. Coburn

In the United States, access to health care services is viewed as a basic human *right* in a way that applies to no other good or service. We ration virtually everything in our society—including food, housing, transportation, and education—according to one's ability and willingness to pay. But not health care. Moreover, our health care "system" apparently offers none of the differing levels of quality that we normally associate with consumer choice. Our society firmly believes that every hospital and every physician should provide and that every citizen, rich or poor, insured or uninsured, should have ready access to the finest health care in the Western Hemisphere.

This has created an extraordinary sense of entitlement that exists in an environment

- With little competition based on quality, service, price, or any other factors normally associated with "value"

- With a vast excess supply of health care providers

- Where this excess supply drives demand to such an extent that neither the poorest-quality nor the most unreasonably expensive providers are driven from business

- Where buyers and sellers of services rarely communicate directly with each other but purchase services through health plans that focus primarily on their own business objectives

- Where the ultimate consumer is largely uninformed but firmly believes he or she is entitled to virtually unlimited services paid for by someone else

A consumer-driven model would address these problems more successfully than virtually any other model. It would afford consumers increased choice and increased discretion about what health care services they buy and when, where, and how they buy them. Providers would become more conscious of quality and service, more price competitive, and more accountable.

A consumer-driven model will represent massive change, and in most communities it is not clear that *any* interested party—whether health care providers, employers, insurers or health plans, government, labor, or consumers—perceives sufficient potential benefit to lead such a change. It will surely evolve, therefore, in the most haphazard fashion.

VISION AND MODELS

The vision of consumer-driven health care is sound and is one of the few models likely to produce true value—satisfied consumers and real price competition. After all, it *makes sense* for buyers and sellers of services to talk to each other. But major hurdles must be overcome.

First, many large employers are reluctant to support this concept:

They believe it would be viewed as a huge benefit loss, and they do not want complaints from irate employees. They helped create a strong sense of entitlement, and a change to a system that is not "employer pays most" would be viewed very negatively.

They have some sense of the level of communication and education that would be required to make employees reasonably knowledgeable purchasers of health care services. Most have not provided this education yet, and they have little confidence that they can provide it to the due diligence level that legal counsel might require.

Large employers *know* the necessary consumer data on provider performance are not available—some have been asking for it for twenty years—and they do not want to be perceived as part of the problem when it does not appear.

The first time that employees who do not buy reasonable coverage for themselves suffer a catastrophic accident or illness, large employers will still look like the deep pockets to plaintiffs' attorneys. And large employers are concerned that providers will take advantage of individual employees and limit or deny access to care to the sickest patients. Every such instance means potential litigation.

Human resource professionals worry that such an approach will make their own roles and jobs superfluous, and they also want the historical benefit levels to be available when they retire.

Despite this reluctance, when annual health care cost increases are now measured in terms of "thousands of FTEs," even large employers can no longer generate sufficient revenue to continue their current benefit structures.

Second, small employers should generally favor this idea. Many genuinely want to provide health benefits to their employees. But to an overwhelming degree their primary need is to minimize operating costs. They are not organized into a market presence nor is health care usually their area of expertise. Many can no longer afford to buy health insurance for their employees,[1] and providing some fixed contribution toward health care coverage may be their only option.

Third, physicians and hospitals will have divergent views on consumer purchasing:

> Most made some price concessions and reduced utilization for health plans, but recent price increases and comparisons of average costs with lowest-observed costs (on a per-unit or per-member basis) reveal they are not close to truly controlling costs. Many are unlikely to be interested in negotiating prices directly with consumers who may well find their prices grossly unreasonable.

> Today neither health plans nor employers hold providers rigorously accountable for quality, service, or price. Physicians and hospitals in virtually every state continue to vigorously oppose efforts to publicly disclose information about their performance or costs. They characterize any change that limits revenue generation as causing "poor quality." They may have little interest in being held accountable by individual consumers who neither understand nor accept their vague concepts of quality, do not appreciate the "value" providers will claim, and demand greater levels of service and responsiveness than they currently provide.

> Other providers, however, believe consumers will demand less accountability, be less knowledgeable about health care processes and outcomes, and have less leverage in fee negotiations than larger organizations. They despise the present health plans and would rather work with literally anyone else.

> In general, increases in patient cost sharing will lead, slowly, to greater transparency. This, accompanied by the extraordinary price variability that already exists, will slowly lead to the beginnings of price competition.

Fourth, most insurers and health plans will actively resist consumer-driven models:

Their efforts to consolidate market share and reduce competition to the point where they can force more favorable arrangements from health care providers and charge employer clients increasingly higher rates, regardless of the actual underlying medical costs, have begun to crumble under the pressure of increasing resistance from providers.

They are greatly concerned about the loss of revenues and profits from administrative services. But because they have failed to control costs on an ongoing basis, provider pressures for increased revenues may render many new products unaffordable.

Fifth, employees have expressed little interest in such an approach:

When employers survey their employees, more than half routinely report they have no personal physician. That means millions of Americans routinely turn to emergency rooms or specialist physicians instead of primary care sites when they seek care, and it is not clear who will lead the massive consumer-education campaign that would be required to change such behavior.

Many consumers already distrust insurers and health plans, and view them primarily as organizations that exist to deny payment and benefits. Consumers may not rush to embrace new products they might create.

Empowering consumers as purchasers will not help to reduce enormous variations in medical practice, especially where there are still too many providers. If General Motors employees are much more likely to undergo cardiac catheterization in Indiana than in Michigan,[2] empowered employees may be able to negotiate price, but they'll have to go against the advice of their physicians (hardly likely) to reduce overall levels of inappropriate utilization.

Sixth, virtually all consumer models require people to select from available health plans that negotiate with providers and offer products to the market. As with current models, this structure may actually limit consumer choice, preclude price negotiation between buyers and sellers, and artificially maintain system costs far above best-practice levels.

Finally, under the existing tax code, cash provided directly to the employee is taxable income. This suggests that employees will be provided *credits,* or *personal care accounts,* which they will continue to recognize as someone else's money and will spend much more freely than if it were their own cash.

CHRONIC PROBLEMS, INNOVATIVE SOLUTIONS

The most complex problems will be difficult to overcome. First, the vast majority of consumers are not ready to pay for information. Most do not use consumer information regularly (advertising, yes; consumer information, less often), and with the advent of the Internet, people expect virtually all information to be free. As in other fields the first information to emerge is likely to be focused on sales rather than education. And when many lower-income employees already cannot or will not make copayments for medical services, it is not likely that they will pay for information about those services.

Second, consumers do not always eagerly embrace change. In particular, "labor unions have been . . . unfriendly to innovative solutions that are attuned to free market principles and greater personal responsibility."[3] But these workers represent precisely the population whose participation will be needed if the consumer-driven concept is to be successful.

Third, consumers uniformly believe their own providers offer the highest-quality care, so they are rarely motivated to seek better care elsewhere. They know that in most other markets (cars, clothes, computers) they can choose to buy different levels of quality for different prices. But in health care, apparently, *there are no differing levels of quality.* Even if there were, what consumer would agree to see a physician designated "second-class"? And what physician would agree to such a designation?

Fourth, academic medical centers and research would be further threatened. Price is a key issue for most consumers. Consumers know that most employers view teaching and research efforts as routine costs of doing business, and have been very reluctant to pay these related health care costs. There is virtually no evidence suggesting consumers will willingly pay high prices to support teaching or research functions,[4] much less to support the sick or the uninsured.

ROLE OF GOVERNMENT

The proposed consumer-driven model would require changes in the tax laws to allow employers to transfer monies to employees to purchase health coverage without adverse tax consequences. And other functions could require extensive government intervention, including interventions that

- Ensure employees actually purchase coverage and do not remain uninsured
- Ensure the unemployed are covered
- Ensure group purchasing pools exist for smaller employers and individuals

- Monitor financial status and ensure that insurers and providers offering these coverages remain financially viable
- Dramatically improve the range, accuracy, and standardization of clinical data reporting
- Audit and monitor the accuracy of the clinical and financial results reported and the consumer advertising information presented
- Review and approve risk-adjustment methodologies
- Hold and disperse cash to subsidize the sickest populations
- Audit balances in patients' medical savings accounts
- Prosecute misleading advertising and sales efforts and cases of provider and consumer fraud, should these occur[5]

Consumers, employers, physicians, hospitals, and insurers *all* distrust government intervention. They may argue, therefore, that there is vastly more government in this consumer-controlled system than is needed to ensure that a market system works according to the market.

CONCLUSION

Consumer-driven health care seems increasingly likely to emerge, because virtually every other nongovernmental attempt to control costs has failed; because it makes no sense that providers of services are not accountable to the ultimate consumer for quality or price or the value of their services; because consumers will continue to insist they are entitled to generous benefits and complete freedom of choice of providers and will not make prudent purchasing decisions as long as they are spending someone else's money; because employers in virtually no other industry can raise revenues per employee as fast as health care costs per employee are rising; and because the latest surge in health care costs, which may continue unchecked for several years, has brought us precipitously close to meltdown of the employer-sponsored health care system.

Of the hurdles to be overcome, several will be especially difficult. Changing society's sense of entitlement could take a generation. Excess supply will be driven from the market only where consumers collectively patronize the most efficient and cost-effective providers, and many would have to do this directly against the advice of their personal physicians. It is not clear who would conduct the massive consumer education initiative or clinical information system improvements that would be required. Perhaps most important, there is no clear leader for this initiative nor an obvious impetus to get it started.

This concept of consumer-driven health care still faces tremendous obstacles. There is no clear leader for this movement because most of the key parties do not want it to happen. It is not likely to be widely tested—there is no time for controlled experiments, and opposition from every principal party is hardly a formula for success. It seems likely to evolve in a random, uncoordinated fashion, in response to the demands of conscientious employers who are no longer able to provide health coverage for their employees. But it does seem likely to happen.

Notes

1. Employee Benefit Research Institute (EBRI). *Health Benefits Survey.* Washington, D.C.: EBRI, Sept. 5, 2000, p. 1.

2. "On the Critical List." *The Economist,* Feb. 13, 1999, p. 66.

3. Thompson, R., and Moran, G. "A Glimpse into the Future of Managed Care." *Minnesota Physician,* Nov. 1998.

4. "An Interview with Paul Ellwood, Jr., M.D." *Managed Care,* Nov. 1997, pp. 53–56, 61–63, 67–68.

5. Herzlinger, R. E. *Market-Driven Health Care: Who Wins, Who Loses in the Transformation of America's Largest Service Industry.* Cambridge, Mass.: Perseus Books, 1999, pp. 267–271.

CHAPTER THIRTY-ONE

Will Consumer-Driven Health Care Work for Employers?

John C. Erb

Employer-sponsored programs continue to serve as the foundation of the U.S. health insurance system, making coverage available to most working Americans. Given the enormous increases in the cost of health insurance over the last twenty years, the fact that most employers continue to provide generally effective and affordable health plans to their employees is remarkable. But inexorable inflation in the cost of health insurance will at some point strain the resources of both providers and consumers to the point where the model no longer provides rational choices. The aging of the baby boomers, the galloping pace of progress in technology, and the dwindling number of competing health plans augers robust growth in the cost of health insurance and, consequently, equally robust growth in the number of uninsured.

The vision driving the consumer-driven health care model is the creation of an economic model in the health insurance marketplace in which consumers will purchase plans on the basis of price and quality. A fair number of large employers have already implemented the model, adapting it to their own demographic environments. In practice the model appears to fulfill the objectives of the employer by capping its portion of the cost of coverage and creating higher employee satisfaction with a benefits menu that offers a variety of plan designs and plan vendors from which to choose. In my experience there is clear evidence that the vision and the models contained in the consumer-driven health care model can produce a rational market.

It seems, though, that the long-term success of the consumer-driven health care model will require that the federal government assume the primary role in creating and administering an effective (and equitable) financing mechanism to properly spread the financial risk among employers, providers, and consumers. At present, however, there appear to be intractable political and economic impediments to such government action, and the assumption of universal coverage used in estimating the model's outcomes is probably not realistic. We can only assume that the federal and state governments will continue to address issues surrounding the entitlement programs, leaving the private sector to fend for itself.

In my opinion the campaign to create a rational economic market in private health insurance will be designed and implemented by employers, either acting alone or in partnership with other companies having a similar vision. These efforts will result in certain pragmatic modifications to the consumer-driven health care model, which may alter the outcomes currently envisioned. Such efforts are likely to include the following:

- A more seamless integration of employer contributions toward benefit programs with employee compensation, both in individual compensation negotiations and in collective bargaining sessions

- Increased use of IRS-sanctioned benefits programs, which allow employees to allocate their fixed employer contribution for benefits among the various benefit choices, including the health insurance benefit

- A sustained appetite for self-funding some or all health insurance offerings

- A growing inclination to outsource employee benefit programs to a third party, such as an employee leasing organization

Each of these circumstances can adversely affect a consumer-driven model, because each weakens at least one of the following critical underpinnings of the model's economic architecture.

First, negotiating employer contributions for benefit programs as part of an employee's total compensation allows employers to leave decisions regarding allocation of those fixed dollars to the employee. Lower-paid workers almost always choose salary over benefits, leaving them, over time, with only enough dollars to purchase the lowest-cost health plan offered and perhaps eliminating coverage for their dependents. Such employees are unable to act as rational purchasers in the current model.

Second, cafeteria plans generally make use of a fixed employer contribution for all available employer-sponsored benefits, often including not only insurance benefits but paid time off as well. Again, lower-paid employees will seek the lowest-cost health plan in order to obtain at least a minimum level of other coverages, such as life and disability insurance. In many cases employees can receive cash compensation from such programs in return for a waiver of health insurance coverage under certain conditions.

Third, self-funding allows employers a significant cash-flow advantage in their health benefit programs. Yet adverse selection is the primary threat to a self-funded program, and adverse selection is a distinct possibility when fully insured health plans are offered along with a self-funded plan. Many employers take steps to limit alternative health plan offerings (and employer contributions to them) to preserve the actuarial integrity of their self-funded plan. This custom, in turn, limits consumer choices and does not allow a truly rational purchasing decision.

Fourth, a growing number of employers, exasperated at the cost and administrative complexity of a health benefits program, have chosen to transfer this function (and expense) to a third-party organization specializing in reducing the cost of human resource administration. Health plan choices in these environments are often limited and inexpensive, denying employees the opportunity to exercise truly rational consumer behavior.

Of course the absence of mandatory employer participation in any health insurance model also means that many small employers (and self-employed individuals, regardless of the tax treatment of health benefits) will simply not offer (or purchase) health insurance because of the expense.

To make the consumer-driven health care model produce the desired outcomes of better coverage, better care, and better prices on a global basis, I am convinced that all the elements outlined in the model must be present. These include

- A financing mechanism created and administered by government with accommodations for low-income participants, risk-laden plan vendors, and local medical market eccentricities
- A mandate of universal participation
- A governmental or quasi-governmental oversight function that ensures patient's rights, provider accessibility, and effective medical practice protocols

The consumer-driven health care model is a viable approach to introducing market forces to our health insurance system if, and only if, it is adopted comprehensively. A piecemeal effort is likely to increase the cost of health care insurance and decrease the availability of coverage.

CHAPTER THIRTY-TWO

The Perspective of an Advocate for the Elderly

John Rother

Health care consumers today face an increasingly confused health delivery environment. Biomedical research and technological advances have added real potential to medical capabilities. Yet, at the same time, growing problems in service quality and restrictions due to managed care are fueling rising consumer frustration. This environment poses real challenges as well as opportunities for proposals that advocate a "consumer-driven" health care system.

Which consumer decisions should be the focus of this approach? Consumers may face three distinct sets of health delivery decisions:

1. Choice of insurer or health plan
2. Choice of provider(s)
3. Choice of treatment or procedure

Each of these decisions is surrounded by its own distinct set of needs and challenges.

CHOICE OF PLAN

About half of working Americans have no choice of insurer—their employer selects a single plan each year on their behalf, or their employer does not provide health coverage at all. For those who do have a choice the predominance of carrier HMOs or PPOs in most markets may reduce the impact of that choice. In such markets, consumer choice of health plan is based on only two key questions:

1. Is my doctor included in the plan?
2. Which plan is less expensive for my family in terms of premiums and likely out-of-pocket costs?

Such choices seem unlikely to promote consumer-driven improvements in health plan organization and delivery.

Any system that promotes individual choice of health plans raises serious problems regarding risk allocation. No adequate risk-adjustment methodology currently exists. A dilemma of health models based on choice is that they depend on this risk adjuster's being developed and applied fairly. Without one, the existence of more plan choices simply increases the incentives and opportunities for "creaming," and inevitably focuses plan energies more on marketing to good risks than on improving care for those at higher risk of actually needing care.

CHOICE OF PROVIDER

By far the most important choice in the minds of most U.S. consumers is the choice of provider. Today most individuals' search for a satisfactory doctor is based on many factors, including reputation and personal chemistry. One of the key challenges for health system improvement is to generate meaningful performance data at the physician level so that consumer choice can be more informed. One of the reasons the original Medicare program is so popular with consumers is that it supports the widest consumer choice of providers. Now the challenge is to enable consumers to make choices based on provider skill and value.

Given the low frequency with which many physicians perform each of the range of available procedures, the need to protect patient privacy, and the cost of data collection, it will be difficult and costly to develop comprehensive outcomes data at the physician level that are statistically valid. Without this or similar information it will be difficult to fit choice of provider into the model for a consumer-driven health system.

CHOICE OF PROCEDURE

Because about 70 percent of all health expenditures in any one year are incurred by the small percentage of individuals with serious illnesses, the care of seriously ill patients should be the focus for health reforms. Treatment decisions involving choice of procedures for such patients may be the area with the greatest potential for consumer-driven care to have significant impact. Patients who have an active diagnosis, particularly those with a chronic illness or disability, will be the most motivated to seek the best comparative information regarding outcomes, risk, and patient satisfaction, and to base treatment decisions on what they learn. As more information becomes available to patients the potential will grow for consumer-driven preferences in chronic care. This dynamic places even greater importance on the need to compensate plans adequately, whether through risk adjustments or other means, such as partial capitation. Without such reimbursement reforms, more consumer information may actually worsen the insurance market by increasing adverse selection.

WINNERS AND LOSERS

One objection to consumer-driven health care proposals is based on egalitarian health care values. To the extent that health care is structured to reward the most aggressive, best-informed, and wealthiest consumers, will consumers without those three attributes become worse off? Current data on health quality and outcomes already reveal differentials that favor the most affluent. Proposals to move in the direction of consumer-driven care must be carefully formulated to avoid worsening these inequities. Health care, after all, is a social good. Changes in health arrangements that benefit the few at the expense of the many—such as medical savings accounts—are hardly to be promoted. Just making more information available about health care choices will not by itself meet this concern. As many as one-third of seniors today are functionally illiterate when it comes to medical or insurance information. Necessary information and individual counseling systems may be expensive to set up and operate. Normal market principles cannot be applied to health care without the development of mechanisms and institutions to offset the tendency of markets to produce losers.

LONG-TERM CARE

One part of health care holds special promise for greater consumer direction. For persons with chronic disabilities our current long-term care patchwork leaves much to be desired. Consumer-directed demonstration programs in this country, along with new programs in Germany and other European countries, show great promise. Consumer-directed long-term care is low-tech, high-touch, and intimately based on consumer diversity in lifestyle preferences. It's the ideal part of the health system in which to incorporate a consumer-driven philosophy.

The basic idea is to restructure long-term care decisions by giving decision-making power to the disabled individual, as opposed to the provider or agency. Once needs are assessed, the disabled person is given cash and counseling and is free to use the cash to make his or her own care arrangements. This approach will not be workable for everyone, particularly for those with dementia, but it promises to strengthen family caregiving, increase patient satisfaction, and lower program costs for the taxpayer.

THIRD-PARTY PAYERS AND PRESCRIPTION DRUGS

There are many areas of health care where consumers lack information and bargaining power and must therefore rely on others. In these areas third-party insurance coverage serves many useful purposes. Insurance and reimbursement policies are also viewed by policymakers as the key tools with which to achieve various health policy goals.

Prescription drug coverage for seniors, as an example, is widely uneven today. Congressional leaders on both sides have called for Medicare coverage of prescription drugs. What is the proper role of Medicare as a third-party payer with regard to prescription drugs? In my view, Medicare should

- Enable seniors to get the benefit of collective bargaining volume discounts on drug pricing
- Allow seniors to elect affordable insurance protection against high out-of-pocket costs
- Promote quality assurance and patient education efforts to improve outcomes

These objectives are not attainable by the individual acting alone in the marketplace. They are achievable for most only in the context of a strong third-party payer that is capable of promoting all three outcomes.

POLITICS AND CONSUMER-DRIVEN CARE

Most health care consumers are opposed to benefit variations that involve some form of health insurance vouchers. Their opposition is easily understood, for most proposals would thrust the consumer into a dysfunctional insurance market, with only poor information and navigation assistance available to them and without adequate financial support. Although accompanied by the rhetoric of individual empowerment, most of these proposals would in fact simply shift risk to individuals and families who already feel at more than sufficient risk. Consumers perceive little potential gain from vouchers.

For this perception to change, consumer-directed proposals must address at least the following three challenges:

1. How to structure health care insurance and delivery choices so that the system works for those with the greatest needs—those in the poorest health

2. How to make excellent information, counseling, and navigation supports available, so the individual has the benefit of knowledge on his or her side

3. How to assure consumers that adequate and stable financial support will continue, so that they will face manageable financial risks going forward

Until these challenges are met, the political resistance to shifting more risk to individuals will continue to be high.

Ultimately, successful innovation in health care will depend on careful balancing of the strengths of insurance with the strengths of individual preferences. This balance may well be different in different parts of health care purchasing and decision making. Policies that encourage more reliance on individual choice must also address the mechanisms—for example, risk adjustment, information about provider performance, and consumer counseling and navigation—that are necessary but that are not in place today. Finally, we must be extremely careful to avoid consumer choice systems that hurt the sickest, the poorest, and the least educated. Whether their situation improves should be the most basic test of the worth of consumer-driven health care.

PART THREE

THE NEW INTERMEDIARIES

Some of those who prefer top-down control of the health care system depict the consumer in a bottom-up, consumer-driven health care system like a child in a haunted house. Strange, venal insurance plans jump out and frighten the consumer into purchase of their fraudulent, slimy wares.

But the fact is that consumers buy all sorts of complicated things, such as cars and computers, in consumer-driven markets. And despite the complexity of these products, ordinary people, like you and me, have driven them to become both better and cheaper. No managed car or managed computer third party needed here, thank you very much.

So why does the consumer-driven market for cars and computers work so well?

And why does the third-party-driven market for health care work so badly?

One reason is the presence of active consumers in one and their nonpresence in the other. And another key difference lies in the availability of intermediaries in the car and computer markets who can help consumers to help themselves. The ample information I can find about the quality of cars and computers in sources such as *Consumer Reports* helps technology-challenged me to buy intelligently. So, although I have only the dimmest idea of how cars and computers work, I can learn enough about the reliability, speed, safety, and cost of different brands and the quality of those who distribute and service them to make me an effective consumer.

For example, a few years ago, when my youngest child learned to drive, I decided to buy a two-seater car. I called it "Mother's Liberation"—no more trips spent hauling basketball teams for me. But after years of driving big buckets, I had little information about two-seaters. So I turned to J. D. Power and *Consumer Reports* publications and narrowed my choices to a Buick, Jaguar, and Saab. After test-driving the models I had identified, I returned to *Consumer Reports* to obtain more information about them, including their cost to the dealer. I called so early in the morning that the only person at work was the editor. He graciously sent me not only the information I needed but also shared his personal views of my choices with me. Not a Jaguar fan for sure. Armed with all this information and support, I bought the Buick and at a darn good price too.

THE NEW HEALTH CARE INTERMEDIARIES

This kind of information and support is almost totally absent in health care at the present time. Part Three of this book discusses the new intermediaries who will provide it in a consumer-driven health care system. The chapters in this part were written primarily by various entrepreneurs, who describe three types of new intermediary firms they have created to

- *Provide information* to help consumers evaluate individual providers and insurers
- *Support* consumers as they use the services of providers and insurers
- *Help consumers to help themselves* in managing their health status

No matter what their functions, these new intermediaries all achieve the following results:

- Increased customer satisfaction, by offering greater choice and convenience
- Increased productivity, by decreasing processing and waiting time
- Decreased costs, by removing layers of administration (a process sometimes described by the jaw-breaking term *disintermediation*)

THE VISION

Part Three begins with seven chapters that illuminate the vision of the new intermediaries. Chapter Thirty-Three presents Bernard Ferrari's vision of the role of information in a consumer-driven health care system. Employing McKinsey & Company's famed 2x2 matrix, Ferrari, a physician who now heads McKinsey's strategic business and who once headed its health care practice, describes the universally optimal matrix quadrant as the one in which empowered consumers receive excellent support and information. Dave Power, also known as

J. D. Power III, the creator of J. D. Power & Associates, explains in Chapter Thirty-Four how health care can benefit from the firm's consumer-friendly ratings and how his company helped to improve the quality of automobiles and to lower their price. In Chapter Thirty-Five, David Lansky, president of the Foundation for Accountability (FACCT), analyzes how FACCT's consumer-oriented data will achieve the same results in health care. Technology-oriented physicians Mark Pearl and Russell Ricci delineate in Chapters Thirty-Six and Thirty-Seven the role of the Internet and other information technologies in facilitating this change, from their vantage points as a venture capitalist (Pearl) and former head of IBM Global Healthcare (Ricci). Last, in Chapters Thirty-Eight and Thirty-Nine, Jon Chilingerian, Arnold Milstein, and Nancy Adler provide us with a framework for and social science insights about structuring the information to be provided.

Some of the new intermediaries use new technologies to provide mass customization. With voice communication and the Internet, they simultaneously offer the economies and consistency of mass production and the virtues of personalization. (See Mark Pearl's chapter for more on this subject.) But the Internet and other new technologies are not the raison d'être of these intermediaries; they merely facilitate their work. The new intermediaries exist fundamentally to help consumer-driven health care. They are consumer driven, not technology driven. Indeed, many of them perform their functions the old-fashioned way, through face-to-face or voice interaction and the mail, without the assistance of digital electronic packages.

INFORMATION TO EVALUATE PROVIDERS AND INSURERS

The next four chapters in Part Three describe some of the new intermediaries, many of them skilled entrepreneurs, who provide the information that enables consumers to select providers and insurers.

Steven Naifeh and Gregory Smith are Pulitzer Prize–winning authors who enable consumers to find the best doctors, especially those who care for victims of rare, devastating problems. Their firm, Best Doctors, was born out of their personal experiences in searching for the best doctors to treat Smith's brain tumor (Chapter Forty). In Chapter Forty-One, Becky Cherney describes how she used the clout of the coalition of large employers she heads to get the data to measure health care quality, and she documents the large resultant savings.

Yet provision of information does not always yield positive results. As described by Katherine Harris, Roger Feldman, Jennifer Schultz, and Jon Christianson, the information provided by the Buyers Health Care Action Group (BHCAG) demonstrated minimal impact (Chapter Forty-Two). This chapter provides a reminder of fact that not all information is created equal. Consumers will respond only to that which is directly relevant to their needs. The artificial intelligence algorithms that help users to select the insurance plans that best meet their needs, described by Asparity Decision Solution's president and CEO Colleen Murphy (Chapter Forty-Three), are examples of the information that fills this bill.

SUPPORT IN USING PROVIDERS AND INSURERS

Yet more remarkable entrepreneurs support consumers as they use providers and insurers. Lawrence Gelb's CareCounsel, as its name implies, provides the expert advice of nurses to consumers as they wend their way through the care process (Chapter Forty-Four). Joseph Tallman founded Access Health Group to provide expert triage during emergencies. As he documents in Chapter Forty-Five, the firm succeeded in directing consumers who need emergency care and those who do not to the services they actually require in a consumer-friendly, cost-effective manner. David Hines's firm, Consumer's Medical Resource, enables consumers to receive expert second opinions of their physician's treatment recommendation (Chapter Forty-Six).

SELF-CARE

The last remarkable group of entrepreneurs consists of those who help people to take care of themselves. In the final three chapters of Part Three, Dean Ornish, president and founder of the Preventive Medicine Research Institute, describes his health-promoting programs (Chapter Forty-Seven); James Fries discusses how the firm he founded, Healthtrac, works with patients through continual feedback (Chapter Forty-Eight), and Donald Kemper and Molly Mettler, CEO and senior vice president, respectively, of Healthwise, present the ways their firm encourages excellence in patient education (Chapter Forty-Nine).

Although all these authors offer compelling evidence of the cost effectiveness of their models, in my view none has yet achieved the broad-based success they all deserve. In his chapter, Dean Ornish reminds us of the reason. In our present system, third parties are understandably not very interested in helping consumers to help themselves. After all, why should they invest in promoting the health of customers who may not be enrolled with the plans when their investment bears fruit in improved health status? But in a consumer-driven health care system, consumers will reverse this paradigm. Unlike insurers, they are vitally interested in their own long-term health status. Consumer-driven health care will enable them to select new intermediaries for themselves when they think they need them.

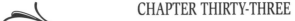

CHAPTER THIRTY-THREE

Where Will Consumer-Driven Health Care Take the Health Care System?

Bernard T. Ferrari

The phrase *consumer-driven health care* reveals more about the changing face of health care than is immediately apparent. Clearly, this phrase tells us that the consumer is gaining importance in the health care industry. But it says more than that. Use of the word *consumer*, that is, one who purchases and uses goods and services, suggests a focus on the economic relationship between buyers and suppliers. And from the word *driven*, we can infer that the supplier will be compelled to react to the consumer's position. Implicit in the complete phrase is that the buy side and supply side of the health care business system will interact in new ways, which will result in a transformed system structure and reconfigured competitive conduct.

If this translation is accurate, consumer-driven health care will fundamentally change the way society manages its health care. In light of the magnitude of such a shift in course, it is important to consider a few basic questions:

What effect will consumer-driven health care have on the efficiency and effectiveness of the health care system? In the United States we now spend over $1 trillion on health care each year, 15 percent of the GNP, more per capita than is spent in other developed countries. However, there is evidence to suggest that we can spend much of it more productively. Therefore it behooves us to understand whether having a "new" consumer at work is a good idea.

What forces will shape this new consumer? If a new consumer is to emerge, then it is important for other key players in the health care system—employers, insurers, government entities, providers—to understand the forces behind this change. These players may want to encourage the forces they see as most beneficial or at least prepare for those they perceive as particularly threatening.

How will the industry change? Certainly, a fundamental change in the way buyers and suppliers interact will cause a meaningful restructuring of the business system and impose a new set of rules about how to compete. This will have implications both for today's players and for new entrants who seek to exploit fresh opportunities.

WHAT EFFECT WILL CONSUMER-DRIVEN HEALTH CARE HAVE ON THE EFFICIENCY AND EFFECTIVENESS OF THE HEALTH CARE SYSTEM?

To understand the extent to which consumer-driven health care is a good idea, we must first establish an objective function by which to measure its impact. When assessing whether a change to a business system will result in greater efficiency and effectiveness, the objective function to measure is productivity. In general, productivity may be defined as the outputs achieved for a given level of inputs. In health care, productivity can be defined as the physical inputs used (labor, capital, and supplies) to achieve a given level of health outcomes. In other words, the concept of productivity can be applied to health care by viewing the management or treatment of a disease as the system's fundamental production process. Although it has been argued that productivity is too simplistic a measure for health care, given the societal entanglements and other complexities of that care, any change to the health care system that reduces productivity is likely pernicious even in the short term and certainly not easily sustainable in the long term.

Because the U.S. health care system has the highest expenditures, whether expressed as a percentage of GNP or dollars per capita, and has mortality data for many conditions and life expectancy data comparable to those for other advanced economies, it has been long thought that the United States is a less productive system. But evidence suggests just the opposite. According to a 1996 McKinsey & Company study comparing the productivity of the U.S. system to that of the systems in the United Kingdom and Germany for four disease states (diabetes, cholelithiasis [gallstones], lung cancer, and breast cancer), the United States is actually *more* productive. The principal findings were as follows:

- The higher spending in the United States was not due to low productivity for these disease states; in fact the United States led Germany in all cases and led the United Kingdom in productivity for lung cancer and gallstones. It trailed the United Kingdom only in diabetes.

The United States led in lung cancer and gallstones because it adopted productive technologies more quickly and broadly and had shorter hospital stays.

Germany was least productive because it used less outpatient care and kept patients in the hospital longer.

- Though the United States spends the most (per capita) on health care overall, followed by Germany and then the United Kingdom, higher spending was largely due to higher compensation for doctors and other personnel and higher administrative costs.[1]

This study uncovered a number of features of the U.S. health care system that contribute to its productivity and promise further gains. For instance, changing from a cost-plus system of reimbursement for hospitals to a prospective-payment system had a significant impact, and other reimbursement plans focusing on outcomes rather than activity are continuing this trend. Creating incentives for providers to use more efficient technologies was another factor in improving the productivity of a health care system. The primary insight gleaned from this study was that the more a competitive market is at work, the more productivity is enhanced. Therefore it is critical that any changes to the U.S. system support a competitive market and do not threaten the progress made toward productivity to date or impede potential gains in the future.

The cornerstone of a competitive market is a well-informed buyer. Such a buyer can accurately judge the value of outputs received for a given level of inputs, comparatively shop among suppliers, and differentially reward those suppliers who give the most and the best for the least. In addition, the informed buyer could knowingly choose a level of productivity for health care at a certain price over a level of higher productivity for a higher price and trade off the savings for other goods or services outside health care.

Given this capability of the informed buyer, it is reasonable to expect that a more consumer driven health care system would be more productive. Understanding the forces that allow the informed buyer to function as critical decision maker also gives us a framework from which to project both the nature and pace of change in today's health care system.

WHAT FORCES WILL SHAPE THE NEW CONSUMER?

Two major forces will shape the evolution and pace of consumer-driven health care. The first is the degree to which consumers, or users, of health care goods and services are empowered to spend their own money and make their own buying decisions. The second is the quality and accessibility of the information relevant to the inputs and outcomes in the care process.

Currently, most consumers in the United States are marginal to the health care purchasing transaction; both price and much choice fall typically under the domain of an intermediary (for example, an employer, a government entity, or an insurer) between consumer and supplier. The major reasons for the existence of these buffers in the purchasing transaction are well known. The tax and other legislative treatments of health care benefits effectively shift the burden of expenditure from the consumer to the employer or government entity. Also, the prevailing societal perspective creates an environment in which some health care is considered a public good or entitlement, allowing the government to become an intermediary.

Shifting the burden of expenditure from consumer to employer or government results in consumers' spending someone else's money when they purchase health care. This has two implications. One is that because someone else's money is being spent, the incentive for getting most for least—the essence of improved productivity—is lost. Under these circumstances other objectives are more likely to influence the buying decision. The other implication is that if someone else's money is being spent, that someone is going to influence or even control the buying decision.

When an intermediary is introduced between buyer and supplier, the agenda of the go-between may not support the productivity objective. For example, in the Medicare program the government is managing and purchasing the benefit package. Here, politically driven objectives may take precedence over the price-choice trade-offs that would be made if productivity were the prime objective. Although Medicare serves as a particularly illustrative example, wherever a go-between exists in the health care transaction, the consumer-driven productivity choices are less likely to occur.

When it comes to the second force at work shaping the evolution of consumer-driven health care—the quality and accessibility of information about the inputs and outcomes in a care process—it is clear that a consumer cannot make choices to optimize productivity if he or she cannot measure that productivity. In the current system we or our intermediaries often make choices (between hospitals, doctors, insurance companies, and so forth) without knowledge of inputs or outcomes.

The most valuable tool we could have to change this buying-blind situation would be accurate, revealing, and up-to-date information, formatted to allow valid comparisons and readily available to a vast majority of consumers. Given these information requirements it is apparent that Internet-enabled communication will alter the information landscape by changing the connections and interactions between today's players in the health care business system. Some might caution that despite such enabled connectivity, the basic information about inputs and outcomes is still missing. The point has merit; however, with greater connectivity, suppliers will have a more compelling reason to develop and make that information available.

HOW WILL THE INDUSTRY CHANGE?

Attempting to predict the exact path and end-state of consumer-driven change in this health care industry would be bold but the prediction itself would likely be flawed. It is more sensible and informative to define a set of the scenarios that could develop over time. One way to define these scenarios is to construct a simple two-by-two matrix, with consumer power on one axis and adequacy of information on the other. The result is the four sectors shown in Figure 33.1. Each sector not only represents a potential scenario but also implies a different direction for the health care business system going into the future.

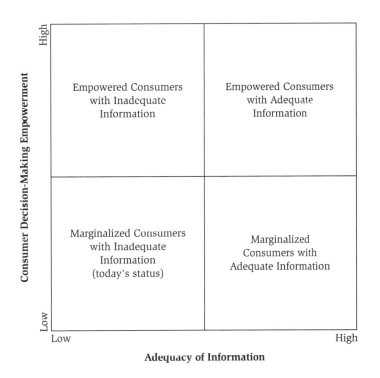

Figure 33.1. Potential Health Care Scenarios.

Marginalized consumers with inadequate information. This scenario defines the state of play today. If we do not move from this position on the consumer empowerment and information dimensions, we can expect continued turbulence and, arguably, very slow progress toward a more productive health care business system. Also, the relationships among consumers, employers, insurers, and providers will remain for the most as they are today, with the fight over economic surplus among the parties playing out in typical fashion.

Marginalized consumers with adequate information. Under this scenario the consumer may be well informed but retains a marginalized role in the buying decision and associated trade-offs. Implicit in this scenario is an unstable relationship among the players, because consumers armed with information will likely seek the power to make their own decisions. Nonetheless, given the resiliency of the employer or government as purchaser in our system, one could foresee this scenario existing for at least a limited period of time. If it were to occur, we might see current or new intermediaries steering consumers to the most productive suppliers. The part of an intermediary's agenda that is not productivity driven would be alterable to the extent that the consumer is not satisfied with the outcomes of the chosen supplier. However, the discipline on the input side could potentially be lax if the go-between purchaser had a non-productivity-driven agenda.

Empowered consumers with inadequate information. In this scenario we would likely see suppliers rushing to establish brand. Without timely, accurate, and understandable information, the consumer would rely on value associated with a brand. Consumers would be taking a leap of faith in their buying decisions. Intermediaries would move from purchasers to interpreters of information. In this capacity they would either try to penetrate the veil of the brand and provide superior information to the consumer or, alternatively, broker the supplier's brand to consumers.

Empowered consumers with adequate information. This scenario captures the spirit of a productive economic system—the educated consumer buying on his or her own account. The implications are profound. Perhaps most significant would be the likely extinction of the intermediaries as we know them today. That is not to say others would not occupy the space. But they would be different. For instance, one can envision provider entities with a marketing and sales front end that would represent the productivity of those providers to the consumer. Or we might see an aggregator of consumers emerge. This aggregator would leverage the volume power of consumers to negotiate a unit price for those who have made like buying decisions.

Although this simple framework begins to outline future scenarios, it raises the question, Will the speed of development of adequate information exceed the speed of consumer empowerment or vice versa? Or, to put it another way, What will the path of change be? If we had to resolve this issue today, the answer would be that information adequacy will outpace consumer empowerment. This answer is informed by lessons learned about the pace and direction of fundamental change in other businesses. There, the so-called high-end, or sophisticated, customer typically defines the leading-edge trend. As suppliers begin to react to the trend, the pace and direction of change are determined. Take financial services as an example. It was the wealthier and more informed investor and borrower who demanded the information and differentiated services that have now become available to a large number of customers over a relatively short time. In health care the Internet has enabled sophisticated patients to know more about their diseases and treatment alternatives than their primary physicians or even their specialists. This sophisticated patient is now quite selective about where care is provided and by whom.

This trend toward informed patients seems to point toward increasingly informed consumers making more of their own health care purchasing decisions. Although shifting the burden of paying for health care onto individuals to a greater extent and challenging deeply embedded societal perspectives seems daunting, the emergence of an informed and empowered consumer appears inevitable. And with the informed and empowered consumer, we can expect an unprecedented change in the services and products offered, not only by suppliers but also by a new breed of consumer-oriented intermediaries. The searching process carried out by the consumer, the bundling and distribution of product, the matching of consumer with supplier, the monitoring of the performance of the supplier—all these processes will change dramatically and create a frenzy of new business ventures in the new space between the consumer and supplier. The greatest risk is that this movement could invite misguided regulatory intervention by the government. However, absent such an intervention, the power of the consumer inherent in the phrase *consumer-driven health care* could lead the U.S. health care system to a new level of productivity.

Note

1. This study provides a more accurate assessment of relative productivity than do most aggregate analyses that compare total health care spending. Many of the total health care spending comparisons fail to make the critical distinction between direct medical inputs used in treatment and their unit costs. In addition, administrative inputs consumed in managing and regulating the health care system are often mistakenly treated as direct medical inputs.

CHAPTER THIRTY-FOUR

The Role of Information

J. D. Power's Paradigm Lessons from the Automotive Industry

J. D. Power III

With more than thirty-four years of experience in capturing, interpreting, and disseminating the voice of the customer, J. D. Power and Associates has gained invaluable insight into the key components of many consumer-driven industries. Best known for benchmarking quality and customer satisfaction in the automotive industry according to the cumulative voice of millions of consumers, my colleagues and I see the health care industry as the battleground for the next consumer revolution. If the industry does not aggressively seek to listen to newly empowered, more information-savvy consumers, there will be untold casualties across the broad spectrum of health care providers.

This chapter focuses on two major and converging trends and their effects on the evolving nature of health care. The first trend is the elevated motivation for the consumer to assume an increasing responsibility for his or her own care. A second trend is the infusion of rapidly advancing technology that provides the opportunity for expanded access to health care information and service providers.

To some extent, John F. Kennedy unofficially declared the beginning of the consumer revolution on March 15, 1962, in a special message to the U.S. Congress on protecting the consumer interest. In his message, President Kennedy declared the following four basic consumer rights:

1. *The right to safety:* to be protected against the marketing of goods that are hazardous to health or life

2. *The right to be informed:* to be protected against fraudulent, deceitful, or grossly misleading information and to be given the facts to make informed choices

3. *The right to choose:* to be assured, wherever possible, access to a variety of products and services, with an assurance of satisfactory quality and service at fair prices

4. *The right to be heard:* to be assured that consumer interests will receive full and sympathetic consideration and fair and expeditious treatment

These rights provided a foundation for the rise of various consumer advocates, and certainly helped to pave the way for J. D. Power and Associates to serve as a catalyst for positive change among industries, based on the voice of the customer.

One industry in which the voice of the customer became paramount was the auto industry. And there are both important parallels and important differences between the auto industry in the 1970s and 1980s and the consumer movement under way today. The differences are found largely in the reasons for the consumer movements; the similarities reside in the necessity and benefit of understanding and embracing the voice of the customer as a differentiating business strategy.

THE CONSUMER REVOLUTION AND
THE AUTOMOTIVE INDUSTRY

In the 1960s and 1970s, there were not many choices for consumers when it came to the mix of automobiles and their features. Big government and powerful labor unions supported the automotive industry. The technology employed by that industry did not permit the quality automakers can produce today, and it showed across the board. The companies with the best technical and manufacturing capabilities dominated the market. The automotive engineers really controlled the industry and made most of the key decisions on what was to be produced. The voice of the consumer was not a high priority in this environment. After all, the auto industry was selling more than ten million vehicles a year, so what could they possibly be doing wrong? Unfortunately, the perception by the industry that the consumer did not have the expertise to judge quality left the door open for major change.

Because U.S. markets allowed more open competition than markets anywhere else in the world, change was finally brought about by the incursion of the Japanese and the energy crisis. The ground rules shifted. The Japanese had a particular focus on reliability and dependability. Taking the lead from Germany's Volkswagen Beetle and moving that concept forward, the Japanese gave consumers an alternative in product quality, with smaller and less expensive vehicles that were dependable and reliable. This had an overriding appeal to the younger generation especially. At the same time, this country began to see the beginnings of an explosion of automotive information available to the average consumer.

It was at this time that J. D. Power and Associates began monitoring consumers, just as they became more inquisitive and assertive. The firm served somewhat as the consumer's conduit to automobile manufacturers. The media played a key role in communicating the consumer's voice to top management in the industry, who finally began to realize that something was wrong with the way they were viewing quality. It took time for domestic manufacturers to change their focus from an inward, *producer* mentality to an outward, *customer-driven* mentality. Resistance to this change became futile because the market-driven effects of the consumer's voice and opinions were now taking control.

THE AUTO INDUSTRY RESPONSE: A QUALITY REVOLUTION

The effects of this change led to an awakening among many manufacturers. Major players in the industry began focusing efforts on improving quality as defined by the customer. Minor players, such as Renault, Peugeot, and the infamous Yugo, could not meet the new quality expectations and were forced to leave the U.S. market. The consumer-led quality revolution had, indeed, led to severe casualties among those who would not listen or could not respond. It also sponsored success for those who embraced the voice of the customer and formally and completely integrated that voice into their decision-making processes. Figure 34.1 illustrates the decreasing rate of problems occurring in cars over the past fifteen years. Today's *average* car exceeds the quality performance of the 1987 industry leader, Mercedes-Benz.

THE CONSUMER REVOLUTION AND HEALTH CARE

In the health care industry today, we are also beginning to see a strong motivation for consumer-centered decision making, although this pressure for change is driven by markedly different circumstances. Employers are in the process of shifting an increasing portion of health care financial responsibility to employees. As employees are being asked to play a more decisive role, they

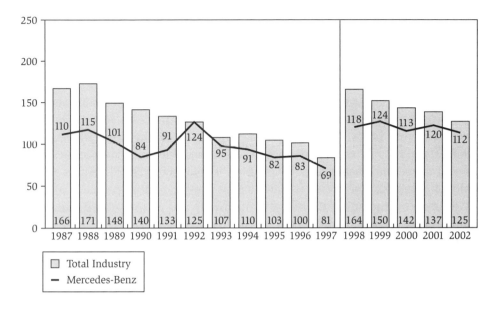

Figure 34.1. The Quality Revolution: Problems per 100 Cars.

Note: The increase in the number of problems reported beginning in 1998 is due to a study enhancement.

Source: J. D. Power and Associates Initial Quality Study. ©1999 J. D. Power and Associates.

pay more attention to what they get. As a result they seek more choice in and control over the diagnostic and treatment resources available to them. Pharmaceutical companies continue to invest heavily in direct-to-consumer promotions that encourage consumers to request specific prescription drugs because they understand the increasing leverage consumers have in today's marketplace.

The Information Society

Technology is providing consumers with opportunities to access an abundance of information about medical conditions. As a result consumers increasingly use the Internet to make health care resource choices and to advance their understanding of health-related issues. How society arrived at this stage deserves a more careful analysis.

In his book *The Third Wave*,[1] Alvin Toffler describes this evolution as occurring in three great "advances," or "waves." The first wave of transformation began several thousand years ago when someone planted a seed and nurtured its growth. With that the age of agriculture began. People moved away from nomadic wandering and hunting and began to cluster into villages and develop culture as a united group. The second wave was the industrial revolution that began in the mid-eighteenth century and took off after America's Civil War.

People began to leave the peasant culture of farming to work in city factories. This wave culminated in the Second World War and the explosion of atomic bombs at Hiroshima and Nagasaki and has been on a decline since.

According to Toffler, the third wave, which has already begun, is based not on muscle but on mind. Best known as the *information age,* or the *knowledge age,* it is powerfully driven by information technology, and its initial effects have been widespread. It is a time when the structure of power that once held the world together is disintegrating and a radically different power structure is taking form. From a business perspective, traditional hierarchical structures such as centralized management, modeled after the military establishment, are gradually phasing out. One reason is that the rank and file (that is, people in all their various roles, including the role of consumer) are gaining more and more knowledge from global information resources.

Today, through satellites and the Internet, global electronic networks instantly spread news and other information to millions of people around the world. One might even speculate that information and knowledge are replacing physical capital as measures of wealth and power. The greatest proportion of value may be generated not from traditional hard assets such as land and equipment but from management talent, brand strength, and organizational knowledge— intangibles that are harder to measure and are not found on the balance sheet.

The Demanding Consumer

In the health care field the dual motivations of wanting greater control over health services and technology-enhanced access to information raise consumer expectations for both health care services and useful decision-making information. When consumers can access highly targeted, real-time information, their expectations are raised, and they come to expect nothing less from product and service providers. In fact they demand even more. Information technology is a significant contributor to the emerging reality of "the never satisfied customer."[2] There appears to be no way to stop the transformation of these rapidly changing consumers, as Internet access enables them to collect and analyze detailed product and service information (twenty-four hours a day, seven days a week) without leaving the comfort of their homes. Today it is not unusual to find consumers more informed about a particular product or service than the salesperson is. In some cases, consumers may be more knowledgeable about treatment options than their physician. The psychological distance between the well-informed seller and the naive buyer is rapidly dissipating, thanks to the Internet.

Managed health care certainly is feeling the effects of this demanding consumer. Internet-savvy consumers looking for health care information on-line are gathering intelligence on specific diseases and their treatment. J. D. Power and

Associates conducts a variety of health-related studies among consumers, employers, and service providers. In a 2002 study, we found that 70 percent of on-line health consumers had sought health-related information on the Internet within the past six months and 52 percent of the same consumers were seeking information on specific diseases. Interestingly, 61 percent of these on-line consumers discussed the information they found on the Web with a family member. In a further demonstration of this new consumer assertiveness, another J. D. Power study found that 97 percent of consumers surveyed "somewhat" or "strongly agreed" with this statement: "I like to have a say in most of the treatment decisions about my care." Among these respondents, 83 percent also agreed with the statement: "I feel uncomfortable when my doctor leaves me out of decisions about my medical care." In a related study conducted among commercial health plan members, we found that only about 57 percent of respondents were "very" or "extremely" satisfied with their health plan and the value they received for the price they paid.

IMPLICATIONS FOR THE HEALTH CARE INDUSTRY

Most industries acknowledge the importance of recognizing and responding to consumer-driven markets. The health care industry can thrive, as other industries have, in times of more demanding and more informed consumers. Although the future structure of the industry is still largely unknown, the information revolution is clearly a catalyst for dramatic change. There are parallels between the auto industry of the 1970s and 1980s and the current state of the health care industry. Consumer-driven health care is as inevitable as consumer-driven demand was for the automotive industry, and as in the automotive industry, there will be casualties. Who these casualties will be will depend on who is best positioned to respond to emerging consumer demands. All constituencies (from employers, providers, and pharmaceutical companies to government and special interest groups) must embrace the response to consumer demands.

It is unrealistic to expect the health care industry to meet all of consumers' demands. There must be a balance between benefits and costs. But that balance must be clearly communicated to consumers who expect not only quick responses to inquiries but also comprehensive information that provides choices. It is in the health care industry's best interest to arm consumers with this information. As a result the consumers' input will increase in value because they will have an appreciation of all the dynamics involved. This is the type of intangible asset that provides a win-win situation for both the industry and its consumers.

POWER PRINCIPLES FOR THE HEALTH CARE INDUSTRY

To provide some guidance for this effort, I conclude with six *power principles,* gained from my firm's experience in helping its customers integrate the voice of the customer into their strategic and daily activities.

1. *Understand issues, preferences, and expectations.* Health care organizations must understand the issues and preferences of their "new" customers. As customers face more choices and decisions, it will be important to understand what consumers are trying to accomplish and how they want to accomplish it. The minivan, for example, was the result of understanding consumers' preference for a vehicle that was more serviceable than the traditional station wagon. As "new" health care purchasers, consumers will likely make decisions different from those made by the employers who once covered virtually all health care–related costs through a predetermined plan. Health care providers must understand the options consumers are actually considering and the reasons for their selections. It will also be important to understand the expectations consumers have for these options. As consumers pay more for services themselves, they will demand more service.

2. *Monitor performance against customer-defined expectations.* Many studies conducted by J. D. Power and Associates reveal a noticeable gap between what is considered important by an organization and what is actually reported as important by consumers. Attention to the elements considered important by the consumer provides a better guide to investment in process and product improvement. Successful organizations adjust performance parameters so that resources are shifted to areas of greater importance to consumers. A classic example of failing to consider consumers' interests closely enough occurs in call centers when performance parameters for the speed with which a call is answered are set at levels beyond what customers expect but do not allow enough time for thorough answers to consumer questions or for asking additional questions to improve the quality of the experience.

3. *Monitor performance against expectations that drive Customer-Delivered Value^{sm}.* Along with monitoring items consumers find important, it is equally important to know which of the items being measured are drivers of behaviors beneficial to the organization, that is, which items have the greatest impact on Customer-Delivered Value (CDV) to the organization. In the auto industry it is not uncommon to find overall satisfaction rates at high percentages, while repurchase rates are at substantially lower levels. The point is to further granulate the organization's attention on the items that are of expressed importance to customers *and* drive their behaviors so they remain loyal, expand their use of products and services, be advocates, and be more compliant with the organization's administrative and clinical requests. These factors all translate to

improved quality and bottom-line performance and should be the ultimate objective of monitoring customer perceptions of organizational performance.

4. *Seek but do not rely only on the customer for solutions.* Customers are best positioned to express their issues and preferences and indicate what is not working well or what would be useful to them. It is the industry's task to create products and processes to meet or exceed those expressions. For example, vehicle owners expressed an interest in being able to fill their gas tanks more quickly and conveniently. Mobil introduced the Speed Pass®, which allowed consumers to wave a key fob at the pump to handle the payment, thus obviating the need to personally execute a transaction and speeding up the overall process even though it had nothing to do with the actual tank-filling process. This is not to say that customers should not be queried about ways to improve services and products. On the contrary, customers feel engaged and tend to be more compliant when their opinions are asked in the context of improving services to them and others.

5. *Recognize that today's exceptional performance will become tomorrow's standard.* Quality is a moving target. J. D. Power and Associates' research shows that expectations will rise as quality improves. As Figure 34.1 illustrated, in 1982, vehicle service performance by Mercedes-Benz led the marketplace and was noticeably higher than the industry average. By 1998, this same benchmark level of performance represented only the industry average. This phenomenon has been witnessed in all the other industries that J. D. Power serves, and we expect the same to be true for the health care sector. We believe it is imperative for organizations to focus attention and investment on the customer in order to increase their opportunities to raise the performance levels that will bring the greatest value to the organization.

6. *Recognize that you are competing with many other industries, not just those in health care.* It is not uncommon to limit benchmarking efforts to performance against competitors. In the emerging environment, where the Internet will frequently be used for health care information and decisions, it is imperative that health care organizations design and compare their capabilities and services against the best models, regardless of industry. For example, if one were helping consumers make decisions among a broad spectrum of providers and packages of services, it would be helpful to review the Let'sTalk Web site (www.letstalk.com), which focuses on wireless telephone service plans. At this site, user answers to relatively few questions about service preferences can winnow the choices down to a relevant handful that can be further explored and compared with ease. More generally, with respect to service performance, my colleagues and I see that consumers increasingly expect service levels similar to those they experience in hospitality and other highly consumer-interactive environments.

CONCLUSION

The health care industry will be characterized by an increasingly consumer-engaged, information-enabled environment. Consumers will be motivated to enter the buying process better informed and more assertive. This will result in a reduction in the psychological distance that has existed between health care in its historical role of expert seller and the individual as the naive buyer. Like the auto industry's consumer the health care consumer will seek conveniently accessible, customizable, and interpretable information about health care service and clinical performance.

The health care industry must therefore be particularly sensitive to today's *information utopia.* Health plans and providers alike must understand the new e-enabled consumers' process of thinking about the semantics and value propositions of health services and products. To stay at least on pace with this movement, organizations must systematically monitor and internalize the perceptions and behaviors of their customers. If health care organizations wish to be the choice of consumers, they must embrace the consumers' voice.

Notes

1. Toffler, A. *The Third Wave.* New York: Bantam Books, 1981.
2. McKenna, R. *Real Time.* Boston: Harvard Business School, Mar. 1999.

CHAPTER THIRTY-FIVE

Providing Information
to Consumers

David Lansky

Consumers and purchasers of health care services are not able to choose doctors, hospitals, or insurance plans based on the quality of care they are likely to receive. They lack the information that can help them evaluate the health care organizations that achieve better results, use proven medical practices, or best meet patients' expectations. Our national failure to publicize quality of care and thus permit the market to reward excellence leaves us with a health system in which competition is founded solely on price and persistently unable to innovate. Entrepreneurs and innovators are not rewarded.

The Foundation for Accountability (FACCT), of which I am president, was established in 1995 by a consortium of large, national health care purchasers and consumer organizations. The members of the FACCT consortium wanted to base purchase decisions on the ability of health care organizations to achieve desirable results for patients. When FACCT was founded, several initiatives were already under way to provide information to help purchasers select among competing health systems. But those programs focused almost exclusively on the performance of health maintenance organizations (HMOs) and examined only the rates at which HMOs executed specified tests and interventions. They did not evaluate whether those activities achieved their intended results (for example, discovered disease) or led to improved health (that is, better functioning or higher quality of life). Nor did they generate information on how well doctors, hospitals, specialized service models, or traditional insurance carriers served their patients. This narrow range of information—focused only on process measures for only one form of health insurance—reduced purchaser and consumer confidence in quality measurement and the viability of a private market.

FACCT was created to overcome these limitations and permit major purchasers to assess the quality of care provided by all their vendors in terms that were important to them and to the people they represented—typically employees or beneficiaries of public programs. Key elements of the FACCT approach include

- Measuring the results of care (outcomes), whether best practices have been followed, and the consumers' experience of care
- Organizing information into categories and terms easily understood by most Americans
- Developing language and stories (messages) that make the quality information relevant and important to most people
- Using state-of-the-art measurement methods for assessing quality
- Coupling expert opinion and published research about quality of care with direct reports from patients about the elements of quality they most value

FACCT INITIATIVES

FACCT initially developed quality measurement systems for public and private sector purchasers. But we quickly learned that purchasers were not able or willing to impose reporting requirements on providers. More recently, many group purchasers have shifted their strategy to emphasize the ultimate importance of the individual consumer as a health care decision maker. The group purchaser is becoming an information broker, providing a menu of choices and informational tools to help employees or beneficiaries make decisions. To help in this process, FACCT is implementing a series of initiatives with three essential elements: a set of consumer-relevant quality measures, a format for communicating measures to the general public, and a series of educational and action messages.

Quality Measures

FACCT's quality measures evaluate how well health care providers help patients achieve desirable outcomes and how well they follow best practices. FACCT measures have been developed, tested, and validated for numerous conditions (breast cancer, diabetes, major depression, asthma, and HIV/AIDS) as well as for the overall health of populations, health of children, and care at the end of life, and for providers' success in helping patients identify and reduce risky behaviors. FACCT's approach emphasizes how people actually live their lives and experience their care, so that it evaluates the health system on dimensions of quality that matter to the consuming and paying public. Many of these measures can be collected by surveying patients directly, avoiding expensive and intrusive data collection in the doctor's office or hospital.

Communications Format

FACCT has conducted qualitative research with hundreds of Americans from all walks of life to determine how best to provide information that will support quality-based decisions. The FACCT communications model has five major categories in which to organize information:

FACCT's Information Categories

The basics: delivering the basics of good care (doctor care, rules for getting care, information and service, satisfaction

Staying healthy: helping people avoid illness and stay healthy through preventive care, reduction of health risks, early detection of illness, education

Getting better: helping sick or injured people recover through appropriate treatment and follow-up

Living with illness: helping people with ongoing, chronic conditions (such as diabetes or asthma) take care of themselves, control symptoms, avoid complications, and maintain daily activities

Changing needs: caring for people and their families when needs change dramatically because of disability or terminal illness, with comprehensive services, caregiver support, and hospice care

Each of these five categories has subcategories that permit consumers to examine more closely specific aspects of a health plan's or medical group's performance. People with chronic illness, for example, may be interested in a specific problem—such as asthma—or a specific kind of skill—such as educating patients and their families in managing daily symptoms. Consumers have expressed strong interest in the ability to drill down to information that is of personal interest. Emerging presentation technologies such as Internet systems make such tailoring possible.

Finally, FACCT has developed a series of presentation formats and tested them extensively with consumers throughout the United States to determine whether they can be easily and correctly understood and whether they are helpful in making health plan and provider selections. This presentation approach incorporates a complete methodology for grouping, scoring, and weighting multiple measures to produce simple summary scores.

Educational Messages

We know that consumers are passionately interested in their own health and in health information. But the concept of informed health care decision making is not familiar to most people. Providers have not routinely collected quality information and have been reluctant to publicize what information is available. Consumers have never been asked to consider that some doctors, hospitals, or health plans provide better care than others, that the selection of these relationships may be vital to their well-being, or that their decisions may influence the functioning of a market for good or ill. They are very interested in such information. In FACCT's qualitative research, consumers have expressed a strong preference for indicators of absolute performance levels. They wish to know whether they are receiving the best possible care as well as which doctor or organization is providing relatively superior care in their community.

FACCT has learned that information about quality of care must be presented in a context that helps people understand its importance, relevance for their lives, and how it can be used. We have developed four simple messages that should accompany any consumer choice information and also be part of a broader educational campaign that precedes and sets the context for obtaining performance information.

First, publishers of data—including group purchasers, governments, health plans, consumer organizations, and mass media—should remind people that *quality matters*—as much as cost or coverage or rules. Second, publishers should help people understand that *quality varies.* If consumers do not appreciate that the quality of care they receive varies by a factor of ten or greater among physicians, hospitals, and health plans, then they will continue to make decisions based solely on cost, coverage, or rules. Third, publishers should explain that *quality can improve.* Consumers must recognize the importance of demanding higher-quality care. Finally, publishers should encourage consumers to understand the importance of their actions for their family's well-being and for society as a whole. Consumers must look carefully at the available information because their personal decisions will affect their personal health and their collective decisions will influence how the health system focuses its resources and defines its objectives.

These three elements—measures, a model, and messages—work together to empower consumers to make important decisions about where to seek their care. As consumers begin to reward superior providers and plans with their business, this society will see the market shift toward consumer-centered health care.

EVIDENCE OF THE NEED FOR CONSUMER CHOICE INFORMATION

Leaders from every sector of the U.S. health system have advocated that rigorous health care quality information should be publicly available. Government efforts abound. Congress, in the Balanced Budget Act of 1997, mandated that the Medicare program begin to publish quality data. The Bush administration began to publish nursing home ratings in 2002. The President's Advisory Commission on Consumer Protection and Quality recommended the creation of both a statutory and a private sector organization to develop reporting standards, leading to the creation of the National Quality Forum. Numerous states have commissioned and published such data (for example, Florida, New Jersey, Pennsylvania, Oregon, and California). Providers have jumped into action too. Health industry trade associations are creating industry-defined standards acceptable to their own sectors. Nor have payers lagged behind. Consortia of private purchasers (for example, the Pacific Business Group on Health, the Central Florida Business Group, and CARS, a consortium of auto manufacturers and autoworkers) have developed "report cards" for their own constituents.

The public's interest in health care information is overwhelming. The annual issue of *Newsweek* that rates HMOs generates the magazine's largest newsstand sales. Public opinion surveys also attest to consumers' demand for this information. In the 2001 Kaiser Family Foundation/AHRQ survey of adults, 87 percent said they wanted a health plan with high quality of care, many more than the 74 percent who wanted a plan that would "keep costs of coverage low" and the 70 percent who wanted "a wide choice of doctors." About 40 percent of those surveyed said they would use quality information to choose a doctor or hospital.[1]

FACCT's interviews and focus groups with over five hundred Americans from a wide range of backgrounds—healthy and sick, affluent and poor, employed and retired, teenagers and people near death—revealed a passionate desire for information that would help consumers make good choices and manage their own care. As the mother of a chronically ill child vividly noted: "I cannot make an intelligent decision on how to choose any health care supplier without some information on quality." And another said: "Results measures would really make a difference in helping people select and then would also give the providers a message that folks are looking at their outcomes."

Information Market Size

At least once a year, virtually every American consumer must make important choices among competing health care options. We choose a personal physician, an insurance carrier, and often a medication, a treatment, a specialist, or a hospital. Over 220 million Americans with some form of health insurance can select primary and specialist physicians and hospitals from those covered under their insurance plan. Today most of those decisions are made with no information about the quality of those services and the organizations that provide them.

In practice, the market for health care decisions can be segmented by decision type, by customer group, and perhaps, by mode of information access. The selection of an insurance *plan*, for example, is a choice available to slightly more than half of employed Americans—about eighty million people. An additional thirty-six million people are insured by Medicaid and similar public programs. The thirty-nine million Americans eligible for health insurance through the Medicare program can choose freely among physicians and hospitals, or if they live in communities where insurers offer managed care plans to Medicare, they must decide whether to join an HMO and, if they do so, which of the HMOs available is best for them.

Evidence of Efficacy and Cost Effectiveness

The critical evaluation question is whether consumers will make decisions that reflect the differences in quality reported to them. When General Motors began sharing performance information with salaried employees in 1996, 22 percent of employees were enrolled in "fair"- or "poor"- quality plans and only 15 percent in "benchmark"-quality plans; by 1998, only 12 percent remained in poorer-quality plans, and 30 percent had chosen benchmark plans.[2] A similar study of Minnesota employees' selection of primary care medical group affiliations showed strong patterns of switching to the groups with higher reported patient satisfaction.[3] In both studies, sponsors created economic incentives to reward higher-quality choices. These quantitative studies have been confirmed by numerous reports from qualitative research that consumers believe they will make more efficacious decisions if quality information is available.[4]

Nevertheless, we cannot yet demonstrate the cost-effectiveness of an informed consumer choice strategy. Because some fear that an uncontrolled informed consumer will drive up health care costs by releasing universal demand for the best care without a corresponding cost consciousness, purchasers are exploring mechanisms to create an economic balance between unrestricted and unaffordable demand.

Other Approaches to Meeting Information Needs

Several initiatives have been launched to help consumers make more informed decisions that reflect quality performance. As mentioned, the Bush administration has announced a commitment to collect and publish measures of nursing home and, eventually, hospital performance. These data are made available in newspaper advertisements and on Medicare Web sites and are supported by federally funded operators through ombudsman programs, and a modest messaging campaign is being coordinated by a national public relations firm. The National Committee for Quality Assurance (NCQA)—an independent agency that accredits HMOs—publishes a set of about sixty *effectiveness of care* indicators. Increasingly, quality of care data are being distributed by both public and commercial Web sites. The Leapfrog Group, made up of employers, publishes lists of hospitals and has adopted practices that increase patient safety (see www. leapfrog.org); on-line doctor directories (such as healthgrades.com and thehealthpages.org) often include patient ratings and give users the opportunity to enter text comments about their doctors; state governments sometimes make information about physician disciplinary actions available (Massachusetts, for example, does this at www.massmedboard.org); consumer advocates are compiling public information about numbers of procedures performed to help people select hospitals and surgeons (see, for example, www.healthcarechoices.org). The next generation of consumer information sites not only will provide performance information but will link it to decision support tools that help consumers understand which health care organizations might be best suited to meet their needs (see, for example, www.accentcare.com and www.subimo.com).

The consumer information industry is evolving, but remains constrained by two limitations. First, in many opinion polls and research studies, consumers have indicated that they are primarily interested in information about the quality of individual physicians, yet physicians do not disclose such information to anyone. FACCT, NCQA, and the Massachusetts Health Quality Partners are developing methods for evaluating individual physician performance through patient surveys and administrative data. Second, individual publishers are not able to undertake a comprehensive approach to education and empowerment. Consumer awareness of quality problems and readiness to use quality information will change only slowly absent a broad national commitment to changing attitudes. The Leapfrog Group has made the most substantial commitment to raising public awareness of the importance of making decisions that recognize quality, but its ultimate impact is not certain.

IMPACT ON SOCIETY

The strategy described in this chapter is intended to have a comprehensive and significant impact on the productivity and cost of the health care system and on the health of all Americans. The aim is to alter the fundamental incentives that shape the behavior of providers, insurers, and consumers themselves. If the public can recognize those providers and plans that outdo others in meeting health needs and consumer expectations, we expect providers and plans to focus their skills and resources on achieving those valued outcomes. Such a quality-focused competition will reward innovation and keep the health system focused on improving the health of those it serves. The most important element of this strategy is that the market reward aspects of quality that consumers value and that reflect the results of care.

BARRIERS TO WIDER DIFFUSION

The greatest obstacle to the diffusion of the FACCT and other consumer information strategies is the lack of consumer-relevant data. Doctors and hospitals and insurers have never been rewarded for knowing what happens to their patients. Understandably, they have made almost no investment in tracking health outcomes or details about clinical services. Few doctors, hospitals, or insurers can even identify groups of patients with common health needs. The information available to providers is of no interest to the public and would not, in any case, provide a sound basis for altering the primary incentives of our vast health system. In the absence of government requirements for collecting relevant information, health plans and providers need only provide information voluntarily. They often argue that the cost of such efforts go unrewarded. No voluntary effort has proven to be of sustained value. A second primary barrier to wide implementation is the inadequately voiced public demand for quality information. Consumers have not known that it is possible to evaluate the quality of those who provide care and have rarely asked for such information. Substantial and sustained public education will be necessary to establish a climate that demands information about quality.

These barriers can be removed through a series of concentrated, collaborative efforts. First, organizations that share an interest in health care consumerism can work together to create a public expectation that care will be high quality and performance information will be available to support choice. State and federal agencies, employers, labor unions, patient organizations, information publishers and vendors, and some health care companies share a vital interest in a quality-seeking public. They can collaborate to shatter the myths that inhibit public demand for quality care.

Second, consumers can ask their government leaders, employers, and others representing their health care interests to provide useful information. Ideally, major public and private purchasers will create contractual requirements that key information be routinely provided and then published. Recent experience does not provide much confidence in the ability of purchasers to make stringent demands of the health system, however. The legislative creation of an SEC-like agency to set requirements for information disclosure may be necessary.

Third, the necessary information about quality must be gathered and shared with the public. We believe that a sound and relevant set of quality measures for health plans, hospitals, and major physician groups could be collected throughout the United States for about $140 million per year—representing .01 percent of our annual health care expenditures. If such an investment would begin the process of focusing the health system on consumer-relevant quality, it would be among the most efficient investments the country could make. Given a sound core database of performance information, entrepreneurs, regional purchasers, and others could build supplementary systems for serving the rich array of public information needs now lying below the surface.

CONTRIBUTION TO BUILDING A CONSUMER-DRIVEN HEALTH CARE SYSTEM

The FACCT strategy is intended to create a high-level, systemic focus on how health care quality affects the consumer and society as a whole. It is one of a number of complementary interventions necessary to reshape the focus, efficiency, and effectiveness of this nation's health system. As other interventions take hold—self-care information, Internet-based delivery, and disease management and specialty service providers—each will expand the number of consumers who recognize their own ability to take charge of their health care, challenge the power imbalance of the current health system, and demand high-quality care from every health care resource.

Notes

1. Kaiser Family Foundation and Agency for Health Care Research and Quality. *National Survey on Americans as Health Care Consumers.* Menlo Park, Calif.: Kaiser Family Foundation, 2000.

2. Bruce Bradley, personal communication to the author, June 9, 1998.

3. Jossi, F. "Money Matters: A BHCAG Update from the Twin Cities." *Business and Health,* Apr. 1998, pp. 41–46.

4. "Making Quality Count: A National Conference on Consumer Health Information." Unpublished conference summary, Foundation for Accountability, Feb. 1999, p. 70. Available from Foundation for Accountability.

CHAPTER THIRTY-SIX

Consumer-Driven Health Care and the Internet

Mark A. Pearl

The use of the Internet is rapidly growing in the United States and worldwide. As the cost of Internet use decreases, it is no surprise that the number of Internet users is projected to increase at a compound annual growth rate of 8.4 percent.[1] Yet, as high as this growth rate is, the growth of the segment of the Internet devoted to health care issues (*health care Internet*) will most likely surpass these projections due to a confluence of two recent trends specific to health care. First, people are taking more responsibility for their health care as access to physicians decreases and out-of-pocket health care costs rise. Second, as personal health care responsibility increases, the demand for health care information also accelerates. The Internet can put the information and tools health care consumers need at their fingertips and empower them to control and participate in their health care decisions.

The current, first-generation health care Internet offerings are crude attempts to meet this accelerating consumer demand. For the most part they are basic, simplistic, and contain very little end-user customization. They are products of the one-size-fits-all philosophy, with little regard for the individual needs of health care consumers or for regional variations in the ways health care is managed and provided.

The future of consumer-driven health care on the Internet should see customized Web sites that offer each individual a personally tailored view (the individual's Internet *front end*). This front end, whether it is a content page or a page on the site of an on-line retailer or a local delivery system, will be based on an individual's personal health care history and risk factors. The personal Web site will be easy to navigate, informative, and entertaining. It will be integrated with layers of information that are relevant to the individual, not merely a series of generic menus strung together. Visiting one's Web site will be a truly rewarding experience—that is, *edutainment.* Once these individualized Web sites are developed, they will become the standard; textbook-style Web sites will quickly become obsolete.

THE GROWTH OF THE INTERNET

The growth of the Internet has been truly staggering. Jupiter Media Metrix estimates that there are currently 141 million U.S. Internet users and that this number should increase to 211 million by 2006 (the result of that compound annual growth rate of 8.4 percent mentioned earlier).[2] The U.S. Department of Commerce estimates that 54 percent of the population currently uses the Internet.[3] Furthermore, the number of worldwide Internet users is projected to grow from 159 million in 1999 to over 509 million by the end of 2003.[4] The Internet is penetrating all aspects of life from shopping to stock trading (now both easily done on-line) and from simple communication between individuals (e-mail) to commerce between businesses (e-commerce). Lower costs to "go on-line" and enhanced ease of use will accelerate the growth in new Internet users.

There are four key reasons for consumer Internet growth:

1. *Ease of information access.* The Internet allows the consumer rapid access to vast amounts of information and commercial resources. Consumers can now have the equivalent of reams of data at their fingertips at very low cost and with little, if any, incremental cost. In-depth product information, comparative pricing information, and consumer satisfaction information can be reached easily and almost instantaneously.

2. *Short learning curve.* The Internet can be accessed via a standard browser, which is now mandatory on all computers. The front-end browser is a simple, clean tool with a short learning curve, the perfect mass-market application. Once a consumer has mastered the use of a browser and a search engine, the full resources of the Internet are available.

3. *Decreasing computer costs.* PC prices are again falling. Companies such as Intel, Compaq, and Hewlett Packard are embracing the low-cost PC movement, and subsequently, PC prices in 2002 are already

hitting the $600 to $800 mark. Such low PC prices will result in further PC penetration into U.S. homes. In effect, the PC has finally become a mass-market tool.

4. *Close relation to work.* The Internet is becoming part of the fabric of business. E-mail is already a mandatory application for all Fortune 1000 companies. Business-to-business electronic commerce is experiencing the same consistent growth as Internet usage overall. According to the U.S. Department of Commerce, in 2000, e-commerce accounted for over $1 trillion of value. And 94 percent of that e-commerce was business to business.[5] Consumers are learning to use the Internet because their work demands that they must.

THE HEALTH CARE INTERNET ENVIRONMENT

Health is one of the most popular topics on the Internet. Interestingly, women and the elderly, who account for the majority of health care costs and decisions, also account for a majority of those who are on-line. Therefore they represent an obvious target for effecting change in health care dollars spent.

User Numbers

Three-fourths of U.S. Internet users between the ages of fifteen and twenty-four have gone on-line to find health or medical information, according to a survey conducted during September and October 2001 by the Kaiser Family Foundation.[6] In a given month, that can translate into as much as 35 percent of all Internet users, as was the case in January 2002.[7] Health information is one of the top content categories that people seek on-line. The only on-line activities in which more people have participated are e-mailing, searching for a product or service, and finding news and entertainment.[8]

User Demographics

The majority of on-line health care information users are women and people aged fifty and over.[9] Jupiter Media Metrix estimates that 80 percent of on-line females search for health information on-line compared to 67 percent of on-line males. It also reports that health content sites report a markedly higher number of female visitors—by a margin of two to one.[10] This fact is important because women exert authority over 75 percent of a household's health care decisions and 66 percent of the health care dollars spent,[11] and the elderly consume the majority of the health care resources in the country. Thus the Internet can become a major influence in consumers' decisions to purchase health care products and services.

THE INTERNET AND TRENDS IN PATIENT EMPOWERMENT

Current trends in health care require the health care consumer to become more involved in the decision-making process. As a result patients need more information regarding their health and health care needs. They are increasingly looking to the Internet for that information.

Increasing Pharmaceutical Copays

Spending on pharmaceutical drugs is rising 13 percent per year, accounting for a significant portion of the 12 to 13 percent increase in national health expenditures.[12] In response to the rapid price increase in pharmaceuticals, employers are now moving their employees to three-tiered copay structures, where the monthly copay per prescription can range from $5 to $50, depending on the drug. Currently, 54 percent of employees are enrolled in these pharmaceutical benefit structures.[13] Increasing monthly copayments will drive consumers to demand more information about their medications and other less expensive alternatives.

Direct-to-Consumer Advertising

From 1997 to 2000, direct-to-consumer drug advertising increased at a compound annual growth rate of 37 percent—from $969 million in 1997 to $2.5 billion in 2000. SG Cowen estimates that that number will rise to $4.0 billion in 2002.[14] As a result of the drug advertising that bombards them (predominately in the television and print media), consumers are now becoming more aware of pharmaceuticals and are more actively seeking answers to their questions regarding health in general and pharmaceuticals specifically. Fulcrum Analytics reports that anywhere from 29 to 31 percent of consumers ask their doctors for information about a drug after seeing a drug advertisement.[15]

Physician Accessibility

The pressure to contain costs has led many physicians to concentrate more on the business side of practicing medicine, detracting from the time they can spend with patients. The average doctor's visit is down to seven minutes,[16] leaving patients dissatisfied with physician office visits and accessibility. A study by Yankelovich MONITOR concludes that consumers feel their doctors are now less accessible than ever.[17] The Center for Studying Health System Change recently reported that 33 percent of patients cited "inability to get an appointment soon" with their physician as a significant barrier to care, an increase from 23 percent in 1997.[18] As a result, patients are looking to the Internet to supplement the information they receive from their physician. (Two-thirds of all U.S. patients do not receive literature about their condition or medication while in their physician's office.[19]) Interestingly, 62 percent of Net-connected physicians reported recommending to their patients that they search for information on the Internet.[20] Ninety percent of on-line U.S. adults want to communicate with their physicians via the Internet. Fifty-six percent said that the availability of on-line communication would affect their choice of physician.[21]

Consumer Empowerment

Managed care's many restrictions on health care services and pharmaceuticals have led to a backlash of patient demands for more choice. Patients learn about the complexities of benefit plans and clinical decisions and are seeking to actively manage and participate in their own health care.[22] In many cases they even bypass traditional medicine and seek alternative therapies. Among on-line health care users, 70 percent agree that the Internet empowers them to make better choices in their lives.[23] The Web is the resource that allows health care consumers access to more health care information in a shorter time frame with greater ease than ever before.

THE CURRENT STATE OF HEALTH CARE ON THE WEB

Health care Internet offerings today are relatively crude and fall into one of four categories: content, community, connectivity, or commerce, as summarized in the following sections.

Content

Currently, health care content offerings in general are simplistic adaptations of reference book-like or textbook-like materials. They are merely factual (at best), offering one-size-fits-all, aggregated (in some cases licensed) health care content. Content sites are more interested in building brand name to capture a large audience than in providing a rich hypertext-linked, multimedia health care experience that is personalized according to medical condition, health interests, risk factors, and so forth. There are currently few differentiating factors among all the on-line health care content offerings. In the majority of cases, health care content offerings aim for a mass market of users through aggregated content in order to drive advertising and sponsorship revenue.

Community

On-line communities provide forums in which users with similar interests can find, exchange, and discuss information with others in the uniquely personal, yet anonymous, environment offered by the Web. Health care communities are often managed by content providers and allow users with particular diseases to exchange information about the disease, treatments, and experiences and to enhance their ability to deal with illnesses.

Like content providers, health care community providers have had the goal of aggregating end-users. Also, like content providers, they have been crude and unsophisticated in their approaches. Community providers have aimed to reach similar-minded Internet users as opposed to similar-minded patients or health care consumers. They have rarely attempted to reach out into the broader community of patients they are targeting, including non-Internet users. They should attempt to truly affiliate and integrate themselves with each illness and each medical specialty that they represent, with the aim of generating a true community of patients. Despite this, the power of Internet-based discussion groups is increasingly appreciated. A recent study found that individuals with chronic back pain who participated in an e-mail discussion group improved on four primary measures of health. Physician visits by participants also declined.[24]

Connectivity

Connectivity in the health care arena is the application of Internet technologies to connect and, more important, automate the entry, transmission, processing, and storage of information. The Internet facilitates the automation of health care processes by connecting all the health care constituents across the continuum of care and providing caregivers with vital information at the point of care.

Physician Connectivity. Today the great majority of health care clinical, financial, and office tasks are performed with the aid of phones, faxes, and paper forms (often in triplicate), resulting in unnecessary redundancy. Internet connectivity allows new electronic transaction sets to remove these inefficiencies by automating many currently manual transactions, such as the ones listed here:

Clinical Tools

Order entry and results: prescriptions (new and renewals), lab tests, radiological studies

Clinical practice guidelines

Physician Practice Tools

Patient eligibility and benefit data; referral requests and authorizations; preadmission certification

Accounts receivable management: billing and claims processing

Capitation and risk management

Some companies now focus on providing business-to-business functionality through localized, physician-centered connectivity. Although they are in their infancy, their focus on the physician and regional implementation show much promise.

Patient Connectivity. The area of patient connectivity—connecting patients to their physicians and to their local hospital—is still underdeveloped. Patients typically cannot make appointments, request referrals, request prescription renewals, or even ask their own doctor or treatment team any questions on-line. This area is being pursued by many local integrated delivery systems in their attempts (often rudimentary) to market their services on-line. In an indication of how immature patient connectivity currently is, a recent survey of Californian hospital Web sites found that only 11 percent allowed patients to make appointments on-line, and only 5 percent allowed users to create on-line health profiles.[25]

Commerce

Health care Web sites devoted to commerce focus either on individual consumers or on businesses.

Consumer Health Care E-Commerce. According to the latest data available, 1999 on-line business-to-consumer health care spending was $0.4 billion. Forrester Research predicts that this figure will rise to $22 billion by 2004.[26] The main problem with health care e-commerce offerings is that they are generic storefronts, no better than on-line catalogs in most cases, not customized to individuals and even not tailored to specific disease categories. However, health care consumers, especially first-time ones, find them easy to use.

Business-to-Business Health Care E-Commerce. The Efficient Health Care Consumer Response Consortium estimates that up to $11 billion could be saved by improved efficiency in health care supply chain management.[27] According to Forrester Research, health care business to business e-commerce is set to rocket from $6 billion in 1999 to $348 billion in 2004.[28] The aim of current Internet offerings in this arena is to develop an on-line marketplace to allow direct communication between sellers and buyers. By pooling buyers and sellers and providing exchanges and auctions to consolidate competitive pricing and information, these sites aim to drive prices lower and squeeze traditional distributors, thereby creating enormous savings.

Unfortunately, many of the current offerings have yet to generate the number of sellers or buyers necessary to create a truly powerful on-line marketplace. Furthermore, many of these on-line marketplaces are trying to import inappropriate models from other industries. The needs of health care buyers and their established contractual relationships (group purchasing organizations and so forth) are so unique that "traditional" on-line marketplaces must be highly modified and even integrated into current computer (legacy) systems to provide real value. Finally, experience in the on-line computer sales arena has shown that such marketplaces may in fact strengthen established distributors and other industry middlemen. In health care, industry middlemen are well entrenched.

Pharmaceutical benefits management companies, for example, are so thoroughly established that on-line pharmacies have for the most part had to align themselves with traditional bricks-and-mortar pharmacy chains, limiting their overall value proposition and market flexibility. Some analysts are saying that the Web is in fact creating another layer of information intermediaries, or *infomediaries.*[29]

CONSUMER-CENTERED HEALTH CARE: THE FUTURE STATE OF HEALTH CARE ON THE WEB

Thus far I have outlined the current state of health care on the Internet and highlighted its shortcomings. Now I turn to the exciting possibilities and future direction of health care on the Web.

Mass Individual Customization

The majority of the current health care Web offerings aim to aggregate users, aggregate buyers, and aggregate sellers. Whether they are content or e-commerce providers, they aim to develop brand franchises and leverage these into real market power. However they are overlooking the real power of the Web. Its power lies *not in its ability to aggregate users and cater to all* but in its ability to cater to individual needs—*to allow users to see uniquely customized views that are specifically tailored for their health care needs and interests.*

A personal page should be easy to navigate, entertaining, and personalized—integrated with information and deep content relevant to an individual's medical conditions, risk factors, and interests. In other words, visiting one's personal page should be a truly rewarding Web experience, not just a selected sample of generic menus and paragraphs of text slapped together. A health care consumer should be able to log onto a secure site and see a personalized, individual front end that includes

- Current health insurance information and options, including all related benefit information.

- Current medications, each of which should be hyper-linked to more detailed information about the drug, the alternatives, the possible interactions, and the side effects.

- A full list of all current diagnoses (including ICD-9 codes) hyperlinked to broad, summary-level content, which itself is hyperlinked to broad and deeper levels of content. This rich, interactive, personalized multimedia content should be integrated to the personal Web page and presented in an entertaining manner (as discussed later).

- An e-commerce offering tailored to the individual's needs, including over-the-counter medications and supplies relevant to the individual's conditions.

In addition, the individual should be able to interact with his or her provider (both physician and hospital), as discussed later.

Wellness

Personalized disease information should be interspersed with personalized wellness information to provide a better understanding of how actions and lifestyles affect the individual's particular disease. The on-line health care consumer's experience should be an uplifting and truly empowering encounter.

Content

Health care content should consist not only of data but also real information, personalized to the end-user. In the language of the Web, it should be *edutainment*—a combination of education and entertainment. Microsoft's *Encarta* controls the CD-ROM encyclopedia market because it was the first resource to fully use the power of the PC. Like *Encarta,* on-line health care information should not be merely factual but contextually rich, not merely the on-line version of a textbook but a true multimedia application. Unlike a standard CD-ROM or textbook, it should move beyond the generic one-size-fits-all to the customized solution, using XML technologies that tag ICD-9 codes and medication lists and then assemble personalized, relevant content from which the consumer can drill down further and further to learn more about every aspect of his or her disease, right down to medical-level reference material—a true web of personalized content.

Provider Connectivity

An individual's Web front end should function like a true on-line call center where information can be obtained about the individual's physician as well as his or her condition or medications. The individual should be able to directly request physician referrals, make appointments, and preregister, allowing the appropriate referral or precertification. If an individual is going to have a procedure, he or she should be able to access information about the procedure, preprocedure preparation, and discharge instructions.

Regional Power

The proximity of patients and providers is key to the delivery of health care services, and so the provision of health care services is centered around local environments. As a result, health care is regulated primarily by individual state and local markets, which has resulted in a wide disparity of delivery models, payment systems, clinical practices, and administrative processes. Therefore, in comparison to other industries, the health care industry will need to do more customizing of its Internet applications to meet the requirements of local markets. Internet health care offerings must address the reality of the needs of patients, their providers, and their communities through local connectivity, implementation flexibility, and software customization.

Other Factors

Myriad other factors will influence the implementation, adoption, and success of Internet health care offerings. Discussion of these factors is beyond the scope of this chapter, but they include various technological issues (for example, bandwidth, security, and application interfaces), clinical issues (for example, physician practice patterns and physician-centered Web offerings), and most important, financial issues (for example, business and revenue models). Further, no discussion of the Internet is complete without mentioning the issue of quality and credibility, an issue of growing significance, especially in health care. We have already seen, for example, the controversies over drkoop.com's policy of "recommending" hospitals that had paid for this recommendation.[30] This highlights the sensitivity and great importance of quality issues for health care Web sites (issues such as full disclosure, especially of conflict-of-interest relationships).

CONCLUSION

The use of the Web is accelerating among the general population, fueled by falling costs and the ease with which users can access reams of data. Internet usage in the area of health care is also accelerating and will continue to do so, driven by recent trends in health care such as increased costs, pharmaceutical advertising, reduced accessibility to physicians, and a desire by consumers to take control of their health care. The Web will accelerate the movement to give health care decision-making power back to the consumer. The information that the Web provides will help health care consumers understand their choices and will allow them to make more informed, cost-effective, decisions.

Current health care offerings are limited in scope and appeal. The long-term success stories in the health care Internet world will likely be Web offerings that have a narrow and deep rather than a broad and shallow focus. They will combine elements of content, community, connectivity, and commerce and be centered on a clearly defined target market and business model. These health care Web models will evolve from hybrids of the current health care Internet offerings. They will enrich the consumer with content personalized by medical condition, health interests, and risk factors. Ultimately, these offerings will become more than a simple educational tutorial or an on-line shopping trip; they will evolve into a truly rewarding Web experience, one that empowers the health care consumer.

Notes

1. Jupiter Media Metrix. "Jupiter Internet Population Model, 10/01 (U.S. only)." Darien, Conn.: JupiterMedia.

2. Jupiter Media Metrix, "Jupiter Internet Population Model."

3. U.S. Department of Commerce. *A Nation Online: How Americans Are Expanding Their Use of the Internet."* Washington, D.C.: U.S. Department of Commerce, Feb. 2002.

4. Russ, C. S., and Cohen, M. *Health Care and the Internet.* Charlotte, N.C.: First Union Capital Markets, June 22, 1999.

5. U.S. Department of Commerce. *E-Stats,* Mar. 18, 2002. [www.census.gov/estats].

6. Kaiser Family Foundation. Reviewed by [www.iHealthBeat.org], Dec. 12, 2001.

7. Jupiter Media Metrix. *The Quality of Care.* Reviewed by [www.iHealthBeat.org], Feb. 14, 2002.

8. U.S. Department of Commerce. *A Nation Online.*

9. Woody, T. "The Trillion-Dollar Opportunity." *The Industry Standard,* Mar. 29, 1999, p. 30.

10. Kaiser Family Foundation. Dec. 12, 2001.

11. Russ and Cohen, *Health Care and the Internet;* Knepper, M. W., and Banaszak, P. *Healthcare Webwatch.* New York: Punk Ziegel & Company, June 1999.

12. McKeever, W., and Fidel, S. *2002 Premium Pricing Survey.* New York: UBS Warburg, Nov. 30, 2001.

13. McKeever and Fidel, *2002 Premium Pricing Survey.*

14. Dolliver, B. K., and Hynes, A. K. *Pharmacy Benefit Management Industry: Major Opportunities in a Changing Landscape."* New York: SG Cowen, Mar. 2002.

15. Fulcrum Analytics. *Cybercitizen Health 2001.* New York: Fulcrum Analytics, n.d.

16. Knepper and Banaszak, *Healthcare Webwatch.*

17. Russ and Cohen, *Health Care and the Internet.*

18. Strunk, B. C., and Cunningham, P. J. *Treading Water: Americans' Access to Needed Medical Care, 1997–2001.* Results from Tracking Study No. 1. Washington, D.C.: Center for Studying Health System Change, Mar. 2002.

19. Knepper and Banaszak, *Healthcare Webwatch.*

20. Knepper and Banaszak, *Healthcare Webwatch.*

21. "Care Delivery Survey: One-Third of Adults Would Pay for Net-Based Communication with Physicians." Harris Interactive Poll, conducted Mar. 27 to Apr. 2, 2002. Reviewed by [www.ihealthbeat.org], Apr. 12, 2002.

22. Russ and Cohen, *Health Care and the Internet.*

23. Russ and Cohen, *Health Care and the Internet.*

24. "Study: Low-Cost E-Mail Discussion Group Improves Health of Back Pain Patients." *Archives of Internal Medicine,* Apr. 8, 2002. Reviewed by [www.iHealthBeat.org], Apr. 12, 2002.

25. *Western Journal of Medicine,* Dec. 2001. Reviewed by [www.ihealthbeat.org], Dec. 10, 2001.

26. Forrester Research Inc. *Sizing Healthcare E-Commerce,* Dec. 1999. Reviewed by T. Chin, *American Medical News,* Jan. 31, 2000.

27. Kearny, A. T. "E + Business: The Rx for Healthcare." *Executive Agenda,* 3(1), 41–50.

28. Boehm, E. W., and others. "Sizing Healthcare E-Commerce." *TechStrategy,* Dec. 1999.

29. Versweyveld, L. "Novel Trends in Internet Health Care Industry Revealed in E*OFFERING's Research Report." *Virtual Medical Worlds,* July 27, 1999. [http://www.hoise.com/vmw/99/articles/vmw/LV-VM-09-99-6.html].

30. Noble, H. B. "E-Medicine—A Special Report: Hailed as a Surgeon General, Koop Is Faulted on Web Ethics." *New York Times,* Sept. 5, 1999, p. 1.

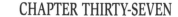

CHAPTER THIRTY-SEVEN

The Present and Future Roles of Information in a Consumer-Driven Health Care System

Russell Ricci

In the past three years, consumerism in health care has grown from an academic theory to a reality. Stakeholders in the health care system have begun to transform their thinking; from payer to provider to manufacturer, there is little talk of the *patient;* rather it is the *consumer* who is the center of attention.

As this transition continues, all constituents in the health care delivery system are attempting to influence the behavior of consumers through targeted information about care delivery and choices. With information ranging from management of diseases to the selection of drug treatment regimens, all parties are reaching out to the consumer in an attempt to encourage specific behavior. Because of the current misalignment of incentives in the health care system, however, the factors influencing health care information today are frequently in conflict. In the near term this conflict is driving increased dissatisfaction and confusion among consumers and providers, threats to quality of care, and potentially, increased costs of care.

IBM believes, however, that over the next five years the increased use of the Internet as a medium for both communication and commerce will enable a rationalization of the care continuum. The unprecedented flexibility and incredibly broad reach of the Internet, coupled with its low cost relative to costs of previous attempts at technology-based solutions, will provide an efficient vehicle for the development of applications and companies that can improve consumer health care while controlling and decreasing society's cost of care.

MEDICAL TECHNOLOGY MANUFACTURERS

Medical technology manufacturers, such as pharmaceutical companies, have historically focused on using information to influence physician behavior. However, as consumers have emerged as significant decision makers in their own care, manufacturers have moved rapidly to deliver information to consumers that will encourage the use of new products. These companies are aggressively using traditional advertising media such as television for the first time and are taking advantage of new channels such as the Internet to reach consumers with their message. These campaigns of direct-to-consumer advertising have been largely aimed at influencing the treatment regimens of patients. Whereas in the past manufacturers would target the physician as the prime decision maker in health care, it is now recognized that the consumer plays a vital role. Pursuing increased profitability, manufacturers are attempting to encourage consumers to make specific choices when receiving care from physicians, in many cases regardless of the care decisions advocated by providers and payers.

HEALTH CARE PAYERS

Health care payers, including governments, employers, insurers, and to a lesser extent providers bearing risk, are interested in managing the cost of care. These constituents are beginning to recognize the power of providing information to consumers that promotes the acceptance of low-cost care alternatives. Through information-intensive disease management and preventive care programs, health care payers are attempting to encourage the well-being and healthy living of the consumers for whose health care costs they are responsible. In addition, payers are attempting to use information to effectively control the expectations of consumers regarding the breadth and depth of the care that will be provided to them as a result of their coverage. Currently, these organizations are in direct conflict with manufacturers who are attempting to encourage the use of new, potentially high-cost drug treatments and to undermine the institutional treatment guidelines designed to maximize clinical cost efficacy.

HEALTH CARE PROVIDERS

Health care providers, especially physicians, are frequently at the intersection of this conflict. As the other stakeholders in the system have begun to use information to influence the behavior of consumers, it is at the expense of the providers' traditionally sole influence on the care of their patients. Increasingly, consumers are approaching their physicians with information and opinions about both their diagnosis and their choice of treatment. This information has made it more difficult for the physician to provide care that satisfies the desires of both the consumer and the relevant health care payer. In addition, consumer-directed information has in many respects undermined the traditional power and authority clinicians have held, resulting in frustration and dissatisfaction.

THE FUTURE

In the near term, pharmaceutical manufacturers appear better able than others to influence the behavior of consumers through the proliferation of information. They have moved quickly to embrace investments in media like the Internet that are well suited to the information and interactivity requirements of consumers. In addition, pharmaceutical companies have the resources at their disposal to invest in national campaigns to disseminate information to a broad group of consumers. In 2000, five pharmaceutical companies were among the top thirty advertisers nationwide. They spent a combined total of more than $7 billion in advertising, much of that in direct-to-consumer ads.[1] In contrast, health care payers have done little to date that has been effective in swaying consumer behavior. However, it is becoming apparent to both payers and employers that an investment in information directed at influencing consumer expectations and behavior and expanding the scope of consumers' dialogues with health care providers is necessary. Increasingly, payers will invest in information sources such as the Internet that will be directed at educating consumers about their choices for cost-effective care.

Although both the rise of consumerism and the proliferation of information have created near-term conflict in the health care system, the widespread availability of credible and thorough information through media like the Internet will ultimately result in a more educated and effective consumer. In addition, over time, health care information and information technology will converge into a medium for improved communication among the various stakeholders and, ultimately, a medium for efficient health care transactions. As this future emerges, efficient information will drive a vastly improved health care system in which cost-effective decisions by all parties involved in health care will result in the delivery of high-quality, evidence-based care.

Note

1. "46th Annual Ad Leadership Report—2000." *Advertising Age.*

CHAPTER THIRTY-EIGHT

Who Has Star Quality?

Jon A. Chilingerian

Consumers can help to transform the way health care is delivered. Indeed, consumers have already effected important changes in the health care system. For example, patient expectations have influenced the architecture of hospital wards, the concerns of the women's movement have led to more family-centered care in obstetrics, and the needs and buying behaviors of individuals with diabetes have changed product-line and research and development strategies in the worldwide insulin business.

Patient expectations are the reason today's hospitals have many small, private rooms. To achieve nursing efficiency and lower construction costs, modern hospitals were originally built with large, impersonal wards, most containing as many as forty beds. However, throughout the world and at different points in time, ward patients complained bitterly about the lack of privacy, amenities, convenience, and information.[1] Despite the benefits of large wards, consumer forces helped to shift the architecture of hospitals. In the United States, hospitals built before 1880 had very large wards only; however, by 1908, private rooms grew to account for 40 percent of all U.S. beds, and large wards declined to account for only 28 percent. By the year 2000, the number of private and semiprivate rooms had grown to account for nearly 100 percent of the

I am very grateful to Dianne Chilingerian, Regina Herzlinger, John Kimberly, and Leon White for their encouragement and thoughtful comments.

beds in almost every economically developed health care system. Owing to consumer feedback, the large *Nightingale wards* have faded into health care's distant past.[2]

The second example of patient behavior effecting change goes back to the 1970s, which saw the blossoming of the consumer movement in the area of obstetrics. Family-centered care was introduced when members of the *women's movement* began to question "routine clinical treatments" that neglected the emotional needs of the family and assigned pregnant women the role of passive recipients of medical care.[3] Within a few years of consumers' raising their voices against standard operating procedures, such things as drugs, general anesthesia, enemas, and surgical incisions became optional medical interventions. The consumer movement allowed fathers to participate during the birth and babies to stay with their mothers after the delivery. Rigid care programs were unbundled, and new choices became available to the new obstetrics consumer.

The *market for diabetes care* is a third example of the consumer movement at work.[4] Eli Lilly, a pioneer in diabetic products, competed by developing purer forms of insulin. Although Lilly was responsive to endocrinologists, it was less responsive to the diabetic consumers who longed for greater convenience and reduced costs. A consumer-oriented company, Novo Nordisk, that made handy disposable insulin injection pens (Novo Pen I, II, and III) began to attract European consumers to its product. Although Eli Lilly knew about injection pens, it was not ready to abandon the time-consuming and less convenient needles and injection kits. Once this implicit consumer movement gained momentum, however, Lilly was forced to rethink an R&D strategy that aimed at perfecting insulin and ignored consumer demand for convenience and reduced costs.

These three examples demonstrate that health organizations do respond to consumers. How fast consumers can effect change, however, depends on the resolution of a great barrier—the lack of consensus on a definition of quality of medical care. Health care providers can help the consumer revolution to improve the delivery of health care by developing a clinically relevant and widely accepted consumer-driven definition of quality. After all, what gets measured gets managed. The remainder of this chapter will focus on a consumer-centered definition of quality.[5]

WHAT IS QUALITY IN HEALTH CARE?

Throughout the twentieth century the ostensible challenge in health care management has been to find a theoretically correct way to assess quality of care, but the real challenge has been to uncover and understand the many factors underlying quality. Although philosophical arguments have seldom delayed business leaders from finding solutions to practical, bottom-line problems, philosophical debates over health care among policymakers, clinical leaders, and managers have paralyzed the measurement of quality.

If quality could be treated as a unidimensional variable, some subjective means of combining multiple measures (or a theory-based mathematical formula that yielded a single, summary measure of quality) could be applied. For example, if variables such as mix of staff, methods of peer review, decision-making efficiency, convenience, patient satisfaction, health status, and mortality were highly interrelated, it would be possible to develop a single concept based on the general features or common elements of quality. But the evidence suggests they are not.[6] Whether these features are unidimensional or multidimensional remains a research hypothesis that requires further empirical work.[7]

Managers know that quality never becomes a simple concept (this is one of the many important lessons they have learned from the economists). Because individuals have widely diverging tastes and preferences, there can never be *one best way* to assess the quality of services.[8] The assessment of service quality is always subjective—people will weigh and rank the characteristics of services in inconsistent ways. Absent a guiding theory of quality, at best we can identify some critical features, components, or underlying dimensions of quality, rank (or grade) them, and report the results. In this sense, measuring quality requires evaluating performance by means of a multidimensional scheme.

The most promising direction is to assume that quality is not as complex as the vast enumeration of variables and indicators that the extant literature implies but rather that quality, as a construct, is best understood in terms of a few underlying dimensions. According to the literature, at least five important dimensions of quality have emerged.[9] These five dimensions are outlined in the following list:

Five Leading Dimensions of Quality of Care

1. Patient satisfaction

    Percentage extremely satisfied and why

    Pain management: discomfort time

    Percentage willing to recommend the provider again

2. Relationships: information and emotional support

    Amount and clarity of information

    Degree of trust

    Time spent encouraging

    Time spent listening

3. Amenities and convenience

    Clean, fast, and timely

    Service available when needed

    Time spent waiting

    Experience of hospitality and respect

4. Decision-making efficiency

    Clinical resources used to achieve constant quality outcomes

    Quick routes to health (diagnosis to treatment)

5. Patient outcomes

    Mortality and morbidity rates

    Readmission rates

    Adverse events and errors

    Falls, nosocomial (that is, hospital-acquired) infection rates

    Changes in functional or health status and severity of illness

Although there is scant evidence to suggest that these five dimensions are highly intercorrelated, they are not mutually exclusive factors, as the following discussion demonstrates.

Patient Satisfaction

Recently, as the orientation to health care began shifting from scientific mandates and medical techniques to markets and the more human side of the health care service delivery system, patient satisfaction became an important dimension of quality of care.[10] In part, the discovery of patient satisfaction was an artifact of clinical work on patient-centered care[11] and of the influence of strategic marketing on health care management. Clinicians learned that throughout the service process, patients and their families experienced hundreds of *clinical moments of truth.* Research on the *satisfied patient* suggested that patients' overall evaluation of quality depends on the results of the processes, as an *experience,* at every point of contact.[12] Quality measurement from this perspective requires mapping and surveying the patient's entire experience with the delivery system.

Medical care tasks produce feelings in patients of satisfaction and dissatisfaction. On the one hand, strong feelings of satisfaction develop when patient (or consumer) expectations are met and exceeded.[13] On the other hand, dissatisfaction may be related to an insufficient rate of uncertainty reduction throughout the care process.[14] There are many different indicators of patient satisfaction, ranging from the patient's overall experience to the patient's willingness to use and recommend the service in the future. To understand the patient's overall experience, we need to pose several questions: Was the patient treated rudely? Did the patient expect less waiting? Did the patient experience unnecessary uncertainty? Was there a focus on the patient as an individual?

Although defection rates (that is, the percentage of patients who change providers) are sometimes used as quality indicators,[15] some critics suggest avoiding such global measures and focusing instead on the specific sources of satisfaction and dissatisfaction that might cause a defection. For example, rather than report a 90 percent satisfaction rate, report that 10 percent of the patients were dissatisfied because their physician never told them what to do or what not to do after they left the hospital and went home.[16] Patient information about extraordinarily good and bad services is captured in satisfaction or dissatisfaction. To avoid losing this information, patient satisfaction should be included in the medical record so all caregivers can regularly monitor each patient's experiences during the service encounters.

Although patient satisfaction is a critical dimension, the knowledge difference between patients and health care providers is so large that *substantial client satisfaction* cannot be the only indicator of quality. The practice of medicine often involves hidden actions and equivocal information, so it is difficult for most patients to know whether diagnostic tests and other treatments were appropriate and the outcomes reasonable. Therefore measures of quality from other vantage points are required to review whether or not a process was adequate and outcomes were acceptable.[17] For these reasons the dimension of information and emotional support and also the dimension of amenities and convenience should be considered.

Relationships: Information and Emotional Support

The second dimension of quality focuses on the relationship between providers and patients in terms of the amount and clarity of information and the degree of emotional support provided. Though related to patient satisfaction, this dimension is treated separately because it gives rise to another fundamental expectation in health services—increasing (or perhaps even optimizing) the patient's control. Good clinical care necessitates task-oriented provider behavior focused on diagnosing symptoms, setting treatment goals, and monitoring recovery. But quality care also requires that providers promote the involvement of the individual and family and support informed choice, offer encouragement, provide clarification, and ensure confidentiality. Therefore good clinical care also requires behavior aimed at building trusting relationships.

Some would argue that caregivers who involve patients and families in decisions, coach patients, and give emotional support reduce uncertainty—the clinical experience then becomes more manageable by the patient and less frightening. Benner reports that teaching patients to prepare them before surgery can actually expedite their recovery.[18] In fact, research suggests that providing better patient information and more effective emotional support can lead to shorter stays, less medication, fewer side effects, better compliance, and higher levels of satisfaction.[19]

Some questions to pose to ascertain quality are these: To what extent do the caregivers educate patients, clarify the treatment regimes, and spend time listening and encouraging? Are patients told when and how to take their medications and what to eat? Are illnesses discussed not only with privacy in mind but tactfully as well? To what extent are the diagnosis, results, and care plan explained? Although some of these factors may be measured by patient surveys, others should be assessed through audits of the medical records.

Amenities and Convenience

Convenience of care and perceived amenities make up a third important dimension of quality of care, and measurements of these items can reflect individual patients' preferences in technology, people, facilities, and coordination behaviors. Measuring these variables implies discovering choices among courses of clinical action and clinical decision making. Herzlinger has stated that there are two new market segments, or new consumers: those who want convenience and those who demand more information.[20] Today's hard-working patients lead busy lives. They demand and deserve convenient and comfortable access to medical services. One could argue that technological advances in minimally invasive surgery were spurred by these demands.

Donabedian has argued that "convenience, comfort, quiet, and privacy" are merely desirable attributes of the health care delivery system.[21] If that position is correct, then they may be covered under patient satisfaction and do not belong in a separate quality dimension. I have separated amenities and convenience from overall patient satisfaction for two reasons. First, researchers have reported that when patients have been asked about their overall satisfaction, they do not emphasize aesthetics, better food and parking, amenities and convenience.[22] Because individual tastes differ, the value of convenience depends on individual needs and preferences. Cultural preferences are also often at work here. A second reason that amenities and convenience should be a separate dimension of quality is that service inconveniences have opportunity-cost implications for patients, and offerings of greater convenience have cost implications for caregivers. As health care becomes increasingly competitive, trade-offs may be necessary to stem the health care cost explosion. By measuring this dimension separately, clinicians can serve the unique needs of individual patients, and patients can request an amenity when it seems to them to add value.

Decision-Making Efficiency

The fourth dimension of quality found in the literature is decision-making efficiency,[23] which is the least developed of the five dimensions of quality and perhaps the most controversial. In the past, physicians were trained to do everything possible for the patient regardless of cost; moreover, physicians tended to equate more intensive medical care with better services. As Harris explains, "doctors have an almost inexhaustible repertoire of things that will make patients better off."[24] But what does "better off" really mean? Providing superior clinical service today requires rapid information processing for diagnosis and treatment. There is growing evidence that quick and accurate diagnosis that expedites treatment increases a patient's chances of success by reducing cycle times for hospitalization, recovery, follow-up treatment, and return to a normal life. Conversely, there is ample evidence that *too many* tests, needles, and x rays may do more harm than good.[25]

Because it makes no sense to evaluate the efficiency of a medical service process that results in morbidity, mortality, or a readmission to a hospital, decision-making efficiency must focus on the resources used in order to *achieve a satisfactory outcome.* Inefficiency in the provision of clinical services occurs when physicians and other care providers use an excessive amount of resources to achieve a satisfactory result. The overutilization of medical services (such as ancillary tests) not only carries patient risks but also increases patient anxiety. This dimension of quality is often overlooked.

Patient Outcomes

Assessment of patient outcomes, the fifth dimension of quality, expresses the degree to which the observed clinical performance approached its potential. According to Donabedian, outcomes record the effects of the care process on the health status of the population.[26] Outcomes include serious clinical results such as death, medication errors, postoperative loss of an organ or limb, and hospital-acquired infection. As one physician has argued, "quality is not how well or how frequently a medical service is given, but how closely the result approaches the fundamental objectives of prolonging life, relieving distress, restoring function, and preventing disability." Many argue that outcomes are the leading indicator of quality and that the outcomes of greatest significance are the changes in health status attainable given current technology, clinical knowledge, and management practices.

Because outcomes vary considerably among clinical providers and systems of care, comparing the outcomes of providers can be difficult. Various reasons have been advanced to explain outcome variations, such as prior health status, poor patient compliance, lack of diffusion of medical technology, poorly coordinated care, lack of provider competence, weak clinical leaders, and ineffective management practices. The development of measures that incorporate these variables, such as case-mix measures or indicators of health status, functional improvement, and severity of illness, has advanced considerably. When case-mix measures are available, it is possible to develop summary measures of the clinical benefits achieved based on changes in functional status or other measures of patient outcomes.[27] For example, measuring the change in severity of illness for a given diagnosis from admission to discharge would be a very good measure of effectiveness of the care process in attaining outcomes in relation to implied clinical objectives.

TOWARD A CONSUMER-DRIVEN DEFINITION OF QUALITY

A few years ago, during a health care lecture I gave for an international audience of clinical leaders, a participant asked, "Is there the equivalent of a bottom line in health care?" The medical profession and the policymakers can enjoy debating this issue for a few more decades, or we can enter the twenty-first century ready to measure quality in ways that allow consumers to ask which providers have star quality and to get meaningful answers. Figure 38.1 summarizes a balanced, consumer-driven approach to the measurement of star quality, based on the dimensions discussed in this chapter. The two legs of star quality are patient outcomes and decision-making efficiency. At the apex, we see patient satisfaction, with information and emotional support on one flank and amenities and convenience on the other. Despite the difficulties of defining and measuring health care outputs, this model can make quality management a more tractable problem. Further progress depends on developing equitable quality *report cards* that make significant comparisons on each of these five dimensions.

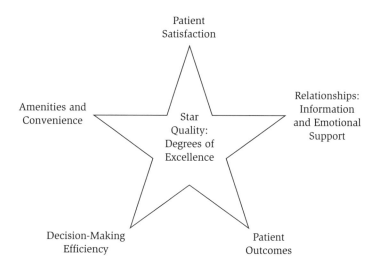

Figure 38.1. Five Dimensions of Star Quality.

Ultimately, the management of quality has one fundamental goal: to benefit patients who need health care services. A consumer-driven definition of quality has a deeper meaning—it can be understood as an indicator of the overall degree of excellence of an individual provider or a care program. Health care delivery systems will change when measurement systems use these five quality dimensions to benchmark providers against the best care observed in practice. When the consumer revolution is armed with appropriate measures of star quality for every provider—individual physician, ambulatory clinic, hospital, nursing home, and so on—at every level of care, the health care system will improve. And perhaps faster than we might otherwise expect.

Notes

1. As one Hungarian chief of obstetrics and gynecology said to me during a recent site visit, "Hungarian citizens no longer tolerated staying in large wards. They demanded private rooms." I have heard this story repeatedly from dozens of clinical leaders in major health care systems around the world.

2. One exception among Western health care systems is the National Health Service in Britain, where one can still find very large wards, with eight to twenty or more beds.

3. Kelley, G. "Special Delivery: A Consumer Guide to Giving Birth in Boston." *Boston Magazine,* Apr. 1978, p. 74.

4. A more complete history of the market for insulin can be found in Christensen, C. M., *Eli Lilly & Co: Innovations in Diabetes Care.* Harvard Business School Case No. 9-696-077. Boston: Harvard Business School, 1996. Much of the information on the market for insulin comes from Christensen, C. M. *The Innovator's Dilemma.* Harvard Business School Press, 1997, pp. 224–226.

5. A mathematical approach to measuring various dimensions of quality by locating best-practice frontiers is discussed in Chilingerian, J. A., "Evaluating Quality Outcomes Against Best Practice: A New Frontier." In J. Kimberly and E. Minvielle (eds.), *The Quality Imperative: Measurement and Management of Quality in Healthcare.* London: Imperial College Press, 2000.

6. Chilingerian, J., and Sherman, H. D. "Managing Physician Efficiency and Effectiveness in Providing Hospital Services." *Health Services Management Research,* 1990, *3*(1), 3–15; Chilingerian, J. "Exploring Why Some Physicians' Hospital Practices Are More Efficient: Taking DEA Inside the Hospital." In Charnes, A., *Data Envelopment Analysis: Theory, Methodology, and Application.* Norwell: Kluwer, 1994; Chilingerian, "Evaluating Quality Outcomes Against Best Practice."

7. Donabedian, A. "The Quality of Care: How Can It Be Assessed?" *Journal of the American Medical Association,* September 23–30, 1988, *260,* pp. 1743–1748; Chilingerian, "Evaluating Quality Outcomes Against Best Practice."

8. Hemenway, D. *Prices and Choices: Microeconomic Vignettes.* (Rev. ed.) Cambridge, Mass.: Ballinger, 1984.

9. See, for example, Donabedian, "The Quality of Care"; Chilingerian and Sherman, "Managing Physician Efficiency and Effectiveness . . ."; Delbanco, T. L., "Enriching the Doctor-Patient Relationship by Inviting the Patient's Perspective." *Annals of Internal Medicine,* Mar. 1, 1992, *116,* 414–418; Herzlinger, R. E. *Market-Driven Care: Who Wins, Who Loses in the Transformation of America's Largest Service Industry.* Reading, Mass.: Addison-Wesley, 1997; Eddy, D. "Performance Measurement: Problems and Solutions." *Health Affairs,* July–Aug. 1998, pp. 7–25; Lang, F., Floyd, M., and Beine, K. "Clues to Patient's Explanations and Concerns About Their Illness: A Call for Active Listening." *Archives of Family Medicine,* Mar. 2000, *9,* 222–227; Shelton, P. *Measuring and Improving Patient Satisfaction.* Gaithersberg, Md.: Aspen, 2000; Chilingerian, "Evaluating Quality Outcomes Against Best Practice."

10. Gold, M., and Wooldridge, J. "Surveying Customer Satisfaction to Assess Managed Care Quality: Current Practices." *Health Care Financing Review,* 1995, *16*(4), 155–173; Berwick, D. "The Year of 'How': New Systems for Delivering Health Care." *Quality Connections,* 1996, *5*(1), 1–4.

11. Delbanco, "Enriching the Doctor-Patient Relationship . . ."

12. Recent research on service organization profitability suggests that the study of satisfaction must focus on the outliers—those who are "*extremely* satisfied" and those who are "*extremely* dissatisfied" (Heskett, J. L., Sasser, W. E., and Schlesinger, L. A. *The Service Profit Chain.* New York: Free Press, 1997). Delivery systems that merely "satisfy" service customers are headed toward mediocrity; in the long run, mere satisfaction is a formula for failure.

13. Heskett and others, *The Service Profit Chain.*

14. Schauffler, H. H., Rodriguez, T., and Milstein, A. "Health Education and Patient Satisfaction." *Journal of Family Practice,* 1996, *42*(1), 62–68.

15. Struebing, L. "Customer Loyalty: Playing for Keeps." *Quality Progress,* 1996, *28*(2), 25–30.

16. Delbanco, "Enriching the Doctor-Patient Relationship . . ."

17. Acceptable outcomes require expert judgments, a priori standards, or explicit expectations (Brook, R. H., McGlynn, E. A., and Cleary, P. D. "Measuring Quality of Care." *New England Journal of Medicine,* Sept. 26, 1996, *335,* 966–969).

18. Benner, P. *From Novice to Expert: Excellence and Power in Clinical Nursing Practice.* Reading, Mass.: Addison-Wesley, 1984.

19. Levitan, S. E. "Providing Emotional Support." *Picker/Commonwealth Report* (Beth Israel Hospital, Boston), Winter 1992, *1.*

20. Herzlinger, *Market-Driven Care.*

21. Donabedian, "The Quality of Care," p. 1744.

22. Delbanco, "Enriching the Doctor-Patient Relationship . . ."

23. Chilingerian and Sherman, "Managing Physician Efficiency and Effectiveness . . ."; Chilingerian, J. "New Directions for Hospital Strategic Management: The Market for Efficient Care." *Health Care Management Review,* 1992, *17*(4), 73–80.

24. Harris, J. E. "The Internal Organization of Hospitals: Some Economic Implications." *Bell Journal of Economics,* 1977, 8(2), pp. 467–482.

25. Eisenberg, J. M. *Doctors' Decisions and the Cost of Medical Care.* Ann Arbor, Mich.: Health Administration Press, 1986.

26. Donabedian, "The Quality of Care."

27. Chilingerian, J. "Evaluating Physician Efficiency in Hospitals: A Multi-Variate Analysis of Best Practices." *European Journal of Operational Research,* 1995, *80,* 548–574.

CHAPTER THIRTY-NINE

Grounding Consumer-Driven Health Care in Social Science Research

Arnold Milstein, Nancy E. Adler

The problem of value shortfall in health care is substantial. The National Academy of Science report on average quality in U.S. health care found defects to be serious and widespread, even in our best delivery systems.[1] Unreliable quality of care, in turn, wastes precious resources. Consistent with several prior projections by individual experts, the Juran Institute estimated that 30 percent of current direct health care costs are wasted due to weak quality management.[2] Intensified consumerism could reduce these shortfalls in value, but there are obstacles to be overcome. The magnitude of gain will depend heavily on how well consumer-driven approaches attend to relevant evidence from social science research in addressing these obstacles.

Health policy analysts have identified a number of threats to optimal consumer health care decisions. They note particularly that health care (1) lacks standardized, publicly reported performance measures; (2) is probabilistic in its value proposition; (3) may reveal its results over long time frames; and (4) is pervaded by scientific unknowns about "what works." These characteristics challenge consumers' ability to discern and capture higher-value health care, whether that care is bundled via the patient's selection of an insurance plan or unbundled via selections among individual provider and treatment options. Social science research suggests several additional, less widely recognized threats to successful consumer value capture in health care.

What are these additional threats and, by inference, promising methods of attenuating them?

454

Information block-out. Herbert Simon documented that when consumers are faced with complex choices, they tend to experience cognitive overload and to choose options that are satisfactory, even if not optimal.[3] Thus they may not seek out additional, potentially important information once they perceive a satisfactory option. For example, the impressive interpersonal manner of a surgeon may cause a consumer to lose interest in investigating the surgeon or hospital's risk-adjusted mortality rate. Information block-out implies a need to simplify the most prognostically important performance information and make it easily available to consumers.

Optimistic bias. Neil Weinstein documented that consumers systematically underestimate personal health risk.[4] In essence, most of us believe that probabilistic health threats, even when calculated flawlessly, do not apply fully to us individually. This implies that extra effort must be made to communicate to consumers the *personal* danger associated with careless selection of health plans, providers, and treatments.

Framing effects. Daniel Kahneman and Amos Tversky documented that consumers attach more weight to avoiding loss than to achieving an identical gain. For example, consumers are more likely to select a surgeon with better outcomes if the outcomes are framed as a reduced mortality risk than if framed as an increased survival gain.[5] This suggests health care performance comparisons should be framed as opportunities to avoid loss.

Availability heuristic. Kahneman and other researchers documented that individuals attach more weight to consequences that are more mentally graphic.[6] As a result, they may be likely to attach more weight to avoiding death from the slip of a surgical knife than from not being prescribed a pill, even when the increased probabilities of death are identical. Particularly in view of optimistic bias, this implies the need for more graphic portrayal of the consequences of suboptimal health care choices.

Stress effects of health danger. Irving Janis documented that consumers may deal with illness-related anxiety by idealizing their providers, who psychologically represent "danger control agents."[7] This interferes with vigilant performance appraisal and objective selection by consumers among best provider and treatment options. It implies the need to offer alternative danger control agents, such as confidence-inspiring consumer advocates, in order to sustain functional consumer objectivity in decision making.

Recent findings by Judith Hibbard, Eric Schneider, and others,[8] document the result that this body of social science research predicts: widespread consumer failure either to use or to attach significant value to available health care quality comparisons. Taken together, these results foreshadow a substantial shortfall in the utility that can be captured from a psychologically naive implementation of a consumer-driven health care market.

What would a psychologically astute implementation look like? Social science research would suggest the following steps: (1) take an approach similar to antitobacco or antidrug abuse advertising and use vivid imagery repeatedly to alert the public to the magnitude of the peril from passive acceptance of average quality care; (2) simplify public performance comparisons of health plans, hospitals, physicians, and treatments, and ensure that the choices are framed for consumers in the language of danger reduction; (3) move consumer deliberations upstream, so that, for example, consumers are encouraged to select an open heart surgeon when an increased likelihood of surgery is identified rather than in the terrifying context of an acute myocardial infarction; (4) create the substance and aura of physician authority around a neutral source of consumer decision support; and (5) ensure that the decision support source offers a spectrum of personalization and emotional support so that it equally serves an eighty-five-year-old's selection of a chest surgeon and a twenty-four-year-old, healthy technophile's selection of a health plan. Several of these ingredients might be concretized in the form of a Web- and telephone-accessible consumer decision support service, operated by a widely trusted sponsor and housing an attractive, easy-to-use decision support tool applied to consumer-conveyed personal health data and provider and plan performance data submitted in accordance with reporting rules similar to those promulgated by the Financial Accounting Standards Board.

Reporting rules for performance data would be needed for five primary categories of health care inputs that may significantly influence a consumer's health care experience and clinical outcome: health plans, hospitals, individual physicians, free-standing care management vendors, and major treatment options. Performance domains should encompass, at a minimum, the six Institute of Medicine–specified aims of health care: safety, timeliness, clinical effectiveness, patients' experience of care, economic efficiency, and equity. The National Quality Forum is the logical home of a national measures endorsement process. Supplemental in-person access to a familiar, financially disinterested, and psychologically trained navigational adviser may be necessary when decision parameters are complex or the patient's cognitive abilities are impaired.

Valid, understandable performance comparisons among health plans, providers, and treatments remain grossly underdeveloped, especially at the levels at which quality and value vary the most—individual physicians, hospitals, and treatment options. Filling this gap will require a multistakeholder push to catalyze the spread of computerized, interoperable health care information systems, especially in physicians' offices.

As aging and biomedical advances accelerate health care cost and likelihood of quality failure, the need to improve health care value via enhanced consumerism will intensify. To avoid disappointment with the yield of consumerism, implementation must address key, relevant findings from social science research and fill large voids in valid public performance comparisons and consumer decision support.

Notes

1. Chassin, M. R., and Galvin, R. W. "The Urgent Need to Improve Health Care Quality." *Journal of the American Medical Association,* 1998, *280,* 1000–1005.

2. Midwest Business Group on Health. *Reducing the Costs of Poor Quality Health Care Through Responsible Purchasing Leadership.* Chicago: Midwest Business Group on Health, 2002.

3. See the chapter "The Failure of Armchair Economics" in Simon, H. A., *Models of Bounded Rationality,* Vol. 3: *Empirically Grounded Economic Reason.* Cambridge, Mass.: MIT Press, 1997.

4. Weinstein, N. D., and Klein, W. M. "Resistance of Personal Risk Perceptions to Debiasing Interventions." *Health Psychology,* 1995, *14*(2), 132–140; Weinstein, N. D., Kolb, K., and Goldstein, B. D. "Using Time Intervals Between Expected Events to Communicate Risk Magnitudes." *Risk Analysis,* 1996, *16*(3), 305–308; Weinstein, N. D. "Accuracy of Smokers' Risk Perceptions." *Annals of Behavioral Medicine,* 1998, *20*(2), 135–140.

5. Tversky, A., and Kahneman, D. "The Framing of Decisions and the Psychology of Choice." *Science,* 1981, *211,* 453–458.

6. Redelmeier, D. A., Rozin, P., and Kahneman, D. "Understanding Patients' Decisions: Cognitive and Emotional Perspectives." *Journal of the American Medical Association,* 1993, *270,* 72–76.

7. Janis, I. L. "Coping Patterns Among Patients with Life-Threatening Diseases." *Issues of Mental Health Nursing,* 1985, *7,* 461–476.

8. Hibbard, J. H., Sofaer, S., and Jewett, J. J. "Condition-Specific Performance Information: Assessing Salience, Comprehension, and Approaches for Communicating Quality." *Health Care Financing Review,* 1996, *18*(1), 95–109; Hibbard, J. H., and Jewett, J. J. "Will Quality Report Cards Help Consumers?" *Health Affairs,* 1997, *16*(3), 218–228; Hibbard, J. H. "Strategically Using the Pathways Through Which Public Reports May Result in Improved Care." *International Journal for Quality in Health Care,* 2001, *13*(5), pp. 353–355; Schneider, E. C., and Epstein, A. M. "Use of Public Performance Reports: A Survey of Patients Undergoing Cardiac Surgery." *Journal of the American Medical Association,* 1998, *279,* 1638–1642; Schneider, E. C., and others. "Enhancing Performance Measurement: NCQA's Road Map for Health Information Framework." *Journal of the American Medical Association,* 1999, *282,* 1184–1190.

CHAPTER FORTY

Providing the Most-Wanted Information When Most Needed

Best Doctors

Steven W. Naifeh, Gregory White Smith

B est Doctors maintains a database of U.S. and international physicians who have been selected by their peers, through detailed, comprehensive surveys of the relevant medical communities, as the best in their respective specialties. The company mines this database to "match" patients with the appropriately skilled providers for the treatment of critical illnesses, catastrophic injuries, and other complex or unusual medical problems.

Some organizations are born of financial necessity, some of market opportunity, some of sheer serendipity. Best Doctors began as a response to a personal need. In 1986, one of the founders, Gregory White Smith, was diagnosed with an inoperable brain tumor and given six months to live. But Smith and his Harvard Law School classmate, Steven Naifeh, had one advantage over other patients. As publishers of *The Best Lawyers in America* they had developed a unique method of assessing the quality of professional services by conducting extensive telephone interviews in which professionals were asked to rate their peers. This peer review method quickly won the respect of the legal community, and today, *Best Lawyers* is in its sixteenth edition and widely regarded as the preeminent guide to the legal profession.

In 1986, the two men not only found a doctor to treat Smith successfully, they also went on to do the same thing for the medical profession that they had done for the legal profession, using the same peer review method of quality assessment. With twenty full-time pollsters, they began exhaustively surveying the medical profession on a regular basis, asking the question: "If you or a loved one needed a doctor in your specialty, to whom would you refer them?" Since then, the company has conducted tens of thousands of interviews and now processes millions of evaluations every year using proprietary software to create ballots and weigh votes. In 1992, as Best Doctors appeared more often in local and national media, the company began responding to individual requests from patients for help in identifying the right doctors for their particular medical problems. In 1997, the company started offering this service through managed care companies, insurers, and others, both in the United States and internationally.

To supplement its unique database of confidential, peer-based quality assessments on, at the time of this writing, approximately 34,000 medical specialists in the United States (and 10,000 internationally), Best Doctors solicits extensive information on each doctor's training and practice.

BEST DOCTORS' U.S. SERVICES

The resulting detailed professional profiles are used to offer the following services in the United States:

AcuMatch

The AcuMatch service provides a list of up to three specialists for a single primary diagnosis. A customer contacts the Best Doctors call center and provides a care coordinator with relevant information (for example, previous treatment, comorbidities, geographical preferences). A preliminary list of appropriate specialists is generated from the database using the company's proprietary search algorithms. Before reporting the results of the search to the customer, the coordinator checks on the recommended physicians' availability to ensure patient access. Where necessary, additional names are drawn from the database. The AcuMatch product also includes medical "concierge" services if the customer chooses to travel for treatment.

For example, a fifty-five-year-old quadriplegic with recurrent urinary tract infections contacted Best Doctors after being treated unsuccessfully for more than five years by a succession of eight urologists, all of whom had prescribed regimens of antibiotics that worked only briefly before the infections returned. A search of the Best Doctors database generated a list of four urologists in the country who specialized in urinary tract infections in paraplegic and quadriplegic patients. The patient chose the specialist at the closest institution. The infections have not recurred in the year since he began treatment with that doctor.

In another typical case an Oklahoma woman called Best Doctors for help in finding a doctor to treat her thirteen-year-old twin sons, both of whom had been diagnosed with HTLV1, an extremely rare adult lymphoma leukemia that virtually never occurs in children. A search of the Best Doctors database turned up a doctor at the University of Nebraska who managed the case, as well consulting specialists at three other U.S. institutions. Best Doctors also located consulting doctors in Japan, where the incidence of HTLV1 is higher than in any other country. The twins were eventually put on a hormone therapy protocol developed at the National Institutes of Health (NIH) and are responding well.

Best Doctors markets its AcuMatch service to individuals both directly, through a membership program, and indirectly, through insurers, reinsurers, self-insured corporations, preferred provider organizations (PPOs), third-party administrators (TPAs), case management firms, and government entities. Both in the United States and abroad the service is attached to supplementary insurance policies, especially critical illness policies, and that is the primary method by which it is made available. However, the only requirement for a suitable "host" policy or plan is that it give the customer freedom to choose a Best Doctors–recommended provider for treatment in the event of a catastrophic or complex medical problem. The company's objective is to make its AcuMatch service available across large populations for a nominal capitated fee.

Interconsultation

In addition to finding doctors for treatment, the company offers the Interconsultation service. This service mines the Best Doctors database to identify the appropriate medical expertise to review the treatment decisions of other doctors or to consult on treatment strategy. Reviews may relate to treatment protocols, diagnoses, or medical or legal determinations, and may be either case specific or disease specific. Consulting includes recruitment of physicians for clinical trials both in the United States and abroad. All reviewers and consultants have been chosen by their peers as the leading experts in their specialties.

A typical Interconsultation case involved a forty-nine-year-old woman in Italy who had been diagnosed with non-Hodgkin's lymphoma. During the grueling chemotherapy regime that followed, she developed severe toxic effects, received multiple transfusions, and was repeatedly hospitalized. After completing twelve cycles of chemotherapy, she showed signs of remission, but her spleen and liver were still enlarged. The woman's Italian health insurer contacted Best Doctors to arrange a second opinion. The U.S. expert identified by Best Doctors reviewed the patient's record and requested additional tests. From the results of those tests, the expert determined that the appropriate diagnosis was follicular lymphoma, not non-Hodgkin's lymphoma, and that the additional chemotherapy regime she was scheduled to undergo would be inappropriate and harmful. Best Doctors accessed its international database to identify a qualified specialist near the patient's home, who worked with the U.S. expert to supervise a new, less-toxic chemotherapy regime that ultimately led to remission.

THE ADVANTAGES

Despite the demand, information on the comparative quality of physicians is extremely rare. Only recently, in response to public pressure, has such information been made available for the low end of the professional spectrum, through listings of doctors with malpractice or other skill-related determinations against them.[1] These "black lists," provided by nonprofit, semipublic, and public entities as a public service, have proven extremely popular with consumers,[2] again demonstrating the unmet demand for this kind of information.

Efforts to create comparable lists at the high end have been undertaken primarily by local media, especially metropolitan magazines, as part of annual "Top Docs" features. Because they are usually done with limited budgets and within limited geographical areas and are subject to advertising imperatives, these lists tend to be neither reliable nor comprehensive. The few attempts at national or even regional lists of "best" physicians[3] suffer from the same problems of limited resources and blunt methodologies (typically a single, vast mailing), as well as from minimal or indiscriminate participation from the medical community.

The three elements essential to information on comparative physician quality are credibility, comprehensiveness, and accessibility.

Credibility. Doctors have confidence in the accuracy and reliability of Best Doctors' referrals because the system the company uses in compiling its database replicates (on a far more comprehensive scale) the peer referral process that doctors themselves use in determining the right specialist for any given case. Consumers have confidence in Best Doctors' referrals because of favorable attention in the media (on *60 Minutes, Today, CNN Headline News,* and *USA Today,* among many other vehicles) and because of the general perception of independence and objectivity. A competitive service rooted in managed care, insurance, government, or professional associations could never be perceived as putting the needs of consumers first.

Comprehensiveness. In the United States, the Best Doctors' database includes over 34,000 physicians in four hundred medical subspecialties and all fifty states. This in-depth information allows the company to identify the right providers in a city, a state, a region, or over the entire country, for virtually any case. Because Best Doctors surveys specialties both nationally and regionally, its database has the depth that regional payers require and the consistency that national payers require.

Accessibility. Best Doctors provides more than just a database. A simple list of superior neurosurgeons, whether in a magazine or a book, no matter how refined the methodology used to compile it, is of little help to a patient with a particular kind of brain tumor or unique set of comorbidities. Patients need help in assessing not just which doctors are best but also which doctors are *right* for their particular case. Best Doctors provides both a credible, comprehensive database and the mining services necessary to give consumers the critical information they need in a form they can use.

In a follow-up, customer satisfaction survey conducted by telephone three months' postservice,[4] 93 percent of respondents said they were "satisfied with the value of the services rendered by Best Doctors"; 83 percent said they were "satisfied with the physician services" rendered as a result of a Best Doctors' referral; 64 percent said they were "more confident about their diagnosis and treatment"; 50 percent said they had "decreased their medication intake for the diagnosis"; 65 percent said they had "a decreased dependence on the health care system"; 71 percent said they had "returned to work or increased level of daily living"; 80 percent said their "quality of health and life has improved"; and 92 percent said they would recommend Best Doctors' services to a friend or family member.

THE MARKET

Best Doctors markets its services to insurers and other intermediaries as value-added services that can be offered as a special benefit to policyholders, enrollees, employees, plan members, affinity group members, and so forth. Although any group, even an ad hoc group, can sign up to receive services, the company's marketing efforts to date have focused on issuers of supplemental insurance policies—policies that in the event of a serious medical diagnosis, put discretionary money in the hands of policyholders. Information about the right doctor allows policyholders to make the most of the monetary benefits of these policies. In the United States, supplemental insurance provides coverage for more than eighty-five million people, generating annual premiums of over $20 billion.[5] Among these supplemental policies, specified-disease (or "critical illness" or "dread disease") policies, which provide lump-sum payments upon specified diagnoses, are the fastest growing.[6] Although relatively new to the United States market, critical illness policies experienced exponential worldwide growth in the 1990s and more recently have colonized the nearby Canadian market.

Best Doctors has positioned itself to take advantage of the expected growth in these and other forms of safety-net private insurance in the next decade, as baby boomers, mistrustful of managed care, demand new solutions that provide more flexibility and better care, especially in the event of a life-threatening illness or injury. The company has already experienced this phenomenon in its business overseas where critical illness insurance products with fixed payouts supplement government-managed health systems that are perceived as inadequate because of poor care, long waits, or both.[7]

As consumers in the United States, too, move away from managed care—except for preventive, standard, low-acuity care—and toward supplementary health care benefits through private insurance for catastrophic events, the company's objective is to follow the model of travel assistance and become an information and facilitation service that is fully capitated, inexpensive, available from multiple sources, and pervasive.

THE CHALLENGES

The greatest challenge Best Doctors faces is the same challenge all consumer-driven health care services face—reaching consumers. By distancing consumers from decisions made about their health care, the third-party payer system has not only insulated consumers from the issue of doctor choice, even in critical cases, it has also prevented them from developing the habit of discernment necessary to make smart choices. Concerns of payers and concerns of patients do not always square and sometimes conflict. In surveys and interviews consumers routinely express concerns about their ability to identify and access an appropriately skilled doctor in the event of a medical crisis. Among third-party payers, information on the comparative quality of doctors is subordinated to the payers' heavy investment in networks and the discounts that are crucial to their profitability. What information does reach consumers over the competing, debased claims of "quality" tends to be either provider-sponsored (hospital referral lines) or advertising-sponsored (magazine "best" lists) and in either case superficial and unreliable.

To enlist third-party payers in offering Best Doctors' information service to consumers requires documenting savings. It is generally acknowledged, in principle, that for a complex case, genuine quality care—an experienced doctor attached to a major medical center—costs less than lower-quality care—a less experienced doctor at a lesser institution. The latter may appear cheaper in a day-to-day or procedure-to-procedure comparison, but if the total cost of care is taken into account, the better doctor at the better institution will prove a better value at a lower cost in almost every case.[8]

Unfortunately, few data are currently available to support this proposition. The comparative data that are available tend to be either institution based or procedure based. Quarterly reporting cycles discourage the kind of long-term effort required to collect comparative cost data for the totality of care in numerous cases, and even where such efforts are undertaken, they face considerable logistical challenges and privacy concerns. Doctor-to-doctor comparative data are even rarer, and their usefulness in determining the most cost-effective provider in a particular case is suspect, especially where the case is unusual or complex. At least one study has shown a correlation between doctors chosen by peer referral and successful outcomes, but the link between such doctors and lower costs has yet to be proven.

Consumer demand, pressing on several fronts, is bringing the concerns of health plans and other third-party payers more into line with the concerns of consumers in a way that will benefit Best Doctors.

- *Lawsuits for inadequate or inappropriate medical care.* Large judgments, and simply the threat of such judgments, are changing the profitability profile of network-driven referrals, especially in rare, complex, and catastrophic cases, and putting a premium on independently verified comparative information about provider quality and appropriateness.

- *Proposed government regulation.* Legislative efforts to enhance consumers' right to choose providers will enhance the value of Best Doctors' services both to consumers and to the payers that market plans to them.

- *New payment mechanisms.* Medical savings accounts and other consumer-driven health care health insurance programs will make it increasingly possible for consumers to circumvent network-driven referrals. Best Doctors' database can fill the resulting information vacuum.

- *Increasing Internet use.* Best Doctors stands to benefit from the increased use of the Internet and the resulting sense of empowerment it gives health care consumers in dealing with their health care plans. The company's unusual history and media profile put it in a unique position both to further this sense of empowerment and to satisfy the demand for information that such empowerment generates.

THE FUTURE

Consumers demand, "Will I be able to find the right doctor in a medical crisis?" and, "Will I be able to access that doctor?" This search for protection and peace of mind is putting pressure on defined benefit plans and spurring the development of insurance mechanisms, both health and nonhealth, that put medical care purchasing decisions in the hands of consumers. The more responsibility consumers have for these decisions, the more they want information to help them make smart decisions.

The combination of discretionary health care dollars and the information to use them wisely will change not only how critical care is marketed in the United States but also how it is delivered. Government's primary role (other than imposing fairness and consistency through regulation) will be to ensure that those who have no health insurance, as well as those insured by the government, are not left behind by this consumer revolution in health care. By encouraging private as well as public insurance solutions that give fixed payouts to individuals who cannot afford first-dollar health insurance for serious illness, the government would not only allow Best Doctors to reach a much broader market by attaching its services to those policies, it would also help relieve the financial drain on hospitals from treating the chronically uninsured.

As more consumers use Best Doctors' services, more complex and catastrophic cases will find their way to the doctors best able to treat them. The referral routes that kept a steady stream of complex cases flowing to the major academic medical centers in the United States, a flow that has been interrupted by network-driven referrals, will be reopened. The hardest cases will get to the best doctors—the doctors who have treated similar cases most often.

Best Doctors believes that the result will be not only better outcomes and lower costs but also better allocation of complex cases to the centers that have developed programs specifically designed to treat them. Without this rational allocation of hard cases and the specialization that results, programs that train succeeding generations of specialists and advance the science of a specialty can never thrive.

Notes

1. See, for example, Wolfe, S., and others. *16,638 Questionable Doctors.* Washington, D.C.: Public Citizen's Health Research Group, 1998; Armstrong, D. "Background Profiles on Massachusetts Physicians Available on Internet," *Boston Globe*, May 1, 1997, p. B2; Kennedy, J. "Law Won't Let State's Doctors Hide Mistakes." *Orlando Sentinel*, May 31, 1997, p. A1.

2. For example, D. Armstrong, "Physician Profiles Faulted" (*Boston Globe*, Apr. 27, 1997, p. A1) reported that the Massachusetts Medical Board's Physician Profile Service is extremely popular among Massachusetts residents, although the writer also reported that the profiles may be dangerous because of missing or misleading information. According to D. Armstrong, "Background Profiles on Massachusetts Physicians Available on Internet" (*Boston Globe*, May 1, 1997, p. B2), the service received 50,000 physician profile requests by telephone between November 1996 and May 1997. See also, McKinnon, J. D. "Consumer Guide to Doctors Isn't All It Was Going to Be." *Wall Street Journal*, Apr. 2, 1997, p. F1.

3. For a sampling of such lists in books and articles, see Castle, J., and Connelly, J. *America's Top Doctors.* New York: Connelly Medical Ltd., 2001; Castle, J., and Connelly, J. *Castle Connolly Guide: New York Metro Area.* New York: Connolly Medical Ltd., 1999; Castle, J., and Connelly, J. *Castle Connolly Guide: Metropolitan Chicago.* New York: Connelly Medical Ltd., 1999; Center for the Study of Services. "The Doctors in South Florida." *Miami Metro Magazine*, Oct. 1998; Center for the

Study of Services. "Top Docs." *Phoenix Magazine,* Apr. 1999; Center for the Study of Services. "Top Docs." *Atlanta Magazine,* May 1999; Tanne, J. "The Doctors in America." *American Health,* Mar. 1996. Best Doctors has registered the trademarks Best Doctors® and The Best Doctors in America.®

4. This survey was conducted in the last quarter of 1998 and the first quarter of 1999, covering patients to whom services were provided in the third and fourth quarters of 1998, respectively. Percentages apply only to respondents; 29 percent of candidates for study were classified "lost to follow-up."

5. Health Insurance Association of America. *Supplemental Health Insurance.* Washington, D.C.: Health Insurance Association of America, 1998, p. 4.

6. Jernstadt, L. "Critical Diagnosis Coverage: Security for the Terminally Ill." *Contingencies* (American Academy of Actuaries), May–June 1997. Jernstadt comments, "Since critical diagnosis insurance was introduced in Europe and Asia, the policies have generated astonishing sales figures" (p. 18).

7. See, for example, for Switzerland, Defeever, C. *Fact Magazine,* Feb. 1, 1997; for Germany, "New Doctor's List of Focus." *Focus Magazine,* Mar. 9, 1997; for Austria, "How You Test Your Doctor." *News Magazine,* July 16, 1998; for Canada, Priest, L. "U.S. Publisher Rates Canada's Best Doctors." *Toronto Star,* Feb. 20, 1999, p. A1; and for Turkey, *Milliyet,* Apr. 13, 1999, center page.

8. In addition to producing direct cost savings, guiding high-acuity cases to the appropriate care generates indirect savings from (1) fewer long-term unresolved medical treatment plans, (2) fewer inappropriate or even harmful treatments, (3) fewer complications, (4) fewer and shorter hospital stays, (5) faster return to work, (6) diminished absenteeism and turnover, (7) diminished frequency and severity of disability claims, (8) fewer and diminished malpractice and other legal claims, and (9) fewer life insurance claims. By way of example, more than 25 percent of the recommendations for back surgery reviewed as part of a Best Doctors service were not confirmed.

CHAPTER FORTY-ONE

The Half-Billion Dollar Impact of Information About Quality

Becky J. Cherney

Nothing is quite as essential or as elusive as information about the quality of health care. It is easier for a consumer to learn about a copay than to determine the appropriateness of an appendectomy. Consumers receive cursory information about the physicians who are in their managed care networks through their directory. But no information exists about which doctors achieve the best outcomes. As a result, patients know more about, say, erectile dysfunction, due to direct-to-consumer advertising, than about the outcomes of doctors who treat prostate cancer.

THE SEARCH FOR QUALITY

When the Central Florida Health Care Coalition,[1] of which I am president and CEO, was founded in 1984, then-popular buzzwords were incorporated into its mission statement: "To seek the highest quality health care at the lowest possible price and educate health care consumers." Although the businesspeople who founded the organization were familiar with terms such as *zero defects* and *white glove customer service*, they quickly learned that these terms were not understood or embraced by the health care industry.

What Are We Buying?

The coalition's employer members spent their initial year trying to find out just what they were buying with their health care dollars. Determining the flow of dollars was the easy part. Claims analysis pointed out where their health care dollars went—so much for inpatient care, ambulatory care, outpatient care, pharmacy charges, and costs such as home health and emergency room care. Small-area analysis identified trends in usage and identified special needs populations. But there was no information to determine the appropriateness, effectiveness, or efficiency of the care. There was a vacuum in the area of clinical quality.

The Trust Walk

Employers knew they could not continue to provide health care to employees if the costs continued to grow at double-digit rates. Their profits were not keeping pace. But no one was responsible for moving the community health agenda forward. Political agendas were determining how managed care developed. Hospitals were focused on market share. Physicians were wary of managed care. Coalition members realized they could not reform an industry to which they did not talk. These employers began to meet with key physician groups, hospitals, emerging managed care plans, and hospital administrators. These early meetings typically revolved around a set of questions and accompanying data that the coalition had abstracted from claim forms and uniform billing statements.

At a meeting with obstetricians, for example, the data indicated the cesarean section rate was three times higher on Friday. Why? After several minutes of silence, one doctor described this scenario: The patient who is nine and a half months pregnant arrives for her 4:30 appointment on Friday. Upon examination, she begins to dilate. The doctor has been called to the hospital every night that week and has never managed to get more than four hours of sleep at one time for the entire week. The doctor is exhausted and really hopes to keep a tee time the next morning to compensate for working a sixty-hour week. The patient is absolutely weary and tired of being pregnant. When the doctor suggests a C-section, they both agree. The physicians in the room nodded in agreement with this scenario. They stated that this happened to each of them only once or twice a year, and they had not known the impact such decisions had. From that day forward, C-section rates have declined, and now they are not any higher on Friday than on any other day of the week.

The lesson was powerful; information is the key to change.

Similarly, hospital administrators were asked why x rays that had been done in other settings were always repeated when the patient was admitted to the hospital. The response was that the hospital's malpractice insurance required it to do the tests on its own equipment because that equipment was inspected regularly to ensure proper operation. Employers with zero-defect programs were quick to realize that the answer was to require the same inspections for everyone using x-ray equipment. Duplicate x rays were eliminated.

Meetings like these picked the "low-hanging fruit" and were critical to progress. The participants understood that their goals were not mutually exclusive. Everyone wanted the best health care for the community. The trust that was built allowed the health care quality agenda to move forward.

The data made some things obvious. The health care professionals could not explain the wide variations in treatment. Employers still did not know what their health care dollar was buying. And employees were never going to be empowered to be true health care consumers without better information. It was important to demystify the delivery of health care.

The Golden Rule

The coalition adopted its own version of the Golden Rule: He who has the gold makes the rules! Faced with double-digit cost increases, the shift to commercial payers of the losses providers sustained from Medicare's inadequate reimbursements, and a near void in actionable information on health care quality, the coalition recognized that more had to be done. With so much of the health care dollar spent on inpatient care, the hospital was a good place to start. Hospital administrators were businesspeople (rather than clinicians) and were perceived as less intimidating by the employers. As the principal payers for health care, the employers decided they had both the right and the responsibility to take the lead in improving it.

COMBINING INFORMATION TECHNOLOGY AND EVIDENCE-BASED MEDICINE

A major problem the coalition encountered in getting started was that costs for hospitalizations were not comparable. When any physician was asked why his or her charges varied compared to those of a fellow physician, the answer was the same, "My patients were sicker." W. Edwards Deming, the guru of quality, always said, "If you cannot measure it, you cannot manage it." However, the few measurement systems found in the hospital setting came from claim forms and other billing systems that were designed for financial measurement, not quality of care. The coalition set out to change this situation.

Rule Number One: Measure

After studying measurement systems for a year, the coalition asked the area hospitals to install a Mediqual Corporation product known as Atlas, a computer-based system that measures quality of care.[2] Clinical information is abstracted directly from the patient's record. Then, using algorithms to adjust for severity, the system measures the patient's response to treatment. It allows the user to drill down and look at all components of care. A procedure validation process ascertains whether care falls within accepted processes. The system also uses the data to determine the appropriateness of procedures. When a financial model is used to measure care, typically the focus is on the total cost of a hospitalization, with so-called discounts being the driver. The availability of an appropriateness measure was key to the coalition's selection of Atlas, because coalition members knew that a 75 percent discount on an unnecessary hysterectomy was still not a good deal for anyone. Atlas also looks at the efficiency of care. What did it cost to deliver care to the patient?

Atlas has a national database that allows a hospital to compare its performance to that of other hospitals. One of the greatest benefits derived from this measurement system is the physician profile. It allows the doctors to see how they are performing and to compare their performance to that of their peers. You will not find doctors who have gone to medical school planning to practice bad medicine. Physicians are smart, competitive, and committed to providing good care. But they do not always receive good information to improve the care they give. With the rapid changes in technology, pharmaceutical products, and other areas of medicine, it is virtually impossible for many physicians to keep pace.

Rule Number Two: Persist

Having found a good measurement tool, the coalition asked area hospitals to install the Atlas system to facilitate community-wide measurement. The hospitals refused, stating that it would add costs and might impair their relationship with doctors. Coalition members, the purchasers of health care, were very discouraged by that attitude. They questioned why any hospital would not want to spend less than a thousandth of a percent per discharge on quality when the beleaguered auto industry was committed to spending about 5 percent of the cost of an automobile on quality. Surely our health must be as important as an automobile!

A breakthrough finally occurred when, after a year, a major hospital system experienced an 18 percent cost increase, yet its primary competitor had only a 9 percent increase. Searching for some answers, the costly hospital decided to respond to the employers' request and use Atlas. That decision forever changed the health care system in central Florida. After a year on the system and an aggressive quality improvement campaign, the hospital's costs were significantly lower than those of its competitor. The competitor decided that it would also use the Atlas system.

Seventeen of the twenty-two central Florida hospitals now track the major diagnosis-related categories with Atlas. Hospitals who have used the system intensively report they recovered their return on investment in about ninety days. Coalition board members meet with doctors from each hospital semian-nually to learn about the progress the hospitals are making and to identify fur-ther areas to be studied.

Empirical Data Document Success

Physicians are unlikely to respond to any information unless they agree that it is evidence-based medicine. The ability to look at their own data as well as other hospitals' data fostered confidence in the applicability of information derived from Atlas. Knowing the purchasers were going to push the quality agenda heightened the importance of cooperating. Because of the purchasing clout of the employers, hospitals and physicians recognized the need to work with them.

Coalition and hospital records indicate that the inpatient quality initiative has saved the community over half a billion dollars in the last seven years. Those savings come from quality improvements—not discounts, cost shifting, or reduc-tions in access. The cesarean section rate for one major system, for example, was 32 percent when the quality initiative began. For 2000, it was 18 percent; the national average is 22 percent.

Many studies have shown that a physician's performance is closely linked to the year of graduation from medical school. That is very evident in this process. Drilling down on coronary artery bypass graft (CABG) surgery data provides an example. Reviews of the use of arterial blood gas tests and x rays revealed that physicians who had been out of school for several years ordered up to five times more of these tests than the newer graduates, without any difference in the out-comes. Many doctors who had completed their residency five years prior had been taught to do some of these tests daily while a patient was hospitalized. They were unaware of more recent research conclusions that it was not neces-sary to continue these tests while the patient was in the hospital unless there was some change in the patient's status. One major hospital system studied its prostate surgery procedures because they were falling outside Atlas appropri-ateness guidelines. The review indicated that some physicians were not aware of several new pharmaceutical interventions that could be tried before resorting to surgery. With this information, the rate for transurethral resection of the prostate (TURP) was reduced by 23 percent.

The sixteen most utilized or costly procedures are the focus of the measure-ments. All hospitals participating in the inpatient quality initiative are continu-ing to track those sixteen procedures, but the physicians and hospitals have expanded the initiative and are now also looking at major areas outside the focus procedures. And the commitment to continuous quality improvement has extended to everyone in the hospital system, not only administrators and doctors. Outcomes have improved dramatically. Costs are down. Charges are down. Length of stay has declined in all areas. But quality has continued to improve.

Rule Number Three: Police Thyself

The hospitals determine how they want to use the Atlas information. In addition to comparing their data to others' data, they provide information to each physician; however, the method of communicating the information varies by hospital. Some have quality assurance staff deliver the reports, others use risk management personnel, and in one large system, the top seven administrators divide the profiles of the top two hundred admitting doctors among them and deliver the profiles in person.

For the hospital's review, physician profiles are ranked from those with the best outcomes to those with the worst outcomes. The national average can be applied to identify anyone performing below that average. The hospitals' internal processes address doctors performing below the national average. Usually a mentor is assigned to help each doctor identify the issues and establish a remedial plan. Although remediation is usually achieved, in the instances when it has not been, the hospitals have asked underperforming physicians to leave the hospital staff because they were putting the coalition business at risk.

Lower malpractice premiums are yet another benefit of the system. A physician profiled by Atlas can supply the insurer with several years of practice patterns. If the physician is sued for malpractice, and it is sad to say that in these litigious times, nearly all of them will be if they practice long enough, this profile information is an excellent defense. The malpractice insurance carrier usually must spend considerable time and money to create a doctor's defense. Because they can provide good historical data for a defense, many central Florida physicians and hospitals using Atlas have successfully negotiated lower malpractice premiums.

The Conclusion and Payoff

Quality is king.

Discounts do not treat patients nor do they provide information to help improve care.

Long-term thinking recognizes that changing the delivery of care has lasting benefits. Those changes provide improvements for the entire community.

The inpatient quality initiative is successful because it is physician driven. Physicians are responsible for admitting and discharging patients. Any measurement system whose purpose is to improve care must be physician driven.

Referral patterns have emerged around the information generated from Atlas. Hospitals can generate lists of physicians by outcomes. Doctors pay attention to who is "best in class."

The Central Florida Health Care Coalition continues to work in partnership with the doctors and hospitals to advance the quality agenda for inpatients. The day is near when all the partners will agree to publish the data so health care consumers can use these objective, empirical data in making health care decisions.

ON TO OUTPATIENT QUALITY

The next frontier is outpatient care. The coalition is now creating outpatient profiles for physicians. Primary care physicians, pediatricians, and several other specialists do not admit many patients to hospitals but they provide care. They need data on their performance in their office setting.

Multiple office settings, multiple specialties, and lack of common computer systems complicate the task. The coalition contracted with MEDecision[3] to use its Practice Review System to create these profiles. Claims for two large employers allowed analysis of over 148,000 episodes of care that cost over $95 million.

The coalition used the data to answer the following questions: Why did employees go to the doctor? What are the most expensive episodes of care? When costs are aggregated, where are the most dollars spent? What are the areas of opportunity, in which education and prevention can be leveraged? Who are the specialists who treat these areas of opportunities? As a result, ten diagnoses became the focus for the outpatient quality initiative: upper respiratory infection, sinusitis, hypertension, lipid and cholesterol disease, abdominal pain, chest pain, lower back pain, diabetes, asthma, and ischemic heart disease and angina. The physician specialists being profiled in the initial phase of the study work in family practice, internal medicine, gastroenterology, cardiology, and obstetrics and gynecology.

Each physician profile shows the number of episodes of care provided for each focused diagnosis, the physician's cost per episode compared to other specialists' costs, and the average network cost. That information can be compared to best practices from evidence-based medicine. Then the profile drills down to show diagnostic tests used per episode compared to the specialists and network averages. Finally, it compares pharmaceutical usage for the physician, other specialists, and network physicians.

The physician now has a template for change. Taking vast databases and extracting actionable information is key. Once that information demonstrates how best outcomes are being achieved, change is inevitable.

PATIENT SATISFACTION

Employers who spend millions of dollars providing health care for their employees need to know how the employees feel about the care their physician provides. Patients who trust their physician are far more likely to comply with the care instructions the doctor gives.

First, the coalition conducted the Consumer Assessment of Health Plans (CAHPS)[4] for three years. That survey did not provide actionable information for the coalition to give to doctors so they could improve their care. And plan-level information was not useful for consumers trying to decide which doctors to use. So, in 2001, the coalition fielded a new study, the Consumer Assessment of Physicians Survey (CAPS). Physicians' patients completed twenty-eight questions about their experiences, including access, care, wellness, and satisfaction. Each physician then received a summary of responses, allowing him or her to determine where patient care should be improved.

Health care does not cost . . . much—until it is used! The coalition will be able to provide consumers with information on physicians' clinical outcomes and patient satisfaction. This information will empower health care consumers to make evidence-based purchasing decisions. The next level of competition for health care providers will be service.

Notes

1. The Central Florida Health Care Coalition (CFHCC) was founded in 1984 by Becky Cherney, then director of human resources for Tupperware International, when she organized the area's ten largest employers to examine rising health care costs. Because fifty-seven cents of each health care dollar was being spent on inpatient care, the coalition used its clout to convince hospitals to install a quality measurement system. In 1989, thirteen area hospitals began using Atlas to measure inpatient quality; today seventeen hospitals use the system. The coalition also uses MEDecision's Physician Profile System to measure a physician's practice in the office setting. Identifying and communicating best outcomes has saved over $500 million as a result of improved quality. The coalition now has 135 members and represents more than one million lives. CFHCC's Quality Initiative has been featured on *World News with Peter Jennings,* on *20/20,* and in the *New York Times.* In 1998, members of the Health Industries Research Council voted the coalition first in the nation in working to improve the health of its members. The coalition is a rollout site for the Leapfrog Group patient safety initiative and a member of the National Business Coalitions on Health and the National Quality Forum.

2. Atlas is a computer-based information system that measures the quality of inpatient care. With over 400 hospitals in its database, it allows hospitals to compare their care internally and externally. For more information, see the Cardinal Information Corporation's Web site [www.cicinfo.com].

3. MEDecision is a data management and analysis company whose proprietary product, Practice Review System, creates a database that allows the user to review all data involved in health care treatment given in the physician's office setting. Users can compare and contrast multiple facets of care including testing, pharmaceutical use, charges, and outcomes. For more information, see the company's Web site [www.MEDecision.com].

4. The Consumer Assessment of Health Plans (CAHPS), which measures patients' satisfaction with their health care, was developed by the Harvard Medical School, Rand Corporation, and Research Triangle Institute, with funding from the Agency for Health Care Policy and Research.

CHAPTER FORTY-TWO

Buyers Health Care Action Group

Consumer Perceptions of Quality Differences

Katherine M. Harris, Roger Feldman,
Jennifer S. Schultz, Jon Christianson

In this chapter we evaluate the success of the Buyers Health Care Action Group (BHCAG) in promoting quality-based competition among local health care providers. BHCAG is a coalition of roughly two dozen self-insured employers in the Minneapolis-St. Paul, Minnesota, area who have created a unique competitive bidding system designed to provide local service delivery organizations with the incentive to compete on the basis of premium cost and quality through risk-adjusted payments, standardized benefits, and the dissemination of quality information to employees.

Economic theory suggests that consumers must perceive and be willing to pay for quality differences if producers of high-quality medical care are to remain in the market.[1] The BHCAG program increases in two ways the likelihood that employees of member firms will differentiate among benefit options on the basis of quality. First, the program increases incentives for individual medical providers contracting with BHCAG to engage in activities that improve outcomes and service quality. Second, unlike typical health plan report cards that aggregate measures of quality across provider groups affiliated with a health plan, BHCAG provides performance measures that allow employees to assess the variation in quality among provider groups.

This work was supported by the Robert Wood Johnson Foundation and, for Katherine Harris, by a National Research Service Award (T32-HS00046) from the Agency for Health Care Policy and Research. The authors would also like to acknowledge helpful comments from Jayanta Bhattacharya, Steven Garber, and Regina Herzlinger.

Efforts to evaluate the success of BHCAG in differentiating its benefit options on the basis of quality are hampered by practical difficulties in measuring provider quality from the consumer's perspective. To address this problem, we adapt an approach developed in the marketing research literature on brand choice—*market mapping*.[2] The idea behind market mapping is that given a measure of attribute importance, the analyst can learn consumers' perceptions of that attribute by observing choices. The more importance a decision maker places on a particular attribute, the more the decision maker will prefer the alternative that is perceived as offering more of that attribute.

We estimate the model with data from a 1998 survey of employees of BHCAG firms. The survey collected information about the health benefit choices of employees and about the importance that employees placed on a number of benefit features in choosing health coverage. We combine these two types of information to estimate parameters representing perceived premium and quality differences across coverage alternatives. We measure the success of the BHCAG system in differentiating providers on the basis of quality and cost by testing whether perceived differences in quality of care, service quality, and premiums influence employees' choices. We validate our approach by comparing estimated perceived premium differences and actual premium differences.

The remainder of the chapter is organized as follows. In the first section, we describe the goals and structure of the BHCAG program and the competitive bidding strategies it uses to control cost and improve the quality of health care services. In the following two sections, we present our empirical results. The last section discusses the implications of our findings for competitive bidding.

BACKGROUND

Increasingly, large health care purchasers use competitive bidding strategies to control costs and improve quality. (Competitive bidding also forms the basis of some Medicare reform proposals.) Two of the longest-running programs are administered by the State of Minnesota for its employees and by the Office of Personnel Management for civilian employees of the federal government. The Minnesota program offers a choice of health plans and pays no more than the premium of the low-cost single coverage plan (or 90 percent of the low-cost family coverage premium). This approach has created price-conscious choice among state employees.[3]

The Federal Employees Health Benefits Program (FEHB) has been suggested as a model for Medicare reform. Proponents of the FEHB model cite low administrative costs and the program's ability to control care costs while providing a broad range of choices for covered employees. However, critics have disputed the evidence on cost control and claim that the indemnity plans in FEHB suffer from severe adverse selection. In reevaluating the FEHB's success in controlling costs, we found that the FEHB has outperformed private insurance programs and Medicare.[4] The program could have performed even better if it had used a level-dollar contribution to premiums. Also, we concluded that the FEHB has suffered some selection problems but not enough to prevent it from offering a wide variety of choices, without standardized benefits or direct risk adjustment.

Competitive bidding systems share several elements: (1) consumers choose among competing care providers; (2) consumers bear the incremental cost of richer benefits and of higher-quality care; (3) purchasers collect and disseminate cost, coverage, and quality information to facilitate comparison among alternatives; (4) choice is limited to annual open enrollments to reduce adverse selection and administrative costs; and (5) providers submit bids based on a standard set of benefits or on minimum standards established in advance by purchasers.

In theory such systems reduce costly inefficiencies in care processes while preserving providers' incentives to maintain and improve health outcomes.[5] Success in achieving these goals depends on the willingness of health plans to compete on the basis of cost and quality and likewise on the ability of consumers to make informed choices among alternative plans on the same criteria. Competitive bidding systems have been credited with slowing the growth of their sponsors' health care expenditures.[6] Nonetheless, as they currently exist, these systems do not address the barriers to aggressive quality competition created by the organization of plans around loosely affiliated groups of physicians and service delivery organizations.

Health plans provide access to a fixed set of providers, often called a *network,* for a predetermined premium and cost sharing in the form of coinsurance and copays. There is a great deal of uncertainty surrounding the quality of network providers. Consumers can reduce this uncertainty to some extent by establishing a relationship with a trusted provider and choosing a plan with which the provider is affiliated. However, accidents and other unexpected illnesses by their nature necessitate encounters with unfamiliar providers. Recent efforts to provide consumers with information about plan quality in the form of report cards are also limited. So far these efforts have focused almost exclusively on nontechnical aspects of care, such as access and interpersonal skills of providers.[7] Moreover, report cards provide average measures of plan performance and convey no information about the distributions surrounding these averages.

Akerlof predicts that if consumers are unable to observe quality differences directly, they will be unwilling to pay more for a good than the price of a good of average quality.[8] Akerlof uses the used-car market to illustrate this point. High-quality used cars cannot command higher prices because consumers cannot differentiate among cars of different quality at the time of purchase. Because higher-quality used cars cannot command higher prices, over time high-quality providers may exit the market, further lowering average price and quality. Economic theory also predicts that producers of high-quality goods will react by engaging in activities that serve as *signals* about underlying quality in order to avert the downward spiral in price and quality described by Akerlof. Educational attainment is a well-cited example of a signal to potential employers of the underlying ability of job seekers.[9] Warranties offered by producers of consumer durables are another well-known example. Hospitals signal quality through staff credentials, staff-to-patient ratios, and specialized clinical services.[10] In principle, health plans in conjunction with participants in their provider networks could signal quality by engaging in activities shown to improve the probabilities of good outcomes of care and patient satisfaction.[11]

There are several disincentives to this type of signaling activity. First, fixed payments based on average costs of care do not compensate network providers for the additional cost of quality improvement activities or for the additional cost of caring for enrollees in poorer than average health status who may be disproportionately attracted as a result of the activities. Second, the many providers who often affiliate with multiple health plans make it difficult for any one plan to internalize the benefits of encouraging network providers to engage in quality improvement.

In a unique effort to overcome this barrier to quality-based competition, the Buyers Health Care Action Group offers a health plan called Choice Plus to employees of its member firms.[12] Instead of soliciting bids from health plans that in turn subcontract with network providers, BHCAG solicits bids directly from service delivery organizations. This method of contracting compensates providers for quality improvement activities to the extent that enrollees recognize their value and are willing to pay higher premiums.

The program consists of fifteen *care systems* in the Minneapolis-St. Paul area, each composed of a group of primary care providers and affiliated specialists and hospitals. Primary care physicians may participate in no more than one care system. Once a year, care systems submit bids, or *claims targets,* based on an average enrollee's cost for a standard package of benefits, and are placed into one of three premium groups, or *tiers,* on this basis. (In 1997, for example, there were three care systems in the high-cost tier, eight in the middle-cost tier, and four in the low-cost tier.) Once employees select care systems the claims target is adjusted on the basis of their demographic characteristics and existing diagnoses, so that payments to providers reflect the health risks of the actual enrollees.[13] Care systems are reimbursed for services by a fee schedule that is adjusted quarterly to reflect the care system's performance relative to the adjusted claims target. If the care system exceeds its target, fees are lowered. BHCAG contracts with an outside vendor for administrative services, such as enrollment, claims processing and member services, case management services, and out-of-area care.

From the perspective of employees with single coverage, the Choice Plus program resembles a choice among three point-of-service plans that are differentiated by their prices. Each of these three has a provider network composed of subsets of the fifteen care systems participating in the Choice Plus program.[14] Each employee must choose a cost tier and a primary care clinic belonging exclusively to one care system. As long as the employee uses providers associated with the chosen care system and follows rules governing referral to specialists, care is considered *in-network* and the employee pays the lowest level of cost sharing. *Out-of-network* care requires higher cost sharing. Employees may switch care systems once per month, but to reduce the potential for adverse selection, they may switch only to a care system in the same or a lower tier. If employees switch to a care system in a lower-cost tier, they continue to pay the higher premium of the tier they originally chose. Employees may switch cost tiers once per year, during an annual open enrollment period.

BHCAG facilitates comparison among cost tiers and care systems in two ways. First, standard benefits reduce the dimensions on which employees compare tiers. Second, BHCAG collects consumer satisfaction information and disseminates the survey results in the form of report cards to employees prior to open enrollment. Because scores are reported at the level of the individual care system, consumers are able to examine the distributions of scores within each cost tier. Each care system receives between one and three stars for each of twelve nontechnical dimensions of satisfaction with quality of care and service quality. (Results are reported separately for adults and children and for clinics in and out of the Minneapolis-St. Paul metropolitan area.) One star means the care system scored below average, two stars that it scored similar to the average, and three stars that it scored above average. A casual reading of the 1997 performance measures suggests that care systems in the high-cost tier only modestly outperform those in the two other tiers. For most dimensions, the care systems in the high-cost tier received proportionately more three star ratings than the middle- and low-cost tiers. However, the low-cost tier outperformed the high-cost tier on two measures of satisfaction with convenience.

In assessing the success of the Choice Plus system in distinguishing care systems on the basis of quality, we want to understand how consumers perceive quality in each system and how these perceptions influence choice. In doing this we face the challenge of measuring quality from the perspective of consumers. Unfortunately, readily available quality measures are not appropriate for inclusion in choice models. One option might be to use the performance information contained in the BHCAG report card as a proxy for perceived quality. However, a number of studies suggest that such report cards are only one source of information consumers use in choosing health care providers and are not particularly influential.[15] Studies of BHCAG member employees have found that even though employees mention using employer-provided information more often than any other source of information, only 47 percent of single employees saw the report card during the 1998 open enrollment period.[16]

Another alternative is to use individual satisfaction ratings in a care system choice model. Despite the wide availability of satisfaction information, the endogeneity between satisfaction ratings and choice of care system makes such data inappropriate for drawing inferences about the effect of perceived quality on choices with cross-sectional data. Even if satisfaction data could be collected prior to the observed choice opportunity, these data would not be appropriate because they refer only to the currently selected alternative in a decision maker's choice set. The perceived quality of the other alternatives remains unobserved.

In our study we solve this problem by treating otherwise unobservable features as choice model parameters representing perceived quality differences across care systems.

DATA SOURCE

The data used in our analysis come from a telephone survey of randomly selected employees of BHCAG member firms. The survey was part of a broader study of BHCAG funded by the Robert Wood Johnson Foundation. It was conducted in early 1998, shortly after the member firms' second annual open enrollment period under the Choice Plus program. During the second year of the program, most BHCAG firms eliminated non–Choice Plus options and established level-dollar contributions based on the low-cost tier premium. The nineteen firms selected for inclusion in the study had full or a very high percentage of enrollment in Choice Plus. If these firms offered another plan, it was a traditional indemnity plan rather than a managed care plan. This reduced the chance that the additional plan was a close substitute for Choice Plus in the eyes of employees.[17]

The telephone survey collected demographic and health status information as well as information about the importance of premiums and various aspects of quality of care and service quality. Bivariate comparisons reveal no statistically significant differences in decision-maker characteristics across the three cost tiers. Nonetheless, several patterns are apparent. Compared to enrollees in the low- and middle-cost tiers, enrollees in the high-cost tier have higher mean incomes, are older, are more likely to have attended graduate school, and have spent the least time with their current employer. Enrollees in the high-cost tier also place more importance on quality of care, convenient hours and location, and short waiting times for appointments with specialists. Enrollees in the high-cost tier place the least importance on low premiums.[18]

RESULTS

We find that consumers do not perceive differences across care systems in quality, convenience, or other subjective attributes. However, they do perceive differences in the number of physicians and in distance to clinics and are strongly attracted to those care system attributes.[19] It is reasonable to think that care systems with providers who have a reputation of providing high quality of care to people in poor health status would attract a disproportionate number of people with chronic health conditions and older people who are at greater risk of using services. But possibly because of the financial protection of a risk-adjusted payment system, there seems to be no evidence of differential selection of health risks across care systems.

Overall, the results suggest either that there were not substantively large differences across care systems in the unobserved attributes for which the personal characteristics are intended to control or that individual preferences for these attributes (however large the differences across care systems) did not differ substantially across decision makers.

To determine whether consumers perceive differences in quality, we analyze the relationship between consumers' stated importance weights for quality and their actual choices. If consumers with high importance weights gravitate toward certain care systems, then we will infer that those care systems have the highest perceived quality.

Our model implies that care systems are not differentiated on the basis of quality. To determine what distinguishes care systems if it is not perceived quality, we use number of physicians and distance to clinics as objective measures of convenience and quality to estimate a care system selection model. Distance is measured in kilometers from the zip code centroid for the individual's residence to each clinic. We found that individuals are more likely to choose systems with more physicians and those that contain clinics closer to their homes.[20]

In terms of choosing care systems in different cost tiers, in addition to the premium importance and firm interaction variables, years in the Twin Cities, job tenure, importance of access to specialists, and importance of short wait times for appointments are all statistically significant. Individuals who rated access to specialists and short waiting times for appointments as important were less likely to choose the middle-cost tier. The estimated parameters for age and chronic conditions are not statistically significant, thus there is no evidence of differential selection of health risks across the two tiers. The intercept term indicates a preference for care systems in the middle-cost tier, other things being equal. Nevertheless, on average decision makers perceive the quality of care given by middle-cost tier providers to be lower than that given in the high-cost tier. This result seems obvious, but it is also heartening. There has been long-standing concern in the health economics and health policy literature that consumers do not understand the structure and relative cost of health benefit options.[21] Consumers perceive the middle-cost tier as having lower premiums than the high-cost tier. In other words, consumer perceptions of premium differences appear consistent with reality.

When we add attribute importance information relating to two aspects of service quality—convenience of hours and location and waiting time for appointments to specialists—the addition improves the model fit. The results suggest that decision makers perceive shorter waits for appointments in the high-cost tier and do not discern convenience differences across tiers. However, the coefficient on quality of care is no longer significant. The reduction in the quality of care coefficient is consistent with the idea that decision makers perceive quality of care and appointment waits for specialists as positively correlated. However, our data do not reveal the source of this positive correlation.

Finally, we examine the effect of controlling for personal characteristics on the perceptual parameters by comparing a cost-tier choice equation with only importance attributes and a constant to one with both importance attributes and personal characteristics. If perceptions of the unobserved attributes are correlated with personal characteristics, we should see changes in the perceptual parameter estimates with the addition of data on personal characteristics. Overall, this comparison suggests that there are not large differences in perceptions of the unobserved attributes related to measured personal characteristics. This finding is consistent with national survey data suggesting that people with health problems and their healthier counterparts do not have different perceptions of changes in quality and access to care.[22]

CONCLUSION

In this chapter we describe an innovative modeling approach we used to evaluate the success of the Minneapolis-St. Paul–area Buyers Health Care Action Group in promoting quality-based competition among local health care providers. The BHCAG program increases the likelihood that employees will differentiate among benefit options on the basis of quality by providing incentives for individual service providers contracting with BHCAG to engage in activities that improve outcomes and service quality and by providing employees with disaggregated performance measures. However, efforts to evaluate the success of BHCAG in differentiating benefit options on the basis of quality are hampered by practical difficulties in measuring provider quality from the consumer's perspective. To address this problem, we treat otherwise unobserved attributes as choice model parameters interpreted as perceived differences in the unobserved attributes across alternatives.

In the care system choice models we find that consumers perceive differences among care systems in the number of physicians and distance to each clinic but do not see differences among care systems in subjective measures of quality of care, convenience, access to specialists, and waiting times. In the cost choice framework we find that consumers perceive differences across benefit options in access to specialists and the waiting time for appointments but perceive no differences in convenience and quality of care. Measured characteristics of individuals do not appear to influence tier choice or care system selection. This is possibly because the risk-adjusted payment system reduces the financial risk to providers of differentiating themselves by providing care that appeals to particular segments of the market.

Our findings suggest that in 1998, the Choice Plus program had not succeeded in differentiating care systems on the basis of quality. How could this have happened? One possible explanation is the ease with which consumers may switch to care systems in the same or lower-cost tiers. The opportunity to switch once per month may lessen consumers' incentives to search for high-quality care systems.

Additionally, the requirement that primary care physicians may belong to only one care system appears to have been weakened by BHCAG's decision to accept any willing care system into the program. More than any other program feature, the single-contracting requirement was opposed by physicians.[23] BHCAG insisted on this requirement to facilitate comparisons among care systems and to reward high-quality providers with more patients. However, by opening the program to any care system that wishes to participate, BHCAG has allowed 95 percent of the primary care physicians in the Twin Cities to participate in Choice Plus. This degree of inclusion may weaken the providers' incentives to compete for patients by improving quality.

It is also unfortunate that the performance measures reported by BHCAG do not allow consumers to compare technical quality of care across systems. Instead, the report card presents measures of consumer satisfaction with quality. Given the way that the information is presented, it is possible that consumers do not have any basis for judging quality differences among care systems from this source. In addition, although our research shows that most employees use some information from the employer, only about half reported seeing the performance results book during the past open enrollment.

Finally, we have a word of caution about our methods. Because of the limited sample size, we focused the analysis on the six largest care systems reported in the survey. It is possible that these popular systems were perceived to have roughly similar quality but were viewed as superior to the less-popular systems.

Despite its inability to create discernable quality differences, BHCAG has been successful in implementing a central tenet of competitive bidding models— consumers are aware of premium differences among competing care systems.

Furthermore, they gravitate toward systems that are closer to their residences and that have more physicians. It is not unreasonable for consumers to value these features of health care choices.

Notes

1. Akerlof, G. "The Market For 'Lemons': Quality Uncertainty and the Market Mechanism." *Quarterly Journal of Economics,* 1970, *84*(3), 488–500.

2. Erdem, T. "A Dynamic Analysis of Market Share Based on Panel Data." *Marketing Science,* 1996, *15*(4), 359–378; Elrod, T., and Keane, M. "A Factor Analytic Probit Model for Representing Market Structure in Panel Data." *Journal of Marketing Research,* 1995, *32*(1), 1–16; Elrod, T. "Choice Map: Inferring a Product Map from Panel Data." *Marketing Science,* 1998, *7*(1), 21–40.

3. Feldman, R., and Dowd, B. "The Effectiveness of Managed Competition in Reducing the Costs of Health Insurance." In R. Helms (ed.), *Health Policy Reform: Competition and Controls.* Washington, D.C.: AEI Press, 1993.

4. Feldman, R., Dowd, B., and Coulam, R. "The Federal Employees Health Benefits Plan: Implications for Medicare Reform." *Inquiry,* 1999, *36*, 188–199.

5. Dowd, B., Feldman, R., and Christianson, J. *Competitive Pricing for Medicare.* Washington, D.C.: AEI Press, 1996.

6. Feldman and others, "The Federal Employees Health Benefits Plan."

7. Lubalin, J., Schanier, J., Forsyth, B., and Gibbs, D. *Design of a Survey to Monitor Consumers' Access to Care, Use of Health Services, Health Outcomes, and Patient Satisfaction.* Final Report (282-92-0045). Rockville, Md.: Agency for Health Care Policy and Research, 1995.

8. Akerlof, "The Market for 'Lemons.'"

9. Spence, M. "Job Market Signaling." *Quarterly Journal of Economics,* 1973, *87*(3), 355–374.

10. Robinson, J. "Hospital Quality Competition and the Economics of Imperfect Information." *Milbank Quarterly,* 1988, *66*(3), 465–481.

11. Improving health outcomes and service quality entails a number of costly activities, including monitoring care processes to ensure compliance with accepted standards; measuring and monitoring outcomes of care, such as mortality and complication rates; rewarding or sanctioning the behavior of individual physicians; and screening physicians seeking affiliation with the plan's provider network on the basis of practice style and interpersonal skills. For a comprehensive discussion of quality improvement activities and health outcomes, see Millenson, M. *Demanding Medical Excellence.* Chicago: University of Chicago Press, 1997.

12. See Chapter Nineteen in this volume for a more complete description of the BHCAG program; also see Robinow, A. "The Buyers Health Care Action Group: Creating a Competitive Care System Model. *Managed Care Quarterly,* 1997, *5*(3), 61–64.

13. Fowles, J., and others. "Taking Health Status into Account When Setting Capitation Rates: A Comparison of Risk Adjustment Methods." *Journal of the American Medical Association,* 1996, *276,* 1316–1321.

14. The analogy is less appropriate for employees purchasing family coverage. Each family member chooses a primary care clinic, and the premium is based on the highest-cost clinic chosen by any family member. In our application we focus on unmarried employees with no dependents to avoid the complications created by multiple decision makers with competing interests.

15. Chernew, M., and Scanlon, D. "Health Plan Report Cards and Insurance Choice." *Inquiry,* 1998, *35,* 9–22; Spranca, M., and others. "Do Consumer Reports of Health Plan Quality Affect Health Plan Selection?" Santa Monica, Calif.: RAND Corporation, 1998; Kaiser Family Foundation, Agency for Health Care Policy and Research, and Princeton Survey Research Associates. *Americans as Health Care Consumers: The Role of Quality Information.* Chart Pack 95-1071-01b. Menlo Park: Calif.: Henry J. Kaiser Family Foundation, 1996.

16. Feldman, R., Christianson, J., and Schultz, J. "Do Consumers Use Information to Choose a Health Care Provider System?" *Milbank Quarterly,* 2000, *78*(1), 44–77; Schultz, J., Call, K., Feldman, R., and Christianson, J. "Evaluation of Consumers' Use of Satisfaction and Quality Information on Health Care Systems." Working Paper, University of Minnesota, Division of Health Services Research and Policy, 1999.

17. A stratified sampling plan was used to ensure that the sample contained employees from all firms. Employees of smaller firms were sampled at a higher rate. In order to obtain the required number of completed surveys, 186 employees were sampled from each firm. The survey response rate was 91 percent for employees with single coverage. We limit our sample to unmarried employees with no dependents in order to eliminate two types of complications arising from employees with family coverage. First, by using single employees, we can be more confident that our model accurately characterizes the survey respondent's choice set. Employees with family coverage often have the option of enrolling in plans sponsored by a spouse's employer. Second, our model is not appropriate for explaining family coverage decisions because it does not account for interdependent utility and varying preferences among family members.

18. For the care system choice models, we limit the sample to care systems within the Twin Cities with more than 50 sampled Choice Plus members. This results in a sample size of 721 for the care system choice models. Care system 6 has the highest enrollment at 329, and care system 4 has the lowest with only 52. Only 86 survey respondents are enrolled in the low-cost tier. The remaining sample members are almost evenly split between the remaining tiers with 467 enrolled in the middle-cost tier and 443 in the high-cost tier. The small number enrolled in the low-cost tier resulted in very imprecise parameter estimates in preliminary analysis of the cost-tier choice model. For this reason we limit our analysis to the 93 percent of employees enrolled in the middle- and high-cost tiers, giving a sample size of 910 individuals for the cost-tier choice model.

19. Detailed data analyses are available from Katherine Harris, RAND Corporation, 1200 South Hayes Street, Arlington, VA 22202.

20. We also estimate a care system choice model with distance, number of physicians, and the premium importance attribute, but excluding the cost-tier index variable. The premium attribute parameter is positive and significant for two care systems in the middle-cost tier.

21. Harris, K., and Keane, M. "A Model of Health Plan Choice: Inferring Preferences and Perception from a Combination of Revealed Preference and Attitudinal Data." *Journal of Econometrics*, 1999, *89*, 131–157; McCall, N., Rice, T., and Sangl, J. "Consumer Knowledge of Medicare and Supplemental Insurance Benefits." *Health Services Research*, 1986, *20*(6), 633–657; Marquis, S., and Holmer, M. *Informing Consumers About Health Care Costs: A Review and Research Agenda.* Santa Monica, Calif.: RAND Corporation, 1985.

22. Knickman, J., and others. "Tracking Consumers Reactions to the Changing Health Care System: Early Indicators." *Health Affairs*, 1996, *15*(2), 21–32.

23. Christianson, J., Feldman, R., Weiner, J., and Drury, P. "Early Experience with a New Model of Employer Group Purchasing in Minnesota." *Health Affairs*, 1999, *18*(6), 100–114.

CHAPTER FORTY-THREE

Helping Consumers Choose Among Complex Insurance Plans

Colleen M. Murphy

In *Market-Driven Health Care,* Regina Herzlinger opines that our insurers do our health care shopping for us and try to provide us with the features we would choose for ourselves and that the insurers (and, may I add, employers) do not know what we want because we have no means of communicating our preferences to them.[1]

Well, now we do.

While conducting market research with thousands of consumers, the founder of Asparity Decision Solutions repeatedly heard that they were "bewildered" by the annual selection process. Many used only three features to choose a plan: cost, the presence of their current doctor in the provider network, and a friend's recommendation. Others spent hours wading through reams of paper or their employer's intranet site in hopes of making the right choice. There had to be a better way.

Asparity, where I am president and COO, is based in Research Triangle, North Carolina, and provides Web- and voice-enabled decision support applications to employers and others who offer human capital products and services to employees and retirees. The company's initial software application helps individuals select health care coverage—one of the most expensive (and important) purchases an individual or family makes every year. Individuals select the health plan attributes (features) that are important to them, rate the relative importance of those attributes, and make trade-offs among them. The software ranks the plans available to each employee in the order that *best fits* the individual's preferences. Use of the tool generates preference data, which can be shared with employers and health insurers and used to improve products and services—thereby increasing employee satisfaction over time.

Asparity decision support experience dates back to 1995, when the company's founder was awarded a series of Agency for Health Care Policy and Research (AHCPR) and Small Business Innovation Research (SBIR) contracts. The contracts funded the development of a Web-enabled decision support tool designed to help employees and retirees choose a health plan in the Federal Employees Health Benefits Program (FEHB). In 1998, the Office of Personnel Management piloted the tool in five states and, in 1999, offered it to FEHB's six million participants. The feedback has been overwhelmingly positive. For example, one federal employee reported that the Asparity software is like "a psychiatrist who understands health plans" in that it extracts employees' preferences and matches them to plans.

Corporate America is catching on. Employers can achieve business objectives by making Asparity's decision support application available to their employees. Charter Communications, for example, offered its employees a choice of plans for the first time, including a consumer-driven health plan, and provided decision support to help employees better understand their health plan options and become better health care consumers. ING Americas used decision support to position its human resource (HR) services to be more responsive to its employees' needs. Given a competitive business climate, the company used the preference data to redesign HR services and health plan offerings. Most important, in both situations, HR could report to company leadership that for the first time, employees who used decision support overwhelmingly enrolled in plans that fit their personal needs.

More than 300,000 consumers have now used Asparity's decision support to help them choose their health care plan. Asparity saves the preference data obtained by these users, aggregates it, protects any personal information, and makes the data available to employers and health plans, which can use it to better understand their customers' needs and improve their products and services.

The data tell quite a story. For example, employees can be segmented into clusters by their key drivers for selecting a health plan. Most consumers are driven by cost, but their specific concerns differ—some want financial predictability (for example, office visit copays) and others financial protection (for example, an out-of-pocket maximum). Yet other consumers are driven by the availability of specific benefit coverage (for instance, chiropractic care) or the accessibility of providers of their choice. Finally, in one population, Asparity found that 15 percent of consumers selected a health plan primarily on the basis of member satisfaction measures.

Consumer-driven health care goes hand-in-glove with Asparity's product. Clearly, consumers are more likely to use the decision support tool when they are shopping for a health care plan. In one situation, 75 percent of consumers who changed plans selected one of the top three best fit plans. Of course, the best fit plan for you may differ from the best fit plan for me. But now that consumers can communicate their preferences to them, my friends in human resources may soon be able to say with confidence that health plans offer products and services that meet their employees' needs. Now, that's progress.

Note

1. Herzlinger, R. E. *Market-Driven Health Care: Who Wins, Who Loses in the Transformation of America's Largest Service Industry.* Reading, Mass.: Addison-Wesley, 1997.

CHAPTER FORTY-FOUR

CareCounsel

Consumer-Driven Health Care Advocacy

Lawrence N. Gelb

Employers are spending lots of money on health benefits, but their employees are increasingly frustrated with the many health plan snafus that they encounter while navigating the complex managed care landscape. After employees' efforts to resolve a health plan claims problem or network access issue have been thwarted, these problems inevitably end up on the Human Resource Department's doorstep. Part of any day in the life of a benefits manager is spent mopping up the flotsam and jetsam of real-world managed care service delivery problems, including lack of timely updates to provider network listings, disconnects between health plans and contracting physician groups, lack of coordination between carve-out coverages, communication breakdowns between health plans and providers, employee misunderstanding of coverage, claims processing errors due to human failures and system problems, and health plan member-service staff who lack the training or resources to make things better.

This chapter describes the market context, service delivery model, and accomplishments of CareCounsel, LLC, where I am president and CEO. In 1997, this San Rafael, California–based firm pioneered the innovative Healthcare Assistance Program, a benefits advocacy service that supports consumers who are using managed care programs. CareCounsel targets employers and other health care payers who want to respond to consumer-driven health care, increase employee and retiree satisfaction with managed care benefits, outsource functions traditionally performed by internal human resource (HR) staff, keep individuals' health information out of their corporate files, and improve their health plan monitoring and data collection capabilities.

THE CONTEXT

This book contains plenty of examples of managed care's hidden costs. At the top of the list is the continuing erosion of employee satisfaction with health benefits, which is coupled with the increasing burden faced by corporate benefits staff charged with responding to and resolving employee complaints. Consider this synopsis of the consumer data:

- Watson Wyatt's *2001 Report on Best Practices in Health Care Vendor Management*, based on a survey of 10,000 employees, found that only 43 percent of employees are satisfied with the overall performance of their health plan. Eighty-three percent of the 255 health benefit managers and HR executives surveyed in organizations with more than four million benefits-eligible employees ranked health plan "problem resolution/advocacy" as an activity crucial to employee satisfaction (and just about half felt they were doing this job well).[1]

- Also, D. S. Howard & Associates reported in June 2001 that 48 percent of employees find health plans too complex and hard to understand and 42 percent had difficulty getting timely answers to benefits questions.[2] A report from the National Committee for Quality Assurance, *The State of Managed Care Quality, 2001*, found that 42.1 percent of health care consumers had a problem getting the help they needed when they called their plan's customer service department.[3]

- Benefits consulting firm Hewitt Associates, in September 2001, released the results of its tracking of over 2,500 health plan issues that employees reported having with a health plan administrator. They discovered that 54 percent of the problems originated with the health plan administrator and 17 percent with the provider of care, and only 29 percent originated with the employee or retiree. The majority of the cases were related to claims problems, and over half required reprocessing by the health plan. Hewitt commented that "the bad news is that these types of issues are very time consuming, emotional and complicated for the employee, which can lead to decreased productivity, morale, as well as overall dissatisfaction with benefits."[4]

- The Kaiser Family Foundation/Harvard University Public Opinion Update survey, released in August 2001, found that 51 percent of adults with health insurance reported that they or someone in their household had experienced at least one problem with a health plan in the past year. For example:

Thirteen percent reported delays or denials of coverage.

Ten percent reported difficulty seeing a physician.

Thirteen percent reported billing and payment problems.

Eight percent reported health plan communication or customer service difficulties.

Of those who had experienced a problem with their health plan, 73 percent experienced increased stress because of the problem, 50 percent said they ended up paying more for care than they should have, 43 percent lost time from work or other important life activities, and 30 percent experienced a resultant decline in their health status.[5]

To date, this country's health plans have not stepped up to the plate to meet these needs. According to Hewitt Associates, "While employers felt that advocacy would be part of basic health plan services, this has not generally materialized. . . . So, while advocacy has been an implied service, the reality is that very few plans succeed in providing service even approaching advocacy."[6]

THE CARECOUNSEL SERVICE

This ongoing failure has created a market opportunity for entrepreneurial ventures such as CareCounsel. The company launched its Healthcare Assistance Program in 1998 and serves more than 100,000 people across the country. Clients include Beringer Blass Wine Estates; Bristol-Myers Squibb; Cost Plus World Markets; eHealthInsurance; Fritz, a UPS Company; Hitachi Data Systems; Nikon Precision; Pillsbury Winthrop; San Diego City Employees' Retirement System; Tetra Pak; the American Cancer Society; and the County of Santa Barbara. CareCounsel's success has attracted much larger firms, such as Hewitt Associates and ADP, to formulate competitive offerings and has led to press coverage on PBS and in the *New York Times, USA Today,* and the *Wall Street Journal.*

CareCounsel's Healthcare Assistance Program provides a bundled service of advocacy, education and information, coaching, and referrals that empowers consumers by providing convenient, expert solutions for their health care needs. These services are high touch, delivered directly to employees and retirees, primarily over the phone by experienced health care professionals, many with master's or R.N. degrees. Areas of assistance include

- Network accessibility issues
- Doctor-patient communication problems
- Quality of care concerns
- Specialist referrals
- Claims problems and collection agency issues

- Eligibility snafus
- Customer service complaints

Advocacy

From an employee relations and risk-management perspective, CareCounsel provides a solution for employers who want to offer confidential, independent managed care troubleshooting and problem resolution for their employees. Care-Counsel helps employees and dependents resolve questions and concerns that arise as they use their health benefits.

Employees call CareCounsel to address a wide range of health plan service and quality concerns, such as

- Provider network accessibility (doctors who are taking new patients and wait time for appointments)
- Physician-patient communication problems
- Availability of specialist referrals
- Health plan customer service complaints
- Claims problems and collection agency issues
- Quality of care concerns

CareCounsel, as the employer's agent, provides information, clarification, and escalated problem resolution in the context of the employer's health plan benefit design. CareCounselors serve as impartial but effective advocates, charged with assisting employees as they use their employer's benefit plans. Interventions range from clarifying plan benefits to engaging in hands-on coordination with a health plan service representative, physician's office, or collection agency about a claim issue to helping members successfully navigate their plan's grievance and appeals process. Because employees call CareCounsel when problems arise, CareCounselors are often the first to identify and help resolve common systems issues, such as eligibility glitches that get passed back and forth between various health vendors before they are addressed. Other calls can result in a referral to a state regulatory agency, medical board, long-term care ombudsprogram, or disease-related support organization. CareCounselors follow up with all callers who require additional or ongoing assistance.

Education and Information

CareCounsel's expert staff provide a single, readily accessible source for guidance about health care issues such as

- Choosing and using a health plan
- Getting the most from doctor visits

- Understanding usual, reasonable, and customary charges
- Choosing a primary care physician
- Selecting a specialist and other health professionals
- Getting answers to disease-related questions

Callers receive supportive counseling accompanied by information relevant to their issue. To ensure consistent, high-quality responses, the firm's automated help desk system provides one-click access to detailed internal protocols, resources, and employer-specific benefit information. During program implementation the employer provides CareCounsel with benefit plan information, including employee health benefits communication materials, health plan evidence of coverage or summary plan description, plan service representative and account manager contact information, and Web links to provider directories. This information becomes part of the client-specific database, so that staff can readily access the structure, benefits, and procedures applicable to each plan (including dental, pharmacy, and behavioral health).

Consumers who access the CareCounsel program also receive proprietary educational material that complements the telephone counseling. The available titles include

"A Consumer's Guide to Medications"

"Advanced Directives"

"All About Dentists"

"Choosing a Primary Care Physician"

"Choosing a Chiropractor"

"Choosing a Hospital"

"Choosing a Specialist"

"Choosing a Mental Health Professional"

"Keeping a Personal Health Record"

"Filing an Appeal or Grievance"

"Health Promotion/Disease Prevention"

"Diabetes: What Informed Patients Need to Know"

"Long-Term Care Alternatives"

"Maximizing Your Healthcare $$$'s"

"Preventive Care Guidelines"

"Questions to Ask Before Surgery"

"Second Opinions"

"Selecting a Health Plan"

"Talking with Your Doctor"

"Understanding Medicare Options"

"Usual, Customary and Reasonable Charges"

"When Someone You Love Has Cancer"

"Investigational Treatments and Clinical Trials"

"Viatical Settlements"

"When You Go to the Hospital"

Most consumers do not know where to find such information. For example, if employees call their health plan and ask how to select a primary care provider, they might be told to consult their provider directory, to ask for recommendations from friends or family, and to call the doctor to see whether slots are available for new patients. Employees who access CareCounsel, in contrast, receive useful tools to make the decision-making process more informed, including

- Physician's credentials, including education and graduation date and board certification
- Primary and secondary areas of specialization
- Licensure actions and malpractice data (in many states)
- A checklist of factors to consider in the PCP selection process, including

  Average wait times for routine and urgent appointments

  Average visit length

  Process for handling after-hours and holiday calls

  Practice style

  Philosophy about prescribing medication over the phone

  Relationships with complementary care providers

  House call policy

  Availability of telephone medical advice

  Health plan reimbursement methodology (for example, capitation)

  Hospital affiliations and continuing education courses taken

Coaching

CareCounselors are also coaches, providing patients with tools so they can adopt a more proactive role in their health care interactions. Research conducted at the Primary Care Outcomes Research Institute in Boston shows that the doctor-patient relationship has a substantial impact on health outcomes, affecting both subjective evaluations of health status and physiological measures, such as blood pressure control for patients with hypertension and blood sugar management in those with diabetes.[7] Talking with a CareCounselor can foster the following patient behaviors that have been correlated with improved health status:

- Taking more control in medical visits by asking more questions
- Becoming more effective in health information gathering
- Learning skills such as medical journal keeping and medical visit agenda planning
- Bringing a supportive friend or loved one to medical visits
- Expressing more emotions during doctor visits (patients who express "negative" affects like frustration or impatience actually have better outcomes)

Resources and Referrals

Many consumers call CareCounsel after they have been diagnosed with a health problem or disease. CareCounselors identify and make referrals to a range of disease-related resources: for example, a support group for parents of diabetic children or a group for cancer patients and their families. Callers receive information about national and local organizations where they can obtain additional educational and supportive resources relevant to their condition. CareCounselors make extensive use of the Internet, helping consumers sort through the maze of disease-specific Web sites to find reputable sources tailored to their information needs.

Automated Systems

The firm's automated system supports CareCounselors, providing comprehensive tracking and management of employee service requests. The call-handling and tracking system gives CareCounselors a single point of entry to

- Employer contract data
- Health plan benefits and contact information
- Employee contact information
- Category-based protocols and guidelines
- Problem-based service request tracking and management
- Problem-based knowledge base and support resources
- Time-based service request notification and escalation
- Request-based quality assurance evaluation and feedback
- Management and program utilization reports

When an employee first contacts CareCounsel, the system generates a service request. Each service request represents an incident or issue, which the

CareCounselor tracks and manages to resolution. The service request application tracks the following data elements:

- Problem category and description
- CareCounselor work log
- Claim information and outcome
- Service request status and status history
- Reminder notice and notification
- Problem complexity level
- Member's emotional state
- Parties involved in resolving the problem (health plan, physician's office, human resources)
- Additional interventions
- CareCounselor analysis of why problem occurred
- Healthcare Tip Sheets and other resources used

CareCounsel provides employers with quarterly reports that track the following data elements:

- Number of service requests generated
- Number of unique members actively using the program
- Utilization by region or division
- Utilization by gender
- Utilization by member type
- Utilization by health plan
- Utilization by problem type
- Utilization by problem detail
- Interventions by type
- Calls generated by type
- Resources utilized by type
- Problem source analysis for claims and network access issues
- Plan design issues and feedback
- Member satisfaction evaluations analysis and a printout of individuals' comments about the program

In addition, text case notes are available in the system documenting the employee's problem, the CareCounselor's interventions, and the outcomes for each service request.

The system generates employer-specific, aggregate utilization reports documenting the issues people encounter as they use their health benefits. While maintaining the confidentiality of program users, the data provide the employer with a snapshot of employee concerns and possible plan quality indicators. The group-specific quarterly utilization reports sort health care assistance requests into over fifty categories. These include intervention categories such as physician access, benefits and coverage, claim issues, quality of care, patient rights, resources, and consumer education as well as employee status and health plan.

In 2001, CareCounsel's utilization rate was 19.4 percent (down from 24 percent in 2000 due to low utilization subsequent to the events of September 11, 2001): 28 percent of service requests involved claims concerns (exclusive of providing general information about the claims process), 27 percent consumer education (including assistance with selecting health plans and health care providers), 24 percent benefits and coverage issues, 10 percent network access issues, 9 percent eligibility troubleshooting, 2 percent quality concerns, and 0.5 percent resources and referrals.

BENEFITS FOR THE EMPLOYER

In marketing this service CareCounsel points to the following valuable benefits for employers. The program

- Supports the employer's commitment to providing quality, cost-effective, and user-friendly health benefits
- Offers enhanced outsourcing support for benefit call center duties, freeing HR staff to focus on recruitment, retention, employee development, and strategy
- Maximizes the employer's health benefits investment
- Provides a mediator for escalated health plan issues, increasing employee satisfaction with their benefits
- Enhances productivity, as employees spend less time on health care issue resolution
- Reduces liability, as sensitive employee health issues and emerging health plan problems are addressed proactively and confidentially
- Fosters improved health status, as patients take a more active role in their health care decisions
- Provides useful quality of service information to support ERISA fiduciary duties related to health care plan selection and performance standards tracking

- Provides a consumer intermediary function for employers moving to a consumer-driven health care benefits environment

RESULTS TO DATE

CareCounsel signed-up its first employer client in February 1998. By March 2002, CareCounsel was providing benefits advocacy services to twenty-one employers and one firm that markets health insurance over the Internet, covering over 100,000 people across the country.

Employer response has been positive. One client stated, "It's probably one of the most appreciated benefits we've been able to provide employees," crediting the program with decreasing employee turnover.[8] Another said, "We've had nothing but positive results since we started using CareCounsel services," adding that "using CareCounsel helps make our [benefits] program stand apart from other companies' programs." Also, the reports provided by CareCounsel gave this client valuable "data to make decisions on the future of the [health] plan as it develops."[9]

Consumers give the program good reviews too. (Individuals who use CareCounsel receive a short questionnaire that evaluates their perception of the service.) Of the 33 percent of CareCounsel users who return their questionnaires, 94 percent "strongly agree" or "agree" that "the assistance provided by the CareCounselor was helpful," and 95 percent "strongly agree" or "agree" that "the CareCounsel program is a valuable benefit for my employer to offer." Employees often volunteer written comments: for example, "My neurologist was unable to diagnose my condition, so he referred me to Mayo Clinic. Mayo is not in my network, so your representative helped me to locate another top-rated facility that would cover my case 100 percent. Without her, I would have been completely lost. Thank you very much for providing this service"; and, "With the complexity of the whole health care process, it would be almost impossible to figure anything out or get any answers without this service."

BARRIERS TO DIFFUSION

The biggest barrier to diffusion of the health care assistance concept has been overcoming payers' reluctance to spend additional dollars on health benefits in an era of double-digit premium increases. Also, many benefits staff regard independent advocacy services as an encroachment on turf traditionally claimed by the HR Department and are reluctant to outsource this function. We expect these barriers to diminish as employers increasingly migrate to a consumer-driven health benefits environment and recognize the need to provide employees with a more robust armamentarium of resources so they can be informed health care consumers.

Notes

1. Watson Wyatt Worldwide. *Maximizing the Return on Health Benefits: 2001 Report on Best Practices in Health Care Vendor Management.* Washington, D.C.: Watson Wyatt Worldwide, 2001.

2. "Health Care 'Consumerism'? Not in the Workplace." Press release. Chicago: Planlinx, Inc., June 12, 2001.

3. National Committee for Quality Assurance (NCQA). *The State of Managed Care Quality, 2001.* Washington, D.C.: NCQA, 2001.

4. "Consumers Not at Fault for the Majority of Escalated Health Plan Issues." Press Release. Lincolnshire, Ill.: Hewitt Associates, Sept. 5, 2001.

5. Kaiser Family Foundation and Harvard University School of Public Health. *New Survey on Consumer Experiences with Health Plans.* Menlo, Calif.: Kaiser Family Foundation and Harvard University School of Public Health, Aug. 30, 2001.

6. Hewitt Associates. "Advocacy and Health Management." White Paper. Lincolnshire, Ill.: Hewitt Associates, Aug. 1999.

7. Kaplan, S., Greenfield, S., and Ware, J. E., Jr. "Assessing the Effects of Physician/Patient Interactions on the Outcomes of Chronic Disease." *Medical Care,* 1989, *27*(3), 10–27.

8. Shinkman, R. "A Growing Concern: Employers' (and Employees') Frustrations with Health Plans Lead to a New Type of Business." *Modern Healthcare,* July 19, 1999, p. 22.

9. DeBare, I. "Frustrated with Health Insurer? New Firm Can Help Sort Out Problems." *San Francisco Chronicle,* Sept. 21, 1998, pp. B1–B2.

CHAPTER FORTY-FIVE

Access Health Group

A Medical Management Perspective

Joseph P. Tallman

Access Health Group exists because of the systemic ineffectiveness that often results in suboptimal cost and quality in patient care. This problem is not caused by a general lack of knowledge or capability—our health care system has exceptional technology and legions of capable providers. The problem is not caused by the money-grubbing, care-denying rules of managed care—practice variation was greater in the days preceding managed care. The problem is certainly not caused by a lack of concern—in studies, individuals regularly rate health as the most important factor in quality of life, and the cost of health care is a significant issue for most corporations and national economies.

HOW ACCESS HEALTH HELPS CONSUMERS: CASE STUDIES

The primary cause of inefficiency and ineffectiveness in health care is the lack of timely, useful information and support. These are the tools that Access Health (AH) provides. To illustrate the offerings, consider the following three actual episodes of care:

A woman in her late fifties called the nurse triage service offered by her health plan, a service operated by Access Health, to help relieve the severe hiccups she was experiencing. Her call went to an intelligent routing system, which identified the next nurse who was qualified to handle this call. The nurse was selected from within a staff of more than three hundred nurses on duty at that time at four geographically distributed telephone care centers. The call was answered within thirty seconds by a registered nurse who confirmed the patient's identity, recorded current symptoms, and then asked a series of structured questions. The appropriate questions were presented to the nurse as she traversed the hiccup algorithm that she had selected out of her clinical tool suite. The algorithm is one of over six hundred binary branch-chain logic algorithms, designed, developed, operated, maintained, and patented by AH.

After asking five questions the nurse recommended that the woman, who was alone in her home, dial 911 and request an ambulance to take her to a specific emergency department (ED). The nurse called back in five minutes to confirm that the patient had taken her advice. The nurse then called the emergency department to forewarn staff there of the arriving case. When the nurse closed this case on her computer, electronic messages were automatically relayed to the woman's designated primary care provider, the health plan medical director, and the health plan claims payment system to authorize the ambulance trip and the ED visit.

Tests later confirmed that the woman was experiencing a myocardial infarction. The accelerated care likely saved her life.

An insurance company contracted with Access Health to provide asthma management services for its beneficiaries. AH medical and pharmacy claims data screens selected candidates for the program, among them a seventeen-year-old male. He had visited the emergency department five times and been hospitalized three times for his asthma in the past six months. During this time he had seen three different providers and had received three different treatment plans. Not surprisingly, his mother was confused about how to manage day-to-day asthma treatment and had special problems in handling her son's frequent asthma attacks.

After physician and member introductory communications, a specially trained AH asthma disease management nurse made the first call to introduce the boy's mother to the program, assess the boy's asthma control, and develop a treatment plan. In the ensuing months, the AH nurse, the mother and son, and the son's most recent provider worked through a variety of educational, treatment, and case management issues. As a result, mother and son gained an appreciation of asthma monitoring, the proper use of medications, and the triggers to avoid, and enhanced their communication with their provider.

During this time the boy's asthma symptoms declined dramatically. Although the asthma was not cured, he was returned to a controlled state. As his doctor wrote, "The asthma support program has been helpful with my patient. The service was instrumental in getting him to go back off cigarettes. He is doing very well now."

An AH utilization management nurse received a request from a doctor for approval for a 360-degree fusion of two levels of the spine using a Ray spinal fusion cage. The primary indication was radicular back pain that was unresponsive to conservative therapy. Using appropriate criteria the nurse determined that the patient met the criteria for a laminectomy but not the criteria for a fusion procedure, as there was no instability of the spine. She immediately passed the case to her team physician for further review and, if necessary, adjudication.

The literature review was clear: although the Ray cage procedure compared favorably to traditional fusion procedures, for this indication it has a higher complication rate and no higher efficacy rate than a simple laminectomy and costs significantly more. In the end the patient received a laminectomy and was therefore spared an unnecessarily invasive procedure with significantly higher risk of complications.

ACCESS HEALTH'S PRODUCT LINE

These three cases are typical of the AH approach and operation. The AH suite of medical management products and services encompasses proprietary clinical process management tools, the software and other technologies that support the large-scale use of these tools, and the delivery of a variety of services by employees. More than forty million people in the United States use one or more of these services, and many more have their care affected by a provider using a licensed product.

AH currently groups its products for management into three broad product categories: (1) acute-care management, (2) population care management (disease management), and (3) utilization management. The products in each of these categories require communication with patients, doctors, and health plans or other clients; documentation of actions and results; and a continual updating of system components so they can maintain their clinical relevance.

Let us examine each of these product groups to see how they address the problems of information and support and to view their documented results.

Acute-Care Management

Acute-care management activities are directed at the time when a patient is about to enter the health care system with a new set of symptoms. AH uses its clinical algorithms to enable its providers, typically registered nurses with physician backup, to make fairly granular recommendations as to the timing, place, and even type of care that should next be sought. Figure 45.1 represents the redirection pattern that is typical for patients who enter the system through this type of process. The 80 percent rate of redirection of care illustrated is indicative of the mismatch between the patients' best assessment of the care they require and the most clinically appropriate care. The typical consequence of this mismatch when there is no redirection is that the first step into most delivery systems results in either too much or too little care. Although the first step may sometimes direct the patient to the appropriate resource, more often, when the process of care starts to go awry, it takes time and considerable expense to get it back on track. Obviously, results like those shown in Figure 45.1 must not compromise a patient's health. AH has never identified harm to a patient resulting from its recommendations and to date has not experienced a lawsuit or threat of one.

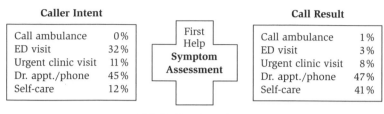

Figure 45.1. Acute-Care Management.

A number of clinical studies have been conducted on these tools to measure their efficacy and safety. Figure 45.2 depicts the outcome of one of these studies. It compares the recommendations of a physician who has just seen a patient and of a nurse who has used AH algorithms to guide her to a recommendation for the same patient. The chart also compares the outcomes of the algorithms to the other nurse triage systems currently in use. It shows that nurses who use AH binary branch chain logic algorithms basically replicate a physician's judgment. It also demonstrates that the other common forms of triage, that is, a nurse using her judgment and clipboard and a nurse relying on guidelines or

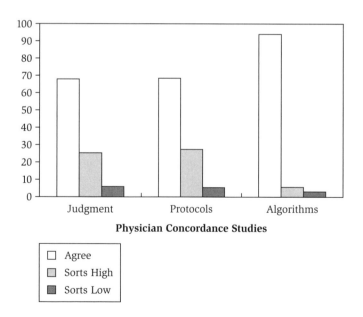

Figure 45.2. Do AH Algorithms Conform to Physicians' Judgments?

protocols as opposed to algorithms, do not compare favorably to the physician's judgment.

Figure 45.3 depicts another study that evaluated the efficacy of AH training. It monitored user variance in terms of recommendation outcomes. The initial scatter of recommendations resulted from a group of nurses who had initial training. After recalibration training, there is much less user variance around a key measurement.

In the end such technology must be deployable by delivery organizations so that it can affect care in a positive and cost-effective way. Figure 45.4 describes the actual impact that a well-regarded health plan realized in its first year of introducing a broad-based AH acute-care management service to its members. When applied appropriately in a delivery system, the service technology can measurably reduce the cost of care.

Population Care Management

Population care management activities identify and assist patients with chronic medical conditions. They optimize the management of these diseases and therefore the state of these patients' health. Table 45.1 represents the findings of one claims-based study of individuals with asthma, conducted by a health plan at the end of a six-month pilot of asthma care management. It shows that the type of systematic, longitudinal management that AH helps plans apply to patients with chronic conditions can markedly reduce service utilization.

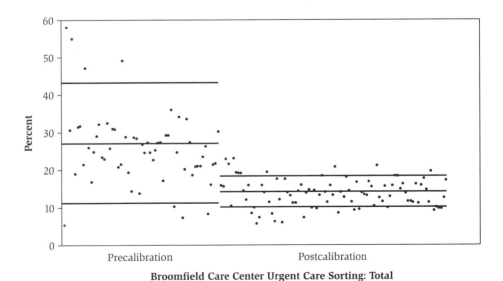

Broomfield Care Center Urgent Care Sorting: Total

Figure 45.3. Does AH Training Reduce Variability in Outcomes?

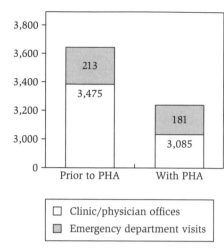

Client: East Coast HMO, with ED claims payment guarantee

RESULTS

- 18.2% fewer emergency department visits
- 15.8% fewer physician office visits
- Over $4 million savings in just one year, with all operational and marketing costs factored in
- 3:1 ROI

Figure 45.4. Are AH Programs Cost Effective?

Source: Data drawn from an Ernst & Young study of health care claims.

Figure 45.5 shows the change in quality of life experienced by the same group of health plan members. Clearly, the patients experienced better health, which came directly from better, more managed health status, because their asthmatic conditions could not actually be cured.

Utilization Management

Utilization management (UM) is an activity that compares standard industry clinical guidelines to the recommendations and requests for treatment made by physicians. This activity results in either approval or further review, research, and ultimate adjudication of each request. A study conducted by a health plan

Table 45.1. Do AH Activities Affect Utilization Rates of Individuals with Asthma?

	Hospital Admits per 1,000 Members per Month	Average Length of Stay	ER Visits per 1,000 Members per Month	Asthma PMPM
Before AH	0.99	2.33	5.69	0.77
With AH	0.43	2.27	3.5	0.48
% Reduction	57%	3%	38%	38%

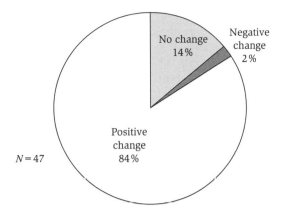

**Changes in Participants' Symptom Frequency,
Nighttime Symptoms, and Overall Functioning**

Figure 45.5. Do AH Activities Affect the Quality of Life of Individuals with Asthma?

showed significant savings in after-hours care at the end of a six-month pilot of the AH utilization management program:

- Bed-days per 1,000 members per six months reduced from 209.1 by 5 percent = 198.6
- Cost per bed-day = $1,325
- 5 percent reduction in bed-days = $706,497 savings on a annual basis

Moreover, this health plan is now experiencing a 10 percent reduction in bed-days, which represents a saving of $1,377,669 on an annual basis.

These reductions in bed-days per thousand members, a commonly tracked utilization measure, and also in the average length of stay per hospital admission, were realized by this health plan even though it had already been implementing variations of UM for a decade.

POTENTIAL IMPACT OF MEDICAL MANAGEMENT

The examples and data given here indicate the tremendous potential to improve the delivery of care to patients through the widespread application of clinical process management products and services like those employed by Access Health. Among the most significant factors these products and services address are these:

- *Health care in the Western world is extremely complex.* Technology and knowledge are expanding at an increasing rate. It is virtually impossible for physicians, human beings all, to stay current without great effort or a narrowing of their focus. Today's patients, who have more access to more health care information than ever before, are typically not capable of sorting through it effectively. The body of knowledge is already overwhelming—and there is so much more to come.

- *Incentives among the various actors in the health care system often are not aligned to optimize the quality and cost of outcomes.* For example, when special interest patient groups lobby effectively to minimize patient responsibility, patients may not work hard at managing the aspects of health care within their control. Also, physician groups that accept capitation of patient risk may reduce access to care as their physicians are financially motivated to spend less time and provide fewer episodes of care per capitated patient. And the politician who prompts an expansion of benefits does not realize that the only way to provide broader service is often to reimburse providers less for each unit of service.

- *Although large amounts of data are captured, relatively little patient-specific information is available to optimize care.* A physician treating a new patient may prescribe new tests, medication, or treatment without knowing about another treatment regime prescribed by another provider. The physician may not ask or the patient may not divulge the information. Further, most health care information databases have historically been developed to support specific functions, often financial. This information often cannot be reinterpreted or reconfigured to provide clinical information to the clinician at the point and time of care. Additionally, there are few centralized clinical information repositories. Credit histories are easily available to many lenders, but health care information is often parceled out into proprietary databases controlled by one provider group or health plan. This information often cannot be coordinated with or even accessed by another system. And the continued proliferation of privacy laws, while justified by the motive of patient protection, will likely serve to further complicate needed distribution and coordination of patient information.

Access Health has been able to achieve and measure improvements in care provided to some patients. In addition to U.S. applications, AH has cautiously entered relationships with clients in Puerto Rico, the United Kingdom, Portugal, and Australia in an attempt to understand the potential for its medical management approach in other cultures and health care delivery systems. Results from a number of these locations indicate that even though these other systems are clearly different, basic patient needs and the inadequacy of existing provider services to meet those needs are essentially the same.

Unfortunately, impediments to much more widespread use of processes like those developed by AH are numerous. Many of these obstacles result from the simple truth that to date, managed care organizations have not actually managed care other than through financial incentives and disincentives to providers. And in this process the managed care industry has disaffected health care consumers and created a frenzied feeding ground for special interest groups and political meddling. The successful application of the types of services that AH offers demands that a health care system embrace clinical process management and integrate it into the fabric of the services the system provides.

CHAPTER FORTY-SIX

Consumer's Medical Resource

Helping Consumers Evaluate
Medical Treatment Options

David J. Hines

Escalating costs. Varying quality. Increased dissatisfaction. The U.S. health care system has fallen into severe decline over the last decade, dramatically bringing into question the future of this trillion-dollar industry. Is a revolution around the corner? Consumer's Medical Resource (CMR), of which I am the founder and president, sees an inflection point in the current health care delivery system, in which the process is becoming consumer, not provider, driven.

CMR sees three key forces accelerating this transformation to a consumer-driven health care market:

- *Renewed escalation of health care costs.* Costs are growing at an estimated 15 percent a year. Double-digit inflation has shown no sign of subsiding. A company employing 20,000 workers may spend $80 million or more per year on health care.
- *Perceived lack of quality and dissatisfaction with the managed care system.* The current managed care system has proven to be a failure. It hasn't demonstrated better quality and efficiencies. Consumer lack of trust is rooted in the fact that many medical decisions have been driven by cost factors not necessarily resulting in the best care. The perception by Americans that managed care will not provide for them in times of need has given rise to consumers who are taking a more proactive, aggressive role in managing their own care. In addition, there is growing consensus that *quality,* the Holy Grail of health care, cannot be achieved without input, active participation, and decision making by patients.

- *The impact of Internet connectivity.* The Internet has fueled an exponential increase in medical information availability, and with it a unique opportunity for consumers to access this information. The advent of consumers who are involved with their own care is a significant, positive development for the U.S. health care system. However, the proliferation of Web sites offering medical information that is inaccurate or out of date and that often conflicts with data on other sites or from other sources impedes the ability of consumers to make well-informed health care decisions. Despite these limitations, consumers have developed an appetite for the Internet as a convenient, inexpensive, and easy-to-use medical information tool and will continue to use it, for better or for worse, in their quest for more knowledge.

In response to these marketplace realities, CMR believes a consumer-driven approach is the best way to ensure that high-quality, satisfactory, cost-efficient health care is delivered in the United States.

SERVICES PROVIDED BY CONSUMER'S MEDICAL RESOURCE

Consumer's Medical Resource provides Medical Decision Support (MDS) services to employees of Fortune 500 and other large organizations, who face serious, complicated, and chronic illness. MDS is a decision support service that offers patients the latest in-depth, objective, and personalized information on their diagnosis and available treatment options. The information is assembled and distributed by a physician-led team. The schematic in Figure 46.1 illustrates the MDS process.

This approach enables patients to fully understand and evaluate their treatment options so they can make the best decisions possible with their doctors. Moreover, MDS helps patients avoid medical mistakes and unnecessary procedures by equipping them to better question their prescribed care. In addition, MDS ensures that a patient's values and personal preferences are incorporated into a final decision.

Currently, patients can access MDS for forty-three types of serious and expensive medical conditions, including cancer, heart disease, diabetes, multiple sclerosis (MS), and attention deficit and hyperactivity disorder (ADHD). Given growing patient and employer needs. CMR is continually adding new diseases to the MDS program. For example, CMR is developing modules for such other difficult and expensive conditions and medical procedures as arthritis, emphysema, and hormone replacement therapy (HRT).

CMR has demonstrated that MDS adds value to today's health care system through the improvements the program has generated in medical decision making. Using a detailed methodology, the company has been able to measure

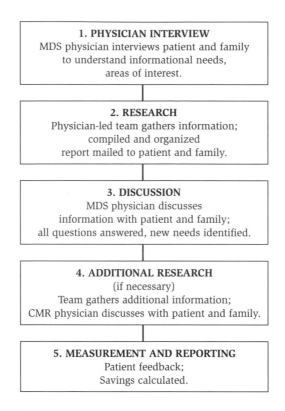

Figure 46.1. MDS Process.

improvements in the quality of decisions a patient and doctor ultimately make based on the information CMR provides.

EMPLOYEE CASE EXAMPLES

Since July 1999, CMR has provided the MDS program to Honeywell International employees in the United States. The following three employee case studies are representative examples of the way a consumer-based approach improves decision making, quality of care, satisfaction, and productivity while lowering costs at a major U.S. company.

A Honeywell employee's child was born with congenital heart defects, including ventricular septum defect (VSD) and a missing aortic valve. At one point a physician recommended a heart transplant "right now or he will not survive the summer." The employee called CMR to get information on heart transplantation, VSD, and other options that might exist. CMR's customized response included information on all treatment options, several of which had not been discussed with the employee. After reviewing the new information with the doctor, the employee decided to seek another opinion. This new opinion confirmed that other, less radical procedures were available and should be attempted before the transplant. Having learned more, the employee decided not to proceed with the heart transplant and to attempt additional repair surgery. Months later, the child, now four, is healthy again and unlikely ever to need a transplant.

Quality of Care Improvements

Sorted out conflicting physician views to achieve best practices
Switched to a higher-quality physician or provider
Discontinued unnecessary treatment
Improved quality of life and comfort

Direct Medical Cost Reductions

Avoided heart transplant: $200,000 (excluding lifelong medications)

A Honeywell employee was diagnosed with diabetes. The doctor put the employee on medications immediately and provided little information about the diagnosis. The employee called CMR to get more information about diabetes and treatment options. The CMR physician was concerned about the quality of care being provided and believed the employee might be on medications unnecessarily. CMR provided information on the kind of specialists who treat diabetes, treatment options, and other ways to regulate diabetes through exercise and nutritional changes. The employee spoke with the physician again and then sought a new opinion for the first time. The new doctor confirmed that the employee was on medications needlessly and recommended only lifestyle changes. The employee changed doctors, discontinued medications, and implemented lifestyle changes. The employee's diabetes is now under control.

Quality of Care Improvements

Sorted out conflicting physician views to achieve best practices
Switched to a higher-quality physician or provider
Discontinued unnecessary treatment
Improved quality of life and comfort
Improved wellness

Direct Medical Cost Reductions

Eliminated diabetes medications, test strips, blood tests: $85,325 (over five years)

A Honeywell employee was diagnosed with multiple sclerosis. At the same time, she began experiencing loud "ringing in the ears" that made it very difficult to hear. The symptoms became so severe that the employee became concerned that her hearing loss was affecting her job performance. The worsening hearing condition also meant she couldn't drive herself to and from work and had to rely on someone else for transportation. When discussing the symptoms with her doctor, the employee was told MS was incurable and that there was "nothing that could be done" to eliminate these side effects. The employee asked CMR for a complete report on MS, treatments available, side effects, and information on hearing loss due to MS. CMR provided information from the medical literature on all known symptoms and complications stemming from MS, none of which included hearing loss. The employee read the report and returned to the doctor and discussed the lack of supporting documentation for hearing loss caused by MS.

Dissatisfied with the doctor's response, the employee sought a new opinion. The new physician confirmed the diagnosis of MS but determined the hearing loss was being caused by something else, Ménière's syndrome, a treatable condition. The employee received treatment for Ménière's, and her hearing returned to normal within two weeks. Although the employee still faces the challenges of MS, she was grateful to have her hearing restored and to be working productively again.

Quality of Care Improvements

Identified a misdiagnosis
Switched to a higher-quality physician or provider
Improved quality of life and comfort

Direct Medical Cost Reductions

Difficult to quantify

RESULTS

Honeywell believes it has significantly improved health care for its employees by using MDS as part of its overall health care strategy. Of the 428 Honeywell employees surveyed over the last two and one-half years, 87 percent rated the MDS program "excellent," and 100 percent said they would recommend it to colleagues.

Also, at a time when health costs are rising 15 percent or more a year, Honeywell found the company saved $2 for every $1 spent on the program because MDS empowered employees and helped them to make better health care decisions.

Most important, quality of care was improved for two out of three Honeywell employees who used the MDS service. Exhibit 46.1 details these measurable improvements in quality of care, satisfaction, and reduced costs.

Exhibit 46.1. CMR's Medical Decision Support Program: Honeywell Results (2 1/2 Years).

I. Quality of Care Improvements

	Improvements per MDS User
Improved quality of life and comfort	1 in 4
Sorted out conflicting physician views to achieve "best practices"	1 in 6
Eliminated or minimized side effects of treatment	1 in 6
Switched to a higher-quality physician or provider	1 in 6
Improved wellness	1 in 9
Discontinued unnecessary treatment	1 in 15
Identified a misdiagnosis	1 in 29

II. Employee Satisfaction

1. How would you rate the overall service offered by Consumer's Medical Resource?

    87%   Excellent

    13%   Very Good

    0%   Average

    0%   Below Average

    0%   Poor

2. Would you recommend CMR's service to other employees?

    Yes   100%   No   0%

3. Do you believe this service is a valuable addition to your employee benefits package?

    Yes   100%   No   0%

III. Return on Investment (Savings-to-Cost)

2.1:1

CHAPTER FORTY-SEVEN

The Cost Effectiveness of Consumer-Driven Lifestyle Changes in the Treatment of Cardiac Disease

Dean Ornish

I used to think that science was the most important determinant of medical practice, but well-conducted scientific research is only one of many factors that play a role in how doctors practice medicine. Equally important are consumer-driven changes, including reimbursement. We doctors do what we are paid to do, and we are trained to do what we are paid to do. When reimbursement changes, then medical practice and medical education often follow. Consumer-driven changes in reimbursement are making a significant difference in these areas.

During the past twenty-five years, my colleagues and I at the nonprofit Preventive Medicine Research Institute (PMRI) have conducted a series of scientific studies demonstrating, for the first time, that the progression of even severe coronary heart disease can often be reversed by making comprehensive changes in diet and lifestyle and without coronary bypass surgery, angioplasty, or a lifetime of cholesterol-lowering drugs. These lifestyle changes include a very low-fat, low-cholesterol diet, stress management techniques, moderate exercise, smoking cessation, and psychosocial support. This was a radical idea when we first began our studies. Now these principles have come into the mainstream and are generally accepted as true by most cardiologists and scientists. Even so, physicians spend most of their time prescribing drugs and surgery, not comprehensive lifestyle changes.

The theme of all of our work is simple: if the underlying causes of a problem are not addressed, then the same problem may recur, new problems may emerge, or there may be painful choices—which is like mopping up the floor around an overflowing sink without also turning off the faucet. When these causes are addressed, then improvement may begin to occur much more quickly than had previously been documented.

Within a few weeks after making comprehensive lifestyle changes, our patients reported a 91 percent average reduction in the frequency of angina. Most of the patients became essentially pain free, including those who had been previously unable to work or engage in daily activities due to severe chest pain. Within a month they showed increased blood flow to the heart and improvements in the heart's ability to pump. And within a year even severely blocked coronary arteries began to improve in 82 percent of the patients. These research findings were published in peer-reviewed medical journals, including the *Journal of the American Medical Association, The Lancet, Circulation, The New England Journal of Medicine, The American Journal of Cardiology,* and others.[1] And they led to further questions and further research trials.

LIFESTYLE HEART TRIAL

We received funding from the National Heart, Lung, and Blood Institute of the National Institutes of Health to extend our study from one year to five years. We found that most of the study participants were able to maintain comprehensive lifestyle changes for five years. On average, these patients demonstrated even more reversal of heart disease after five years than after one year. In contrast, the patients in the comparison group who made only the moderate lifestyle changes recommended by most physicians (that is, they adopted a 30 percent fat diet) worsened after one year, and their coronary arteries became even more clogged after five years.[2]

Also, after five years the incidence of cardiac events (for example, heart attacks, strokes, bypass surgery, and angioplasty) was 2.5 times lower in the group that made comprehensive lifestyle changes. A one-hour documentary of this work was broadcast on *NOVA*, the PBS science series, and it was featured on Bill Moyers's PBS series *Healing and the Mind*.[3] These findings have particular significance for women. Heart disease is by far the leading cause of death in women in the Medicare population. Women also have less access to bypass surgery and angioplasty, and when they do undergo these operations, they have higher morbidity and mortality rates than men. However, women seem to be able to reverse heart disease even more than men when they make comprehensive lifestyle changes.

MULTICENTER LIFESTYLE DEMONSTRATION PROJECT

The next research question was, How practical and cost-effective is this lifestyle program?

There is bipartisan interest in Washington, D.C., in finding ways to control health care costs without compromising the quality of care. Many people are concerned that the managed care approaches of shortening hospital stays, shifting from inpatient to outpatient surgery, forcing doctors to see more and more patients in less and less time, and so forth may compromise the quality of care because they do not address the lifestyle factors that often lead to illnesses like coronary heart disease.

Beginning in 1993, my colleagues and I at PMRI established the Multicenter Lifestyle Demonstration Project. It was designed to determine (1) whether we could train other teams of health professionals in diverse regions of the country to motivate their patients to follow this lifestyle program, (2) whether this program might be an equivalently safe and effective alternative to bypass surgery and angioplasty in selected patients with severe but stable coronary artery disease, and (3) what the resulting cost savings would be. In other words, can some patients avoid bypass surgery and angioplasty by making comprehensive lifestyle changes and can they do this at lower cost and without increasing cardiac morbidity and mortality?

We trained a diverse selection of hospitals around the country to implement our program. In brief, we found that almost 80 percent of the individuals participating in the program and eligible for bypass surgery or angioplasty were able to avoid it safely for at least three years by making comprehensive lifestyle changes. Mutual of Omaha calculated an immediate savings of almost $30,000 per patient. These patients reported reductions in angina comparable to what can be achieved with bypass surgery or angioplasty without the costs or risks of surgery. These findings were published in 1998.[4] We also found that patients who had received bypass surgery or angioplasty were able to reduce the likelihood of needing another operation by making comprehensive lifestyle changes after surgery.

In addition, several patients with such severe heart disease (ischemic cardiomyopathy) that they were eligible for heart transplants improved sufficiently that they no longer needed to be considered for transplantation. This improvement was clinically significant and verified by cardiac PET scans or echocardiograms. Each patient who can avoid a heart transplant saves approximately $500,000.[5]

In the past, lifestyle changes have been viewed only as *prevention,* increasing costs in the short run for a possible savings years later. Now this program of lifestyle changes is offered as a scientifically proven alternative *treatment* to many patients who were otherwise eligible for coronary artery bypass surgery or angioplasty, thereby resulting in an immediate and substantial cost savings. For every patient who chooses this lifestyle program rather than undergoing bypass surgery or angioplasty, thousands of dollars are immediately saved that would otherwise have been spent. When one includes the cost of likely complications from these procedures, even more is saved. (And of course there is also the benefit of sparing the patient the trauma of undergoing cardiac surgery.)

In addition, providing lifestyle changes as a direct alternative for patients who would otherwise receive coronary bypass surgery or coronary angioplasty may result in significant *long-term* cost savings. Despite the great expense of bypass surgery and angioplasty, up to one-half of bypass grafts reocclude after only five to seven years, and 30 to 50 percent of angioplastied arteries restenose after only four to six months—another example of mopping up the floor around the overflowing sink without also turning off the faucet. When this occurs, then coronary bypass surgery or coronary angioplasty is often repeated, incurring additional costs.

Over fifty insurance companies are covering this approach as a defined program either for all qualified members or on a case-by-case basis at the sites PMRI has trained. One of these, Highmark Blue Cross Blue Shield, was the first insurer to both cover and to provide this program to its members, now at several sites. Highmark has now established a new company, Lifestyle Advantage, to make this program more widely available.[6]

MEDICARE

These research findings have particular significance for Americans in the Medicare population. One of the most meaningful findings in our research was that the older patients improved as much as the younger ones. The primary determinant of change in their coronary artery disease was neither age nor disease severity but adherence to the recommended changes in diet and lifestyle. No matter how old they were, on average, the more people changed their diet and lifestyle, the more they improved. Indeed, the oldest patient in the study (at age eighty-six) showed more reversal than anyone else. This is a very hopeful message for Medicare patients, because the risks of bypass surgery and angioplasty increase with age, but the benefits of comprehensive lifestyle changes may occur at any age.

Over 500,000 Americans die annually from coronary artery disease, making it the leading cause of death in this country. Approximately 600,000 coronary artery bypass operations and approximately 700,000 coronary angioplasties were performed in the United States in 1999 at a combined cost of over *$30 billion,* more than was spent on any other surgical procedure. Over $20 billion of this expense is paid for by Medicare each year, so the potential cost savings of avoiding bypass surgery or angioplasty are significant. Not everyone is interested in changing lifestyle, and some people with extremely severe and unstable disease may benefit from surgery, but billions of dollars per year could be saved immediately if only some of the people who were eligible for bypass surgery or angioplasty were able to avoid it by making comprehensive lifestyle changes instead. Another $30 billion is spent each year on statin drugs, much of which could also be avoided by making comprehensive lifestyle changes instead.

Unfortunately, for many Americans on Medicare, the denial of coverage is the denial of access. Our program of comprehensive lifestyle changes can contribute to a new model for lowering Medicare costs without compromising the quality of care or access to care. It is a model that is caring and compassionate as well as cost effective and competent. This approach empowers the individual, may immediately and substantially reduce health care costs while improving the quality of care, and offers the information and tools that allow individuals to be responsible for their own health care choices and decisions. It provides access to quality, compassionate, and affordable health care to those who most need it.

Because of the success of our research and demonstration projects, we asked the U.S. Centers for Medical and Medicare Services (then called the Health Care Financing Administration [HCFA]) to consider providing Medicare coverage for this program. We believed that our work could provide a new model for lowering Medicare costs without compromising the quality of care or access to it. Coverage was to be limited to people who choose this program of comprehensive lifestyle changes as a direct alternative to bypass surgery or angioplasty. These are the patients in whom cost savings are the most dramatic and immediate. My colleagues and I hoped to work with an outside group (for example, the American College of Cardiology) that could certify that a comprehensive lifestyle program has sufficient scientific evidence of medical effectiveness and cost effectiveness to justify coverage. This certification could be offered on a nonexclusive basis and would meet the need for credentialing of programs to avoid fraud and abuse, thereby making the program available to the people who most need it.

I first met with officials from HCFA on June 9, 1994, and have met with them many times since then. Then, as now, they expressed concern that if HCFA were to cover the program, then a Pandora's box would be opened. They worried that everyone who had any kind of alternative medicine program would demand coverage from HCFA.

I understand this concern. In my first meeting with HCFA, in 1994, I was accompanied by the medical director of Mutual of Omaha. In response to this concern, he explained that Mutual of Omaha decided to provide coverage for this program because of the scientific data from many years of randomized controlled trials demonstrating the program's safety and efficacy. If other programs develop this scientific evidence of safety and efficacy, then Mutual of Omaha would consider providing coverage for those programs as well. The other insurance companies that are providing coverage for this program in the sites we have trained have expressed similar ideas. As an editorial in *The New England Journal of Medicine* has stated: "There cannot be two kinds of medicine—conventional and alternative. There is only medicine that has been adequately tested and medicine that has not, medicine that works and medicine that may or may not work. Once a treatment has been tested rigorously, it no longer matters whether it was considered alternative at the outset. If it is found to be reasonably safe and effective, it will be accepted."[7]

Medicare is now paying for 1,800 patients to go through this lifestyle program, in the sites that PMRI has trained, as a direct alternative to bypass surgery or angioplasty or, in those who have already undergone these procedures, to reduce the likelihood of needing another one. This is the first time that Medicare has ever paid for an alternative medicine intervention. If Medicare validates the cost savings shown in the Multicenter Lifestyle Demonstration Project, then Medicare administrators may decide to cover this program as a defined benefit for all Medicare beneficiaries. If this happens, then most other insurance companies may do the same, thereby making the program available to the people who most need it.

In summary, increasing evidence indicates that comprehensive lifestyle changes can be both medically effective and cost effective. Consumer-driven demand for reimbursement for lifestyle programs such as the one described in this chapter is having a significant impact on both medical practice and medical education.

Notes

1. See, for example, Ornish, D. M., and others. "Effects of Stress Management Training and Dietary Changes in Treating Ischemic Heart Disease." *Journal of the American Medical Association,* 1983, *249,* 54–59.

2. Ornish, D. M., Brown, S. E., Scherwitz, L. W., and others. "Can Lifestyle Changes Reverse Coronary Atherosclerosis? The Lifestyle Heart Trial." *The Lancet.* 1990, *336,* 129–133 (reprinted in *Yearbook of Medicine.* New York: Mosby, 1991; *Yearbook of Cardiology.* New York: Mosby, 1991); see also, Ornish, D. and others. "Intensive Lifestyle Changes for Reversal of Coronary Heart Disease: Five-Year Follow-Up of the Lifestyle Heart Trial." *Journal of the American Medical Association,* 1998, *280,* 2001–2007; Ornish, D. *Dr. Dean Ornish's Program for Reversing Heart Disease.* New York: Random House, 1990; Billings, J., Scherwitz, L., Sullivan, R., and Ornish, D. "Group Support Therapy in the Lifestyle Heart Trial." In S. Scheidt and R. Allan (eds.), *Heart and Mind: The Emergence of Cardiac Psychology.* Washington, D.C.: American Psychological Association, 1996.

3. Published as "Changing Life Habits: A Conversation with Dean Ornish," in Moyers, B. *Healing and the Mind.* New York: Doubleday, 1993.

4. Ornish, D. "Avoiding Revascularization with Lifestyle Changes: The Multicenter Lifestyle Demonstration Project." *American Journal of Cardiology,* 1998, *82,* 72T–76T; see also, Ornish, D., and Hart J. "Intensive Risk Factor Modification." In C. Hennekens and J. Manson (eds.), *Clinical Trials in Cardiovascular Disease.* New York: Saunders, 1998; Ornish, D. "Concise Review: Intensive Lifestyle Changes in the Management of Coronary Heart Disease." In E. Braunwald (ed.), *Advances in Cardiology.* New York: Saunders, 2002.

5. Gould, K. L., and others. "Changes in Myocardial Perfusion Abnormalities by Positron Emission Tomography After Long-Term, Intense Risk Factor Modification." *Journal of the American Medical Association,* 1995, *274,* 894–901.

6. For more information visit the company's Web site [www.lifestyleadvantage.org].

7. Editorial. *New England Journal of Medicine,* 1998, *339,* 839–841.

CHAPTER FORTY-EIGHT

Healthtrac

*Proven Reduction of
the Need and Demand
for Medical Services*

James F. Fries

Healthtrac, Inc., was established by me in 1984 as a private corporation with three goals: first, to improve health; second, to reduce medical care costs; and third, to prove the company's effectiveness in meeting the first two goals. The business plan was formed around the belief that the only reason not to purchase a program that improved health and saved money for the sponsor would be the absence of convincing proof. For this reason, and helped by the development of Healthtrac from an academic background, extremely rigorous product evaluation has been a part of all activities. These three goals have shaped product development because they constrain the types of products offered to those that can be both effective and cost effective. These goals also dictate content, presentation, program cost, and delivery mechanism.

Healthtrac's endeavors are based on a large body of science, some of which is specifically elaborated in the previous chapters, with substantial contributions from my research group at the Stanford University School of Medicine. Some central postulates establish the mandate. Eighty percent of illness in the United States is chronic. Seventy percent of this illness is preventable. There is wide variability in the use of costly medical resources between states, between cities, between physicians, and most important, between patients. Health care in United States is extremely costly by international standards, and yet this is not the healthiest nation. Minimum attention to prevention and maximum attention to technologically based "cures" characterize our health system.

Consumer autonomy in the United States is potentially extremely important but is generally unexercised. When we queried patients about what they want from the health care system, they answered with the famous "five D's": to avoid death, disability, discomfort, drug toxicity, and dollar cost. They want to be alive as long as possible, they want to function normally, they wish absence of pain and other symptoms, they don't want side effects from the treatment, and they wish to remain solvent. The system, however, is based on appropriate medical responses to acute episodes, not to preservation and maintenance of long-term health. It pays little attention to any of the D's except death.

Yet health is consumer determined in the final analysis. All of the most important decisions are made ultimately by the consumer. What to eat, how to exercise, whether to smoke. When to see the doctor, what type of doctor to see, whether to be active or passive, whether to sign a release for the surgery, whether to take the medicine, how to die. The autonomous consumer, exercising the rights and responsibilities available, represents the strongest possible force for a healthier population.

In 1984, a scientific literature gaining in strength suggested that behavioral interventions designed to improve health could be successful. A smaller literature suggested the possibility of cost reduction through prevention of disease. The self-care movement, led in part by the Healthtrac publication "Take Care of Yourself," coauthored by me, had proved successful. Worksite programs by Johnson & Johnson and others had shown promising results. But the adequacy of the scientific proof still could be challenged by skeptics.

Thus my colleagues and I saw an opportunity to improve the national health and to allocate medical care more effectively through consumer activation, and set before ourselves these goals:

Specific Goals for Products: Choosing the Large Targets

- To improve personal self-efficacy and increase autonomous consumer behavior
- To increase self-management skills
- To increase chronic disease self-management skills
- To decrease behavioral health risks, particularly those associated with smoking, lack of exercise, and high-fat diets
- To increase the intensity of interventions for high-risk individuals as compared to low-risk ones
- To decrease the number of very low birthweight babies
- To decrease the frequency of inhumane and undignified care at the end of life

Each of these goals deals with important, high-cost medical areas. Population-based approaches, we believed, were feasible and would prove more cost effective than approaches based in the clinicians' office.

PRODUCT DEVELOPMENT: AN INTERACTIVE DISCUSSION WITH YOUR DOCTOR

We sought to develop direct-to-consumer health assistance, paid for by the employer, government, or health plan. Programs would be driven by consumer-provided questionnaire data on individual health risks and health problems, provided by mail, and supplemented by telephone. These data would lead to an individualized, focused recommendation letter and report from a physician, computer generated and tailored precisely to the needs of the particular individual, together with self-management materials selected for the individual. Serial questionnaires at three- to six-month intervals would provide feedback, allowing an interactive conversation and using computer data linkages to reinforce positive changes and to evaluate the results in particular groups (group reports).

PRODUCTS

The first Healthtrac program was standard Healthtrac, with questionnaires completed at six-month intervals generating physician recommendation letters and reports and with "Take Care of Yourself," other self-management materials, and newsletters provided to the individual. The individualization (many millions of responses were possible) and the serial reinforcement, together with the power represented by an intervention over a doctor's signature, were characteristic even of these early interventions. The following program, Senior Healthtrac, extended these same concepts into the senior population and dealt additionally with the particular problems of particular age groups. Reading level was tailored to education level, size of type to participant age, and so forth. Subsequently, Babytrac was introduced, with questionnaire and report cycles completed by mothers prior to conception, during each trimester, and postpartum. The program was designed to reduce the number of very low birthweight babies by actively involving the prospective mother in the health behaviors important to carrying babies to term.

In 1994, Healthtrac presented its first High-Risk programs, with an even greater individualization. An algorithm applied to the initial questionnaire identified those individuals expected to be most costly over the next twelve months and channeled them to specific high-risk programs in fourteen areas including arthritis, diabetes, asthma, congestive heart failure, cigarette smoking, and obesity. The self-management materials were individualized to the problem and detailed chronic disease self-management recommendations were provided at three-month intervals. The stand-alone, chronic disease self-management programs in arthritis, in Parkinson's disease, and more recently in stress, follow the same general sequence. Information is requested and received from the participant, individualized recommendations are made, positive changes are subsequently reinforced, and negative changes receive additional attention.

The self-management materials are updated annually and have been based on "Take Care of Yourself," "Taking Care of Your Child," "Living Well," and "The Arthritis Helpbook," among others. Materials are selected for their enhancement of personal self-efficacy, the soundness of their medical recommendations, and the degree to which they empower the consumer. More recently, Web interfaces to these Healthtrac programs are becoming available.

PROOF

The definitive standard of proof in clinical science is the randomized controlled trial. To date, only about twenty such trials have been performed for health promotion, disease prevention, and cost-reduction programs. Healthtrac has been associated with nine of these, including the ones generally considered the strongest and best performed, and published in major, peer-reviewed medical journals.

Healthtrac self-management materials were evaluated in three randomized controlled trials. First, a large study in a Medicare population showed a 15 percent reduction in total medical visits, with a return on investment (ROI) of 2.19 to 1.[1] Second, a workplace health education program used self-care books with 5,200 employees and controls and noted a 17 percent reduction in total medical visits for not only the employees but their entire households—a highly significant result.[2] Third, Vickery and colleagues provided "Take Care of Yourself" or "Taking Care of Your Child" to a population of 2,833 households, with randomized controls, and observed that households provided with these books experienced 17 percent fewer total medical visits and 35 percent fewer minor medical visits compared with the control group.[3]

Four randomized controlled trials and two observational controlled studies are among the major reports on the Healthtrac program itself. In the California Public Employees Retirement System (PERS) study, a randomized controlled twelve-month trial was conducted to measure the impact of health risk assessments and accompanying interventions provided to participants at six-month intervals. Approximately 57,000 participants were studied. Claims data were used to measure program impact. Additionally, self-reported data were used to analyze changes in health habits and costs. The program participants experienced a reduction in health risk scores of approximately 12 percent at twelve months, a reduction in self-reported medical service use of 20 percent, and declining claims growth compared with control subjects. Claims costs saved were three to six times more than the program cost.[4]

In the Bank of America trial, 4,712 retirees were randomized into three groups and followed for twenty-four months. The intervention group received the full Healthtrac program with health risk assessment, feedback letters and reports, and self-management materials. The second group received a modified intervention with health risk assessment only for the first twelve months and the full program for the subsequent twelve months. The third group received nothing and was followed only by medical claims. Overall health risk scores improved 12 percent after twelve months and 23 percent at twenty-four months. Costs for the intervention group were reduced by more than 20 percent as measured by self-report and more than 10 percent as measured by claims experience. The return on investment for the full program group was 5.4 to 1.[5]

The Parkinson's disease trial of the PROPATH intervention involved approximately 400 subjects, randomized to full-program or questionnaire-only groups.[6] The intervention group had significantly increased exercise, reduced drug side effects, and improved Parkinson's disease scores that remained improved for a period of over two years. Doctor visits, hospital days, and sick days were significantly reduced for this group. They had improved quality of life as measured by their self-reported global self-efficacy scores and their spouse or caregiver assessments.

The Healthtrac arthritis program studied about 800 individuals by randomized trial, similar in design to the Parkinson's trial.[7] At six months, physical function had improved, pain had decreased, global vitality had improved, and fewer inflamed joints were present in the program group compared with controls, with an average effect of improvement of from 5 to 20 percent. Costs were decreased 16 percent in the program group, and days of missed work or confinement at home decreased by over 50 percent in the program group as compared with controls. Health improvement continued after the first year. The control group, when provided with the program subsequently, showed improvement similar to that of the original program group during the first six months.

An observational study of 103,937 consecutive Healthtrac participants over a minimum of six months to a maximum of thirty months showed continued health improvement over thirty months.[8] Improvement in computed health risk scores over eighteen months was 15 percent for those sixty-five years of age and over and 18 percent for those under sixty-five. After thirty months, improvement had extended to 19 percent and 26 percent, respectively; results were highly statistically significant. The program was equally effective in those who had not completed high school and in college graduates.

In an observational study of 2,586 persons computed to be at high risk, entered into the High-Risk program, and compared with standard Healthtrac experiences, each of the high-risk disease modules was compared against each other and against employee and senior groups.[9] Health risk scores had improved by 11 percent in the overall high-risk group at six months, compared with 9 percent in the employee group and 6 percent in the senior group. Physician use decreased by 0.8 visits per six-month period in the high-risk group compared with smaller changes in the other groups. The return on investment was about six to one in the high-risk group compared with four to one in comparison groups. These results indicate that programs directed at health improvement in high-risk individuals yield a greater return on investment and larger health gains than do programs for already healthy individuals.

Finally, Ozminkowski and others of the MEDSTAT Group published two classic studies: the first identifying a high ROI of five to one for the Healthtrac program and the second documenting major effects on health risks.[10]

These nine studies have been highly rated in a number of reviews[11] and have resulted in five C. Everett Koop National Health Awards for Healthtrac (no other program has received more than two). In summary, Healthtrac programs reduce health risks by an average of 10 to 12 percent per year and reduce medical care costs by in the first program year, with return on investment multiples of two to eight.

Development of programs of this quality has been both expensive and time consuming. Over $10 million has been expended in research and development, and the time required for performance and publication of even a single major clinical trial is four years.

SOCIETAL IMPACT

The potential impact on society is large. These programs can improve the national health, delay the development of disability with age by in excess of seven years, reduce medical care costs by 20 percent or more over time, and contribute to saving Medicare from insolvency. The programs are generalized, involve only moderate costs, and provide a return on investment of four to one or greater. Healthtrac is well positioned to achieve extremely wide diffusion, having well-documented programs, multiple best-in-class awards, and leadership in every systematic review.

BARRIERS TO WIDER DIFFUSION

Healthtrac has been ahead of its time. When it began its work, other cost-saving approaches had not yet failed. Demand-side approaches were neither well articulated nor well understood. Consumer initiatives were not popular. Strangely, the industry in which Healthtrac resides is often referred to as *health risk appraisal*, or HRA, as though the questionnaire were the product. (It's the intervention, stupid!) Instead, it's the results. It's the health improvement. It's the lower costs. The HRA "industry" was perceived as a field filled with fluff, leading to skepticism. The need- and demand-reduction field is greatly underdeveloped.

The fallacious perception that health improvement programs take years to have effects has posed a barrier. In fact, as documented in this chapter, major health and cost benefits may accrue in the first twelve months of a properly designed and executed program. This has been a Healthtrac goal from the inception of the company, but this perceived barrier has been difficult to overcome. The sales cycle for Healthtrac products to large organizations is long, and over the sales development period internal champions may move on, bureaucracies may be stifling, and middle managers may need immediate results. Healthtrac programs provide positive twelve-month results, but still there are barriers here, with a hard-to-eradicate perception that it might take a decade or more to obtain health savings from behavioral changes. The relevant scientific literature is in medical and health care research journals, with relatively little in policy journals or the economic or business literature, hence many have been underinformed about progress. Capital has not been readily available for service corporations. The Healthtrac sales staff has always been small, without sufficient entry into organizations at the CFO level or higher. (For need- and demand-reduction programs, the internal champions must be highly placed, otherwise one corporate division pays for the program and another gets the cost savings.) The market is capricious. The academic strengths of Healthtrac are formidable but have been hampered by business and marketing weaknesses.

REMOVING BARRIERS

The times are catching up. The failures of managed care are now well understood. Medical inflation has resumed and there is a paucity of new cost-containment approaches. There is fear and even desperation among the leadership of health maintenance organizations. The empowered consumer, voting for those health plans that are directed at improvement in present health and lifetime health, will be playing an increasing role.

The presence of proof acts to remove many barriers. There is now increasing recognition that peripheral benefits such as decreased workers' compensation claims, decreased absenteeism, improved morale, and decreased employee turnover are important. Professional management is now in place at Healthtrac, and software efficiencies are being developed. Interfaces to the Web are being created. Yet the future remains a difficult vision.

More recently, a number of major initiatives directed at similar goals have begun, serving to open the field. The Centers for Medicare and Medicaid Services (CMS) has created the Health of Seniors surveys, which focus on improving health outcomes. RAND has performed an evidence review of senior health promotion programs, has identified Healthtrac as the leader in the field, and has recommended large-scale demonstration projects. Healthier seniors can save Medicare financially. Only a few Medicare HMOs would need to have success in pilot need- and demand-reduction programs to result in a rapid surge in implementation among the rest. Broad Medicare approaches are now in discussion phases. "Healthy senior" bills have been introduced in both Houses of Congress. The health improvement field can now well justify investment of $100 per person per year, or approximately $30 billion per year. Health plans and corporations must learn to practice health risk management, and those that do will have a better chance of survival.

Notes

1. Vickery, D. M., Golaszewski, T. J., Wright, E. C., and Kalmer, H. "The Effect of Self-Care Interventions on the Use of Medical Services Within a Medicare Population." *Medical Care,* 1988, *26*(6), 580–588.

2. Lorig, K., Kraines, R. G., Brown, B. W., and Richardson, N. "A Workplace Health Education Program That Reduces Outpatient Visits." *Medical Care,* 1985, *23*(9), 1044–1054.

3. Vickery, D. M., and others. "Effect of a Self-Care Education Program on Medical Visits." *Journal of the American Medical Association,* 1983, *250*, 2952–2956.

4. Fries, J. F., and others. "Randomized Controlled Trial of Cost Reductions from a Health Education Program: The California Public Employees Retirement System (PERS) Study." *American Journal of Health Promotion,* 1994, *8*(3), 216–223.

5. Fries, J. F., and others. "Two-Year Results of Randomized Controlled Trial of a Health Promotion Program in a Retiree Population: The Bank of America Study." *American Journal of Medicine,* 1993, *94*, 455–462.

6. Montgomery, E. B., Lieberman, A., Singh, G., and Fries, J. F. "Patient Education and Health Promotion Can Be Effective in Parkinson's Disease: A Randomized Controlled Trial." *American Journal of Medicine,* 1994, *97*, 429-435.

7. Fries, J. F., Carey, C., and McShane, D. J. "Patient Education in Arthritis: Randomized Controlled Trial of a Mail-Delivered Program." *Journal of Rheumatology,* 1997, *24*(7), 1378–1383.

8. Fries, J. F., Fries, S. T., Parcell, C. L., and Harrington, H. "Health Risk Changes with a Low-Cost Individualized Health Promotion Program: Effects at up to 30 Months." *American Journal of Health Promotion,* 1992, *6*(5), 364–371.

9. Fries, J. F., and McShane, D. J. "Reducing Need and Demand for Medical Services in High-Risk Persons: A Health Education Approach." *Western Journal of Medicine,* 1998, *169*(4), 201–207.

10. Ozminkowski, R. J., and others. "A Return on Investment Evaluation of the Citibank Health Management Program." *American Journal of Health Promotion,* 1999, *14,* 31–43; Ozminkowski, R. J., and others. "The Impact of the Citibank Health Management Program on Changes in Employee Health Risks over Time." *Journal of Occupational and Environmental Medicine,* 2000, *42,* 502–511.

11. Pelletier, K. R. "A Review and Analysis of the Health and Cost-Effective Outcome Studies of Comprehensive Health Promotion and Disease Prevention Programs at the Worksite: 1991–1993 Update." *American Journal of Health Promotion,* 1993, *8*(1), 50–62; Aldana, S. G. "Financial Impact of Health Promotion Programs: A Comprehensive Review of the Literature." *American Journal of Health Promotion,* 2001, *15,* 296–320; Chapman, L. S. "The Role of Demand Management in Health Promotion." *The Art of Health Promotion,* 1998, *2*(4), 1–7.

CHAPTER FORTY-NINE

The Healthwise® Approach

Reinventing the Patient

Donald W. Kemper, Molly Mettler

Imagine belonging to a health care plan that will assign a special health manager to you twenty-four hours a day, seven days a week. This manager is well informed about medical science and is familiar with your personal values, preferences, and special needs. The manager's job is to help you promote health and prevent disease, make good self-care decisions at home, and work with you and your doctors to decide on which medical treatments are best for you. This personal manager is, of course, you.

THE HEALTHWISE PERSON

Think of yourself as a *Healthwise Person*. A Healthwise Person acts, competently and confidently, as a bona fide health care provider in seven areas of care:

- *Disease prevention and health promotion.* The person chooses wellness and health behaviors so that personal health risks and lifestyle preferences are clearly balanced.

- *Self-care.* The person chooses personal care for minor illnesses and injuries wherever and whenever it is needed.

- *Self-triage.* The person decides when and where to seek professional services. The decisions are based on skillful observation of symptoms and clear guidelines for assessing the urgency of care.

- *Visit preparation.* The person comes to every clinical visit well prepared to participate fully with the doctor in diagnosis and treatment.
- *Self-management.* The person takes primary responsibility for managing daily care of chronic illness.
- *Shared decision making.* The person understands the likely risks and benefits of each treatment option, factors in personal preference, and shares in making treatment decisions with the doctor.
- *End-of-life care.* The person maintains control of decisions around end-of-life care as it is needed or through advance directives.

A Healthwise Person with skills and confidence in these seven areas of care will reap significant benefits in better health outcomes, overall lower costs, and greater satisfaction. A health system that embraces this model will reap the same.

To move individuals and whole populations to this model requires a fundamental shift in the way the patient's role is perceived and practiced. The new vision reframes the traditional divide between "patient" and "provider." Rather than being seen as a passive recipient of medical services, the new health care consumer is recognized as a capable, and essential, member of the health care team, acting in partnership with physicians. Simply put, we must reinvent the patient.

THE HEALTHWISE MISSION AND MESSAGE

Healthwise, Inc. is a not-for-profit organization that has committed itself to reinventing the role of the patient. It was founded in 1975 as a consumer health information organization, and its mission is "to help people do a better job of taking care of their health problems and their health." From its beginning, its focus has been to help people and their doctors accept the role of the patient as a full partner in health care.

Believing that the health care consumer is the greatest untapped resource in the health care system, Healthwise set out to understand what consumers needed and wanted to become more actively involved in their own care. After interviews with hundreds of consumers, a clear message came through. Consumers needed and wanted

- Information on how to handle minor health problems at home
- Guidelines on when to call or visit doctors
- Instructions on how to get full value from each doctor visit

That was twenty-seven years ago. Today's consumers want much more. Consumer expectations of choice, control, and information require shifting the consumer's role from patient to partner. To effectively achieve this shift, three things are needed: a new mind-set, a new skill set, and a new tool set of information.

The Healthwise Mind-Set: Embracing the Patient-As-Partner Role

A change in role begins with mental perception. As a foundational step, people must see themselves as equipped and empowered to help make meaningful decisions. They must feel they have the ability and society's "permission" to make a difference. Creating a new mind-set in a vacuum is difficult, but the process can be accelerated once factors encouraging change are in place. Advancing this change is the emergence of the *new consumer.* According to Regina Herzlinger,[1] a new consumer is someone with analytical sophistication (at least one year of college coursework), financial flexibility, and access to a variety of health information resources. Since 1978, the percentage of the American population that can be described as new consumers has grown from 25 percent to 45 percent. New consumers are expected to be a majority, 52 percent, by 2005.[2]

Changes in the medical professional mind-set are also expected. Studies conducted by Healthwise indicate that two-thirds of health care providers support working with engaged and involved patients, up from one-third twenty years ago. Healthwise's physician seminars and continuing medical education courses in doctor-patient partnerships are key in gaining provider buy-in and support for the patient-as-partner role. Physicians see these expectations expressed by more of their patients each day, and they are moving toward a shared decision-making model (some more rapidly than others).

The Healthwise Skill Set: Self-Care and Shared Decision Making

Once people accept the patient-as-partner role, they need to develop skills to play it out in a way that has impact. People can develop their self-care, self-triage, and shared decision-making skills through workshops, written guidelines, interactive tools, and other communications. Ideally, these skills are developed and used over a lifetime for both major and minor problems. When people begin practicing self-care and shared decision making for minor and acute problems, they can build on that experience later if more significant health problems develop. It is more challenging (but by no means impossible) to develop the skills required once one is facing a life-threatening diagnosis of cancer, heart disease, or a similarly serious condition.

Physicians, too, must learn a skill set of communication approaches to reinforce and support patient partnership. For example, in the health care of today and tomorrow, skills for prescribing information are becoming as important as skills for prescribing medications.

The Healthwise Tool Set: Access to Evidence-Based Information

People need access to reliable and bias-free health information to complete the transition from passive patient to active partner. Since 1976, Healthwise has published basic self-care guides, the *Healthwise Handbook* and *Healthwise for Life,* to increase the level of medical information in the home.[3] Millions of copies of these books are in print—enough for one in every ten households in America. Special editions are also used in Canada, South Africa, and the United Kingdom. The books provide user-friendly guidelines to help with self-care and self-triage decisions for most common symptoms.

However, today's patient-as-partner wants and needs far more information for the myriad of health problems than can be covered in a single book. The Internet provides a partial solution. However, even though the Web has made boatloads of health resources available to anyone with a computer and modem, not all medical information is created equal. On the thousands of Internet resources for cancer, for example, treatment advice can range from psychic surgery to the evidence-based guidelines from the National Cancer Institute. The Internet's boundless information is not coupled with boundless quality.

For laypeople the challenge rests in getting consumer-friendly, evidence-based information for each *decision point* that arises in the treatment and management of a health condition. Healthwise began the daunting task of building such a database in 1992. The *Healthwise Knowledgebase®*, a comprehensive, electronic, consumer-health database, now includes many succinctly written consumer health entries covering virtually all symptoms, conditions, medical tests, and medications. The *Knowledgebase* is used on the World Wide Web, in nurse call centers, and on intranet systems.

Putting It All Together: Using Information as Therapy

The emergence of the new medical consumer with new information technologies provides us with the capacity to treat information as therapy. Consider *prescription information:* the delivery of specific medical information to a specific person, at a specific time, for a specific purpose. Like prescriptions for medications, information prescriptions can be written at different dose levels, presented in different forms, and repeated at different frequencies. They can also be written as standard orders that are executed whenever the patient criteria match the criteria specified in the orders.

Healthwise has developed the concept of *information therapy* to help physicians and health care systems assist patients in getting the information most likely to help them make better decisions. Information therapy is "the prescription of specific, evidence-based medical information to a specific patient, caregiver, or consumer at just the right time to help them make a specific health decision or behavior change."[4]

There are three ways to get information therapy: via physician to patient communication through hand-held order-entry computers and secure messaging, via systems applications piggybacked on lab reports, medication prescriptions, scheduling confirmations, or preauthorization notices, and of course via the effort and input of the consumer herself. Once the electronic medical record and physician order-entry systems are in place, information prescriptions can be launched with only a few taps on a PDA (personal digital assistant). The ease and effectiveness of supplying such information prescriptions will redefine the role of information from being *about* care to being an essential *part* of care.

THREE CHANNELS FOR DEVELOPING THE PATIENT-AS-PROVIDER

Healthwise employs three channels for reaching consumers with its patient-as-partner message: institutional markets (health plans, hospitals, and employers), the community, and the Internet.

The Institutional Channel

To date, most consumers access Healthwise services via their health plan or self-insured employer. The mission of Healthwise is often aligned with both the desires of the consumer or employee for better information and the goals of the plan or payer for improved utilization decisions. The rise of capitated care has provided the impetus for payers and plans to redefine the role of the patient. Kaiser Permanente, for example, has purchased *Healthwise Handbooks* for every member household nationwide. Similar commitments to providing handbooks to members have been made by Group Health Cooperative of Puget Sound, Aetna/US Health care, Medica, CIGNA, Harvard-Pilgrim Health Plan, and many other health insurers and HMOs. Some clients have integrated the self-care books with the *Healthwise Knowledgebase* through telephone-based nurse care counseling services and Web-based interactive information sources. Icons in the text of the books refer readers to plan-sponsored call centers and Web sites when additional information is available to support improved decision making.

The Community Channel

Working with health plans enables Healthwise to reach millions of people quickly and efficiently. However, that approach leaves out many uninsured people who could also benefit from access to good consumer health information. In 1996, Healthwise began a three-year demonstration project with a quarter of a million Idahoans living in four counties. The purpose of the program was to "create the best informed, most empowered medical consumers on earth" and to show the impact a "patient partnership" program could make on a community-wide basis. With funding from the Robert Wood Johnson Foundation, regional health plans and hospitals, and local employers, the Healthwise Communities Project (HCP) set out to create the mind-set, skill set, and tool set needed for self-care and shared care. The program began with a distribution of handbooks to the 126,000 households in the area. Six months later, access to the *Healthwise Knowledgebase* was made available through a nurse call center, a Web site, and computer kiosks set up in libraries and physician offices.

Because the project was population-wide, we could use mass communication tools (billboards and radio, TV, and newspaper ads and editorials) and direct contact with physicians to engender support. All sectors of the community embraced the goal of helping to create the smartest health care consumers on earth. Successes from this project have encouraged replication efforts in South Carolina.

The Internet

Healthwise also distributes its evidence-based content via popular public Web sites. On the Internet the content can be linked to self-help groups, interactive assessments, personalized home pages, and customized medical news services in order to fully meet the needs of the new health care consumer.

COST AND QUALITY OUTCOMES

The three most critical questions about the outcomes of the Healthwise program are: Do people use the resources (books and electronic database)? Are costs reduced? Is quality increased?

Do People Use the Resources?

The answer to the first question is "definitely" for the books—client studies show that 69 to 75 percent of *Healthwise Handbook* recipients use the book within the first six months of receiving it.[5] This number increases (up to 90 percent) as the program continues.[6] The rate of use is affected by the degree to which providers and mass media can be employed to reinforce use of the book, as shown by the community-based programs piloted in Idaho and South Carolina. By the end of the project in 1999, out of every ten Idaho households in a six-month period:[7]

- Nine reported having a medical reference book.
- Seven used the book to self-treat a symptom or health problem. The average number of uses was 3.5 per six-month period.
- Four households reported saving at least one visit to the doctor.
- Two households saved at least one emergency room visit.

The Partners Health Initiative in Anderson, South Carolina, reported similar findings from its community-based project, which supplied 154,000 families with Healthwise information.[8] Among the general population:

- Twenty-three percent reported saving an unnecessary trip to the doctor.
- Thirteen percent saved an unnecessary visit to the ER.
- An estimated $21 million was saved in eighteen months, through reductions in unnecessary doctor and emergency room visits.
- Sixteen percent of sponsoring organization employees said they saved a sick day from work.
- The underinsured and uninsured were the greatest users of the Healthwise information.
- Use of the Healthwise information increased over time, from 36 percent at six months to 40 percent at eighteen months.

Industry reports on triage-type, call center services indicate a standard 10 percent usage rate among the target population. With the HCP community-based care counseling line, calls were taken from over 20,000 families, or 15.8 percent of the population. The books, which were linked graphically to the Web site, were distributed twelve months into the study. With this added enhancement the rate of Web use increased by 2.44 percent.[9]

Also, a survey of local Idaho physicians showed that 91 percent wanted the *Healthwise Handbook* in their exam rooms and that 83 percent wanted their patients to have access to the *Healthwise Knowledgebase.*[10]

Are Costs Reduced?

Costs associated with utilization are clearly affected. In a review study of many self-care program models, visits to physician offices were reduced by 7 to 24 percent.[11] Healthwise programs have been associated with reductions in total clinic visits of 9 to 13 percent.[12] One study tracked a 31 percent decrease in visits for time-limited symptoms.[13] Another saw a reduction of 12.2 percent for primary care visits and 17.1 percent for urgent care visits.[14] Emergency room usage is affected as well. In the community model, Blue Cross of Idaho tracked an 18 percent reduction in ER claims;[15] Kaiser recorded a 15.4 percent reduction in ER visits.[16]

Is Quality Increased?

Quality is enhanced when patients obtain the right level of care, at the right place, at the right time. For some that means taking care of a minor problem at home; for others it means getting to professional care early enough and quickly enough to avert larger problems. Overall, reductions in phone calls to clinics and in urgent care, primary care, and ER visits seem to indicate that educated patients are handling their health issues with a greater degree of confidence and competence. In light of customer satisfaction, Kaiser polled its membership on their overall opinion of the plan after receiving their self-care book—58 percent of respondents indicated that their overall opinion of Kaiser increased after receiving the *Healthwise Handbook*.[17]

CHALLENGES TO MAINSTREAM REPLICATION

We have observed at least four major barriers that will have to be overcome before approaches of the Healthwise type can become widespread.

Patient and Physician Resistance

Change in the traditional doctor-patient relationship will come slowly to some. Although many new consumers are demanding a more central role in decision making, others are content with the status quo. Physicians cannot abruptly shift paradigms for fear of leaving many patients behind. Any transition must allow for patient-specific flexibility. Physicians, too, are spread out on a continuum of readiness for change. Moreover, moving too far, too fast can create resistance.

Money

Health care budgets are under siege. Even when substantial savings are proven, if the benefits fall to one group in an organization and the costs go to another, the organization may not be able to find a compelling reason to implement the program. Health plans working under capitation agreements with physician groups, for example, have few short-term incentives to reduce costs. To overcome these barriers, additional evaluation studies must show that the savings are substantial, continuing, and relevant to the economic success of program sponsors.

Reimbursement Models

Provider incentives are still tied largely to volume, not quality, and to efficiency, not consumer empowerment. As long as reimbursement is based on episodes of care, encouraging providers to maximize patient volumes, there will be significant barriers to adopting a patient-as-provider model.

Employment-Based Health Care Coverage

Because U.S. health care coverage is neither universal nor portable, there is little incentive to invest in prevention or early intervention for employees who are likely to drop their enrollment before long-term savings can be realized. And what is the likelihood of our seeing more community-based models, in which everyone, insured or not, participates? It remains to be seen whether such models can be sustained without a heavy infusion of exploratory, foundation-based funding.

THE NEW GENERATION

Self-care and shared decision making are important to today's health care. As they evolve, the patient is placed at the center of his or her own health care system. As the individual consumer gains mastery over health and medical choices and behaviors, the health care system will become a *system of one*, which will adjust to each patient's individual profile, learning styles, special needs, interests, risks, and past history.

Clearly, the role of the patient will be far different from traditional models and also more complex as we proceed into the twenty-first century. The themes of patient-as-partner, information as therapy, and patient mastery over health will define a reinvented role for the patient—and with that role, a reinvented health care system.

Notes

1. Herzlinger, R. E. *Market-Driven Health Care: Who Wins, Who Loses in the Transformation of America's Largest Service Industry.* Reading, Mass.: Addison-Wesley, 1997.

2. Herzlinger, *Market Driven Health Care.*

3. Kemper, D. W., and Healthwise Staff. *Healthwise Handbook: A Self-Care Guide for You.* (15th ed.) Boise, Idaho: Healthwise, Inc., 1997; Mettler, M. K., and Kemper, D. W. *Healthwise for Life: Medical Self-Care for People Age 50 and Better.* (4th ed.) Boise, Idaho: Healthwise, Inc., 2000.

4. Kemper, D. W., and Mettler, M. K. "Information Therapy: Prescribed Information as a Reimbursable Medical Service." Boise, Idaho: Healthwise, Inc., 2002; also see [www.informationtherapy.org].

5. Hibbard, J., and Greenlick, M. *Idaho Community Health Survey Follow-Up.* Portland: Oregon Health Sciences University, 1997; PacifiCare of Colorado. *Healthwise Medical Self-Care Program: Executive Summary.* Englewood, Colo.: PacifiCare of Colorado, 1995; Health Net. *Healthwise Medical Self-Care Program Executive Summary.* Woodland Hills, Calif.: Health Net, 1994.

6. Larson, P. "The Kaiser Permanente Self-Care Program." In *17th International Conference Official Proceedings.* Reading, U.K.: International Federation of Health Funds, 1998.

7. Oregon Health Sciences University. *Final Grant Report.* Healthwise Evaluation Project: Robert Wood Johnson Foundation Grant ID #027929, May 1, 1996, to November 30, 1999. Portland: Oregon Health Sciences University, 1999.

8. Except as discussed in this note, these consumer-reported data were supplied by Partners Health Initiative, Anderson, South Carolina. The six-month figure was provided by Clemson University; the eighteen-month figure by InSights Consulting.

9. Healthwise. *Final Grant Report.* Healthwise Communities Project, September 1, 1995–August 31, 1998. Boise, Idaho: Healthwise, Inc., 1998.

10. Hibbard, J., and Greenlick, M. *Healthwise Evaluation Physician Interviews: Summer 1997 Detailed Report.* Portland: Oregon Health Sciences University, 1997.

11. Kemper, D. W., Lorig, K., and Mettler, M. "The Effectiveness of Medical Self-Care Interventions: A Focus on Self-Initiated Responses to Symptoms." *Patient Education and Counseling,* 1992, *21,* 29–39.

12. Elsens, V. D., Marquardt, C., and Bledsoe, T. "Use of Self-Care Manual Shifts Utilization Patterns." *HMO Practice,* June 1995, pp. 88–90; Larson, "The Kaiser Permanente Self-Care Program."

13. Elsens and others, "Use of Self-Care Manual Shifts Utilization Patterns."

14. Larson, "The Kaiser Permanente Self-Care Program."

15. Sternberg, L. "Healthwise Handbook Impact Study." Boise, Idaho: Blue Cross of Idaho, 1998.

16. Larson, "The Kaiser Permanente Self-Care Program."

17. Larson, "The Kaiser Permanente Self-Care Program."

PART FOUR

INNOVATIVE CONSUMER-DRIVEN SOLUTIONS TO CHRONIC PROBLEMS

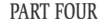

The failures of the health care system are legion: unwarranted variability in the delivery of services, lack of focus on chronic diseases and disabilities, insufficient consumer involvement, inappropriate use of technology, and hard-core managerial shortcomings.

For many years, these problems have been documented and countless solutions have been proposed.

But the solutions have not worked.

Why do I make this bold statement?

Because the failures continue inexorably. Just read today's newspaper. It is filled with health care failures, no?

The authors of the chapters in Part Four of this volume not only document the problems but also illustrate the effective, consumer-driven solutions they have studied or implemented to correct them. The problems they analyze are of the chronic variety: unexplained variability in care; inattention to consumer-driven health promotion, especially for chronic care; and indifference to managerial concerns. The solutions they present are innovative. They fall into the categories of focused health care factories that concentrate on treating all the manifestations of one disease or disability and thus reduce variability in treatment; providers and executives who concentrate on managerial issues in various organizational settings; and visionary scientists and engineers who create patient-centered drugs.

These innovative solutions reduce variability, support self-care, and emphasize the role of management. Innovations like these will be widely supported in a consumer-driven health care system that will enable consumers to seek out the reliable, well-managed delivery systems and technologies that focus on their needs.

THE PROBLEMS

The three chapters that begin Part Four document the problems. Michael Millenson, author of *Demanding Medical Excellence*, dramatizes the extent and impact of the unreasonable variability in the process of delivering health care (Chapter Fifty); Jessie Gruman, CEO of the Center for the Advancement of Health, and her colleague, Cynthia Gibson, delineate the need for consumer-focused solutions to chronic diseases (Chapter Fifty-One); and Harvard Business School professors Richard Bohmer, Amy Edmondson, and Gary Pisano discuss the role of mismanagement in causing the medical errors usually attributed to the adoption of new technologies (Chapter Fifty-Two).

Many health policy experts turn up their noses at the work of these innovators. To them, only a centrally controlled system can right these wrongs. For example, at one meeting, a health policy expert doubted the managerial accomplishments of the chain hospitals, claiming that they only knew how to raise their prices. I hope that the persuasive details contained in these chapters will help to reverse such dismissive views of the powers of management.

These problems are pervasive and solutions, as the chapters throughout this book demonstrate, are clear. So why do the problems persist? Because the current typical solutions require the imposition of one person's ideas on another person. Consider the following vignette:

We were eating dinner in an elegant restaurant in the suburbs of one of the great cities of the United States—the brilliant CEO of the country's most successful health insurance company, the able head of his small-group division, and me. The CEO, daringly bucking conventional opinion, had introduced a large variety of health insurance plans for small-employer groups and individuals. They had been enormously successful. But my interests were not only on this area.

"How can you help to control the underlying costs and quality problems of health care?" I asked. "After all, most of these are with chronic diseases."

"Oh, we can do it," he answered readily. "We have guidelines and protocols for virtually all chronic diseases. We have carve-outs too, for those who want to take them on."

"How well do they work?" I asked.

"The doctors, nurses, and patients should comply with our guidelines, but frequently they do not.

"But I'm sanguine about the future," he noted. "I think Web-based disease management will help considerably with the compliance problem."

His statement turned on two of my red alerts:

The *should* alert.

The *compliance* alert.

In the real world, solutions that work are not *imposed* on the sources of the problem. Instead, they are developed *organically* by those suffering the problem and those who created it. For example, the U.S. automobile industry did not re-create itself by *complying* with *should*s promulgated by the insurance sector. It re-created itself through massive internal restructuring, led by feedback from tough consumer groups and ferocious competition.

THE SOLUTIONS

In a consumer-driven health care system, consumer-provider teams will evolve solutions that

- *Reduce unwarranted variability in medical practice.* The reduction in the unwarranted variability in health care treatment must come from providers—not from those who seek to impose guidelines on them—and from the consumers who evaluate the success of different solutions for themselves.

- *Implement effective integration in the management of chronic diseases.* The focus on chronic diseases must come, not from outside microman-agers, but from providers who can stitch together integrated, focused factories, guided by the individuals who have catastrophic or chronic diseases and who long for a focused approach.

- *Enable joint decisions on the appropriate use of technology.* The appropri-ate use of technology must be resolved by those employing the technol-ogy and by those who evaluate the technology's access and price.

- *Reward well-managed providers.* As the problems of managed care illus-trate, the mismanagement of health care organizations can best be cor-rected by a bottom-up approach involving providers and the consumers of their services, not by hectoring, top-down consultants and auditors.

The bulk of the chapters in Part Four address the vision behind the neces-sary solutions, the service providers who are already organizing focused facto-ries and other focused models of health care, and the technology providers.

The Visions

The vision of collaborative, focused health care services is illuminated in three chapters. Alfred (Al) Lewis, executive director of the Disease Management Purchasing Consortium and founder of the Disease Management Association of America, explains how to reduce the barriers standing in the way of innovative solutions (Chapter Fifty-Three). Physician entrepreneur Bernard Salick, chairman and CEO of Bentley Health Care, and his colleague Seth Yellin, an associate director at UBS Warburg, describe visionary solutions for health care for the chronically ill (Chapter Fifty-Four); and Robert Levine, a physician and the volunteer chair of the Juvenile Diabetes Research Foundation, and his colleague Laura Adams, a consultant and a faculty member at the Institute for Health care Improvement, discuss how to drive the medical research that can provide high-quality care for catastrophic illness (Chapter Fifty-Five). For example, future health care consumers will play new, pivotal roles in prioritizing a medical research agenda that focuses on their needs, rather than solely on the researchers' professional priorities, and will serve as screeners and evaluators of research outcomes.

Focused Factors—Innovative, Consumer-Driven Health Care Service Providers

The next twelve chapters by providers and respondents offer many examples of provider-led initiatives that have reduced variability, focused on chronic diseases, and revamped management approaches, all while working in conjunction with the customer.

One of the most pressing present-day health care problems lies in the treatment of chronic diseases. Management of these diseases is unnecessarily inefficient and ineffective because providers are not integrated and focused on the needs of the patient. The problem is of great financial significance because chronic diseases account for around three-quarters of U.S. health care costs, an amount that in 2002 hovered around one trillion dollars. The creators of organizations that specialize in the treatment of diseases or on performing specific procedures as effectively and efficiently as possible, *focused health care factories* in my nomenclature, are working to remedy this problem.

In Chapter Fifty-Six, world-renowned heart surgeon Denton Cooley, president and surgeon-in-chief of the Texas Heart Institute, and John Adams Jr., president and CEO of CardioVascular Care Providers, describe how they lowered the cost and improved the quality of cardiovascular procedures by providing bundled, focused care. They emphasize the key role of doctors in creating this system.

In Chapter Fifty-Seven, Lynn Taussig, president and CEO of National Jewish Medical and Research Center, and David Tinkelman, vice president of health initiatives at National Jewish, explain how focus and consumer empowerment revolutionized their hospital's care. For example, the hospital's consumer-focused asthma program includes nurses who visit patients in their houses.

In Chapter Fifty-Eight, Daryl Urquhart, health care management consultant at Shouldice Hospital, and Alan O'Dell, managing director at Shouldice, document how the hospital's focus on hernia procedures and patient-empowering techniques (*mental medicine* in their term) lowered costs, increased quality, and caused such unequaled customer loyalty that "alumni" annually throng a reunion that celebrates their hernia operations.

And in Chapters Fifty-Nine and Sixty, respectively, Stuart Lovett, chief of obstetric and gynecologic service at Hill Physicians Medical Group, a California IPA, and Robert Stone, executive vice president of American Healthways, a disease management firm, explain how their associations achieve goals that participating members likely could not have achieved on their own. Lovett explains how his IPA reduced costs and raised quality (as measured in reduced suffering, pain, and days of work missed) by focusing on specific gynecological diseases within its network. Stone, in turn, details how patient- and physician-empowering techniques dramatically helped the cardiovascular and diabetic outcomes of his firm's patients.

Currently, providers of focused services are not favored by insurance firms. The insurers fear that if they cover care by these experts in the management of chronic diseases, they will draw the chronically ill to their fold (as Alfred Lewis explains in Chapter Fifty-Three). But a consumer-driven health care system will reward such experts—through the risk-adjustment mechanisms described in Parts One and Two and because empowered patients will naturally seek them out.

But is a focus on health care needs from the consumers' point of view sufficient to guarantee higher quality and lower costs?

Apparently not.

In discussing management issues in Chapter Fifty-Two, Richard Bohmer, Amy Edmondson, and Gary Pisano illustrate that the usual explanations of high-quality health care—volume and academic medical center affiliation—do not predict the success rates of the new, complex surgical procedure they studied. Ironically, the highest success rates were achieved in a small community hospital. The secret? Managerial focus, as demonstrated by an intense interest in the surgical process. Managerial detail piled on managerial detail led to success: a surgical team devoted solely to the process, continual measurement of the results, debriefing sessions to learn from the success and failures, and constant training and improvement.

What organizational settings can provide the managerial resources needed to replicate the successes of focused organizations? A number of large, management-intensive settings commend themselves: horizontally integrated chains, multi-specialty physician practices, group HMOs, and academic medical centers are the four most natural environments in which to replicate focused factories.

In Chapter Sixty-One, Thomas Frist Jr., the cofounder and retired CEO of Hospital Corporation of America (HCA), the country's largest hospital chain, presents dramatic examples of the power of a chain and lucid explanations of how these results are achieved. HCA's chain structure enables substantial economies of scale in information, human resources, purchasing, and capital, as well as expansion to new services that are not feasible in a stand-alone setting.

In Chapter Sixty-Two, then–associate medical director Les Zendle explains how Southern California Kaiser Permanente uses vertical integration to manage the care of people with chronic diseases and to empower patients. For patients with diabetes, kidney and heart disease, asthma, and HIV/AIDS, Kaiser's programs have raised quality of care and decreased costs. All the programs have a major emphasis on education, self-care, and information dissemination.

The management task faced by Vanderbilt University Medical Center was to bring medical research and training to bear on health care delivery in order to reduce variability of care, improve care quality, and lower care costs. In Chapter Sixty-Three, Harry Jacobson, vice chancellor for health affairs at Vanderbilt, describes the role played in this effort by excellent care management and information systems.

And in Chapter Sixty-Four, Brandeis University assistant professor Jody Hoffer Gittell provides statistical evidence that focus in health care service delivery results in quality and efficiency. She also theorizes that providers working in focused environments with defined patient populations develop relationships among themselves that improve care coordination.

Are physicians aware of the burdens that consumer-driven health care will place on them? Three respondents address this issue. James Rodgers, vice president of health policy at the American Medical Association, feels that consumer-driven health care will prove helpful to physicians and is widely anticipated by them (Chapter Sixty-Five). Roger Bulger, a physician and CEO of the American Association of Academic Health Centers, explains how this association can promulgate consumer-driven health care among its member academic medical centers with the vision of a "learning integrated delivery system" that can correct the health care system's chronic problems (Chapter Sixty-Six). And investment banker François Maisonrouge, co-head of the Global Health Care-Life Sciences Group at Credit Suisse/First Boston, predicts an enormous, viable investment opportunity in the shift to consumer-driven health care, although he also raises concerns about the timing of this shift and about the cost-controlling efficacy of consumer-driven health care (Chapter Sixty-Seven).

Innovative, Consumer-Driven Health Care Technology Providers

Last, technology can also help ameliorate the problems associated with treating chronic disease. Because the etiology of most chronic diseases is typically unknown, therapies are broadly based and not tailored for the individual. As a result they may be unnecessarily forceful or timid. For example, some percentage of those who take a given drug will not find it effective, and the chemotherapy drugs used to poison cancer cells should in some cases optimally be administered in much smaller doses. The new science of genomics offers hope not only of discovering the genetic origins of chronic diseases but also of developing drugs tailored for the specific genetic metabolic needs of the individual.

Two leaders of medical technology firms demonstrate how technology can enable a consumer-driven health care system. In Chapters Sixty-Eight and Sixty-Nine, respectively, Tony White, chairman and CEO of Applera, a firm that helped to unravel the human genome, and Mark Levin, chairperson and CEO of Millennium Pharmaceuticals, Inc., write of the promise of genomics to tailor diagnosis, therapy, and technology to our unique characteristics.

CHAPTER FIFTY

The Role of Providers

Michael L. Millenson

Popular misconceptions notwithstanding, variation from the *right care* is not the sole province of physicians who are either unskilled or poorly trained. Rather it is the natural consequence of a health care system that systematically tracks neither processes nor outcomes, preferring to believe that good facilities, good intentions, and good training lead ineluctably to good results. Many physicians remain more comfortable with the habits of a guild, where each craftsman trusts his fellows, than with the demands of the information age.

A veteran internist who consults on quality improvement recalled his experience when putting together a care guideline for physicians at a four-hundred-bed hospital in California:

> We sat down with the cardiologists, a small group. They said, "We're high quality, we're all doing everything right." Then you do the [patient medical] chart audit, and you discover only 30 percent of the congestive heart failure patients who should be getting ACE inhibitors are getting them.
>
> And that [problem] didn't include the unnecessary tests and redundant tests the doctors were ordering.[1]

Research for this chapter was supported in part by an Investigator Award in Health Policy Research from the Robert Wood Johnson Foundation.

If variation is hard for doctors to see, it is well-nigh invisible to patients. In the absence of hard data, ignorance is bliss. The physician firmly believes that "quality of care is what *I* provide," and the patient is equally convinced that "*my* doctor provides good care." Indeed, whatever the failings of doctors in general, "to distrust one's [own] doctor is to be vulnerable in the most fundamental and undesirable of ways."[2] Yet variation remains a central problem of U.S. medicine. It surfaces in study after study, in disease after disease. Because patients do not write their own prescriptions or order their own surgery or tests, providers must take the lead in addressing the problem. Their role is to move the system to a *best-care* state by eliminating inappropriate variation.

This does not mean treating patients like interchangeable parts, nor does it imply an expectation of perfect results. *Inappropriate* variation is variation unrelated to scientific uncertainty, individual patient needs, or so-called common cause variation within defined parameters. Inappropriate variation can also involve a failure to include the patient's preferences or values in a decision. Put simply, the right care will balance physician autonomy with equally necessary physician accountability.

Unfortunately, physicians have historically believed that attempts to standardize practice pose a bigger threat to patients than unchecked autonomy. That belief is deeply rooted in economic and cultural factors.

PROVIDER BARRIERS TO CHANGE: "IN MY HEART, I KNOW I'M RIGHT"

The Flexner Report has been called the most important document in the history of American medicine.[3] Issued in 1910, it called for overhauling medical education as it existed then and for basing that education on a standard scientific curriculum. The Flexner Report "insisted on the fundamentally scientific nature of medicine, on the pursuit of excellence and on the inadmissibility of ignorance, sham and fraudulent claims," wrote Jeremiah Barondess, president of the New York Academy of Medicine, in 1990.[4]

Of course, most patients of the time presumed that *their* doctor was scientific already. As playwright George Bernard Shaw acidly put it in the 1913 introduction to his play, *The Doctor's Dilemma:* "I presume nobody will question the existence of a widely spread popular delusion that every doctor is a man of science. . . . To a sufficiently ignorant man, every captain of a trading schooner is a Galileo, every organ-grinder a Beethoven. . . . As a matter of fact, the rank and file of doctors are no more scientific than their tailors; or, if you prefer to put it the reverse way, their tailors are no less scientific than they."

Still, standardizing medical education was very different from trying to standardize how doctors practiced. Around the same time Flexner was active, Ernest

Amory Codman proposed to have all U.S. hospitals measure the "end results" of their care. Codman, a Harvard-trained surgeon, even wanted hospitals to share those findings with patients(!). For his troubles he ended his days as an ostracized and penurious gadfly. Codman's insights into his failure are relevant even today. Although he saw what we would call best care as a prerequisite for hospital "efficiency," he also understood the economic disincentives for those whose actual results might belie their reputations. He wrote: "For whose *interest* is it to have the hospital efficient? Strangely enough, the answer is: No one. . . . There is a difference between interest and duty. You do your duty if the work comes to you, but you do not go out of your way to get the work unless it is for your interest."[5]

That economic wisdom from the early twentieth century remains important at the dawn of the twenty-first. In addition, Codman faced, as today's crusaders for best care still do, substantial cultural barriers. Doctors act as a consulting profession, not a scholarly one. As medical sociologist Eliot Freidson has pointed out, their training emphasizes personal intuition rather than the careful testing of assumptions and biases: "The model of the clinician . . . encourage[s] individual deviation from codified knowledge on the basis of personal, first-hand observation of concrete cases. This deviation is called 'judgment' or even 'wisdom' . . . since it is intimately bound up with the personal life of the knower . . . it is no wonder it has a dogmatic edge to it, resisting contradiction by embarrassing facts and contorting itself to reconcile contradictions."[6] And he added, "So long as [the profession] emphasizes good intentions rather than good performance . . . the profession cannot really regulate itself."[7]

And it has not. Personal preferences still reign supreme. Back in 1934, the American Child Health Study showed that "variation is not so much due to the differences in the conditions of the children as to differences in the viewpoint and standards of the [physicians]."[8]

Some sixty years later, in 1991, "only" one in four tonsillectomies was still inappropriate.[9]

In 1953, an article reviewing more than 6,000 hysterectomies presented a horrifying picture of hundreds of women of childbearing years who received no preoperative diagnosis or were diagnosed with a vague symptom such as "pain." Overall four in ten hysterectomies were inappropriate.[10]

Although the overall hysterectomy rate is now down, large pockets of doubtful surgery remain. A review by General Motors Corporation of areas in which it has plants found that the 1995 hysterectomy rate in Anderson, Indiana, for women aged forty-five to sixty-four was nearly twice that for GM employees as a whole and 60 percent greater than the rate for a similar population in the Flint, Michigan, area. Although the rate has declined somewhat, in 1997 the GM hysterectomy rate overall was 8.5 per 1,000, the Anderson rate was 13.2 per 1,000, and the National Committee for Quality Assurance (NCQA) benchmark rate was 9.2 per 1,000.[11]

In 1984, leaders of the medical profession promised to make practice variation a major priority after Congress and the news media focused on the variation studies of Dartmouth's John Wennberg.[12] But when public pressure faded, "interest" reverted to "duty," a synonym for apathy. In 1999, the third edition of Wennberg's *Dartmouth Atlas of Health Care* still concluded that "geography is destiny" when it comes to determining the likely treatment for a particular condition. Other data buttress those conclusions: even in Department of Veterans Affairs hospitals, with salaried doctors and similar patients, there are widespread geographical differences in both inpatient and outpatient care.[13]

Practice varies both when the treatment evidence is inconclusive and when it is not. A review of the recent medical literature by RAND Corporation researchers found that just half of patients receive the preventive care the literature recommends. Only 60 percent of those with chronic conditions get the treatments recommended by the medical literature, and 20 percent get contraindicated care. Even for patients with acute conditions, where our health care system takes particular pride in its performance, the numbers fall far short of any reasonable definition of excellence: 70 percent of acute-care patients receive the treatments the medical literature says they should, and 30 percent receive contraindicated care.[14]

In light of this and other evidence, a series of expert panels and commissions have sounded the alarm about both the prevalence and depth of quality problems in U.S. medicine. The drumbeat began in 1998 with the Institute of Medicine (IOM) National Roundtable on Health Care Quality and President Clinton's Advisory Commission on Consumer Protection and Quality,[15] and it has grown louder with the 2001 release of the IOM report *Crossing the Quality Chasm.* "Health care today harms too frequently and routinely fails to deliver its potential benefits. . . . Between the health care we have and the care we could have lies not just a gap, but a chasm," said the IOM report. It added, "Millions fail to receive effective care."[16]

The effect on patients of providers' cultural and economic barriers to change has been exacerbated by provider unwillingness to share information or decision-making power. However, patient power is an evolving, and accelerating, phenomenon.

PATIENT EMPOWERMENT

The "beneficence" of the physician toward the patient has often worked better in theory than in practice, as Jay Katz relates in his classic work *The Silent World of Doctor and Patient.*[17] It took a 1905 decision by the U.S. Supreme Court to establish a patient's right to know in advance what surgical procedure a doctor was planning to perform. The case involved a forty-eight-year-old woman with epilepsy whose surgeon removed her uterus and ovaries without telling her because he feared she would resist. Although the surgeon said he acted for her own good, the court ruled that the rights of a free citizen forbid "a physician or surgeon, however skillful or eminent . . . to violate without permission the bodily integrity of his patient . . . and [to operate] on him without his consent or knowledge." Nonetheless, it was not until 1957, in a ruling by the California Court of Appeals, that patients acquired the legal right to be told not only what the doctor was going to do but also the possible adverse effects. The case involved a fifty-five-year-old man whose legs were left paralyzed after a diagnostic procedure. Only in the 1970s did court rulings compel physicians to disclose in plain English not just what they were going to do (the process of care) but also the evidence about its likely effect on the patient's life (the outcome).

Adding insult to injury has been the insistence by some physicians that it is they who are controlled by patients. Decades of unneeded tonsillectomies? A response to patient demand. Decades of questionable hysterectomies? "Often time patients prefer to be operated upon; they get well quicker if an operation is done which is not really necessary," one surgeon explained.[18]

The mechanisms by which patients in the 1970s began to take back power offer insights into ways to overcome the present barriers to provider behavior change and move toward best care.

CHANGING BEHAVIOR

Eisenberg has written that physicians, like other adult learners, quickly slip back into old habits when reinforcement stops.[19] And so the question quickly becomes how to induce best performance among the great mass of physicians already possessed of best intentions, as Freidson might put it.

One way, of course, is to provide a steady stream of information that supports change. For example, since 1997, the Agency for Healthcare Research and Quality (formerly the Agency for Health Care Policy and Research) has funded twelve evidence-based practice centers that review the clinical literature and then produce reports and recommendations for the profession and for policymakers. In a similar vein, professional societies have regularly begun churning out evidence-based recommendations to their members on everything from beta blocker use after a heart attack (the American Medical Association) to the use of patient-generated information to improve the appropriate use of prostate surgery (the American Urological Association).

It is possible that the dead trees needed to produce the paper these efforts will consume will also produce fewer dead patients. Possible, but not likely, absent some other reinforcing mechanism. Fortunately, a number of these mechanisms exist.

Legal Actions

In the 1970s, newly formed consumer organizations such as the Public Citizen Health Research Group fought back against physician-sponsored laws that prohibited "information that would point out differences between doctors." Since then the possible causes of action have advanced. In 1999, a photographer-artist who had displayed her mastectomy-scarred chest on the cover of the *New York Times Magazine* won a $2.2 million legal judgment because her doctor had not disclosed that a lumpectomy might have been adequate treatment.[20] Interestingly, a study presented to the American Society of Clinical Oncology in early 1998 found that just 44 percent of women with breast cancer received breast-conserving surgery (BCT)—a synonym for lumpectomy—even though 75 percent of women were likely eligible. The study concluded that surgeons' "misunderstanding" of professional society guidelines on lumpectomy appropriateness "is a major factor responsible for low national rates of BCT."[21]

Lumpectomy versus mastectomy is not the only area in which misunderstanding guidelines might raise legal issues. For instance, although some doctors blame patients for pushing them to prescribe unneeded antibiotics,[22] patients' pleadings often seem curiously ineffective when it comes to chronic pain control. Angry activists have already begun Web sites.[23] Might legal action follow? Similarly, NCQA notes that more than 875 cases of blindness would be prevented each year "if all health plans were performing at the 90th percentile benchmark" for providing eye exams for diabetics.[24] How long might it be till failure to reach a benchmark level is actionable?

On the downside, lawsuits are a blunt instrument that can have negative consequences that ultimately retard progress. Moreover, legal mandates can be finessed. Doctors seeking legally required informed consent routinely seek to influence the patient's choice. Notes medical ethicist Howard Brody: "Talking *with* patients about medical facts remains rare."[25]

Corporate Activism

When Congress created Medicare and Medicaid in 1965, employer contributions for health insurance amounted to less than a tenth of pretax profits. By 1983, employer expenses for health benefits equaled half of pretax profits. Chrysler Corporation, struggling to stay alive in the late 1970s, embraced the concepts of medical auditing and computerized analysis as a way of examining both the cost and quality of care. That concept has since become commonplace as companies look more closely at the link between appropriate treatment of medical problems and employee performance on the job. Increasingly, benefits managers talk of the need for an *absence management strategy, productivity management,* or *managed time loss.* That is particularly true in the chronic care realm.

Chronic disease is now the major cause of illness, disability, and death in the United States, affecting almost 100 million persons and accounting for 70 percent of all medical expenses.[26] That in turn is having a large impact in the workplace. By way of example, diabetes alone accounted for $44.1 billion in direct medical and treatment costs in 1997. Moreover, individuals with diabetes, aged eighteen to sixty-four, lost an average 8.3 days from work, or almost five times the missed days of other workers.[27] Obviously, employers and patients have a shared interest in eliminating inappropriate variation from best practice. One strategy is to conduct the type of medical audit mentioned in the second paragraph of this chapter. Another strategy is to set up workplace education and outreach programs. Delta Air Lines, for example, in cooperation with the National Institute of Mental Health, offers a workplace program focused on depression.[28]

Health Insurer Pressure

In the 1970s, the primary function of insurers was to pay quickly "usual, reasonable, and customary" charges. Thirty years later that function has radically changed. Of those Americans working for a company with ten or more employees, 93 percent were in some sort of managed care plan by 2001,[29] as were 58 percent of Medicaid recipients, according to other data, and 13 percent of Medicare beneficiaries were in HMOs. For better or worse, the managed care movement has pushed doctors toward some sort of standardization, even if different plans still have different standards.

Like employers, plans have a financial interest in improving chronic disease care. Now that both employers and consumers are asking more pointed questions about chronic care, disease management programs have proliferated. For example, half of managed care plans say they offer diabetes disease management.[30]

Media Pressure

On June 30, 1973, the Long Island daily *Newsday* revealed that the death rate for bypass surgery at Nassau County Medical Center was nearly triple that of the area hospital with the second worst rate. The story marked the end of the news media as mere cheerleaders putting out a steady stream of "medical miracle" reports and the beginning of their critical examinations of community care. Today, there is a cadre of journalists informed about health care system issues. NCQA reports are featured on the network news, and national publications such as *Newsweek* and *U.S. News & World Report* put out provider and plan ratings of their own.

The Internet is both supplementing and leading the traditional news media. So, for instance, ratings of physician groups in California and the Pacific Northwest that are compiled by the Pacific Business Group on Health appear in traditional news outlets when first released. At the same time, the results are placed on the Web and remain permanently accessible to patients at www. healthscope.org. In contrast, a consulting firm in Colorado went directly to Web publishing with its risk-adjusted rankings of hospitals for a number of procedures, using Medicare claims information. The media have since found their way to the site, www.Healthgrades.com, which for copyright reasons is in a format that can be read but not printed out. In both traditional and electronic form, this kind of information spotlights the difference between actual and possible performance. As time passes, such educational efforts will steadily supplant the patient's ignorance—once lampooned by George Bernard Shaw—of the lack of science in medicine. The publicity may also motivate providers. At a private meeting of a nonprofit hospital group, for example, a physician described an event at an institution whose heart surgery department had been ranked lower than four competitors on the health care report card Web site. After seeing that, the institution's doctors had gone to the administration and had asked for improvement assistance. Before the doctors saw the Web site, the administration's own attempts to interest them in quality improvement had had little effect.

Government Actions

Until the 1970s, Congress treated the medical profession with deference. Then, in 1974, a House subcommittee held the first hearings on inappropriate surgery. As medical costs increased, the government established what are now called PROs (peer review organizations) to review care on behalf of Medicare patients. PROs have continued to evolve, with many now preferring to call themselves QIOs (quality improvement organizations) and emphasizing partnership rather than oversight. There are a number of other actions government might take, which are enumerated in chapters elsewhere in this book (see Part Five).

Patient Empowerment

The feminist movement began a talk-back-to-the-doctor trend. Gay activists have carried it to its logical conclusion, immersing themselves in the clinical details of AIDS research and treatment in an effort to secure both more research funding and quicker operationalization of research results. As AIDS evolved into a chronic condition, nonphysician patients often became the acknowledged information equals (or more) of doctors. The gay community also has rejected the dependency implicit in the terms *AIDS sufferer* and *AIDS victim.* The preferred term is PWA, or *person with AIDS.* The phrase unmistakably asserts that the disease, no matter how deadly, is less important than the individual harboring it. Other disease groups have since embraced the same terminology and activism.

Ultimately, the goal of patient empowerment is not to supplant physician judgment but to enter into a partnership with it. Eliminating inappropriate variation in care requires acknowledging the values of the person who lives with a disease. Moreover, physicians must encourage some activism in the many patients whose sickness understandably fosters dependency. As an organization that has researched patient-centered care puts it: "Patients need information, skills and support in order to handle the experience of illness and adjust to the rigors of medical treatment."[31]

Of course some patients, particularly those who are not hospitalized, are quite able to act on their own. The child whose mother daringly read Dr. Spock as a declaration of independence has grown up to become a patient with a consumer version of the *Physician's Desk Reference* on the bookshelf and a Web browser bookmarked to a host of general and disease-specific medical sites. Estimates of the number of people surfing the Net for medical information continue to grow exponentially. In mid-2002, Harris Interactive put the figure at 110 million, up from 60 million only four years before.[32] Just as the Protestant Reformation and the newly invented printing press shattered the monopoly of the Catholic Church in Western Europe and changed forever the average person's relationship with God, today's greatly increased spread of information, and an audience of consumers prepared to use that information, is altering the relationship between physicians and those in the world outside their profession.

INFORMATION AGE MEDICINE

Outsiders—attorneys, employers, insurers, the media, and patients—will be understandably skeptical of provider assurances that *this* time they have really changed. The challenge for providers is to demonstrate that they can provide the best care without being micromanaged. To do that, they must demonstrate improvement. As quality measurement pioneer W. Edwards Deming put it: "In God we trust, all others bring data." Or better yet, "information." "Before information can be useful it must be analyzed, interpreted and assimilated," says Donald Wheeler, in *Understanding Variation: The Key to Managing Chaos,* "[but] even highly educated individuals can be numerically illiterate."[33] Using data requires a leap of faith, Wheeler adds; that is, it is only through use that true understanding of usefulness emerges. However, physicians have traditionally resisted quantification fiercely. "The certitude that is found [in medicine is] most often that of an artist," declared the French physician Pierre-Jean-Georges Cabanis in 1788. That attitude, if not widely stated in public, still persists.

Certainly, outsiders must take actions to assure providers that data will not be used punitively and that change will be encouraged financially. In a discounted fee-for-service environment, an aggressive effort to reduce unneeded clinical services can be economically fatal.[34] In addition, some health plans still use the term *managed care* to characterize actions more accurately categorized as *managed cost.*

Nonetheless, technological and social changes are inexorably pushing medicine to bid farewell to the old guild mentality. It is only by embracing accountability that providers can protect essential autonomy. After all, if providers cannot be differentiated based on clinical performance, then purchasers are free to differentiate on price alone. If that happens, the dreaded commoditization of medicine will have become a reality.

A 1994 editorial in the *British Medical Journal* phrased the challenge to physicians this way: "to promote the uptake of innovations that have been shown to be effective, to delay the spread of those that have not yet been shown to be effective and to prevent the uptake of ineffective innovations."[35] Patients and others outside the health care profession will be encouraging physicians and hospitals to take on that task.

Notes

1. S. Garber, personal communication to the author, Apr. 13, 1999.

2. Malmsheimer, R. *"Doctors Only": The Evolving Image of the American Physician.* Westport, Conn.: Greenwood, 1988, pp. 1, 45.

3. Stoline, A. M., and Weiner, J. P. *The New Medical Marketplace.* Baltimore: Johns Hopkins University Press, 1988, p. 15.

4. Barondess, J. A. "Medicine and Its Mandate: Reasons for Change." Paper presented at the Centennial of Johns Hopkins Medical Institutions, "Doctoring America: The Last 100 Years and the Next 100 Years," Feb. 23–24, 1990.

5. Codman, E. A. *The Shoulder.* Boston: Thomas Todd, 1934, p. xviii.

6. Freidson, E. *Profession of Medicine: A Study of the Sociology of Applied Knowledge.* New York: Dodd, Mead, 1970, p. 347.

7. Freidson, *Profession of Medicine,* p. 366.

8. American Child Health Association. *Physical Defects: The Pathway to Correction.* New York: American Child Health Association, 1934, p. 82.

9. Millenson, M. L. "Many Medical Procedures May Be Unneeded." *Chicago Tribune,* Mar. 21, 1991. This article describes a review performed by Value Health Sciences, Santa Monica, California, of the records of eleven million insured workers and their families belonging to five indemnity Blue Cross Blue Shield plans and one Blue HMO.

10. Doyle, J. C. "Unnecessary Hysterectomies: Study of 6,248 Operations in Thirty-Five Hospitals During 1948." *Journal of the American Medical Association,* 1953, *151,* 360–365.

11. G. Nastas, senior data analyst, Health Care Initiatives, General Motors Corp., personal communication to the author, June 28, 1999.

12. Wennberg, J. E. "Dealing with Medical Practice Variations: A Proposal for Action." *Health Affairs,* 1984, *3*(2), 6–32.

13. Ashton, C. M. "Geographic Variations in Utilization Rates in Veterans Affairs Hospitals and Clinics." *New England Journal of Medicine,* 1999, *280,* 32–39.

14. Schuster, M. A., McGlynn, E. A., and Brook, R. H. "How Good Is the Quality of Health Care in the United States?" *Milbank Quarterly,* 1998, *76*(4), 517–563.

15. President's Advisory Commission on Consumer Protection and Quality in the Health Care Industry. *Quality First: Better Health Care for All Americans: Final Report to the President of the United States.* Washington, D.C.: U.S. Government Printing Office, 1998.

16. Committee on Quality of Health Care in America, Institute of Medicine. *Crossing the Quality Chasm: A New Health System for the 21st Century.* Washington, D.C.: National Academy Press, 2001, pp. 1, 3.

17. Katz, J. *The Silent World of Doctor and Patient.* New York: Free Press, 1984, pp. 48–84.

18. Williams, L. P. *How to Avoid Unnecessary Surgery.* Los Angeles: Nash, 1971, p. 215.

19. Eisenberg, J. M. *Doctors' Decisions and the Cost of Medical Care.* Ann Arbor, Mich.: Health Administration Press, 1986, pp. 116–117.

20. "New York: Artist Wins Suit for Unnecessary Mastectomy." *Chicago Tribune,* Mar. 28, 1999, sec. 1, p. 12.

21. Morrow, M., and others. "Factors Responsible for the Underutilization of Breast Conserving Surgery (BCT)." Paper presented at the annual meeting of the American Society of Clinical Oncology, Los Angeles, May 1998.

22. Mangione-Smith, R., and others. "The Relationship Between Perceived Parental Expectations and Pediatrician Antimicrobial Prescribing Behavior." Pediatrics, 1999, *103,* 711–718.

23. Foreman, J. "Ow! Ow! Ow! Chronic Pain Often Goes Untreated Because Some Doctors Don't Believe Their Patients." *Boston Globe,* Mar. 22, 1999, p. E1.

24. National Committee for Quality Assurance. *The State of Managed Care Quality, 1998.* [www.ncqa.org/pages/communications/state%20of%20managed%20care/report98.htm], 1998.

25. Brody, H. *The Healer's Power.* New Haven: Yale University Press, 1992, pp. 88–89.

26. Millenson, M. L. *Demanding Medical Excellence: Doctors and Accountability in the Information Age.* Chicago: University of Chicago Press, 1997, p. 331.

27. American Diabetes Association. "Diabetes Facts and Figures." [www.diabetes.org], Sept. 2, 2003.

28. The Business Roundtable. *Quality Health Care Is Good Business: A Survey of Health Care Quality Initiatives by Members of the Business Roundtable.* Washington, D.C.: The Business Roundtable, Sept. 1997, pp. 56–57.

29. William M. Mercer, Inc. "Health Benefit Cost Up 11.2 Percent in 2001." Press Release. [www.mercerhr.com/pressrelease/details.ihtml?idContent = 1011125], Dec. 10, 2001.

30. InterStudy. "The InterStudy Competitive Edge, Part II: HMO Industry." Industry Analysis: HMO Disease Management Initiatives. St. Paul, Minn.: InterStudy, Oct. 1997, pp. 63–72.

31. Gerteis, M., Edgman-Levitan, S., Daley, J., and Delbanco, T. L. (eds.). "Through the Patient's Eyes: Understanding and Promoting Patient-Centered Care." San Francisco: Jossey-Bass, 1993, p. 96.

32. Harris Interactive. "Cyberchondriacs Update." Harris Poll No. 21. [www. harrisinteractive.com/harris_poll/Index.asp?PID = 299], May 1, 2002.

33. Wheeler, D. J. *Understanding Variation: The Key to Managing Chaos.* Knoxville: SPC Press, 1993, p. vi.

34. Millenson, *Demanding Medical Excellence,* pp. 272–281.

35. Haines, A., and Jones, R. "Implementing Findings of Research." *British Medical Journal,* 1994, *308,* 1488–1492.

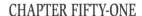

A Disease Management Approach
to Chronic Illness

Jessie C. Gruman, Cynthia M. Gibson

Rapid-fire technological and scientific advances in recent years have fueled the perception that most, if not all, illnesses and conditions can be readily cured. Since the 1920s, however, the number of people with chronic conditions and diseases that are not easily treated with high-technology diagnostic and therapeutic interventions has sharply increased. These conditions create persistent and recurring health consequences over a long period of time, and most have no cure.

Given the prevalence of chronic disease, as well as its enormous cost, health care systems traditionally focused on offering acute care and heroic interventions as disease cure-alls must now find new ways to help growing numbers of chronically ill patients manage their conditions so they can lead full and active lives for as long and as well as they can. Meeting this challenge requires massive changes, not only in the way health care is provided to chronically ill patients and their families but also in the attitudes and perceptions of consumers who refuse to accept modern medicine's limitations. Patients with chronic illness must be willing to assume greater responsibility for their own health care, and health care institutions must facilitate this process.

Collaborative management is a model that can help us meet both goals by strengthening and supporting self-care among people with chronic illness while ensuring that effective medical, preventive, and health maintenance interventions take place. It is also a model that many health care researchers, providers, and administrators increasingly view as more effective than current models in addressing the needs of chronically ill patients. What follows is a description of the elements of collaborative management—which together make up a common core of services for chronic illness care that need not be reinvented for each disease—and a discussion of what health care systems can do to institute this model and, ultimately, provide better care for the many chronically ill patients they serve.

WHY DO WE NEED TO FOCUS ON CHRONIC DISEASE?

There are at least major five reasons why we all ought to be working toward better ways to manage chronic disease.

It Is All Around Us

Currently, chronic conditions such as cancer, diabetes, AIDS, heart disease, arthritis, and emphysema affect approximately ninety million Americans. Although the elderly are far more likely to have a chronic condition than are members of other age groups—nearly 88 percent of the elderly have at least one—they account for only about a quarter of all persons living with these illnesses. More than one-third of young adults, ages eighteen to forty-four, and two-thirds of middle-aged adults, ages forty-five to sixty-four, have at least one chronic condition. In fact, working-age adults, ages eighteen to sixty-four, account for nearly 60 percent of all noninstitutionalized people with chronic conditions.[1]

It Is Expensive

Chronic disorders account for a major portion of the nation's health care expenditures; in 1987, for example, costs of health services and supplies for noninstitutionalized persons with chronic conditions totaled $272.2 billion, accounting for 76 percent of the direct medical care costs in the United States. Annual health care costs for people with chronic conditions average about $3,074, compared to $817 for people with only acute conditions. Those with chronic conditions account for a disproportionately large share of health care use, both in services and supplies. Almost all home care visits (96 percent), 83 percent of prescription drug use, 66 percent of physician visits, and 55 percent of emergency department visits are made by people with chronic conditions.[2]

Nearly half of all people with chronic conditions have more than one,[3] which adds considerably to the costs of chronic illness. Moreover, the likelihood of comorbidity increases with age. One study shows that among those eighty years of age or older, 70 percent of women and 53 percent of men have two or more of nine common chronic conditions.[4]

There are also hidden costs associated with chronic disease, including the costs of lost productivity and independence, of institutionalization, and of support provided by caregivers, on whose shoulders the day-to-day responsibilities of these illnesses fall most heavily. Currently, one-quarter of all Americans provide some degree of personal care for friends or family members with chronic health conditions.[5]

It Is Influenced by Behavior

Behavioral and psychosocial factors influence the onset of some diseases, the progression of many, and the management of nearly all. Smoking, dietary habits, drug and alcohol abuse, and physical activity levels are the precursors of a number of chronic conditions and can also exacerbate their cause. Behavioral factors also largely determine patients' adherence to medication and illness management regimens—such adherence is critical to preventing disabling complications and crises. Estimates of noncompliance rates with prescribed medical regimens, for example, range from 30 to 60 percent. Most researchers agree that at least 50 percent of all patients fail to receive the full benefits of their prescribed medication because of inadequate adherence.[6]

It Is Not Going Away

Decreasing mortality rates, improved lifestyles, and longer life expectancies across all age groups augurs continued growth in the number of people with chronic conditions. Moreover, the population is rapidly aging—by 2030, one in five people in the United States will be age sixty-five or older—and as chronological age increases, so does the likelihood of having one or more chronic illnesses.[7] One study estimates that by 2030, the number of people of all ages with chronic conditions will rise to 148 million—a 65 percent increase from the current number of chronically ill people.[8]

It Is Not Addressed by the Current System

Like most health care, chronic illness care is oriented toward and organized around acute crises or episodes. This approach emphasizes the diagnosis and treatment of symptoms and physiological abnormalities rather than prevention and long-term self-care. Insurance, for example, will pay for the amputation of a limb for diabetes-related gangrene but not for the sustained diabetes self-management and monitoring that can lessen the probability of needing more costly interventions later. Moreover, because the chronically ill often have one or more providers, depending on their needs, their care is frequently fragmented, which can result in duplication or unnecessary treatments.

Even among systems that recognize the need for better management of chronic illness, numerous barriers exist to the full implementation of services that will improve health outcomes for people with chronic illness. Among these barriers are rushed practitioners who fail to adhere to established practice guidelines, a lack of care coordination and follow-up to ensure optimal management and outcomes, and patients inadequately trained and supported in the management of their illnesses.

WHAT DO CONSUMERS WITH CHRONIC CONDITIONS NEED FROM HEALTH CARE SYSTEMS?

According to considerable evidence, patients and caregivers who successfully manage a chronic condition are able to (1) engage in activities that promote health, build energy and strength, and prevent the likelihood of future complications; (2) interact with health care providers and adhere to recommended treatment protocols; (3) monitor physical and emotional status and make appropriate health-related decisions based on the results of such self-monitoring; and (4) manage the effects of illness so that they can function in their work, family, and day-to-day roles.[9]

Increasingly, research has shown that health care can play a powerful role in helping people with chronic conditions perform these tasks and that providing this help results in improved medical, emotional, and functional outcomes. These outcomes are particularly enhanced when providers and patients work together toward shared goals. In fact *both* self-care and medical care are enhanced by effective collaboration among chronically ill patients and their families and health care providers. A review of the evidence[10] regarding chronic condition care found that the interventions and practices that best supported such collaborative management emphasized

- Collaborative definition of the problem: that is, patient-identified problems are acknowledged and recorded along with physicians' medical diagnoses.

- Targeting, goal setting, and planning that enables both patients and the physician or health care team to focus on specific problems, set realistic objectives, and develop action plans for attaining those objectives when patients say they prefer or are ready to do so.

- Provision of a continuum of self-management training and support services to which patients readily have access and that help them carry out medical regimens. Examples include learning how to use devices (for example, asthma inhalers), quitting smoking, understanding and using pain management skills, and making use of available community services for transportation, food, social support, and the like.

- Active and sustained follow-up through which patients are contacted at specified intervals to monitor health status, identify potential complications, and check and reinforce progress in implementing the care plan.

Notwithstanding numerous studies demonstrating the effectiveness and improved health outcomes of collaborative approaches that incorporate these principles as part of primary care programs, these approaches continue to be in short supply for several reasons.

First, many health care systems continue to view self-care as competing with, rather than complementary to, traditional medical care.

Second, some perceive these approaches as difficult to implement because they require multidisciplinary teams of health professionals to work in systems that may not have traditionally supported the care of patients with long-term needs. Even health care systems that have developed their own integrated care management strategies to address chronic illness tend to have a specialized, fragmented focus, that is, they either refer care to specialists, use disease management or carve-out programs to handle this care, or implement condition-specific programs.[11]

Although these kinds of efforts may be easier to implement, because they involve a small number of providers with a narrow focus, they continue the current failure to provide adequate patient accountability and care coordination— a gap that contributes to high health care costs.[12] Thus, as the number of people with two or more chronic conditions continues to increase, health care systems may have no alternative but to develop and incorporate more comprehensive and collaborative models. By offering a common core of services that cut across all chronic diseases, such models eliminate the need to reinvent programs for each condition.

In the meantime, recent developments indicate a gradual movement toward providing consumers with the kind of chronic illness care they need and want. A Center for the Advancement of Health survey of HMO medical directors in seven states,[13] for example, found that nearly all had in place evidence-based guidelines for most of the major chronic conditions (although the extent to which these guidelines are being used by health care professionals is yet unclear).

WHAT SHOULD WE DO TO BETTER SERVE THE CHRONICALLY ILL?

Although the availability of condition-specific programs is a positive step in providing better care for people with chronic conditions, it is not enough to ensure that they receive the *best* possible care. Ultimately, this will be achieved only through broad systemic change.[14]

A Practice Design That Better Meets Chronic Illness Needs

Recognizing that standard medical practice is not designed to meet the needs of chronically ill patients, health care organizations can reconsider the ways in which they deliver care—including assessing who the primary caregiver is and what the role of specialists is; how the organization makes appointments, allots clinic time, delegates tasks, and manages clinical data; and the extent to which it conducts follow-up activities—and then redesigning practices to better reflect the needs of the chronically ill.

Greater Patient Participation in Care

Health care organizations should provide opportunities for patients to become active participants in their care by designing and implementing interventions that facilitate behavioral change and self-management skills. This recommendation is based on considerable research that shows the most effective chronic disease programs are those that increase patients' knowledge about their condition, help them adhere to a proscribed medical regimen, and make adaptations to this regimen as each patient's disease state changes. Whether they are classes, one-on-one counseling sessions, psychosocial support services, or computer programs, educational interventions not only help patients learn about and adopt behavioral changes that improve their health outcomes but also enhance their sense of self-efficacy, which can reduce the likelihood of future disease complications.

Willingness to Diffuse Expertise Across Providers

Rather than relying on specialists—an approach that tends to fragment care and contribute to increased medical costs—health care systems should expand efforts to distribute health care expertise among all providers. Training local experts or health educators, for example, and then making that expertise available to primary care practices or using a combination of specialists and generalists to manage patient care in primary health care settings are particularly effective strategies to achieve better health outcomes with chronically ill patients. In addition, training should be available to help providers learn how to better communicate with patients and respond to their questions or information requests in a consultative, personalized, and hands-on style.

Coordinated Patient Information Systems

Information about patients, their care, and their outcomes must be readily available to, as well as coordinated and systematized for, health care providers, caregivers, and patients. Health care systems, for example, can compile patient registries (lists of all patients with a particular condition). With such lists providers are not restricted to communicating with patients at the times they present for care but can make opportunities to communicate with them regularly about their progress and to provide support and advice for identifying problems before they become crises. A shared care plan made available through computerized clinical information systems is another form of information that can be quickly accessed and used by several providers, as well as by caregivers and patients.

IMPLEMENTATION BARRIERS AND OPPORTUNITIES

Encouraging wider acceptance and use of this kind of model in the treatment of chronic illness will require overcoming several barriers and exploiting new opportunities.

Formidable barriers, for example, continue to exist at the insurance and purchasing levels. Insurers have traditionally avoided risk-adjusted payments for the chronically ill, a decision that has virtually eliminated health plans' incentives to offer more coordinated and comprehensive care for these patients. Health care purchasers' tendency to focus on the bottom line and employers' reluctance to finance what are widely perceived as expensive and long-term treatments also have made it extremely difficult to advocate for better coverage of these services.

At the same time, health plans are realizing that simply restricting the amounts and types of services available to people with chronic conditions is short-sighted, especially in markets where member turnover is slow or there is only one plan available. In addition, employers and other health care purchasers want all employees, even those who are chronically ill, to be productive workers. These trends should provide incentives to researchers and practitioners to demonstrate more concretely how collaborative approaches can lead to better health outcomes, meet consumers' needs, and perhaps save money in the long term. Such information must then be made more widely available to administrators, insurers, providers, and consumers.

The assumption that consumers will want to shoulder greater responsibility for their care and that providers will permit them to do so represents both barriers and opportunities for each constituency. Most health care professionals, for example, continue to be educated and trained under, and thus oriented to, acute-care or specialist models, with little or no training in the multidisciplinary, collaborative approaches that are more effective in meeting the needs of chronically ill patients. Nevertheless, a shift toward these approaches is slowly occurring, especially in the training of new professionals. As more institutions offer this kind of training, the greater the likelihood that it will become a standard facet of core health care curricula, not only for new students but also for existing professionals enrolled in continuing education programs.

Ultimately, in a market-driven health care system, these programs and services will most likely be offered when consumers demand them. On the positive side, consumers appear to be open to new health care approaches, as evidenced by their extraordinary levels of use of alternative medicine and other interventions that require more self-care and self-monitoring. On the downside, this trend may be nothing more than a reflection of consumers' frustration with the care they are currently receiving or the desire to find cures for chronic conditions.

Moreover, consumers with chronic conditions and consumers who are healthy have very different views of collaborative care. In a recent series of focus groups with people with chronic conditions, participants enthusiastically embraced the idea of physician-patient partnerships that could help them manage their condition, teach them about the disease, problem solve, and so forth. When healthy people were asked their impressions of this same approach, they said they found it intrusive, infantilizing, and a possible violation of confidentiality. Despite these differences, the two groups also shared some fundamental similarities—among them, an increased willingness to entertain alternatives to traditional care and a sense of their growing clout in a fiercely competitive health care market. Given these circumstances, there is an unprecedented opportunity to mobilize consumers to advocate for services and programs that have been shown to be more effective in addressing the needs of people with chronic conditions. However, achieving this mobilization will require clarifying chronically ill patients' incentives for embracing collaborative approaches and educating healthy consumers about their benefits.

These are just a few of the issues that must be addressed if collaborative approaches are to be adopted broadly and in ways that better serve millions of Americans with chronic conditions. With greater attention to helping them manage their conditions and live as well and as long as they can, full implementation of collaborative models of care can help the chronically ill achieve better health outcomes over the long term. With no cure in sight for the majority of chronic conditions, their exorbitant cost and growing prevalence demand nothing less.

Notes

1. Hoffman, C., Rice, D., and Sung, H. Y. "Persons with Chronic Conditions: Their Prevalence and Costs." *Journal of the American Medical Association,* 1996, *276,* 1473–1479.

2. Hoffman and others, "Persons with Chronic Conditions."

3. Hoffman and others, "Persons with Chronic Conditions."

4. Guralnik, J., LaCroix, A., Everett, D., and Kovar, M. *Aging in the Eighties: The Prevalence of Comorbidity and its Association with Disability, Advance Data.* Washington, D.C.: National Center for Health Statistics, 1989.

5. Schroeder, S. *Chronic Health Conditions.* Annual Report. Princeton, N.J.: Robert Wood Johnson Foundation, 1993.

6. Rogers, P. G., and Bullman, W. R. "Prescription Medication Compliance: A Review of the Baseline of Knowledge: A Report of the National Council on Patient Information and Education." *Journal of Pharmacoepidemiology,* 1995, *2,* 3.

7. Hoffman and others, "Persons with Chronic Conditions"; Day, J. C. *Population Projections of the United States, by Age, Sex, Race, and Hispanic Origin: 1993–2050.* Current Population Reports, Series P-25, No. 1104. Washington, D.C.: U.S. Bureau of the Census, 1993.

8. Hoffman and others, "Persons with Chronic Conditions."

9. Clark, N. M. and others. "Self-Management of Chronic Disease by Older Adults: A Review and Questions for Research." *Journal of Aging and Health,* 1991, *3,* 3–27; Clark, N. M., and others. "Impact of Self-Management Education on the Functional Health Status of Older Adults with Heart Disease." *Gerontologist,* 1992, *60,* 552–568; Lorig, K. "Self-Management of Chronic Illness: A Model for the Future." *Generations,* 1993, *17,* 11–14; Wagner, E. H., Austin, B. T., and Von Korff, M. "Organizing Care for Patients with Chronic Illness." *Milbank Quarterly,* 1996, *74,* 511–544; Von Korff, M., and others. "Collaborative Management of Chronic Illness." *Annals of Internal Medicine,* 1997, *127,* 1097–1102.

10. Korff and others, "Collaborative Management of Chronic Illness."

11. Wagner, E. H., Austin, B., and Von Korff, M. "Improving Outcomes in Chronic Illness." *Managed Care Quarterly,* 1996, *4,* 12–25; Wagner, E. H. "Chronic Disease Management: What Will It Take to Improve Care for Chronic Illness?" *Effective Clinical Practice,* 1998, *1*(1), 2–4.

12. Wagner and others, "Improving Outcomes in Chronic Illness"; Wagner, "Chronic Disease Management."

13. Center for the Advancement of Health. *Health Behavior Change in Managed Care: Medical Directors Survey.* Washington, D.C.: Center for the Advancement of Health, 2000.

14. Wagner, E. H., and others. "Quality Improvement in Chronic Illness Care: A Collaborative Approach." *Journal of Quality Improvement,* 2001, *27,* 23–80; Wagner, E. H., and others. "Improving Chronic Illness Care: Translating Evidence into Action." *Health Affairs,* 2001, *20*(6), 64–78.

CHAPTER FIFTY-TWO

Consumer-Driven Health Care

Management Matters

Richard M. J. Bohmer, Amy C. Edmondson, Gary P. Pisano

Technology occupies a precarious position in health care—at the same time vilified as the cause of cost increases and untimely patient deaths and hailed as a savior that will improve treatments and thereby reduce expenditures in the care of individual patients. Few new technologies in recent years have been more controversial than minimally invasive heart surgery. High expectations were first fueled by aggressive marketing by a young company whose founders were drawn from the ranks of the Stanford Medical School and then dashed by early reports of patient deaths.[1] The subsequent debate pitted surgeon skill against technology design. Did patients die because surgeons were not good enough or because the intra-arterial balloon catheter, the centerpiece of the new technology, was too stiff? The research we discuss in this paper suggests that even though new medical technology plays a role in early adverse outcomes, the nature of that role is more subtle than it first appears. We argue that to assess a new technology's impact on adverse events, patient health, and even cost, understanding how the technology adoption process is managed is as important as understanding the nature of the technology itself.

In this chapter we argue that the clinical and economic impact of a new medical technology depends heavily on how the adoption process is managed. We argue that the successful adoption of a new technology and the realization of its full benefits require substantial learning by both individual physicians and the organizations in which they practice—learning that must be actively managed. We propose that the characteristics of any new technology demand different kinds of learning of individuals and organizations and that the technologies that pose the greatest learning challenge are those that disrupt existing professional boundaries, status relationships, and communication patterns. Thus we argue that the decision to adopt a new technology should take into account the ability and incentive of the individual provider organization to learn.

PRIOR RESEARCH

Prior to the era of managed care the decision to adopt a new technology lay primarily with the individual physician. Reimbursement to the provider was on a cost-plus basis, and the capital costs of new equipment could be passed on directly to insurers. In general, the adoption decision for a new technology was based solely on the degree of incremental benefit the technology provided for patients. Accordingly, research has assumed that technical merit and communication by opinion leaders determine the diffusion of innovations, and has paid less attention to the intricacies of realizing the full benefit of an innovation after the adoption decision has been made.[2] In particular, the literature has assumed that the full burden of learning to utilize a new technology falls on the individual adopting physician and that the effects of the team or organization in which he or she works can be ignored.[3] Past research has regarded this learning as a simple function of cumulative experience measured as number of cases undertaken. Not surprisingly, the ways in which specific characteristics of an individual technology may influence the learning challenge have not been studied; instead, new technologies have been treated as uniform, just as adopting them has been seen as straightforward.

Our perspective differs from that of traditional research. Without attention to the need for management and organizational learning, adverse consequences are likely to result from adopting new technology, ranging from failure to realize the technology's full potential to adverse clinical outcomes. To explore this view, our research examined the factors that influence the rate at which an individual adopting center realizes the full benefit of a technology.

In the following sections we review the results of our research examining the adoption of minimally invasive cardiac surgery and then discuss the management issues we identified. We go on to review literature relevant to new technology adoption, and finally we discuss the implications of our findings for health care providers and consumers.

LEARNING AND NEW TECHNOLOGY ADOPTION: THE CASE OF MINIMALLY INVASIVE CARDIAC SURGERY

To further understand the issues in technology adoption in health care, we studied the adoption of an innovative minimally invasive cardiac surgical technique at sixteen hospitals nationwide. Minimally invasive cardiac surgery differs from conventional cardiac surgery in a number of subtle yet important ways. A conventional operation on the heart is divided into three phases: accessing and stopping the heart, performing the actual surgical procedure (for example, a coronary artery bypass graft [CABG] or heart valve replacement), and restarting the heart and closing the chest (in CABG, the vein to be used to bypass a diseased coronary artery is harvested by some team members while others are accessing the heart). In the first phase the breastbone is split and the chest is opened. The patient is hooked up to the heart-lung bypass machine (the *pump*) via tubes that carry unoxygenated blood from the patient to the pump and carry oxygenated blood under pressure back to the patient. Once this is done the heart can be stopped. A clamp is then placed over the aorta, near the heart, so that blood does not flow back into the heart during the second phase, the bypass or valve repair operation. When this cardiac procedure is completed, the third phase begins, in which the process in the first phase is reversed, allowing the heart to fill with blood, recommence beating, and eventually take over full responsibility for maintaining blood pressure. Only then is the patient weaned from the pump and the chest closed.

The major difference between minimally invasive surgery and the conventional approach is that the breastbone is not split apart. The heart is accessed via a small incision between the ribs, and the tubes that carry blood to and from the pump are placed in the artery and vein in the groin. A balloon that is fed up from the groin to the aorta and then inflated serves the purpose of the clamp. The well-being of the heart is monitored with sensors that read the pressure at various points in the circulation system. The rest of the operation is largely unchanged. This different route of access to the heart has some important implications. First, the surgeon cannot visualize and touch the heart with ease and must perform the cardiac procedure in a greatly restricted space. Direct visual and tactile information is replaced by digital data, displayed on monitors that hang from the operating room ceiling. Second, the anesthesiologist has an expanded role in placing the various catheters that measure pressure, delivering fluids, and monitoring the position of the aortic balloon. Third, the perfusionist (the technician who operates the pump machine) also has an expanded role in managing the aortic balloon clamp. Finally, all members of the team rely more heavily on communication with one another because none has a good view of the patient's heart. Surgeons must rely on the other team members (anesthesiologist, perfusionist, and scrub nurse) to watch the monitors that display the critical blood pressures and report any danger signs to them.

Technological Innovation Categories and Their Impact on Organizations

Researchers in innovation have articulated a distinction between component and architectural innovations.[4] A *component* innovation is one in which there is a change in a basic component, but the system in which the component is placed remains unchanged. An example is the antilock brake. The basic car is the same; its conventional brake is simply replaced with an antilock brake. A good example of a component innovation in health care is a me-too drug, such as a new ACE inhibitor with a slightly different side effect profile. The basic process of care for congestive heart failure remains the same, and the new drug is simply substituted for the older generation one. The new drug causes relatively little disruption to the care delivery process. In contrast, *architectural* innovations are ones in which the basic components remain unchanged but are configured differently, forming a new system. Front-wheel drive is an example of an architectural innovation. All the components of the car are the same, but they are reorganized so that their relation to each other is changed significantly.

Architectural innovations pose particular challenges because they require the greatest amount of organizational change for successful adoption. As Henderson and Clark note, architectural innovations may be deceptive.[5] Radical innovations that change both the components and their relationship to one another tend to be obviously radical. However, because the components remain the same in an architectural innovation, organizations may underestimate the extent of change that the new relationship among the components implies. Even when an organization recognizes the extent of change, it may not be able to adapt to it if the current organizational structure does not support the new architecture or if the organization has difficulty gaining the new knowledge required to successfully adopt it. Architectural innovations place a premium on an organization's ability to learn—to seek, organize, and act upon new knowledge. Sometimes those organizations that have experienced the greatest difficulty in responding to architectural change are those that have been most successful with the old technology, because they are the most committed to the current way of viewing the problem and its solution (the *competency trap*[6]).

Minimally invasive cardiac surgery is an interesting case because it can be categorized as an architectural innovation. None of the equipment or techniques used is particularly new. Using an intra-aortic balloon clamp, performing a heart-lung bypass via the femoral artery rather than through a central chest wound, and operating via a small incision are three techniques that have been available for many years. What is new to the surgical team is the way these components are organized into a surgical process and the new relationships among the team members that this reorganization implies. For example, adopting minimally invasive cardiac surgery requires more learning by the whole surgical team than by the individual surgeon, as she may already be competent in one of the three techniques. Like other organizations adapting to architectural innovations, some adopting hospitals in our study failed to recognize the need for organizational change. Current clinical processes and status relationships among professional disciplines are often reflected in hospital organizational structures (such as having separate departments for anesthesiology, surgery, perfusion, and nursing) and can be hardwired in an institution. These current processes and relationships erect a barrier to learning new surgical processes that are dependent upon highly integrated teamwork.

The experience of hospitals adopting this technology helps to identify the critical issues in managing new medical technologies.

The Findings

When they adopted minimally invasive cardiac surgery, all the hospitals in our study experienced an initial worsening in performance, as indicated by the amount of time taken to complete a case. Although a detailed examination of mortality rates was beyond the scope of our study, mortality did not increase, and thus this decrease in efficiency was not associated with deteriorating clinical outcomes.[7] Typically, a conventional CABG takes anywhere between three and six hours, depending on the illness of the patient, the complexity of the procedure, and the presence of trainees. Early minimally invasive cases in our sample took three times as long, from ten to twelve hours. The direct cost of $1,200 per hour for a cardiac surgical operating room (which includes the costs of staff, drugs, and disposable equipment but not surgeon's fees) means that a tripling of operating room time for a given case presents a significant cost increase. For some this case time increase means the difference between one and three cases a day in an operating room, thus suggesting even greater losses in revenues beyond the direct cost to the hospital of the operating room time (under the diagnosis related group [DRG] reimbursement system, the payment for a cardiac surgical admission is the same regardless of procedure length). This capacity constraint can be a disincentive to adopt the new technology, and the ability to come down the learning curve rapidly is an important consideration in the decision to adopt.

Adopting hospitals improved their procedure times but varied considerably in the rate at which they achieved this improvement after the initial worsening, despite all receiving the same standardized training prior to undertaking their first cases.[8] Some hospitals were able to halve their case times over the first fifty cases, whereas at the other end of the spectrum, some experienced no improvement in case-mix-adjusted procedure time. This conflicts with the commonly held belief that improvement in the performance of procedures is predominantly a function of case number and that (holding volume constant) it is unlikely to vary from one hospital to the next.[9]

Hospitals also learned on dimensions other than procedure time. Over time, surgical teams learned to take on more complicated cases, going from a predominance of single vessel bypasses early in their experience to triple and quadruple bypasses later. Reductions in time in the ICU and overall length of stay were not the focus of most of the hospitals in our study, either because they had already dramatically shortened length of stay for cardiac surgical patients or because they were not yet faced with an incentive to do so.

Importantly, hospitals also varied in their approach to managing the adoption of the new technique. Some institutions managed it proactively, treating it like a project. They did such things as holding multidisciplinary training sessions and dry runs (in which the entire operating room team practiced the procedure, beginning to end, in the operating room, using all the equipment but without the patient) prior to the first case, briefing the referring cardiologists on the ideal patient characteristics for the early cases, deliberately selecting simple cases for their first experience, insisting on stability in the operating room team for the first ten to fifteen cases, debriefing after each early case to reflect on what went well and what did not, and keeping the surgical procedure constant by not varying any of the steps for the first fifteen to twenty cases.[10]

Other institutions apparently did not identify the technology as particularly new and made no deliberate attempt to manage the adoption process. In some of these institutions, for example, there was no discussion of the way in which the team would work together with the new technology. In others the team that performed the first case was not the team that went to training. Thus, for some team members, the first case was the first time they had seen the procedure. Some institutions significantly changed the procedure they had been taught as early as the first or second case. Finally, there was often no process for sharing learning among the various members of the surgical team.

The institutions adopting minimally invasive cardiac surgery also differed in their preadoption characteristics, most notably in the culture of the operating room. Learning in a team setting is a potentially threatening activity. It requires individual team members to publicly reveal their ignorance, ask for guidance, and give and receive advice. Psychological safety, the sense that one can comfortably speak up about one's own uncertainty or the potential errors of others, is associated with increased rates of learning on work teams.[11] Cardiac surgical operating rooms, which tend to conform to a hierarchical social and professional structure with autocratic surgeons at the head,[12] can in fact differ substantially in their cultures. Some adopting teams exhibited a high degree of psychological safety. Surgeons welcomed comments and corrections, apparently reasoning that the more eyes looking out for mistakes in this highly complex procedure the better. Furthermore, these teams viewed open communication as essential, relying as they did on the pressures displayed on overhead screens to monitor a patient's well-being. In contrast, other surgical teams did not welcome expressions of concern by lower-status team members.

MANAGEMENT ISSUES IN NEW TECHNOLOGY ADOPTION

This study identified four important management issues for the adoption of new medical technology: the management of learning prior to the first case, during the early experience, and later in the institution's experience, and management of the institution's decision to adopt.

Learning Prior to Adoption

Learning begins prior to the first case. This is not simply formal training by the manufacturer's clinical specialists but also includes assignment of tasks, redefinition of communication patterns and information flows, practice sessions, and reengineering of care processes to accommodate the new technology. For example, although all hospitals in our study were encouraged to undertake a dry run after returning from training, only some hospitals approached this practice session in a detailed way. In an effort to learn-before-doing in the most systematic way, staff in two of the study hospitals undertook a formal failure modes and effects analysis (FMEA) of the new operative process prior to the first case.[13] Thorough dry runs give staff an opportunity not only to become familiar with new equipment and the associated tasks but also to explicitly discuss and plan mechanisms for communication and information sharing. As this description implies, all members of the surgical or other implementation team should be present. The content of the dry run should include not only technical aspects of the procedure, such as the placement of new equipment in the operating room, but how team members will communicate with one another about the details of the operative process and about actual or potential adverse events.

Finally, as other members of the wider care team in the hospital also have an impact on the learning prior to the first case, it is important to communicate broadly about plans for the new technology. For example, some of the study hospitals went to great lengths to inform the referring cardiologists of the plans for the new procedure and to suggest characteristics of patients who were ideally suited for it.[14] In so doing they helped ensure that surgeons would gain early experience on cases that were less challenging. As one surgeon commented, "I want to start with a case in which the surgery is not the problem." Similarly, in these hospitals, clinicians responsible for delivering postoperative care, such as the physicians and nurses working in the intensive care unit and the postoperative care wards, were briefed about the new procedure and its likely effects on the elements of care for which they were responsible.

Learning During the Early Cases

Next, a number of specific strategies can be used to increase the learning potential in the early cases. Deliberately keeping the adopting team and the new process of care stable gives team members enough time not only to become comfortable with the new technology but also to develop a sufficiently deep understanding of its underlying principles to solve problems in real time. Evaluating early experience on a case-by-case basis is another component of active learning management, akin to the technique of *after action review* used by the military to maximize the potential learning from a limited number of experiences. Case-by-case debriefing treats an individual case as a detailed history rather than a single data point[15] and allows users to learn from experience long before sufficient cases have been amassed to reach statistical significance. Individual case analysis is a complement to, not a substitute for, the retrospective analysis of aggregated outcomes data. The techniques of statistical process control have been well validated in health care as mechanisms for identifying significant trends in outcomes while sample sizes are still relatively small.[16]

A culture that supports learning behaviors is even more important than specific learning processes.[17] For example, when the team culture supports speaking up about actual or potential errors, the reported error rate increases, thereby enabling timely corrective action.[18] The culture in cardiac operating rooms can be anything but supportive. For example, a perfusionist at one site in our study reported in an interview that "once, when we were having trouble with the venous return and I mentioned it, the surgeon said, 'Jack, is that you?' I said 'yes.' He said, 'Are you doing this case?' I said, 'No, I'm assisting.' 'Well in the future, if you are not doing this case I don't want to hear from you.' You see, it's a very structured communication."

Later Learning

In the later phases of learning it is critical to reflect on the patterns emerging from aggregate experience with a new technology. At this stage, teams no longer need to focus on how to do the procedure; instead they need to learn more about for whom, among the usual types of patients seen by the institution, the new technology is best suited. In this way institutions develop a sense of what do they do well and what they do not do well. For example, a team could note that in its hands and with its usual patients, the technique of minimally invasive cardiac surgery was better suited for mitral valve repair and replacement than coronary artery graft procedures, or perhaps was particularly suited for reoperations. These lessons can change over time. As the team gains experience, more complicated types of patients can become eligible for the technique. The distinction between learning how and learning when (or for whom) is analogous to that made by Argyris[19] between single- and double-loop learning, in which single-loop learning involves detecting and correcting errors in a given process, whereas double-loop learning involves reflecting on the nature of the process and considering alternative processes, goals, or frameworks. In new medical technology adoption, both kinds of learning are important. The accumulation of aggregate data allows an organization to reflect on its progress in the adoption process and to suggest alternative next steps. This helps the organization avoid the trap of *superstitious learning*—the dangerous process of drawing inferences from individual cases or anecdotes.[20]

Technology Assessment: The Adoption Decision

Technology assessment is the process of evaluating the safety, efficacy, effectiveness, feasibility, and indications for use of new technologies. Although the Food and Drug Administration (FDA) is charged with the responsibility for evaluating safety, efficacy, and indications, hospitals often undertake their own additional technology review before allowing new technologies to be used. The technology assessment process typically focuses on the *efficacy* of a new technology—that is, its performance under ideal clinical trial conditions, using data from the published scientific literature. In contrast, the *effectiveness* of a technology—its performance under average conditions of routine use—must consider the characteristics of the local environment, including the skill level of users, the level of supporting resources, and the types of patients and conditions usually treated. It can be extremely difficult, if not impossible, to predict how many nuances of the use environment will affect the performance of the technology. Under most circumstances it is not feasible to "do it right the first time." This phenomenon has been well documented in a range of industrial settings as well as in health care.[21]

The fact that the definition of patient eligibility for the procedure can change over time at adopting hospitals highlights the need for technology assessment to be a local process. However, the pace at which an organization or team can learn to use a new intervention, and the risks inherent in the institution's learning process, are not usually part of a provider organization's technology assessment process. Learning-by-doing must be considered a critical element of the adoption process. Provider organizations less frequently take the learning curve into account when planning the adoption of a new technology and thus tend not to assess the conditions and processes that support rapid learning in the organization or the costs that will be involved during the learning process.

The Role of Leadership

Consistent with research on organizational change,[22] the results of our study suggest that leadership plays a central role in the adoption of new technology in health care. Leadership involves a different set of tasks in each of the stages of new technology implementation described previously. Prior to the first case the leader (for example, an adopting surgeon) can play a critical role in putting together a team that has the appropriate mix of skills, not only technical skills and relevant experience but also interpersonal skills. The kind of leadership that promotes team learning combines a deep understanding of the science that underlies the new technology with the abilities to coach other team members, to give and receive criticism, and to encourage communication across disciplinary boundaries. Next, the leader plays a critical role in facilitating early learning once implementation is under way, by putting structures in place to support learning (for example, ensuring team and process stability, or organizing debriefing meetings), creating an atmosphere of psychological safety to foster open communication of concerns and questions, and coordinating with other departments who play direct or indirect roles in the broader process of care. In the final stage of implementation, leadership is needed to initiate systematic review of both short- and long-term outcome data, including relevant hypothesis testing, which allows the implementation team and the larger organization to learn from the team's accumulated experience.

DISCUSSION

Our findings differ from mainstream research into technology adoption in health care. This literature reports on innovation diffusion and views medical practice as a social activity, defined by social structures and norms of behavior, in which users are organized into local communities.[23] It examines the way in which innovations are communicated among members of this society.[24] This literature also stresses the role of local opinion leaders in leading changes in practice. Opinion leaders are found to be more influential than the published scientific literature in shaping physicians' attitudes to particular new technologies.[25] The significant variation in the utilization of medical technologies among different geographical regions[26] is found to be a function of individual physician behavior[27] but is also powerfully influenced by the norms of communities of physicians, unified either by geography, site of practice,[28] or subspecialty.[29] Despite this emphasis on social factors in diffusion, this literature has not paid attention to the microdynamics of the adoption of a given technology at individual sites.

The characteristics found to influence the rate of spread of an innovative technology through a community of potential users are relatively independent of the users and ignore the way in which a new technology and existing organizational routines interact. In short, the innovation diffusion literature treats technology adoption as an essentially *passive* process and does not recognize the role played by individual and organizational learning in performance improvement in technology adoption. Our research, in contrast, treats technology adoption as a dynamic process that continues after the decision to adopt has been made.

Understandably, the medical literature virtually ignores the role of organizational learning in the adoption of new technologies. It focuses predominantly on the relationship between individual cumulative volume and the outcome of procedures. At the center of the debate in the medical literature about this relationship is the observation that institutions that do more of a given procedure tend to have better results. The two possible explanations for this phenomenon are that practice does indeed make perfect or, conversely, that causality runs in the other direction, so that institutions with better outcomes attract more referrals. Neither of these approaches recognizes that different institutions may have different learning potential. Rather than identify the characteristics of a good learner, this literature seeks to answer the question, How many procedures must an institution or an individual physician perform to be considered competent? Usually the answer to this question is "quite a lot"—ranging from 20 for surgeons performing laparoscopic fundoplication,[30] to 45 to 60 for anesthesiologists performing spinal and epidural blocks,[31] to 180 for gastroenterologists performing endoscopic retrograde cholangiopancreatography (ERCP).[32]

The possibility that improvement of performance with increased experience is mediated by organizational learning is rarely addressed in the medical literature. For example, in the aforementioned study, researchers found that complication rates for surgeons learning the procedure of laparoscopic fundoplication were notably higher in the first twenty cases. They also found that adverse outcomes were less likely for those surgeons that began their training later in their organization's experience—implicitly suggesting an organizational learning effect. In contrast, evidence from our study suggests that new technologies that disrupt existing routines or professional boundaries—that is, architectural innovations—will affect the ease with which adopters learn to use them, the speed with which reliably good results will be achieved, and therefore the rate at which the technology will be adopted. Furthermore, all cases do not have uniform learning potential, and all hospitals are not equally skilled learners. In sum, some hospitals manage the process of learning to use a new technology more effectively than others do.

IMPLICATIONS

Device and pharmaceutical technologies are multiplying and advancing at an ever-greater rate. The FDA reviews over 4,000 original device applications annually.[33] New technology has brought important changes, fundamentally altering the way medicine is practiced and health care is delivered. The various participants in the health care industry—patients, doctors, managed care companies, and hospitals—tend to treat technology adoption as an all-or-nothing phenomenon to be facilitated or retarded. They have failed to attend to the *process* of technology adoption and to recognize the effects of this on the outcomes of the use of all the various technologies. Our findings point to the importance of this process.

Implications for Providers

New technologies have redefined the art and science of medicine—what tasks make up medical care, who performs them, and where. Physical examination, for centuries the essence of medical practice, has been replaced by x rays, MRIs, ultra-sounds, and blood tests, often with a substantial increase in accuracy.[34] Interventions such as coronary angioplasty have allowed cardiologists to treat conditions previously reserved for cardiac surgeons. The development of the intra-arterial stent has allowed radiologists to treat vascular surgical conditions. New technologies have the potential to shift the boundaries of medical subspecialties—boundaries that currently represent a balkanization of the human body based on the technology and understanding of anatomy and physiology available at the end of the nineteenth century.

New technologies require an updating of this map, so that subspecialties that have not previously worked together as a team must learn to collaborate. For example, intra-coronary radiotherapy requires a cardiologist and a radiation oncologist to collaborate. New bodies of knowledge, such as genomics, have the potential to further alter roles and relationships in the health care delivery process.[35] For example, oncologists treating patients with breast cancer are increasingly likely to collaborate with companies specializing in genetic testing to interpret results of sophisticated genetic tests and to define treatment plans for individual patients. Finally, many procedures once regarded as requiring a prolonged hospital stay, such as cholecystectomy (removal of the gallbladder) or knee surgery, now have very short lengths of stay or are even performed in outpatient day surgery centers where the composition of the team and the way team members collaborate is usually very different from what is found in general hospitals. Hence new technologies are increasing the importance of managing learning among members of a multidisciplinary team, characterized by increasing numbers of specialized roles and a redrawing of traditional professional boundaries. What is being learned is not simply the specific details of the new technology itself but a new way of working together in a team to realize the full potential benefit the technology offers—in essence to align effectiveness with efficacy.

We can speculate that in the future new professions may have an effect similar to that of the new technologies discussed here. In particular the rise of new roles such as nurse practitioner and case manager has forced delivery organizations to rethink care processes and redefine status and working relationships in the care delivery team. In one sense the nurse practitioner is an architectural innovation—appearing similar to the old "technology" of the registered nurse—but in reality being very different. Nurse practitioners are highly trained, able to make medical decisions, and authorized to prescribe a limited range of drugs. Hence, they function very differently from registered nurses when they are members of the health care team and eventually may have status, authority, and expertise approaching that of a primary care practitioner.

To illustrate, Oxford Health Plans allows its New York City members to identify a nurse practitioner as their primary care practitioner.[36] Large numbers of nurse practitioners are being trained—the number of nonphysician clinicians (predominantly nurse practitioners, nurse midwives, and physician's assistants) is expected to grow by 60 percent between 1995 and 2005,[37] and those currently in practice increased the number of prescriptions they wrote by 66 percent from 1997 to 1998. Consumers find nurse practitioners a very acceptable alternative to primary care physicians.[38] The rise of the nurse practitioner has the potential to change the face of health care delivery and force physicians and hospitals to rethink the optimal structure and function of the health care delivery team, much in the same way that minimally invasive cardiac surgery does.

A similar innovation in professional roles has been the development of hospitalists. Initially the focus of some disagreement—on the grounds that these dedicated inpatient physicians would further fragment the care delivery process, increase costs, and decrease quality—hospitalists have become accepted in some of the nation's best hospitals and are credited with significant reductions in cost without a commensurate reduction in quality.[39] Additionally, adherents to this new medical specialty of *site-focused* care have the potential to become leaders in hospital quality improvement initiatives by reducing the risk of nosocomial infections and advancing end-of-life care.

Implications for Consumers

For consumers, new technology represents a double-edged sword. On the one hand new technologies offer previously unavailable health care solutions or reduce the morbidity associated with existing solutions. For example, arteries can be unblocked and gallbladders removed without much of the long-term pain once associated with these procedures. These innovations have the effect of making care more available to consumers. For example, when laparoscopic cholecystectomy was introduced in 1989, open cholecystectomy did not disappear.[40] Instead the total number of cholecystectomies being performed increased substantially, suggesting that some patients who might not have considered their symptoms bad enough to justify an operation when the old technology was the only option were willing to undergo the new, less invasive procedure.[41]

A cautionary note is needed here. Media coverage enhances consumer awareness of new diagnostic and therapeutic interventions and often inflates consumers' expectations of achievable outcomes. For example, cardiac surgeons performing minimally invasive surgery reported increased patient demand after the technique was depicted on the television show *Chicago Hope* as extraordinarily quick and painless.[42] One recent study found that media coverage of new technologies was biased in favor of positive interpretation because relative, rather than absolute, risks and benefits were preferentially reported and in many cases information about potential harms was not included.[43]

On the other hand some new technologies carry additional risks because of their very novelty. Although health care providers and technology manufacturers are committed to minimizing these risks, neither has an incentive to publicize them. Further, hospitals in which new technology is a fact of life may not even notice the increase in risk.[44]

For consumers, the lesson from the case of minimally invasive cardiac surgery may simply be, if possible, to avoid being among the early candidates for a new technology. Of course someone has to be the first at any institution, and for some patients it may be impossible to wait. However, the patient is not always told that the hospital has limited experience with a new technology. Existing quality report cards do not yet offer a solution to this problem because current metrics do not provide consumers with any insight into the risks they run when being treated with new technologies. The volume of a given procedure at an institution generally has been used as a proxy for the quality of care delivered at that institution.[45] Our results indicate, however, that the relationship between volume and outcome is complex and that the quality of care cannot be inferred from surgical volume alone.[46] Nor do current report cards make it possible to identify which institutions have robust processes in place for managing new technology adoption. Attempts to accredit hospitals based on the presence or absence of essential processes has thus far not protected patients from adverse events. For example, the two Boston hospitals at which well-publicized, preventable patient deaths occurred in 1994 and 1997 were both accredited by the Joint Commission on the Accreditation of Healthcare Organizations (JCAHO), one with commendation.[47] This suggests a need for more sophisticated measures of quality than we currently have and has important ramifications for the consumer-driven health care model, which has as one of its central tenets the free availability of reliable information that consumers can use to inform their choices. In short, information in the health care sector, unlike that in the financial services sector, is not always readily available or reliable. Even the Internet, the focus of a vibrant market for health care information[48] for consumers, is not reliable.[49] In this study we focused on just one of the many important characteristics of providers—their ability to safely adopt new technologies—and our results show that this feature is not yet sufficiently accurately measured to enable consumers to make the critical choice of which provider to use. It may be possible in the future to validate measures, such as use of practice sessions and early team stability, which would broaden the scope of report cards and further enhance their value to consumers. In the interim, what prudent consumers can do is discuss with their caregivers before treatment the prior experience an institution and an individual physician have had with a new technology.

Beyond consumer awareness of new technologies and their risks and benefits is another, societal implication. Whether or not a new technology will ultimately become broadly available to the patients who can genuinely benefit from it depends as much on the skill of the managers, both medically trained and not, responsible for its adoption and implementation as on the specific performance capabilities of the technology itself. Simply put, if the adoption of even an excellent new technology is not well managed then consumers will not receive its benefits. Minimally invasive cardiac surgery is a case in point. Even though cardiac surgeons agree that some form of minimally invasive cardiac surgery will ultimately be a standard of care,[50] the specific technology marketed over the last five years has fallen out of favor and is now infrequently used.

CONCLUSION

The concept of architectural innovation, in which the components of a product remain the same but their relationships to one another are reconfigured, has an exact analogy in the process of health care delivery. When relationships among disciplines contributing to the process of care change, the resulting new processes can be deceptively difficult to manage. In the same way that producers of an architectural innovation may have difficulty diagnosing the level of change and learning the new skills required to adapt to it, adopters of medical technologies that change the relationships among clinical disciplines may also underestimate the amount of learning these technologies require. Furthermore, they may fail to actively manage this learning, thereby reducing the likelihood that they will realize a technology's full potential and, worse, putting their patients at risk.

For the benefits of consumer-driven health care to be fully realized many providers will need to learn how to implement innovations—whether new technologies or new processes for managing patient care. That is, some of the most important innovations are new models for serving consumer needs. Both new technologies and new service delivery models can require reconfigured clinical care processes and new relationships among care providers (who constitute an expanding pool). Moreover, both kinds of innovations can foster a reconceptualizing of the relationship between providers and consumers as a partnership of equals. Our study highlights provider learning that involved new processes and relationships, and shows that this reconfiguration was neither automatic nor straightforward. Some innovative providers will find new ways of meeting the needs of lead consumers; however, widespread change in the way providers deliver care and serve consumers will not simply follow increased consumer expectations of service and technical excellence. Provider learning and change must be managed.

In this chapter we have proposed that to achieve better outcomes, adopters of new technologies must actively manage three phases of the adoption process—learning before doing, learning during early cases, and later learning. We have highlighted different factors and activities that must be managed at these different phases of adoption. Furthermore, we have suggested that in the design and marketing of new technology, developers must take into consideration the ability of adopting organizations to learn and change. Finally, when choosing health care providers, consumers must be aware that organizations may vary in their ability to adopt new technologies safely, and thus consumers may need to critically evaluate their providers' experience with a given technology before agreeing to certain new treatments.

Notes

1. King, R. T. "Second Opinion: Keyhole Surgery Arrived with Fanfare, but Was It Premature?" *Wall Street Journal,* May 5, 1999, p. A1.

2. Greer, A. L. "The State of the Art Versus the State of the Science: The Diffusion of New Medical Technologies into Practice." *International Journal of Technology Assessment in Health Care,* 1988, *4,* 5–26.

3. See, for example, Kopacz, D. J., Neal, J. M., and Pollock, J. E. "The Regional Anesthesia 'Learning Curve': What Is the Minimum Number of Epidural and Spinal Blocks to Reach Consistency?" *Regional Anesthesia,* 1996, *21*(3), 182–190.

4. Henderson, R. M., and Clark, K. B. "Architectural Innovation: The Reconfiguration of Existing Product Technologies and the Failure of Established Firms." *Administrative Science Quarterly,* 1990, *35,* 9–30. Note that Henderson and Clark use the term *architectural innovation* predominantly to describe new relationships among components of a product. We consider new relationships among participants in a health care process to be architectural innovations also.

5. Henderson and Clark, "Architectural Innovation."

6. Levitt, B., and March, J. G. "Organizational Learning." *Annual Review of Sociology,* 1988, *14,* 319–340.

7. A national study in 121 hospitals similarly found no excess mortality. See Galloway, A. C., Shemin, R. J., Glower, D. D., and others. "First Report of the Port Access International Registry." *Annals of Thoracic Surgery,* 1999, *67,* 51–58.

8. Pisano, G. P., Bohmer, R.M.J., and Edmondson, A. C. "Organizational Differences in Rates of Learning: Evidence from the Adoption of Minimally Invasive Cardiac Surgery." *Management Science,* 2001, *47,* 752–768.

9. The volume-outcome hypothesis has been a focus of debate, most notably in the cardiac surgical literature. See Luft, H., Garnick, D. W., Mark, D. H., and McPhee, S. J.

Hospital Volume, Physician Volume and Patient Outcomes: Assessing the Evidence. Ann Arbor, Mich.: Health Administration Press, 1990; Hannan, E. L. "The Relation Between Volume and Outcome in Health Care." *New England Journal of Medicine,* 1999, *340,* 1677–1679.

10. Edmondson, A. C, Bohmer, R.M.J., and Pisano, G. P. "Disrupted Routines: Effects of Team Learning on New Technology Adoption." *Administrative Science Quarterly,* 2001, *46,* 685–716.

11. Edmondson, A. C. "Psychological Safety and Learning Behavior on Work Teams." *Administrative Science Quarterly,* 1999, *44,* 350–383.

12. Helmreich, R. L., and Schaefer, H. "Team Performance in the Operating Room." In M. S. Bogner (ed.), *Human Error in Medicine.* Mahwah, N.J.: Erlbaum, 1994.

13. FMEA is a tool frequently used in industry to calculate the probability of (systemic, process, or human) failure and the impact of that outcome. The results are used to identify those points in a system or process that should be improved in order to minimize adverse outcomes. Human factors analysis is a related technique, use to gauge the likelihood of human error.

14. Note that these characteristics changed over time as the surgical team gained experience, so that a patient who may not have been a candidate for the procedure early in the hospital's experience may have become eligible later on.

15. March, J. G., Sproull, L. S., and Tamuz, M. "Learning from Samples of One or Fewer." *Organization Science,* 1991, *2*(1), 1–13.

16. Blumenthal, D. "Applying IQMS to Physicians' Clinical Decisions." In D. Blumenthal and A. C. Scheck (eds.), *Improving Clinical Practice: Total Quality Management and the Physician.* San Francisco: Jossey-Bass, 1995.

17. Edmondson, A. C. "Learning from Mistakes Is Easier Said Than Done: Group and Organizational Influences on the Detection and Correction of Human Error." *Journal of Applied Behavioral Science,* 1996, *32*(1), 5–28.

18. Edmondson, "Learning from Mistakes . . ."

19. Argyris, C. *Reasoning, Learning and Action: Individual and Organizational.* San Francisco: Jossey-Bass, 1982.

20. Levitt, B., and March, J. G. "Organizational Learning." *Annual Review of Sociology,* 1988, *14,* 319–340.

21. Pisano, G. P. *The Development Factory: Unlocking the Potential of Process Innovation.* Boston: Harvard Business School Press, 1997, chap. 2.

22. See, for example, Kotter, J. P. *Leading Change.* Boston: Harvard Business School Press, 1996.

23. Greer, "The State of the Art Versus the State of the Science."

24. Rogers, E. M. *Diffusion of Innovations.* (4th ed.) New York: Free Press, 1995.

25. Greer, "The State of the Art Versus the State of the Science."

26. For a review of physician practice variation and its determinants, see Bohmer, R.M.J. *Changing Physician Behavior.* Harvard Business School Case No. N9-699-124. Boston: Harvard Business School, 1998.

27. Leape, L. L., and others. "Relation Between Surgeons' Practice Volumes and Geographic Variation in the Rate of Carotid Endarterectomy." *New England Journal of Medicine*, 1989, *321*, 653–657.

28. For example, after adjusting for differences in patient mix, the rate of repeat cesarean section is higher in teaching than nonteaching hospitals. See Stafford, R. S. "The Impact of Nonclinical Factors on Repeat Cesarean Section." *Journal of the American Medical Association*, 1991, *265*, 59–63.

29. For example, interventional and noninterventional cardiologists treat the same types of patients very differently. See Di Salvo, T. G., Paul, S. D., Lloyd-Jones, D., and others. "Care of Acute Myocardial Infarction by Noninvasive and Invasive Cardiologists: Procedure Use, Cost and Outcome." *Journal of the American College of Cardiology*, 1996, *27*(2), 262–269.

30. Watson, D. I., Baigrie, R. J., and Jamieson, G. G. "A Learning Curve for Laparoscopic Fundoplication: Definable, Avoidable, or a Waste of Time?" *Annals of Surgery*, 1996, *224*, 198–203. Laparoscopic fundoplication is a procedure in which the stomach is prevented from sliding up into the chest, so reducing the incidence of heartburn.

31. Kopacz and others, "The Regional Anesthesia 'Learning Curve.'"

32. Jowell, P. S., Baillie, J., Branch, M. S., and others. "Quantitative Assessment of Procedural Competence: A Prospective Study of Training in Endoscopic Retrograde Cholangiopancreatography." *Annals of Internal Medicine*, 1996, *125*, 983–989.

33. Food and Drug Administration, Office of Device Evaluation. *Annual Report.* Washington, D.C.: Food and Drug Administration, Office of Device Evaluation, 2001.

34. Zuger, A. "Are Doctors Losing Touch with Hands On Medicine?" *New York Times*, Jul. 13, 1999, p. F1.

35. The propensity of new technologies to redraw professional boundaries and change professional relationships is well known. A well-documented example is the CT scanner, which had a significant effect on the relationship between radiologists and radiology technicians. See Barley, S. R. "Technology as an Occasion for Structuring: Evidence from Observations of CT Scanners and the Social Order of Radiology Departments." *Administrative Science Quarterly*, 1986, *31*, 78–108.

36. Galewitz, P. "Nurse Practitioners and Physician Assistants Prescribing More Drugs." Associated Press, Aug. 17, 1999.

37. Cooper, R. A., Laud, P., and Dietrich, C. L. "Current and Projected Workforce of Nonphysician Clinicians." *Journal of the American Medical Association*, 1998, *280*, 788–794.

38. Freudheim, M. "As Nurses Take on Primary Care Physicians Are Sounding Alarms." *New York Times*, Sept. 30, 1997, p. A1.

39. Wachter, R. M., and Goldman, L. "The Hospitalist Movement 5 Years Later." *Journal of the American Medical Association*, 2002, *287*, 487–494.

40. Steiner, C. A., and others. "Surgical Rates and Operative Mortality for Open and Laparoscopic Cholecystectomy in Maryland." *New England Journal of Medicine*, 1994, *330*, 403–408.

41. Legorreta, A. P., Silber, J. H., Costantino, G. N., and others. "Increased Cholecystectomy Rate After the Introduction of Laparoscopic Cholecystectomy." *Journal of the American Medical Association,* 1993, *270,* 1429–1432. For a discussion of this issue, also see Herzlinger, R. E. *Market-Driven Health Care: Who Wins, Who Loses in the Transformation of American's Largest Service Industry.* Reading, Mass.: Addison-Wesley, 1997, chap. 9.

42. Several cardiac surgeons interviewed by the authors for their Managing Medical Innovation research project volunteered this observation.

43. Moynihan, R., and others. "Coverage by the News Media of the Benefits and Risks of Medications." *New England Journal of Medicine,* 2000, *342,* 1645–1650.

44. For a discussion of the normalization of risk in high-risk environments, see Vaughn, D. "The Trickle Down Effect: Policy Decisions, Risky Work and the Challenger Tragedy." *California Management Review,* 1997, *39*(2), 80–102.

45. Green, J., Wintfield, N., Krasner, M., and Wells, C. "In Search of America's Best Hospitals: The Promise and Reality of Quality Assessment." *Journal of the American Medical Association,* 1997, *277,* 1152–1155.

46. Pisano and others, "Organizational Differences in Rates of Learning."

47. See Bohmer, R.M.J., and Winslow, A. *The Dana Farber Cancer Institute.* Harvard Business School Case No. 9-699-025. Boston: Harvard Business School, 1999; Tye L. "Clashing Evaluations of Hospital Spur Worry." *Boston Globe,* Aug. 20, 1997, p. A1.

48. Herzlinger, R. E., and Burroughs, A. *Note on Health Care Accountability.* Harvard Business School Case 1-198-065. Boston: Harvard Business School, March 1998.

49. Biermann, J. S., and others. "Evaluation of Cancer Information on the Internet." *Cancer,* 1999, *86,* 381–390.

50. King, "Second Opinion."

CHAPTER FIFTY-THREE

Consumer-Driven Health Care for the Chronically Ill

Al Lewis

The old joke about health maintenance organizations is that they are a great place to receive health care—unless you are sick. Whatever the validity behind this joke in years past, the opposite is true today. HMOs have successfully developed or contracted for disease management programs specifically targeted at the chronically and severely ill segments of the population. These programs are almost invariably free to the HMO member because better health pays for itself in reduced member claims. They are also always voluntary—no precertifications or reviews necessary, and no denials. Most important, their effectiveness, according to virtually all published studies, has been dramatic enough to motivate *Newsweek* to conclude that HMOs now offer "some of the country's finest programs" for managing the chronically ill.[1]

As one would expect, patients responded to the lure of more services—education, home visits, free equipment, and more—by enrolling in droves: by 1980, nationwide enrollment exceeded 3.1 million.[2]

And yet Washington continually complicates or threatens to complicate the administration of these programs—both by impeding access to data and by perverting health plan incentives to improve member health.

On the data front, Congress overresponded to legitimate concerns about medical privacy by regulating even appropriate uses, such as using medical records to identify people who would benefit from disease management programs. As of this writing, the regulations are acceptable, but this level of acceptability was achieved only through intensive lobbying.

On another front, the midlevel civil servants at the Centers for Medicare and Medicaid Services (CMS)—despite the best intentions of the people who run this agency—are not easily able to accommodate state initiatives in disease management. One regulator wanted to define a disease management company as a provider, which would mean that any disease management company could serve patients, a wholly impractical approach. Another regulator wanted to define a disease management company as a health plan because such organizations "take risk," a rather tortured interpretation of the fact that they guarantee their fees.

One can only conclude from these two government initiatives that the regulatory system at worst has broken down and at best is ill-suited to oversight of disease management. Clearly, a new paradigm is needed to deliver disease management services.

FAST FORWARD: THE CONSUMER-DRIVEN DISEASE MANAGEMENT FOCUSED FACTORY

In a consumer-driven model of chronic disease management, four factors should be scrutinized to determine how much regulation is needed to make a consumer-driven disease management model function efficiently:

1. Privacy of data

2. Pricing of health care for chronically ill people

3. Employer-funded health care for high-cost employees

4. Outcomes measurement

Privacy of Data

Because privacy of data is a timely topic, it is worth exploring first. Some believe that individuals have a "right to privacy" that extends to their medical data, even within a health plan. Others point out that when individuals join a health plan, they voluntarily acquiesce to the needs of a system that, like any organization, uses information to make decisions. Their medical data are part of that information base, within reason of course.

The government's initial reaction to those concerned about privacy was that almost all uses of data should be made illegal, which would have driven up the cost of health care and denied millions of people access to disease management programs. However, only about 3 percent of the people who are enrolled in disease management programs automatically and are given the opportunity to opt out actually do so. Even if every one of those 3 percent opted out for privacy reasons, government regulation of privacy would have satisfied only a tiny fraction of people while potentially affecting the health of many more.

In contrast, a consumer-driven health plan marketplace would find an elegant solution on its own. A few health plans would advertise, as one of their benefits, the absolute privacy of their medical information. These health plans would attract the people who valued their privacy above all else, including their health. Presumably these health plans would cost more, if one assumes that plans that use member medical data well to identify candidates for disease management programs save money by doing so and that health plans that give up their ability to use these data thereby lose some of their ability to manage the diseases of their population of members.

The difference with a consumer-driven solution is that rather than share the cost burden of privacy across the entire plan membership, it focuses the cost, appropriately, on those who value privacy above health. Although the cost would not be trivial, one can nonetheless imagine a market for such plans among people who have AIDS, depression, or other conditions for which they would prefer anonymity. Whether such plans are profitable will depend on whether they are fairly compensated for taking on those high-cost patients (with the privacy premium). And that question leads naturally into the next major disease management issue of consumer-driven health care.

Pricing for Chronically Ill People

Here's what does *not* work, regardless of one's viewpoint on the subject of government intrusion in the marketplace: pricing according to a formula that does not differentially reimburse patients according to diagnosis and severity—as is the case today in Medicare except for end-stage renal disease patients and institutionalized patients and also some payment variation according to geographical area.

Insurance executives and benefits managers are well acquainted with the concept of adverse selection: the more attractive an insurance plan is to people who are sick, the more sick people will apply for it. A health plan that becomes widely known for its management of congestive heart failure patients will attract more congestive heart failure patients. This is a recipe for financial disaster, barring what Medicare refers to as *risk-stratified pricing*. (In risk-stratified pricing, the health plan receives extra reimbursement for sicker patients.)

There are two ways that this extra reimbursement level can be calculated. The first is to examine recent *claims history* and infer a patient's health status from it. This approach penalizes health plans that spend money effectively to improve a patient's health status and thereby reduce a patient's claims. The reimbursement will follow the claims downward, thus negating financial rewards for the improvement that the insurers achieved. If the goal of stratifying people is to give health plans incentives to improve the care of members, this method is dead wrong. From a disease management perspective, it is worse than no stratification at all.

The second way is to examine *independent* variables—mostly diagnoses, because severity is much more subjective. Perhaps there could be a simple "with complications" qualifier in some cases to capture severity. Although this severity-adjusted diagnosis approach is subject to some degree of gaming, a well-designed arbitration system with penalties for reversals of classifications could provide a sentinel-based system for preventing diagnosis inflation. These prices would be revised frequently, of course, but that is no different from today's practice in Medicare's reimbursement of health plans.

With the second methodology, if prices were set reasonably, health plans would actually *compete* to enroll people with congestive heart failure, diabetes, and the like if they thought their disease management programs were sufficiently effective to allow them to manage these patients better than the pricing assumed. This is precisely the system one would want to see, allowing a match between consumers with regular or special needs and health plans with broad or specific expertise. Niche health plans would serve as *focused factories* for the chronically ill.

Employer-Funded Health Care for High-Cost Employees

So far, so good—for any government-funded health program. But what about group health? How could employers possibly work within a system that required them to identify and pay differently for people with chronic disease? As described previously, the system would simply not work in an employer situation in which confidentiality of individual medical data (meaning protection from scrutiny by the employer, not by the employer's health plan) is a well-established principle. Experience rating would not work either, for the same reason that stratification based on utilization would not work: using previous claims experience to set future premiums effectively removes any incentive to reduce those premiums, making disease management a financially disastrous undertaking.

There are a number of potential solutions. Probably the cleanest is a simple regulation that all employers over a certain size that offer health insurance must include all accredited health plans, or at least one accredited health plan in every major disease category, and allow employees to choose. (One can assume, as is the case with disease management companies today, that many health plans will offer care for multiple chronic diseases in their focused factories, so this requirement is nowhere near as onerous as it might appear.) This can be done on an administrative services only (ASO) basis, as many employers prefer to do today, or else be premium based. Employers that elect not to follow this requirement would lose the ability to pay for health care on a pretax basis.

To solve the problem of data confidentiality, an individual employee's choice of health plan would have to be subject to much stricter confidentiality standards than those that exist today, because an employee would be telegraphing his or her condition through health plan selection. That is one irony of a consumer-driven model: if it is so efficient in market creation that the chronically ill have options specific to their needs, the choice of health plan will necessarily reveal one's health status. The need for greater privacy protection may increase the trend toward outsourcing human resource (HR) functions, because it will be much easier to create a wall between an outsourced HR function and the employer than between an internal HR function and the rest of the company.

Outcomes Measurement for Chronically Ill Members

It is generally well accepted in managed health care that some kind of standardized outcomes measurement tool must be established industrywide, rather than relying on health plans' or providers' own reports of successes. For example, it has been the universal experience of the Disease Management Purchasing Consortium in looking for end-stage renal disease vendors that all dialysis companies can compare their "outcomes" to the national averages and demonstrate the Lake Wobegon ideal—according to these companies they are all better than average. It would appear that some more objective outcome measurement tools are needed. Although such tools for chronically ill patients have not been universally accepted yet, several important principles are generally accepted in the industry and endorsed by the Disease Management Purchasing Consortium:

- The impacts should be population based, not based on whoever voluntarily participates.
- Certain disease-specific quality measures, such as hemoglobin A1c test results in diabetes, can serve as proxies for overall health status.
- Changes in frequency of emergency room visits and inpatient admissions are a proxy for access and quality (as long as no change has occurred in the amount that enrollees pay for emergency visits).
- Self-administered health status assessments are valid, if they are done on as close to a population-wide basis as possible.

Counterintuitively, it will probably be easier to develop outcomes measures for chronic disease focused factories than for health plans as a whole, for three reasons:

- There are not many items on the previous list, and all are clearly measurable.
- Because the people involved are sick and the health plan is spending considerable sums on relatively few people, it is cost effective to obtain close to 100 percent patient compliance on completing health status surveys.
- No one can claim "my members are sicker" if an entire industry of focused factories is competing for the same target segment of sick people

CONCLUSION

A major attribute of a consumer-driven market is that some health plans will migrate from avoiding sick enrollees to actively recruiting them. In a consumer-driven health care system, people will be able to choose among alternatives that reflect their health status, health needs, and preference for privacy in a way that today's marketplace does not accommodate. The barriers to doing this are, in the scheme of things, fairly minor pricing policies for government-funded health care along with some confidentiality issues for employer-funded health care and outcomes standards for both employer- and government-funded care, standards that are already evolving.

Even with these changes taken into account, this consumer-driven system will require far less regulatory intrusion into the marketplace than the current system does. And the regulations that are necessary to effect a consumer-driven health care system will not contradict one another or penalize the 97 percent in order to comply with the vocal demands of the organized 3 percent.

Notes

1. Spragins, E. "Outsmarting an Illness." *Newsweek*, Mar. 29, 1999, p. 82.

2. U.S. Census Bureau, *Statistical Abstract of the United States: 2002.* Washington, D.C.: U.S. Census Bureau, 2002, p. 101.

CHAPTER FIFTY-FOUR

A Cost-Effective Model for High-Quality Catastrophic Care

Bernard Salick, Seth M. Yellin

The world faces a crisis of uncontrolled cost increases in health care services. Although health care reform and managed care approaches have attempted to control health care expenditures through resource management and rationing, most of these approaches have failed.

The single most significant target of health care spending is the treatment of catastrophic illness—HIV/AIDS, end-stage renal disease, solid organ transplantation, heart disease, and diabetes—which accounts for roughly 80 percent of annual U.S. health care expenditures.[1] Bentley Health Care, Inc., where the lead author is chairman and CEO, has developed a health care delivery model to control health care expenditures in cancer and HIV/AIDS, two diseases that together account for more than 12 percent of annual U.S. health care costs.[2] Cancer and HIV/AIDS are unusual because they can be carved out of the health care spectrum and treated independently, a characteristic that exists for few other catastrophic diseases. The carve-out leads to better and more cost-effective care.

Bentley was established to provide comprehensive, high-quality, and cost-effective care to a diverse geographical population across the entire continuum of care. The Bentley model controls expenditures through comprehensive management of the quality of care provided. The model utilizes a constantly evolving database, evidence-based protocols, comfortable and convenient patient settings, and other appropriate support services needed to achieve optimal patient care outcomes. This model supports a uniform approach to health care delivery, regardless of the financing structure. It can be applied universally.

THE CRITERIA FOR SUITABLE CATASTROPHIC ILLNESSES

The Bentley approach is based on disease management—the coordination of resources across the entire health care delivery system and throughout the life cycle of a specific disease. Bentley targets diseases that meet the following criteria:

High percentage of health care costs. Diagnosis and treatment of the disease must consume a large percentage of total health care costs. Only a disease that represents a significant portion of health care expenditures can justify the cost of developing specialized facilities to manage the disorder; cancer, for example, consumes $100 billion per year (direct and indirect costs), or 10 percent of all health care expenditures.[3]

Outpatient utilization. A significant portion of the diagnosis and treatment services employed to manage the disease can be performed on an outpatient basis. Shifting services from large inpatient facilities to disease-focused outpatient centers optimizes the cost and outcomes of diagnosis and treatment and offers a more comfortable and convenient setting for the patient. Specialized outpatient facilities and highly trained clinical staff provide core services, augmented by an affiliated hospital, satellite facilities, and home care services.

Definable. There must be a definitive method of diagnosis for the disease in question. Cancer tissue diagnosis and the HIV antibody test unambiguously determine whether a patient has the disease in question, at which point the patient is entered into the Bentley system, and the appropriate treatment regimen is begun. Because other chronic diseases, such as Alzheimer's, hypertension, and diabetes, are less definable, a clear course of treatment is more difficult to determine.

Clinical guidelines. The outcome of care must be enhanced by standardization. The course of the disease must be generally predictable and a definitive plan of diagnosis, treatment, and palliation identifiable. Clinical guidelines and outcome measurement create a uniform, consistent approach to disease management, which enhances efficiency by reducing redundancies and inappropriate variations. For example, cancer management and treatment is optimal when generally accepted and appropriately applicable treatments are administered.[4]

Reliance on specialty care. For this model to be cost effective and deliver consistent high-quality care, it must focus on diseases in which a subspecialist treats the entirety of the disease. For example, this model is not as successful for chronic cardiac disease as it is for cancer. In congestive heart failure a patient may require treatment not only from a cardiologist but also from physicians in other specialties, such as nephrology. In a cancer program, however, the treatment of the patient has historically been managed by an oncologist. This characteristic of the disease creates two benefits for the model: every patient with cancer flows through the cancer program, thus creating continual patient volume, enabling total oversight of patient treatment, including adherence to clinical guidelines and maintenance of the appropriate level of quality assurance and control.

Cancer, HIV/AIDS, end-stage renal disease, and solid organ transplantation fit our disease management model; heart disease does not. Although heart disease consumes a large percentage of health care costs, the wide variation in cause, diagnosis, and prescribed treatments is inconsistent with a highly defined treatment approach. Cancer, in contrast, is a disease that has been managed with great success in outpatient centers. HIV/AIDS, a catastrophic illness that until recently was treated primarily in a hospital or in a doctor's office during business hours, is now manageable on an outpatient basis with the advent of protease inhibitors and combination antiretroviral therapies.[5]

THE SYSTEM FOR TREATING CATASTROPHIC ILLNESS

Bentley develops comprehensive health care delivery systems that integrate all levels of diagnostic and treatment services. The delivery system is composed of a wide network of diagnostic and treatment facilities and specialty providers linked together, nationally and internationally. It provides services predominantly on an outpatient basis, which is more convenient and less costly than inpatient hospital-based care. An important element of the Bentley program is the affiliation of the outpatient facilities with major academic medical centers and university-based health systems, under thirty-five-year exclusive agreements to provide all elements of the diagnosis and treatment of cancer and HIV/AIDS for these affiliated institutions. This network contributes to a continually evolving clinical database specific to cancer and HIV/AIDS. This advancing database, in turn, supports the evolving Bentley treatment guidelines.

Comprehensive Outpatient Tertiary Care Facilities

In the Bentley model, outpatient facilities are located in major metropolitan areas and provide a comprehensive spectrum of outpatient services for the diagnosis and treatment of a single disease. These centers are located near affiliated academic medical centers, to which patients requiring sophisticated and experimental care tend to gravitate for treatment, and house the full array of services required for the management of a particular disease.

For example, the five major approaches to treatment of cancer—surgery, radiation, chemotherapy, biologic response modifiers, and potentially, gene therapy—are all provided in Bentley's comprehensive cancer centers. These centers typically include physician offices, a twenty-four-hour *day hospital* treatment facility, infusion therapy, stem cell and bone marrow transplantation, radiation oncology, diagnostic radiology, screening and detection, ambulatory surgery, laboratory services, pathology services, pharmacy services, psychosocial counseling, biologic response modifiers, pain management, patient education, nutrition counseling, gene therapy, data measurement, and clinical trials.

To enhance the quality of care and the patient's comfort, these facilities offer patients and their physicians access twenty-four hours a day, seven days a week. Such accessibility allows patients to schedule appointments at their convenience and to manage emergencies or complications as needed. These facilities also house disease-focused "centers of excellence," specializing in high-frequency disorders such as breast and prostate cancer as well as gynecological oncology. Additional patient-oriented support amenities are also provided, such as pickup and drop-off shuttle service, valet parking, and child care.

Satellite Treatment Centers

An internal component of the Bentley model is to surround the tertiary care centers with a regional network of satellite treatment centers. These outpatient facilities offer a more limited array of services: infusion therapy, chemotherapy, stem cell collection and mobilization, screening and detection, laboratory services, pain management, basic radiology services, patient education, and pharmacy services. The satellite facilities enable patients to receive high-quality care in a nearby location, reducing their need to travel to the tertiary facilities. All satellite facilities are coordinated with the tertiary facilities and the provider network to create a continuum of care and expertise that reduces duplicative tests and procedures and enhances results.

Home Care Services

The home care unit provides basic services performed by nurses at the patient's home. These include the management of complications such as febrile neutropenia and treatments such as hyperalimentation and, importantly, pain management.

Specialty Provider Network

A specialty provider network of cancer and HIV/AIDS specialists has been established and covers a broad geographical region. All the physicians and their patients are integrated into the Bentley program, following the approved treatment guidelines and tracked by the information system. This provider network enables Bentley to service broad regions of patient populations while monitoring quality of care, resource utilization, and costs.

THE INFORMATION SYSTEM

A fundamental aspect of the Bentley model is a sophisticated and powerful integrated information network. All elements of the program, nationally and internationally, are networked and linked—all tertiary care facilities are linked to the system of satellite treatment facilities and the entire physician network. This is not merely an electronic medical record system but a continually evolving database of all patient demographic data, encounter data, and laboratory and diagnostic data, as well as detailed utilization and cost information. This information system enables Bentley to provide detailed outcome analyses; to further improve and refine diagnosis and treatment guidelines; to enrich third-party payer databases, whose demographic data lead to improved population coverage; to provide consistent and reliable coordination and administration for large, national clinical trials with pharmaceutical and biotechnology companies; and to prepare detailed utilization and cost analyses for disease-specific care. The complete and efficient recording, retrieval, and exchange of diagnostic and treatment information among physicians around the world enables Bentley to refine diagnosis and treatment protocols continually as well as evolve more accurate and equitable pricing structures.

Some critics claim that the bricks-and-mortar aspect of this delivery model is capital intensive and thus prohibitively expensive and that the length of time required to develop a full-scale program is a deterrent to the model's increased use. The development of highly sophisticated tertiary care facilities, outpatient satellite centers, a provider network, and an integrated medical information system is indeed expensive, requiring significant financial sponsorship. The Bentley model, however, balances this cost with significant health care benefits and the economic value of a thirty-five-year exclusive agreement with the affiliated academic medical centers. The overall benefits derived more than balance its up-front costs.

PRICING STRUCTURES

A model that is effective in controlling costs requires a competitive pricing structure. A capitated pricing system suits the Bentley model. The capitation is carefully developed. Breast cancer capitation, for instance, begins with an analysis of clinical outcomes by an independent panel of breast cancer experts. Based on the outcome data, this panel outlines the most effective treatment protocols for various types of breast cancer. Multiple protocols are developed that account for every aspect of breast cancer treatment, from surgical, chemotherapy, and radiation therapies to autologous bone marrow transplantation when and if indicated. All levels of care are included in the pricing model, including currently experimental protocols, because these modalities may become mainstream treatments in the near future. For example, although interleukin is currently considered an experimental treatment in the treatment of kidney cell cancer, in two to three years it may account for the treatment of a large number of kidney cell cancer cases. Therefore, a five-year pricing model accounts for use of this protocol from the initiation of coverage.

The information system is then used to analyze the guidelines and to determine the total cost of providing each of the services outlined in those guidelines. A careful evaluation is then performed of the patient population to be covered to determine the historical incidence of breast cancer, weighted for age, gender, and particular incidence irregularities of the population. This analysis determines the total number of breast cancer cases expected to occur over the next several years. A price is then calculated on a per-member per-month (PMPM) basis to provide cancer treatment for the entire patient population over the next five or more years.

One of the significant risks of using a capitated pricing model is adverse selection, the phenomenon in which the incidence of a disease treated by a provider increases beyond historical numbers as a result of the quality of care provided. For example, assume that a provider initially sets a capitation rate of $10.00 per member per month based on the assumed costs of providing care for a 1 percent historical incidence of cancer in the provider's existing population. However, say that a large number of patients with cancer enroll in this program soon after initiation of coverage due to the high quality of care provided, and the incidence rate rises to 5 percent. The provider, however, still receives the agreed-upon rate of $10.00 PMPM, a price that covers the cost related to the treatment of one-fifth of the total number of cases. The very quality of care provided has adversely affected the demographic makeup of the patients being treated.

There are several solutions to the adverse selection problem that do not reduce the quality of care or the level of patient coverage. For one, coverage of a large population is extremely important; for example, coverage of a population of one million lives reduces the effect of an additional one hundred patients. Additionally, long-term contracts, of five or more years, that are reevaluated at regular intervals to renegotiate price structures based on population shifts must be used. Over the long term, a single event of patient increase can then be offset in later years by adjustment to the pricing structure of the capitation rate. The last method of reducing capitation risk is the use of *risk corridors.* The cost of health care is extremely unpredictable because new technologies and modalities can quickly increase the costs of providing treatments. Risk corridors create a floor and a ceiling to the maximum profit or loss that can be experienced by either the payer or the provider; they thus provide security to both in an unpredictable arena.

CONCLUSION

The goal of Bentley Health Care is to provide the highest-quality disease-specific care in the most cost-effective manner. Bentley achieves this through advanced outpatient delivery facilities staffed by dedicated and highly trained specialists who use a state-of-the-art information system. This information system provides the basis for a rational and equitable pricing structure for altogether irrational diseases. Bentley is an evolving model for twenty-first-century medical care.

Notes

1. Hoffman, C., Rice, D., and Sung, H. Y. "Persons with Chronic Conditions: Their Prevalence and Costs." *Journal of the American Medical Association,* 1996, *276,* 1473–1479.

2. American Cancer Society. *Cancer Facts & Figures—1999.* Atlanta, Ga.: American Cancer Society, 1999, p. 3.

3. American Cancer Society. *Cancer Facts & Figures—1999.*

4. Hewitt, M., and Simone, J. (eds.). *Ensuring Quality Cancer Care.* Washington, D.C.: National Academy Press, 1999, pp. 164–175.

5. U.S. Department of Health and Human Services, Centers for Disease Control and Prevention. *HIV/AIDS Surveillance Report,* 2000, *2*(2); also see Haburchak, D. "The Economics of AIDS in America." *The AIDS Reader,* 1997, *7*(5), 155–160; Becker, S. "The Economics of AIDS and Cost Effective Antiretroviral Therapy." *Medscape HIV/AIDS,* 1997, *3*(3) [www.medscape.com/hiv-aidshome]; Moore, R. "Update on the Cost of HIV/AIDS Care and Cost Effectiveness of New HIV Therapy." *The Hopkins HIV Report,* May 1997 [www.hopkins-aids.edu/publications/report/may97].

CHAPTER FIFTY-FIVE

Collaborating with Consumers to Advance Health Knowledge and Improve Practice

S. Robert Levine, Laura L. Adams

Viktor Frankl tells us, "Man's search for meaning is the primary motivation in his life."[1] Choosing a health-related career offers the opportunity to find that meaning by helping people improve their health. However, the overwhelming pace of scientific advances, the increasingly specialized demands of science and medicine, and our health care system's sometimes perverse incentives, make it difficult to sustain the capacity and drive to achieve this ideal. Professionals are less able to ask and answer the questions required to progress along the path from discovery to cure, to overcome every resource obstacle, and to apply new knowledge rapidly and consistently to benefit their patients. Furthermore, the collaborative activities required for success often go unconsummated, and the time, energy, and expertise needed to synthesize new knowledge and apply it for the benefit of people is unavailable or lost.[2]

WE'RE IN THIS TOGETHER

Health is the ultimate enabler. It is the vital force that propels us through our today and promises us a better tomorrow. Increasingly, we define health through the lens of scientific process—through research. Research is at the core of our understanding of health, of what we expect from our health care system, and what we anticipate for our future and that of our children. When we lose our health, research is our hope. And when we seek help, we rely on the health care system to properly apply new knowledge—the outcome of research.

Health Is Personal

Consumers' expectations of providers and researchers are very personal. Sandra Silvestri, whose eight-year-old son Joey was diagnosed with Type 1 diabetes six years ago, is a Juvenile Diabetes Research Foundation volunteer. (Founded by the parents of children with Type 1 diabetes, and led by volunteers, including myself as chairman, JDRF is the world's largest private, nonprofit funder of diabetes research.) She writes: "A mother's or father's connection to the health care system begins the moment their child is diagnosed with diabetes. They carry their child into the emergency room and literally place them in its arms. The health care system is the lifeline that keeps the family and child alive. Research is an extension of this lifeline. The family reaches out to be connected to their future through gaining information about research. Supporting research fulfills the need to do something positive in the face of the threats on one's life that diabetes brings."[3]

Health Is Collaborative

Health researchers and providers can reconnect with their idealism and join consumers in a collaboration focused on achieving personal, family, and community health goals. Consumers can be effective partners in all aspects of the health research enterprise. JDRF's nearly thirty years of experience in supporting biomedical research affirms this. Furthermore, the experience of organizations committed to health practice improvement, like the Foundation for Accountability (FACCT), is also that consumer engagement and leadership are key to the success of outcomes improvement.

The Proposition

We must learn from these experiences and welcome consumers as collaborators in the research and practice improvement enterprise. Consumers provide context, energy, and insight. Consumers are the interested party who will most consistently and passionately seek accelerated distillation, synthesis, application, and translation of scientific advances. Consumers will force the reassembly of knowledge gained through reductionism scientific methods. They will cheer innovation and will insist on its rapid and broad application. Although consumers may not know how to answer their most pressing health questions, they can provide the drive that challenges research to result in better health for all.

PATH TO A CURE

The *path to a cure* is a framework for understanding the stages of medical research and practice improvement as they move from the laboratory bench to the patient's bedside. It teaches us how what was once unknown and only a research question can become a treatment answer.

The path to a cure for any specific clinical problem is neither exclusive nor linear. It develops along a multidimensional weblike *continuity* (Figure 55.1) from the creation of fundamental knowledge (basic research) to progress in understanding the cause and course of illness (epidemiology and disease-oriented basic research) to patient-oriented application of new knowledge (clinical research) to translation of new knowledge into innovations in health care practice (health services research) to wide adoption of new knowledge by practitioners (professional behavior change) and finally to analysis of the impact of practice change on health (outcomes research).

The path to a cure framework reminds us that it is not basic research alone that must be our hope. Even as we are thrilled by an amazing laboratory discovery with the potential to lead to a "cure," we must recognize that laboratory "cures" must also be clinically tested, translated into an intervention usable across a wide spectrum of circumstances, performed cost effectively and consistently (from a quality standpoint), and evaluated over the long term.

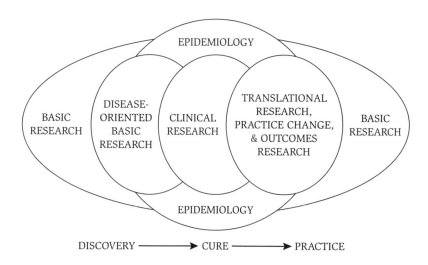

Figure 55.1. Path to a Cure.

A Path Taken

Eileen Gelick, another JDRF volunteer, reflects: "I have been a careful recorder of the promise of islet transplantation as a potential cure for diabetes [islet cells produce insulin]. The peaks and valleys of the research have been a wild and somewhat depressing experience. More than twenty years ago, I remember being in a laboratory at a leading research institution, and the energy and excitement was almost overwhelming. There was a 'breakthrough' in the transplantation of islets in animals. It seemed as if it was only a six month 'walk across the street' for this research to be applied to humans."[4]

Sadly, islet transplantation has yet to be proven successful. The families and researchers who were so hopeful twenty years ago were not naive. But researchers and families alike failed to anticipate the many complexities and obstacles of moving from an animal model to human intervention. However, despite their disappointments, the group of parents who were first captivated by the idea of a cure through islet transplantation never stopped prodding the research community to solve these problems. They remained good partners in soliciting, selecting, and supporting scientifically meritorious related research. Happily, in 2002, JDRF, in partnership with the National Institute of Allergy and Infectious Diseases, launched a $120 million, seven-year clinical trial to test the efficacy of islet cell transplants.

A Journey Not Yet Complete

Even a successful clinical trial does not complete the journey along the path to a cure. If a technique is proven to work, doctors must become familiar with it, properly identify and counsel candidates for intervention, refer these patients to qualified centers, and follow up closely. Unfortunately, if current performance is a guide, doctors cannot be uniformly relied on to accomplish these steps.[5] Further, the data systems for widespread collection and analysis of information regarding outcomes of everyday practice do not exist. Yet such data are critical to answering key questions: Once used widely, has the new intervention really mattered? Who gets the best results? Who is most likely to benefit? These are the final necessary steps along any path to a cure.

Consumers as the Catalyst

In JDRF's experience the catalyst for advancing from basic to clinical research was the families of people affected by diabetes and the community of committed researchers they helped build. These families, and families like them, must also be the change agents for the wide adoption and proper use of new knowledge in the everyday practice of medicine.

ACCOUNTABLE HEALTH RESEARCH

With a budget that will exceed $15 billion this year, the National Institutes of Health (NIH) is the world's most important supporter of academic experimentation along the path to a cure. But even though there is widespread agreement that funding biomedical research should be a top national priority,[6] there is animated disagreement about how these research dollars should be allocated. This disagreement has been the genesis of a number of recent reports, including those by the NIH,[7] the Institute of Medicine (IOM),[8] and the Progressive Policy Institute (PPI).[9] Each report tries to address the fundamental challenges posed by how we prioritize and spend public contributions to biomedical research. But how can NIH be more accountable in balancing scientific opportunity with public health needs, if, as Nobel laureate Arthur Kornberg asserts, "though it seem[s] unreasonable and impractical, counter-intuitive even to scientists, [the way] to solve an urgent problem of disease [is] by exploring apparently unrelated questions in biology, chemistry and physics."[10]

The solution goes beyond the steps articulated in the NIH, IOM, and PPI reports. It includes mechanisms that simultaneously recognize the unpredictability of the scientific process and need to encourage innovation and the legitimate urgency of the public's expectation that science can help them solve the health problems they face. It requires the engagement and full participation of all stakeholders, especially consumers, who must be present and valued at every stage of decision making.

Science Roadmaps

NIH adoption of *science roadmapping,* an inclusive, dynamic, and flexible strategic planning and evaluation process, would be constructive. Science roadmapping would identify research goals and establish the "potential to reduce future disease burden" as the lens through which prioritization decisions are made for all but the most basic research.[11] As Robert Galvin puts it:

> A "roadmap" is an extended look at the future of a chosen field of inquiry composed from the collective knowledge and imagination of the brightest drivers of change in that field. Roadmaps can comprise statements of theories and trends, the formulation of models, identification of linkages among and within sciences, identification of discontinuities and knowledge voids, and interpretation of investigations and experiments. Roadmaps can also include the identification of instruments needed to solve problems. Roadmaps communicate visions, stimulate investigations, and monitor progress. They facilitate more interdisciplinary networking and teamed pursuit.[12]

Science roadmaps are not equivalent to directed research. Roadmaps establish a vehicle for public communication and accountability—they do not say,

"do *this* research," but rather, "show how you are trying to solve *this* problem."
In addition:

- Roadmaps are dynamic. Roadmaps can be publicly posted in the same
  way as data from GenBank, a worldwide repository of genetic sequence
  information, is posted on the Web.[13] This information is universally
  accessible for real-time review and updating.

- Roadmaps are scalable, analytical tools. They can be a framework for
  trans-NIH, transagency, and trans-sector portfolio review and planning.
  Roadmaps can be scaled to accommodate the needs and interests of
  different users.

E-Biomed

If adopted, an NIH science roadmapping process would be substantially
enhanced by implementation of NIH director Harold Varmus's bold *e-biomed*
proposal,[14] which would establish an Internet-based, electronic space for
the posting of peer-reviewed or credentialed research. Such a site would
(1) democratize access to scientific reports; (2) allow the assembly of personalized, cross-disciplinary journals; (3) improve the format for publication of
modern biology; (4) allow more rapid dissemination of scientific information;
and (5) reduce costs. Science roadmaps and e-biomed are not panaceas, but they
are important enablers of full and productive public participation in research
decision making and assessment as well as facilitators of research progress.

CONSUMER-DRIVEN PRACTICE IMPROVEMENT

If the promise of the path to a cure is to be fully realized, once research has produced new knowledge, that knowledge must be widely, rapidly, and consistently
used and its effect evaluated. This is easier said than done. As far back as 1910,
the Flexner Report, a seminal publication on the status of U.S. medicine, suggested, "One of the problems of the future is to educate the public itself to appreciate that very seldom, under existing conditions, does a patient receive the best
aid which it is possible to give him under the present state of medicine."[15]

Quality Counts

For example, Stephen Soumerai and his colleagues have documented that
although prescribing beta-blocker drugs after a myocardial infarction is solidly
grounded in science, only 20 percent of eligible patients received this therapy. The
consequences were devastating—with those not receiving the drug demonstrating a 20 percent greater rate of rehospitalization and a 43 percent greater mortality rate.[16] In 1996, the *Dartmouth Atlas of Health Care* revealed many indefensible

patterns of health care delivery in the United States, such as a thirty-fold variation in the rate of breast-conserving surgery for breast cancer. This led the atlas editors to suggest that "geography is destiny."[17] These reports are hardly unique in the medical literature. Nearly a century after Flexner, it is clear that consumers are still not consistently receiving the best health care that science has to offer.

Overcoming Obstacles to Accountability

The effort to promote health system quality measurement and process and outcomes improvement is also not new. In 1912, Ernest A. Codman, a physician and founder of the American College of Surgeons, adamantly espoused his "End Results Idea,"[18] advocating the measurement of the ultimate results of health care services. But despite short-term advances, Codman saw a confluence of factors halt the diffusion and acceptance of his idea. The lack of funding, the threat to those who held the power in medicine and health care, the lack of pressure for external accountability, and the absence of any real reward for improvement were a toxic mixture. The problem continues today.

Recent efforts have tried to shift the forces that preserve this unfortunate status quo. One of the most notable was the formation of the Foundation for Accountability (FACCT), in 1995. FACCT president David Lansky recalls that

> FACCT felt that the quality of American health care was the most serious and yet least seriously addressed health problem facing the public. Just to illustrate: 180,000 Americans die each year as victims of avoidable errors in U.S. hospitals and only 21% of Medicare beneficiaries with diabetes have simple screening tests (eyes, feet, blood sugar) performed on a regular basis.
>
> Our original strategy was to use the sheer economic power of large employers and government purchasers of health benefits to demand improvements in the quality of health care. We have been fortunate to have very influential partners in this effort—the Medicare, the Federal Employees Health Benefits Program, General Motors, AT&T, AARP, the AFL-CIO, and so on. Together, the organizations that governed and largely funded FACCT represent the health care needs of over 80 million Americans. With this much market power, we thought we could introduce significant changes into U.S. health care and create an environment that demanded quality.
>
> We were wrong. It has become clear to us that even thoughtful and committed organizations—a significant smattering of doctors, health plans, employers, government officials—are incapable of leading us towards a higher quality health care system.[19]

Even objective measures that demonstrate the cost-effectiveness of quality care cannot promote change.

Consumers Are the Missing Ingredient

Decades of effort have failed because the remedies for the toxic mixture that felled Codman's idea have all lacked a key ingredient: a compelling demand for accountability by the only group with the power to effect real change—consumers.

Consumers are those whose daily lives are most affected by health research, the dissemination and use of new knowledge, and the outcomes of the processes of care. Consumers are the engine for change that can drive the broader use of research advances and create the mechanisms to evaluate the effect. They alone are fueled by the passion and energy that results from living with the effects of illness.

David Lansky and FACCT have come to the same conclusion: "The health system will not improve until the American public understands it and demands it. Yet they have neither the understanding nor the tools to force change in how medical care is organized, financed, and delivered."[20]

Get the Damn Data

The challenge is to create a system that facilitates consumers' understanding and provides the tools they need to effect change. It begins by positioning the consumer as a collaborator in assessing whether health care sources are fulfilling the promise of scientific advances. The view of consumers as passive recipients of health bestowed on them by a knowing, kindly other cannot survive. It must evolve to a view of consumers as informed partners with a responsibility to participate. Universal access to new knowledge is critical. Consumers must be empowered with personalized analyses of information that make it useful for individual decision making. Further, the system must establish a secure environment in which consumers can give researchers and providers feedback on outcomes and experience, thus enabling prospective evaluation of health system effectiveness.

The Benefits of Sharing

Implementation will require reconciling legitimate privacy concerns and recognizing that achievement of a better system and better health for everyone requires all parties to share their experiences. The context in which this information exchange takes place must be a positive one of learning for improvement, as opposed to a negative one of judging for blame.

The Internet as Platform

The Internet, through its unique capacity to connect all stakeholders, is the logical platform for such a system. It creates opportunities for the real-time generation of outcomes data of which Codman could only dream. Within the confines of secure, personal *health management accounts,*[21] consumers will be able to connect to leading experts, access information on self-care and best practices, and share with their personal health providers what they have learned and how they are doing. This collaborative approach not only promotes continuity and quality of care but also allows consumers to meet their obligation to consistently provide feedback regarding the outcomes of care, thereby contributing to process improvement.

COLLABORATION AS CURE

Collaborating with consumers will render the work of health researchers and professionals more personally fulfilling. Rapid advances in understanding the fundamental bases of health and illness and in the capacity for real-time global exchange of new knowledge create extraordinary opportunities to achieve shared goals. But the complexities inherent in this progress demand greater interaction across disciplines of science and with all stakeholders.

Valuing consumer collaboration at every step along the path to a cure is the key to our mutual success. We must

1. Establish mechanisms to provide a relevant context for productive consumer participation and cross-disciplinary collaboration in research prioritization, allocation, and evaluation (for example, science roadmapping)

2. Facilitate more timely, universal access to new knowledge, scaled to user needs (for example, e-biomed)

3. Use the Internet to create the secure personal spaces and connectivity required for consumers to access new knowledge and share, with confidence, personal health information and outcomes of care (for example, health management accounts)

4. Defend intellectual property and personal privacy when necessary but value and provide incentives for information sharing

5. Establish outcomes of care, evaluated through consumer self-reporting and the systematic assessment of everyday practice, as the principal metric by which we evaluate the success and value of health research and care delivery

Collaboration gives us the opportunity to find meaning in our lives while serving the mission of health research—"to uncover [and apply] new knowledge that will lead to better health for everyone."[22]

Notes

1. Frankl, V. E. "Man's Search for Meaning." New York: Simon & Schuster, Washington Square Press, 1985, p. 121.

2. Goldstein, J. L., and Brown, M. S. "The Clinical Investigator: Bewitched, Bothered, and Bewildered, But Still Beloved." *Journal of Clinical Investigation,* June 1997, *99,* 2803–2812.

3. Sandra Silvestri, personal communication to the author, May 1999.

4. Eileen Gelick, personal communication to the author, May 1999.

5. Dartmouth Medical School, The Center for the Evaluative Clinical Sciences. *The Dartmouth Atlas of Healthcare.* (J. Wennberg and others, eds.) Chicago: American Hospital Publishing, 1996; National Committee for Quality Assurance. *The State of Managed Care Quality, 1998.* [www.ncqa.org/pages/communications/ state%20of%20managed%20care/report98.htm], 1998.

6. Research! America, a nonprofit advocacy organization, reports that more than two-thirds—68 percent—of respondents back a proposal to double federal funding for medical research over a five-year period. See Research! America, *America Speaks: Poll Data Booklet,* vol. 4. Alexandria, Va.: Research! America, 2002, p. 23.

7. National Institutes of Health (NIH), Working Group on Priority Setting. *Setting Research Priorities at the NIH.* Washington, D.C.: NIH, Sept. 1997.

8. Institute of Medicine, Health Sciences Policy Program, Committee on the NIH Research Priority-Setting Process. *Scientific Opportunities and Public Needs: Improving Priority Setting and Public Input at the National Institutes of Health.* Washington, D.C.: National Academy Press, 1998.

9. Tengs, T. O. *Planning for Serendipity: A New Strategy to Prosper from Health Research.* Health Priorities Project Policy Report No. 2. Washington, D.C.: Progressive Policy Institute, July 1998.

10. Kornberg, A. "Of Serendipity and Science." *Stanford Medicine,* Summer 1995, *12,* 42–43.

11. Tengs, "Planning for Serendipity."

12. Galvin, R. "Science Roadmaps." *Science,* May 8, 1998, *280,* 803.

13. For Genbank, see [www.ncbi.nlm.nih.gov/Web/Genbank/index.html].

14. Varmus, H. "E-Biomed: A Proposal for Electronic Publications in the Biomedical Sciences." [www.nih.gov/welcome/director/ebiomed/ebi.htm], May 1999.

15. Flexner, A. "Medical Education in the U.S. and Canada." Bulletin No. 4. Menlo Park, Calif.: Carnegie Foundation for the Advancement of Teaching, 1910.

16. Soumerai, S. B., and others. "Adverse Outcomes of Underuse of Beta-Blocker in Elderly Survivors of Myocardial Infarction." *Journal of the American Medical Association,* 1997, *227,* 115–121.

17. Dartmouth Medical School, The Center for the Evaluative Clinical Sciences. *The Dartmouth Atlas of Healthcare.*

18. Donabedian, A. "The End Results of Health Care: Ernest Codman's Contribution to Quality Assessment and Beyond." *Milbank Quarterly,* 1989, *67*(2), 257–267.

19. David Lansky, personal communication to the author, May 1999.

20. Lansky, personal communication.

21. Kendall, D., and Levine, S. R. *Creating a Health Information Network.* Health Priorities Project. Washington, D.C.: Progressive Policy Institute, July 1997.

22. National Institutes of Health (NIH), Working Group on Priority Setting. *Setting Research Priorities at the NIH.* Washington, D.C.: NIH, Sept. 2002.

CHAPTER FIFTY-SIX

Package Pricing at the
Texas Heart Institute

Denton A. Cooley, John W. Adams Jr.

Founded in 1962, the Texas Heart Institute (THI) has developed into the largest cardiovascular diagnostic and treatment center in the United States. Patients from all fifty states and more than ninety countries have traveled to Houston for cardiovascular services. Physicians affiliated with THI have extensive experience in diagnosing and treating heart disease. More than 100,000 open heart procedures, 45,000 vascular procedures, and 220,000 catheterization procedures have been performed at the institute's clinical partner institution, St. Luke's Episcopal Hospital. In addition, THI is one of the most successful transplant centers in the world; thus far, it has performed more than 850 heart transplants.

The mission of THI is to advance the understanding and treatment of cardiovascular disease through innovative and progressive programs in research, education, and patient care. THI is involved in basic and clinical research and education through the work of its four divisions: cardiology, surgery, anesthesiology, and pathology. The institute's ultimate purpose is the delivery of improved patient care.

Many pioneering surgical procedures have been performed at THI, including the first successful human heart transplant in the United States and the first total artificial heart implant in the world. However, the achievement that may have the greatest impact on health care did not occur in the operating room or in the research laboratory. It happened on a piece of paper, in 1984, when we at THI created the first-ever package pricing plan for cardiovascular surgical procedures.

This plan, administered by an organization we called CardioVascular Care Providers (CVCP), Inc., incorporated the concepts of bundled services, shared risk, and single payment for professional services, thereby embodying a radical new approach to health care delivery.[1]

FORMATION OF CARDIOVASCULAR CARE PROVIDERS

By 1984, managed care provider networks had become extremely popular, and THI physicians were being inundated with requests to participate in such networks. About that time, a large, self-insured, Houston-based company approached us about the possibility of providing cardiovascular services for its employees and their dependents. In comparing claims data with patient outcomes data, the company had determined that THI provided the highest-quality cardiovascular care in the United States, at the least cost. Meanwhile a large managed care organization recognized that THI was performing more open heart operations than any other single facility in the world and asked us whether a flat-fee arrangement could be implemented. In response to these requests, an organ-specific, all-inclusive payment package, initially covering sixteen selected cardiovascular surgical procedures, was established.

The development of package rates required careful analysis of the population to be covered and was facilitated by the extensive patient database maintained at THI. This database contains information on more than 160,000 cardiovascular patients and procedures, dating from the time of the first coronary artery bypass in the late 1960s. For every cardiovascular operation performed at THI, the patient's diagnosis, surgical procedure, postoperative course, and other medical information, as well as personal demographic data, are recorded. In addition, long-term follow-up studies are conducted. For large patient population subgroups, additional data of a highly specific medical nature are maintained.

Analysis of the data in 1984 revealed that the majority of patients clustered around a central mean; however, two distinct patient subpopulations could be identified: those who underwent technically successful operations but died either in the operating room or in the intensive care unit after one to three days of care and those who had a postoperative complication resulting in extensive additional resource utilization.

These two subpopulations added significant risk to the negotiation of flat-fee arrangements. Rather than marginally increasing the packaged rates to account for these outliers, we adopted the concept of shared risk among the participating physicians, that is, in cases requiring a high use of services, the physicians would share equally in the financial loss. Conversely, should the physicians maintain their usual cost efficiency in all other cases, they would share in the financial gain, which would offset the outlier case losses. With this approach the payers were assured that expenses would be fixed and predictable and that quality care would be provided at a cost savings.

As interventional cardiology evolved, global pricing was developed for cardiac catheterization, percutaneous transluminal angioplasty, electrophysiologic studies, and other nonsurgical procedures. Today, there are forty-seven separate packages in the CVCP program, covering everything from an initial office visit to a heart transplant procedure.

Some skeptics of our packaged pricing policy have suggested that the program excludes higher-risk patients and patients for whom extended care and cost may be anticipated before surgical or interventional procedures. That has not been the case in our practice. All patients are accepted regardless of risk or the possibility of extended care. Our patients are actually much sicker than the average because we are a tertiary care center and take many patients who have been turned down by other centers. We believe that the extra cost of treating such patients is adequately covered by the modest profit made from the routine or less complex cases.

HCFA DEMONSTRATION PROJECT

In November 1985, on the basis of CVCP's early success, CVCP proposed that the Office of Research and Demonstrations in the Health Care Financing Administration (HCFA) investigate the feasibility of a similar plan for Medicare patients who were to undergo coronary artery bypass graft (CABG) surgery.[2] At the time, the combined facility and physician fee for CABG under the CVCP plan was $13,800, in contrast to the national average Medicare payment of $24,588.[3] In a 1987 study, the inspector general of the U.S. Department of Health and Human Services, Richard P. Kusserow, showed that HCFA could decrease its annual bill for CABG by more than $192 million if it paid THI's price for the surgery.[4] Citing THI as one of the nation's best and least expensive centers for CABG, Kusserow pointed out the irony of the fact that CVCP patients received the very best care at such a low price.

In November 1988, the Office of Research and Demonstrations endorsed the plan proposed by CVCP and requested proposals for participation in the Medicare Participating Heart Bypass Demonstration Project from U.S. hospitals that performed more than 250 CABGs per year.[5] Hospitals were chosen to participate on the basis of quality outcomes, facilities, years of physician and support staff experience, number of CABG operations performed per year, marketing plans, global price, and long-term follow-up of patients.

In July 1991, HCFA selected four sites for the project. In 1993, it added three more sites, including THI and St. Luke's Episcopal Hospital in Houston. THI and

CVCP wanted to participate with St. Luke's in the project not only because we had initiated the concept but also because the project offered us an opportunity (1) to gain additional experience in managed care, (2) to continue developing the working relationship between physicians and the hospital in the context of global pricing, (3) to maintain our leadership in performing CABG procedures, and (4) to participate in research designed to examine the possible cost and quality benefits of such a program.

During the first year of participation in the program, the costs per case for St. Luke's Medicare patients in DRG 106 (CABG with catheterization) decreased 5 percent from the previous year, and the costs for DRG 107 (CABG without catheterization) decreased 11 percent. Much of the cost reduction was the result of a 14 percent decrease in fixed direct costs, which was due in part to an increase in the number of patients and to a decrease in the average length of stay. During this period the average length of stay decreased by 15.8 percent for DRG 106 and by 11.4 percent for DRG 107. Pathology and pharmacy services for this patient population were also reduced. At the same time, the satisfaction rate for patients enrolled in the project was 89.1 percent compared with St. Luke's overall satisfaction rate of 85.1 percent. These rates were measured by Press Ganey, a consulting firm that specializes in marketing and patient satisfaction programs for health care organizations.[6]

At the seven involved centers, the HCFA demonstration project continued beyond the planned five-year period, extending until December 31, 1998. In a letter addressed to the participants, Michael A. Hupfer, director of the Division of Demonstration Programs, stated HCFA concerns regarding reimbursement:

> Results from this demonstration showed an estimated savings to Medicare of $38 million for 9,900 CABGs at these seven sites. These savings were largely the result of changes in patient management, such as shorter length of stay, substitution of generic drugs, standardization of equipment, and other changes. Although this demonstration has been successful, it has created reimbursement difficulties for its participants. This has resulted in a large amount of time from HCFA staff, the hospitals, and carriers to process demonstration claims.[7]

In contrast, although our site did experience some operational problems, they were minor. We had benefited greatly from the experience we had previously gained through CVCP, particularly in the areas of claims processing and adjudication.

As a physician-driven organization with more than fifteen years of experience in adjudicating physician claims under package-pricing arrangements, CVCP assumed the responsibility of processing physician claims and payments, not only for the HCFA demonstration project but for all managed care contracts. The assumption of payment responsibility gave our participating physicians more control over their destiny; as a result we had more physician buy-in at the organization.

CVCP TODAY

Our organization is a network of independent, private-practice physicians that was formed to provide cardiovascular services. When we founded CVCP, we had three goals: (1) to give employers or payers a simple, predictable, and cost-effective method for providing cardiovascular services to employees or members of insured groups, (2) to provide easy access to the finest quality of care for each patient at a guaranteed price, and (3) to avoid unnecessary diagnostic and treatment procedures, which prolong a patient's hospital stay or otherwise increase costs.

CVCP is a 5.01(a), certified nonprofit health care organization, as designated by the Texas Medical Practice Act and approved by the Texas State Board of Medical Examiners. It is a taxable, not-for-profit entity, which serves as the exclusive managed care contracting organization for the physicians affiliated with THI. The program currently involves 141 THI physicians, including 42 cardiologists and 8 cardiovascular surgeons. The remainder are hospital-based physicians and consultants who are routinely involved in the care of cardiovascular patients.

There are established fee schedules for each specialty in each of the forty-seven packages, and all the physicians in a given specialty are treated equally from a reimbursement perspective. CVCP currently has sixty-one managed care contracts, including forty-five PPO or HMO agreements, nine direct employer arrangements, and nine international agreements. Of these contracts, forty-eight are package agreements, one is a capitated cardiology carve-out, and the remainder are fee-for-service agreements. In each of these payer agreements, CVCP has been delegated credentialing responsibilities.

CVCP has proved successful because it is physician-driven and directed. The board of directors consists of eight physicians: three cardiovascular surgeons, one cardiovascular anesthesiologist, and four cardiologists affiliated with THI. The organization has a very active committee structure. (The standing committees include the Contract Committee, Medical Management/Quality Management Committee, Credentialing Committee, and Financial and Reimbursement Committee.) The membership of each committee includes physicians from a variety of specialties. The Contract Committee establishes the parameters for each managed care contract and approves each contract before it is presented to the board of directors. The Medical Management/Quality Management Committee establishes and monitors patient care guidelines and develops physician profiles for the entire network. The Financial and Reimbursement Committee holds the tremendous responsibility of negotiating the provider fee schedules for each of the specialties involved in CVCP. A key governance success factor has been maintaining the proper balance on the board and in the committee structures, allowing each participant to feel fairly represented.

An integrated physician network such as CVCP requires a comprehensive claims administration system as well as a clinical information system. During its first ten years of operation, CVCP used a proprietary claims system, which was developed internally. We eventually outgrew this system. In 1995, after an extensive search, CVCP made a substantial capital investment in a practice management system (Medical Manager System) with an integrated claims-adjudication system (ProClaim). This proved a very good choice for two reasons. First, Medical Manager and CVCP agreed to partner in the development of package-pricing software to meet our specific needs. Second, ProClaim proved to be the most extensive claims-adjudication system then on the market. It had three modules: repricing, packaging/bundling, and standard capitation. The Medical Manager System was fully automated, allowing CVCP to handle more than 7,500 claims and 4,000 referrals per month. Along with a sophisticated reporting capability, CVCP can generate a variety of utilization reports based on the claims information received from the network. CVCP has since outgrown the Medical Manager System and has invested in the MD Serve Managed Care System. This Internet-based system contains all the latest technology that enables contemporaneous physician-to-network connectivity. The system currently has over 10,000 loaded, defined benefit plans mapped to each of our payer contracts—all linked to internal fee schedules.

SUMMARY

The overall success of CVCP during the past eighteen years is the result of

- A shared vision among the physician participants of making the highest-quality cardiovascular services accessible and affordable
- A history of THI physicians' working together as an efficient team
- A physician network that provided the necessary capital to acquire the systems, management expertise, and infrastructure needed to support the network

During the last six years, CVCP revenues have more than tripled. This trend is projected to continue. Although capitation is not as dominant as it once was projected to be, package pricing for cardiovascular services will continue to offer payers and employers a viable option for controlling costs. Whether the market demands package pricing, capitation, or fee-for-service arrangements, CVCP offers the participating physicians maximum flexibility in negotiating with payers.

Because of our local success, other physician networks around the nation began to inquire about using our services. As a result, in 1997, the CVCP board of directors formed a for-profit network management company called Global

Health Care Alliance, Inc. Global is owned by the physicians affiliated with CVCP. It acquired the operating assets of CVCP and signed a twenty-year management services agreement to manage the CVCP network. Its mission is to provide network organization, integration, and management services for existing physician networks and to develop cardiovascular networks in other viable markets. With the information system capabilities and the infrastructure we currently have in place, we believe that we can offer expertise to other physician networks that share our goal of providing the highest-quality care in the most cost-efficient manner. Global has provided management services to specialty and multispecialty physician networks in New York, Louisiana, North Carolina, and Texas. Global also provides network management services to the MD Anderson Physicians Network in Houston, Texas.

Notes

1. Edmonds, C. H., and Hallman, G. L. "CardioVascular Care Providers: A Pioneer in Bundled Services, Shared Risk, and Single Payment." *Texas Heart Institute Journal,* 1995, *22,* 72–76.

2. Nangle, M., and Duncan, J. M. "The Medicare Participating Heart Bypass Demonstration Project in Houston, Texas: The Experience of St. Luke's Episcopal Hospital, Texas Heart Institute, and CardioVascular Care Providers, Inc." *Texas Heart Institute Journal,* 1995, *22,* 77–80.

3. Edmonds and Hallman, "CardioVascular Care Providers."

4. Stevens, C. "Is This the Beginning of DRGs for Doctors?" *Medical Economics,* 1989, *16,* 27–36.

5. U.S. Department of Health and Human Services, Health Care Financing Administration, Office of Research and Demonstrations. "Request for Proposal: Medicare Participating Heart Bypass Demonstration." Bethesda, Md.: U.S. Department of Health and Human Services, 1988.

6. Nangle and Duncan, "The Medicare Participating Heart Bypass Demonstration Project in Houston, Texas."

7. Hupfer, M. A. Letter to Michael K. Jhin, St. Luke's Episcopal Hospital, Dec. 15, 1998. Department of Health and Human Services, Division of Demonstration Programs, Center for Health Plans and Providers, Bethesda, Md.

CHAPTER FIFTY-SEVEN

Helping Patients Manage Their Asthma

The National Jewish Approach

Lynn M. Taussig, David Tinkelman

The belief that patients are the best managers of their asthma has led National Jewish Medical and Research Center to develop and implement an innovative and cost-effective telecommunications-based program to help people deal with their respiratory problems. National Jewish, which opened its doors in 1899 as a non-profit, non-sectarian haven for indigent tuberculosis patients, now researches and treats various respiratory, immunologic, allergic, and infectious diseases.

An estimated 17 million Americans suffer from asthma, which is the sixth most common chronic condition in this country. More than 5,400 people die every year from asthma, which disproportionately strikes minorities and inner-city residents. Among children, asthma accounts for ten million lost school days every year. For adults over age eighteen, three million workdays are lost. Asthma is the number one cause of hospitalization among children under the age of fifteen, and it accounts for one in six of all pediatric emergency room visits.[1]

Patients with asthma have a profound effect on the costs associated with health care:

- A very small percentage of the estimated 17 million asthma sufferers account for the majority of the total cost of treating asthma.

- In 1999, asthma caused nearly 2 million visits to emergency rooms.[2]

- Asthma accounts for approximately 3 million doctor visits and 200,000 hospitalizations annually among those under eighteen years of age.[3]

- The annual direct health care costs of asthma are approximately $8.1 billion; indirect costs (for example, lost productivity) add another $4.6 billion, for a total of $12.7 billion dollars.[4]

These statistics indicate that the classic acute-care approach to chronic disease, although appropriate during actual episodes, often does not provide the support needed by asthma patients as they try to manage their disease on a daily basis. At National Jewish Medical and Research Center we contend that with appropriate care and monitoring we can lower many of these costs while simultaneously improving health.

The National Jewish outreach programs have two major components. First, we make it possible for people to gain access to our knowledge and expertise through telecommunications. Second, we offer our Disease Management Program to health care organizations as a means of improving the care of asthma patients while simultaneously lowering the costs of care. This program enhances the relationship between the primary care physician and the patient by assisting them to collaborate on the development of an asthma management plan and helping them with the continued implementation of that plan.

TELECOMMUNICATIONS

National Jewish maintains three telephone services, supplemented by Internet and mail services, that help patients obtain appropriate care and also care for themselves.

LUNG LINE

In 1983, National Jewish established LUNG LINE (800-222-LUNG), a toll-free, no-charge service that allows callers to talk (Monday through Friday, 8 A.M. to 4:30 P.M. MST) to registered nurses who are specially trained to answer questions about the newest asthma medications and how to cope with seasonal allergies, asthma, emphysema, and other ailments. The nurses also have information on tuberculosis and immune diseases such as rheumatoid arthritis, chronic fatigue syndrome, and lupus. Although our nurses do not diagnose disease or prescribe treatment, they provide information—by phone, Internet, and mail—that helps people make informed choices about their own health.

The printed information, which is sent at no cost, includes educational booklets such as "Your Child and Asthma," "Management of Chronic Respiratory Disease," and "Understanding Allergy." Since LUNG LINE's inception, its nurses have fielded more than 700,000 calls from people throughout the country. In 2001 alone, they answered almost 40,000 calls and e-mails and mailed over 50,000 pieces of literature. LUNG LINE can also be accessed on the Web at www.njc.org or by e-mail at lungline@njc.org.

Lung Facts®, established in 1987, is a free, automated information service that operates twenty-four hours a day, seven days a week. It was developed to enhance LUNG LINE and increase our specialty services to the public and to organizations. Lung Facts receives 10,000 calls per year. Presently, Lung Facts offers a total of seventy one- to two-minute messages that address asthma, emphysema, and other lung ailments as well as allergic and immunologic diseases. For example, two of the titles offered are "Nocturnal Asthma" and "Asthma Triggers." This information line is constantly updated so that information will be current. In addition to listening to the messages, callers can have printed materials, most of which are the same as those used by LUNG LINE, mailed to them.

Physician Line

Doctors around the world who need advice about respiratory, allergic, and immunologic diseases can avail themselves of Physician Line, 800-NJC-9555, which provides a free telephone consultation with a National Jewish pulmonologist, allergist, or immunologist. When a physician calls, a nurse records his or her questions and refers the query to the appropriate National Jewish physician, who returns the call within three days. Although our physicians do not treat cases over the phone, they can serve as a valuable resource because of their clinical experiences and research. There are approximately 7,000 calls per year to the Physician Line.

Managed Care Consult Line

National Jewish maintains the Managed Care Consult Line for physicians or case managers who work with an insurance company, health maintenance organization, or any other managed care entity and who need assistance in getting a patient to National Jewish or in obtaining the services of a National Jewish physician.

DISEASE MANAGEMENT

Individual patients and physicians benefit from the tremendous amount of expertise offered by National Jewish over the telephone. In addition six health care organizations with total enrollment of over 2.5 million people around the country are realizing considerable benefits by taking advantage of our Disease Management Program: Asthma (DMP:Asthma). At the time this chapter was written, a total of 7,496 people were enrolled in this disease management program.

An estimated 90 to 95 percent of the health care decisions that affect chronically ill populations are made by the patients themselves.[5] Thus DMP:Asthma was developed on the assumption that the best way to treat asthma is to help patients or the parents of patients make the best possible decisions. The goal of

DMP:Asthma is to assist organizations and individuals to manage asthma better. The program does this both by reinforcing management plans developed by primary care physicians and by enhancing patients' relationships with their physicians. National Jewish works closely with each health care organization and physicians to identify patients with asthma who would benefit from DMP:Asthma.

Patients who meet one or more of the criteria for *disease management referral* are referred to DMP:Asthma. Once the patient or parent agrees to enroll in DMP:Asthma, we take a *proactive* approach. We ask the primary care physician for a copy of the patient's asthma management plan. One of our nurses then makes two visits to the patient's home. Participants are given educational materials and flow meters in an effort to guide them into monitoring their asthma. During subsequent calls the nurse educates the patient or parents of a patient about managing asthma and discusses ways of minimizing specific situations that can trigger the patient's attacks. That same nurse, having established a relationship with the patient, makes additional telephone calls four times a year to monitor compliance and to encourage and reinforce the family's asthma management efforts. Although the nurse will call four times a year, there is no limit to the number of times the patient can call for help. Patients have twenty-four-hour-a-day telephone access to nurses who can provide additional information and assistance. Patients are also encouraged to call or visit their primary care physician.

This personal and persuasive approach works with large numbers of those with asthma and the parents of asthma patients. Those who follow the management plan outlined by their physician usually find that their health, or that of their children, drastically improves. With improved health comes lower costs—as much as 70 percent lower in some cases.

Results in Terms of Quality of Life

For consumers, the advantage of National Jewish's DMP:Asthma can be summarized in three words: *quality of life.* When a patient or his or her parent manages asthma properly, there are fewer days of missed work or school and a significant reduction in trips to the emergency room. Patients now enjoy lives that approach normality.

We measured quality of life for adult patients through the Asthma Quality of Life Questionnaire[6] and for pediatric patients through the Paediatric Asthma Caregivers Quality of Life Questionnaire.[7] During the enrollment process, baseline quality of life surveys were administered to all patients. In addition, baseline utilization data, covering experiences from zero to six months prior to enrollment, were collected. Because this baseline data pool reflected standard asthma management in the studied population, it served as the control to which we later compared our six- and twelve-month experimental data.

After patients had participated for six months in DMP:Asthma, all utilization indices for these patients showed substantial reductions from baseline, and adult workdays missed dropped by over 85 percent. When utilization data for twelve months of participation were gathered, both adult workdays missed and care-taker workdays missed dropped by over 90 percent.

For physicians and health care organizations, DMP:Asthma reduces the amount of time spent on asthma patients and thus the costs of managing their disease. This was best shown by a study in which National Jewish assumed the management of a high-risk, high-utilizer Medicaid population in western Pennsylvania. Patients were selected to participate based on several factors: an analysis of their hospitalization and claims data for the previous year, their current clinical status and utilization of services, and physician referral. Three hundred and seventeen patients with moderate to severe asthma stayed with the program for at least six months, and when their program experiences were compared to their experiences in the six months immediately prior to enrolling in the National Jewish program, their improvement was substantial:

- Adult days of work missed decreased from 879 to 131 ($p < .001$).
- Adult days of work missed to care for a sick child fell from 312 to 90 ($p < .001$).
- Emergency room visits fell from 546 to 180 ($p < .001$).
- Hospitalizations declined from 157 to 62 ($p < .001$).
- Unscheduled doctor visits decreased from 1,083 to 413 ($p < .001$).
- Prescriptions for oral steroids decreased from 343 to 185 ($p < .001$).

In just six months the National Jewish program saved the organization $445,833. After paying for the program—an average of $303 per patient—the savings totaled $349,782.

Follow-up data were available for sixty-two patients at twelve months. The drop in numbers occurred because patients either refused to participate further in the program (10 to 15 percent), could not be reached, had switched plans (25 percent), or had not reached the twelve-month mark. We found that Medicaid patients tend to move more often than other patients. Among those we were able to reach, improvement was remarkable:

- Adult days of work missed decreased from 288 to 2 ($p < .039$).
- Adult days of work missed to care for a sick child fell from 158 to 12 ($p < .001$).
- Emergency room visits fell from 140 to 33 ($p < .006$).
- Hospitalizations declined from 52 to 33 ($p < .028$).
- Unscheduled doctor visits decreased from 171 to 58 ($p < .001$).
- Prescriptions for oral steroids decreased from 100 to 50 ($p < .001$).

The quality of life for patients improved significantly as well. Factors such as "mood disturbance" and "breathlessness" showed a significant positive change over both six- and twelve-month periods, and all factors improved as a result of the DMP:Asthma program.

Obstacles to Success

In our studies, several obstacles to a program such as DMP:Asthma have become immediately apparent. As mentioned earlier, asthma disproportionately affects the poor and minorities and, as one nurse put it, "families of any status who do not have their act together." A 2000 study, for instance, revealed that 41.6 percent of children in New York City homeless shelters had been diagnosed with asthma, compared to 25 percent in primary care populations.[8] Patients must volunteer for the program, and for a variety of reasons some people will not do so, even those who would realize immediate benefits from it. About 60 percent of some of the subjects appropriate for enrollment actually participated in the program.

For the ones who do wish to take part, other pitfalls remain. Because much of our approach rests on reaching patients or their caregivers by telephone, families who have no phone, who have intermittent telephone service, or who move and leave no forwarding number tend to fall through the cracks. Similarly, patients who change jobs frequently or for some other reason cannot stay enrolled in a long-term program cannot receive program benefits. A high percentage of some of the subjects did not stay in the program, for this was a very transient population.

Language and literacy barriers are also present, although these can be reduced by using nurses who speak Spanish or other languages and by providing appropriately translated printed materials. In addition to brochures written at the eleventh- or twelfth-grade level, DMP:Asthma offers low-literacy brochures aimed at patients with a third- to fourth-grade reading level.

Far harder to overcome is resistance to the notion that patients should manage their own asthma. Families who have fallen into a pattern of ignoring a child's asthma until it becomes so critical that a trip to the doctor's office or the emergency room is necessary sometimes have a hard time assuming the responsibility for using a flow meter and complying with maintenance doses of medications. Taking advantage of preventative care and routine office visits is encouraged by our program, yet some families prove difficult to convince.

Among physicians a barrier to implementation of the National Jewish approach is the perceived potential for loss of income. However, the decline in unscheduled office visits among our 317 Pennsylvania patients during the first six months of the DMP:Asthma program actually increased the cash flow for their capitated primary care physicians. Some practitioners also fear—unjustifiably, we believe—that National Jewish's program and similar approaches are trying to steal their patients. In addition, some physicians are not entirely convinced of the wisdom of self-management of chronic diseases. They do not want to give up their control of the total management of the disease to the patient or family. Only 10 to 30 percent of the physicians in our various plans completed the necessary forms, including the care plan.

As for health care organizations, some of them have not acknowledged the extent of the costs that people with moderate to severe asthma create, and thus do not recognize the benefits of a program like DMP:Asthma.

THE OUTLOOK FOR DISEASE MANAGEMENT PROGRAMS

Among consumers the movement toward attaining increasing self-management of diseases is compatible with DMP:Asthma and similar efforts. Patients who can sit down with their physicians and develop a plan to manage a disease and who are able to implement that plan and adhere to it will obtain considerable benefits. When they have asthma, they can see a rapid improvement in quality of life.

Among physicians, those who embrace the concept of a more equal partnership between doctor and patient and who support initiatives that enhance that partnership will thrive with the new disease management approach. As new paradigms of care become more accepted across the United States, more physicians will abandon their fears and resentments and accept this facilitated approach as a standard part of their practice. However, changing the prevailing culture and demonstrating that reducing the time spent with patients with asthma will mean more time to care for additional patients will not occur quickly.

Perhaps the most willing supporters for disease management approaches like that of National Jewish's DMP:Asthma will be health care organizations, especially when they observe how a program such as DMP:Asthma can reduce their costs while enhancing care and the quality of life for patients.

Notes

1. American Lung Association. [www.lungusa.com], May 17, 1999.

2. American Lung Association. [www.lungusa.com], May 17, 1999.

3. Taylor W., and Newacheck, P. "Impact of Childhood Asthma on Health." *Pediatrics*, 1992, *90*, 657–662.

4. American Lung Association, [www.lungusa.com], May 17, 1999.

5. Vinicor, F. "Diabetes Mellitus and Asthma: 'Twin' Challenges for Public Health and Managed Care Systems." *American Journal of Preventive Medicine*, 1998, *14*, 87–92.

6. Marks, G. B., Dunn, S. M., and Woolcock, A. J. "An Evaluation of an Asthma Quality of Life Questionnaire as a Measure of Change in Adults with Asthma." *Journal of Clinical Epidemiology,* 1993, *46,* 1103–1111.

7. Juniper E. F., and others. "Measuring Quality of Life in Children with Asthma." *Quality of Life Research,* 1996, *5,* 35–46.

8. Bernstein, N. "Asthma Is Found in 38% of Children in City Shelters." *New York Times,* May 5, 1999, p. B1.

CHAPTER FIFTY-EIGHT

A Model of Focused Health Care Delivery

Shouldice Hospital

Daryl J. B. Urquhart, Alan O'Dell

The delivery of health care has long been plagued by the conflict between medical ethics and fiscal expenditure. Doing what is best for the patient is a doctor's innate objective. However, what is best for the patient is often limited by the fiscal capabilities of the general hospital, which must allocate its funds among a multitude of needs. One resolution of this conflict is to specialize in, or focus on, a particular disease or procedure. The mission of delivering specialized care can facilitate high-volume centers that develop superior skills through their high frequency and deliver care at a greatly reduced cost. A general mandate, in contrast, may limit a facility's experience in individual disciplines, to the detriment of the levels of skill.

Shouldice Hospital is an example of specialized care.[1] It is a private, acute-care hospital in Thornhill, Ontario, with eighty-nine beds and five operating theaters. The entire facility and staff are exclusively dedicated to the surgical repair of external abdominal wall hernias without complication, in a manner that provides safety, comfort, and respect for the patient. The hospital is built to handle a high volume of cases and to facilitate care that meets the specific needs of hernia patients. It is strategically situated on twenty-three acres of landscaped grounds designed to enhance a successful recovery process. Through consistent, high-frequency exposure to hernias and repetition of a specific surgical technique, its surgeons and staff maintain superior competency in the care of their patients and the successful repair of abdominal wall hernias.

The Shouldice approach to hernia repair and to the delivery of health care addresses the following issues found among the general population:

- A high volume of hernia occurrence
- A high postsurgical hernia recurrence rate
- The rising costs of health care delivery
- A high rate of postoperative complications
- Consumer demand for quality, holistic health care and patient involvement

EVIDENCE OF NEED FOR THE SHOULDICE APPROACH

Estimates of the incidence of inguinal hernias without complications range from 3 percent to 13 percent of the population. The Lichtenstein Hernia Institute suggests that 50 percent of middle-aged men will develop a hernia.[2] In general community surgery, recurrences of hernias and other complications are reported to exceed 10 percent of cases.[3]

Hernias are among the most frequent surgical challenges and yet are most commonly repaired by general surgeons with comparatively little focused exposure. For example, in the province of Ontario, with a population of approximately nine million, the average annual number of hernia repairs, excluding those performed at Shouldice, is 32,000[4] and the number of general surgeons is approximately 750.[5] Therefore the average surgeon's exposure to hernia surgery is forty-three cases per year, or less than one case per week per surgeon.

Historically, abdominal wall hernia surgery has been fraught with complications. It is estimated that in excess of 10 percent of cases result in a recurrence of the hernia;[6] up to 6 percent experience infertility, and 26 percent subfertility;[7] sepsis has been reported in up to 4 percent of the cases; and ischemic orchitis and testicular atrophy rates are as high as 5 percent.[8] Up to 16 percent of the cases present a secondary hernia,[9] which is undetectable without complete dissection and exploration. Because many hernia repair techniques do not require extensive exploration, these secondary hernias can present at a later date and require additional surgery, which in itself can be considered a complication.

When these complication rates are applied to the reported 700,000 hernias repaired each year in the United States,[10] the numbers are staggering. Secondary hernias alone would cause 112,000 potential cases of redundant surgery. The average charge for individual primary hernia repair in one state, Michigan, is US$4,000 (including surgeon's fees, anesthetist, and an outpatient one-day hospital stay).[11] At that charge, 700,000 cases cost approximately US$2.8 billion per year. And this does not include the cost of patients' downtime or the follow-up health care required for any postoperative complications.

TYPICAL APPROACH TO HERNIA SURGERY

Hernia surgery is typically performed in a general hospital by a general surgeon or surgical resident. The continual search for a simple and effective hernia repair technique has brought about experimentation with a mesh prosthesis and with plugs that are implanted to patch the hernia defect. The prostheses are used with either open surgical or laparoscopic techniques. General anesthetic is common. The objective is a quick repair requiring minimal time in the operating room suite and enabling outpatient status for the patient. Comprehensive dissection and exploration of the anatomy cannot be presumed. Traditional open techniques such as the Bassini and Shouldice repair are also used. They do not use mesh. Outpatient status and general anesthetic are often characteristic of these traditional techniques also.

Typically, U.S. insurance companies now suggest that payment for basic hernia surgery be offered primarily for outpatient procedures. Outpatient treatment places the recovery process in the hands of the patient and available family or home care services.

SHOULDICE'S PRIMARY PRODUCT

In contrast the Shouldice procedure is a natural tissue repair that combines the surgical technique with the body's natural ability to heal. It is performed in 95 percent of cases under local infiltration and a light sedative. The procedure demands a comprehensive dissection and exploration of the region before strengthening the anatomy. The actual operation takes forty-five minutes on average to complete. It involves imbricating (overlapping) the individual layers of the abdominal wall and securing them with one continuous, permanent, 32-gauge, stainless steel suture to address any weaknesses discovered during the dissection. It was determined that stainless steel was most effective because of its integral longevity, which gives the natural tissues of the abdominal wall time to regenerate adequate structural integrity. The skin is approximated with Michel clips, 50 percent of which are removed twenty-four hours after surgery, and 50 percent forty-eight hours after. The wound has then healed sufficiently to remove all bandages.

The technique does not use artificial prosthetic material such as mesh because mesh can introduce unnecessary complications such as infection or migration,[12] dramatically increasing the cost of the operation. It does not use laparoscopic technology because of the potential for bile duct injuries and intestinal punctures, which may lead to infection and peritonitis.[13] Laparoscopic technology also requires the use of general anesthesia and increases the cost of disposable items per surgical procedure by over US$600.[14] Surgical outcomes for the majority of cases that use these two technological innovations show no improvements over the Shouldice technique.

The operation is performed by surgeons who are employed exclusively by Shouldice, devoting 100 percent of their surgical practice to the repair of external abdominal wall hernias.

SHOULDICE'S SECONDARY PRODUCT: MENTAL MEDICINE

Mental medicine is the application of noninvasive, holistic procedures and routines that improve patients' condition before, during, and after surgery. Shouldice provides preoperative management of patients to ensure that they are best prepared for surgery and successful recovery. Patients with colds and flus are not admitted until their symptoms are eliminated. (The reasons for this are explained to the patient.) Obese patients are given selected diets and managed weekly until their weight and general condition will result in successful surgical results. (This also is explained to the patients, so that they can actively participate in their treatment.) The patients' involvement in their own health care helps to build their confidence in the process. When these patients are admitted, they have partially prepared themselves for surgery. They have also spoken twice to a specialized surgeon who has confirmed the diagnosis, explained the procedure, and answered any questions.

As they begin their inpatient stay of 3.2 days on average, all patients live in semiprivate rooms (two beds) to promote interaction and ambulation through a "buddy" system. Patients' background, age, gender, and personal interests or profession are considered in making room assignments.

The approximately thirty new admissions each day participate in an on-site group orientation made possible by the fact that they all share a common condition. Dinner is then served at group tables in the dining room. Here they meet more patients (there are eighty-nine in the hospital at any time), those who have already been through the procedure. Conversation among preoperative and postoperative patients provides a degree of empathy not available from any surgeon. The result is a reduction in apprehension or fear and an improvement in the patient's readiness and preoperative condition.

Postoperative patients go through daily routines that include wake-up, medication, breakfast in the dining room, exercise class, rest periods, lunch in the dining room, more exercise activities, rest, and dinner, served once again in the dining room. All meals are freshly prepared and nutritionally balanced, and special diets can be accommodated. To promote ambulation the dining room is down a flight of stairs. The stairs are designed with low risers, to ease the climb while building confidence. To further encourage mobility and interaction with other patients, televisions and telephones are not placed in the rooms but in common areas.

The putting green and walking paths on the grounds are designed with appropriate inclines for the physical challenges faced by a hernia patient. Pool tables, shuffleboard, and exercycles are also in place to stretch specific muscles in a manner conducive to speedy recovery.

Every patient and every staff member, doctor, nurse, administrator, and housekeeper knows exactly why he or she is there. Each of them knows what to expect at every moment. The more than seven thousand patients a year who go through this environment at a rate averaging thirty a day all feel the effects of being cared for in a facility designed, built, and staffed exclusively for the purposes of caring for people with their condition. The result is confidence.

This is mental medicine.

EVIDENCE OF EFFICACY

To test the efficacy of the Shouldice approach, many studies into recurrence rates of hernias repaired at Shouldice as well as frequency of complications have been conducted. The data have been collected over fifty-five years of annual follow-up with approximately 280,000 patients. Comprehensive, retrospective studies as well as random samplings reveal that

- The recurrence rate in the first ten years postoperatively is less than 0.5 percent
- The recurrence rate over fifty-three years is less than 1 percent
- The complication rate is 0.5 percent
- Patients return to work in eight days on average
- Patient satisfaction with the quality of care is rated on a scale from 1 (low) to 5 (high). Ninety-eight percent of patients rated the quality of care at 5. The remaining 2 percent rated quality of care at 4.

With respect to patient satisfaction regarding the surgical outcome, the studies also reveal that over 96 percent of responding patients had no complaints of any sort.

SOCIETAL IMPACT

Shouldice costs per procedure are substantially lower than costs at other institutions.

- According to recent publications from the Ontario Ministry of Health, the average hospital cost per diem in the province of Ontario is approximately $800.[15] Current estimates are closer to $850. The comparable average cost per diem at Shouldice Hospital is $290.

- In Ontario the average community hospital cost per case for hernia surgery is $2,339,[16] compared with $997 at Shouldice.
- General community hospital costs for disposable items per hernia operation range from CDN$148.00[17] to US$600.[18] Disposable costs per hernia operation at Shouldice are CDN$24.50, on average.

When these cost savings are applied to the 7,500 hernia repairs at Shouldice Hospital in 2000, the savings to the Ontario Ministry of Health hospital funding budget are approximately $10 million. The total savings to the ministry if all cases were handled in the Shouldice model would be approximately $43 million.

In addition, a reduction in hernia recurrences following community-based surgery in the United States, from the published average of 10 percent to the recorded average of less than 1 percent at Shouldice Hospital, would mean a reduction of 63,000 cases per year. Based on the cost of a procedure in the State of Michigan (US$4,000), annual national savings in the United States would be US$252 million.

Last, nosocomial infections at Shouldice are low (< 0.5 percent) as a result of the exclusive focus on elective, clean hernia surgery. This not only reduces cost but also helps to create a healthy environment that assists in building patient confidence and willingness to participate in the process.

BARRIERS TO DIFFUSION

Volume of cases is the predominant barrier to replication of the Shouldice model. Enough cases must exist to merit the creation of a specialized facility. The effectiveness of the model depends on sufficient volume to achieve competency as well as financial stability. Therefore locations close to major population centers as well as focus on a common elective procedure are two critical factors.

THE SHOULDICE MODEL AND CONSUMER-DRIVEN HEALTH CARE

As clearly outlined in Regina Herzlinger's *Market-Driven Health Care*,[19] the consumer will drive the cost and quality of health care to preferred levels of acceptability. The Shouldice model demonstrably reduces costs and increases quality in a manner appealing to the consumer. Consumers prefer to be served by "experts" and will participate more actively in their own health care when they believe that the guidance they receive is rooted in depth of experience.

Notes

1. Shouldice Hospital was founded in 1945 by Edward Earle Shouldice, M.D., for the sole purpose of providing a facility in which he could practice his method of repairing external abdominal wall hernias. It was located in the city of Toronto until 1953, when the need for expansion forced a move to Thornhill, Ontario, just eleven kilometers north of Toronto. The staff of the hospital have always believed in the benefits of treating patients with personal respect and dignity during their stay at Shouldice. This has been rewarded in the past fifty-five years at the annual Shouldice reunion. It is a celebration, paid for and attended by up to 1,400 patient alumni to honor the staff and the institution. A mandatory hernia examination is part of the evening, which also includes dinner and entertainment.

2. Devlin, B. H. "Trends in Hernia Surgery in the Land of Astley Cooper." *Problems in General Surgery,* 1995, *12*(1), 85–92; Lichtenstein Hernia Institute. Home page. [www.American-HerniaInstitute.com], July 2002; Ponka, J. L. *Hernias of the Abdominal Wall.* Philadelphia: Saunders, 1980.

3. Rutkow, I. M., and Robbins, A. W. "Groin Hernia." In J. Cameron (ed.), *Current Surgical Therapy. St Louis: Mosby,* 1995.

4. Canadian Institute of Health Information. *Incidence of Hernia Procedures in Ontario,* 1996. Ottawa: Canadian Institute for Health Information, 1997.

5. Professional Target Marketing. *Demographic Report of Canadian Health Care Professionals & Institutions.* Toronto: Professional Target Marketing, 1997.

6. Rutkow and Robbins, "Groin Hernia."

7. The Royal College of Surgeons of England. *Report of a Working Party Convened by the Royal College of Surgeons of England: Clinical Guidelines on the Management of Groin Hernia in Adults.* London: Royal College of Surgeons of England, July 1993.

8. The Royal College of Surgeons of England. *Report of a Working Party . . .*

9. Urquhart, D.J.B. *Shouldice Hospital, Retrospective Study: Incidence of Secondary Hernias.* Ontario, Can.: Unpublished study, 1999.

10. Devlin, B. H. "Trends in Hernia Surgery . . ."; Rutkow and Robbins, "Groin Hernia."

11. Edward J. Gorin, personal communication to the author.

12. Wantz, G. E. "Complications of Synthetic Prostheses in Hernia Surgery." *Problems in General Surgery,* 1995, *12*(1), 79–83.

13. Schurz, J. W., Tetik, C., Arregui, M. E., and Phillips, E. H. "Complications and Recurrences Associated with Laparoscopic Inguinal Hernia Repair." *Problems in General Surgery,* 1995, *12*(2), 191–196; Lichtenstein Hernia Institute. Home page. [www.American-Hernia.com], July 2002.

14. Hammond, J. C., and Arregui, M. E. "Cost and Outcome Considerations in Open Versus Laparoscopic Hernia Repairs." *Problems in General Surgery,* 1995, *12*(2), 197–201.

15. Ontario Health Insurance Plan. *Ontario Case Cost Project.* Ontario, Can.: Ontario Health Insurance Plan, 1998.

16. Ontario Ministry of Health. "Case Mix Group—269, 271." Ottawa: Ontario Ministry of Health, Nov. 2001.

17. Urquhart, D.J.B. "Research on Cost of Disposable Items in Community Based General Hospitals." Ontario: Unpublished manuscript, 2002.

18. Hammond and Arregui, "Cost and Outcome Considerations . . ."

19. Herzlinger, R. E. *Market-Driven Health Care: Who Wins, Who Loses in the Transformation of America's Largest Service Industry.* Reading, Mass.: Addison-Wesley, 1997.

CHAPTER FIFTY-NINE

Chronic Problems, Innovative Solutions

Paving the Way to the Focused Factory

Stuart Lovett

The last decade has produced enormous change in the structure of our health care system. Managed care has become the dominant mechanism for overseeing health services in the United States, and health maintenance organizations (HMOs) have become the dominant private reimbursement vehicle. As in other industries, in health care the past ten years have been a time of major consolidation, resulting in a dramatic reduction in the number of entities who influence *how* care is delivered.

Has the consumer benefited from this consolidation? The answer is no.

Have the consolidators benefited as expected from their acquisitions? Again, no. Projected cost savings have failed to materialize.

What is the reason for this failure? Experts offer a number of theories, but they are generally off target. This consolidation has failed because it did nothing to further the interest of the consumer.

The future of health care belongs to the entity that reinvents itself as the consumer's champion, as an expert facilitator that directs its customers to integrated teams of physicians providing disease-specific care in settings designed explicitly to support the treatment regimen. In this brave new world the consumers' needs are paramount.

This chapter details

- The need to reinvent medicine to reflect the needs of the consumer
- The demise of physician-focused medicine

- The ways in which informational, clinical, and technical innovations are forcing the evolution of a disease management, or *focused factory,* model
- The characteristics of the emerging integrated delivery system that will implement the focused factory model
- The efforts of a Northern California independent practice association, Hill Physicians Medical Group, that has pioneered focused factory programs
- The way in which focused factory evolution will move forward

REINVENTION

The significant shift to managed care did more than introduce the terms *discounted fee for service* and *capitation* into our vocabulary. It brought *oversight* into a profession that had none. It required physicians to ask permission to do what *they* had already decided was best for the patient. Faced with history's first assault on their clinical autonomy, physicians responded in kind. Reaching out to their patients, they railed against this new system of "interference," noting the Orwellian implications of Big Brother getting between physicians and their patients. Although this counterattack did little to slow the growth of managed care, it did have one long-lasting effect: it forever branded managed care as the *enemy.*

We continue to characterize patients by the specialty or subspecialty of their physician. That designation merely identifies the training of the attending physician, *not* the patient's disease. This is precisely where our health care system fails the consumer. A "medicine" patient may be really a *diabetes* patient. A "surgery" patient, a *cancer* patient. A "pediatric" patient, an *asthma* patient. Optimal treatment of each of these diseases demands the full attention of an integrated clinical team, expert in management of the specific disease. In this reinvented world, education and training does not define the physician's role. Instead, physicians are defined by the diseases they manage. In the new world of health care, specialty training identifies only a physician's initial skill set. The important question is *which* disease management teams will the physician join?

SEA CHANGE: FROM INDEPENDENT PHYSICIAN TO MEDICAL TEAM

The explosion of information (new technology, surgical techniques, drug and treatment regimens, research findings) is overwhelming the individual physician. One of the greatest challenges faced by those of us in the medical profession is developing the tools to share clinical and technological breakthroughs with our colleagues. And yet, as the information and administrative demands of medicine intensify, we remain committed to a structure of care that places at its core a single physician.

Why the emphasis on one doctor? How can any one physician stay current? Would not patients be better served by a team of doctors, with complementary skills, managing major treatment decisions?

This is not to suggest that the role of that one doctor, the primary care physician (PCP), is not an integral one, merely that it is overemphasized. The PCPs have been required to oversee *all* care. It is unfair to ask them to do it alone. We have reached the stage where the informational demands are so great that the responsibility for devising treatment plans should be shouldered by health care teams.

Patients do need a point of entry into the health care system, which PCPs provide. And PCPs can also help in optimizing the health status of their patients and in managing chronic disease after the acute problem is addressed. As we move toward a disease management model, PCPs will be a crucial link in coordinating care between the patient and the focused factory.

DIRECTION

A new kind of facilitating organization will emerge to shape the next generation of health care delivery. Positioned between HMOs and their members, this entity will provide access to an integrated network of disease management teams, or focused factories. The entity's mission is twofold: (1) direct care to the most appropriate team of clinical experts in the most advantageous setting, and (2) bridge the administrative functions among the payer, the consumer, and the focused factory.

The entity must have the intellectual resources and clinical savvy to develop elite medical teams for the treatment of specific diseases, a process that will require excluding recalcitrant or less qualified physicians. Some facilitating organizations may choose to build their own focused factories and others may decide to purchase services from existing disease management organizations. Some entities may choose to combine these two approaches.

As an integrated delivery system, this organization must demonstrate the ability to manage each of its key functions in an expert and cohesive fashion. Successful implementation of this model *demands* equal expertise in the clinical, administrative, financial, information, and marketing arenas; it also requires an unprecedented integration of these functions. Development and maintenance of a first-rate network of focused factories will depend on

- Financial and administrative leadership that supports clinical initiatives
- Information systems that support the clinical network and measure key outcome parameters

- A marketing arm that can communicate the organization's success directly to the marketplace

The first entity to successfully structure a seamless focused factory with a full range of disease management options will enjoy a tremendous marketing advantage over traditional managed care organizations. The *patient-first* orientation of the linked focused factory concept will have great appeal for the health care consumer.

IMPLEMENTATION

Can the focused factory approach work in a traditional managed care setting? There are examples where small-scale applications of the disease management concept are succeeding. With 360,000 members and more than 2,000 affiliated physicians, the Northern California–based Hill Physicians Medical Group is one of the largest independent practice associations (IPAs) in the country. (HMOs contract with IPAs to provide physician services for their subscribers.) Founded in 1983 by CEO Steve McDermott and COO Darryl Cardoza, Hill Physicians has established a reputation for excellence in both fiscal management and clinical innovation, making it a prime candidate for early-stage development of the focused factory model.

In 1992, Hill introduced the first phase of a three-tiered women's health initiative, which has evolved into a small-scale focused factory for obstetrics and gynecology. Its three program elements include

- Enhanced detection of major fetal congenital anomalies
- Treatment of women's gynecological cancer
- Management of benign uterine disease

For Hill, development of the OB-GYN program fit comfortably within its organizational philosophy. Some ask why Hill has prospered when large, highly capitalized entities like MedPartners have failed. CEO McDermott contends that it is Hill's focus on clinical programs that sets it apart. "We do almost no marketing. We realized long ago that the consumer judges us by the quality of their care *experience.* Our job is to facilitate access to quality health care, not to hinder it," he explained. "If consumers view Hill as their advocate, then we're achieving our organizational objectives."[1]

Evolution of Women's Health Focused Factory

In 1992, in my role as medical director of the senior perinatology group (high-risk obstetrics) at East Bay Perinatal Medical Associates, I met with Hill COO Darryl Cardoza to discuss a plan to use the services of the perinatologists to improve obstetrical outcomes.

I proposed directing *all* pregnant Hill patients to a perinatologist for a fetal anatomic ultrasound survey (an obstetrical ultrasound) performed between the sixteenth and twenty-second weeks of gestation in a State of California–designated prenatal diagnosis center. The idea was to take advantage of the perinatologists' expertise in prenatal diagnostic testing to raise the level of obstetrical care for all OB patients, regardless of their risk status. I noted that the specialist—the perinatologist—was often the best person to determine whether a seemingly low-risk pregnancy was in fact progressing normally.

When Cardoza questioned the need for the program, I described how third-trimester patients were frequently referred to our practice and then diagnosed with a major fetal anomaly, despite multiple "normal" ultrasounds performed by their OB-GYN. Many of these anomalies would have been detected in the second trimester by more specialized providers. For the expectant parents, the finding often was devastating. Earlier detection would have increased the range of treatment options, including access to tertiary care services. These findings were *not* isolated incidents; major fetal congenital anomalies occur in 2.3 percent of all pregnancies.[2] I detailed for Cardoza several studies[3] that documented an anomaly detection rate of nearly 75 percent when obstetrical ultrasound was performed by perinatal experts[4] as compared to a rate of 13 percent when the procedure was performed by OB-GYNs or radiologists.[5] My point was simple: Hill would never allow its radiologists to continue to perform breast cancer screenings if their detection rate was 13 percent. Why not put the procedure in the hands of the most competent practitioner and improve both Hill's detection rate and consequently its obstetrical outcomes?

"I was drawn to the idea of the specialists rolling up their sleeves to improve care," commented Cardoza. "We use a solitary measuring stick for each new proposal: we ask if it is in the best interest of the patient. If the answer is yes, we move forward, despite the predictable political ramifications."[6]

With the second-trimester ultrasound program in place, I discussed with Hill the possibility of expanding the disease management approach beyond obstetrics and into gynecology. Hill's OB-GYN medical management team identified two diseases that warranted a collaborative approach: cancer of the reproductive tract and benign uterine disease. They were appropriate choices because treatment of both diseases was highly variable, with little agreement on the preferred treatment methodology.

Cancer of the Reproductive Tract

Surgical procedures used to treat cancer of the uterus or ovaries are routinely performed by either OB-GYNs, general surgeons, or gynecological oncologists. Recent studies have shown significantly improved outcomes when gynecological oncologists (experts in treating cancer of the reproductive tract) perform these procedures.[7] With the support of its medical management team,

Hill required all gynecological cancer cases to be referred to a gynecological oncologist for consultation.

Hill's reasoning was simple: practice makes perfect. As Ronald Kimball, a gynecological oncologist at the Women's Cancer Center of Northern California, notes: "Each member of our group does 200–300 of these procedures a year. An extremely busy gynecologist or general surgeon may do five to ten. We are much more aggressive in debulking [removing] the tumor. Because of our training and experience, we are more familiar with the characteristics of the cancer's growth and that takes us into areas where other surgeons won't go."[8]

Kimball believes that the specific protocols that now govern treatment of Hill patients and that mandate referral to a gynecological oncologist have saved or extended patients' lives: "In many cases, Hill patients have *greater* opportunity for a successful recovery than patients with indemnity or PPO coverage. There are three keys to maximizing outcome: (1) discover the cancer early; (2) remove as much of the tumor as is possible during the initial surgery; and (3) properly ascertain the stage of the cancer during surgery so that the subsequent adjuvant treatment (radiation and chemotherapy) is appropriately matched to the progress of the disease. This program gives patients the best chance of achieving these treatment goals."

Benign Uterine Disease

In late 1997, Hill Physicians teamed with Ethicon Endo-Surgery, a Johnson & Johnson subsidiary, to design and implement GYN-Care, a program that addresses treatment of benign uterine disease (polyps, fibroids, endometriosis, and so forth). The GYN-Care program may be the most widely debated of Hill's three women's health care initiatives. The controversy stems from Hill's willingness to direct surgeries *to* physicians with specific procedural skills and *away* from those without them.

Hysterectomy is the most common surgical approach to treating benign uterine disease. Sixty to 70 percent of hysterectomies performed are total abdominal hysterectomies, the most invasive form of the procedure with the longest recovery period. Although it is an effective procedure, it is often not the most efficient. Other less invasive types of hysterectomy are available, including vaginal hysterectomy and laparoscopically assisted vaginal hysterectomy. For some patients, a new and very simple procedure called endometrial ablation (a ten-minute procedure with a two-day recovery) is a viable alternative to major surgery. So why are these employed less often than total abdominal hysterectomy? Because few physicians can perform these more technically complex procedures. Some doctors, driven by ego or financial imperatives, choose to perform the more invasive surgery rather than refer the patient to a physician with proven expertise in these more efficient,[9] less invasive procedures.

After diagnosing a Hill patient with benign uterine disease, the OB-GYN submits a therapeutic treatment plan to the medical management team for its approval. The team may disagree with the plan, recommending instead a less invasive procedure or perhaps a more complex one. If the physician is not trained in the recommended procedure, he or she will be paired with a mentoring physician (often the gynecological oncologist) skilled in the recommended surgical approach. If the physician balks, the medical management team directs the patient to another physician for a second opinion, to ensure that she is fully informed of her treatment options and can make an educated decision.

Program findings have demonstrated a significant increase in the rate of minimally invasive surgery associated with the treatment of benign uterine disease. The findings further supported a reduction in the length of hospital stays, a reduction in patient pain and suffering, a quicker return to work and normal activity, and increased patient satisfaction.[10]

"Our approach is to recommend the procedure that is the best solution for the patient. We want the problem fixed the first time," said Cardoza. "We routinely challenge our physician leadership to develop programs that enhance the care we offer. We don't ask how to do it for less money; we ask how to achieve the best results, because, ultimately, the most effective course of care proves to be the most economical as well."[11]

For Hill, the success of the women's health program has raised a number of possibilities. "We realized that we had a unique infrastructure that *enabled* our physician leadership to devise and implement innovative clinical initiatives," said Steve McDermott, CEO. "Why not challenge the physician leadership in other specialties to develop similar disease-management programs? We asked our leadership to look at disease management within their own specialties and evaluate whether we're providing optimal care in an ideal setting. Are we doing all we can for the patient?"[12]

The response of Hill's physician leadership has been impressive. To date, Hill has implemented numerous disease management programs, which address chronic health issues ranging from pediatric asthma to congestive heart failure.

THE FUTURE

Medicine is being reinvented to reflect the needs of its consumers. The shift to a disease management, or focused factory, model is a crucial step toward delivering care that places the needs of the consumer first. The future of health care belongs to the entity that reinvents itself as a fully integrated network providing access to linked focused factories. I have examined how one organization, Hill Physicians Medical Group, has made strides toward implementation of this model. How do we move from the theoretical to the actual implementation of a focused factory model? How will the health care consumer move into and out of focused factories? Who empowers the disease management model to function?

Clearly, it takes an organization like Hill Physicians to *enable* the focused factory. As Hill's Cardoza observed, "Hill Physicians keeps everyone focused on the patient, *not* the doctor. We pave the road to the focused factory and create the distribution system for its services to be delivered."[13]

Hill did not choose reinvention because it was easy. Clearly, it is not. Its leaders realize, however, that Hill's future depends on the organization's ability to define itself in a way that makes sense to the health care consumer. That is a valuable lesson for the entire industry.

Notes

1. Steve McDermott, communication to the author, 2002.

2. VanDorsten, J. P., Hulsey, T. C., Newman, R. B., and Menard, M. K. "Fetal Anomaly Detection by Second-Trimester Ultrasonography in a Tertiary Center." *American Journal of Obstetrics and Gynecology,* 1998, *178,* 742–749.

3. Saari-Kemppainen, A., Karjalainen, O., Ylostalo, P., and Heinonen, O. P. "Ultrasound Screening and Perinatal Mortality: Controlled Trial of Systematic One-Stage Screening in Pregnancy." *Lancet,* 1990, *336,* 387–391.

4. VanDorsten and others, "Fetal Anomaly Detection . . ."

5. Ewigman, B. C., and others. "Effect of Prenatal Ultrasound Screening on Perinatal Outcome." *New England Journal of Medicine,* 1993, *329,* 821–827.

6. Darryl Cardoza, communication to the author, 2002.

7. Eisenkop, S. M., and others. "The Impact of Subspecialty Training on the Management of Advanced Ovarian Cancer." *Journal of Gynecologic Oncology,* 1992, *47,* 203–209; American College of Obstetricians and Gynecologists. "ACOG Educational Bulletin: Ovarian Cancer." *International Journal of Gynecology and Obstetrics,* 1998, *63,* 301–310.

8. Ronald Kimball, communication to the author, 2002.

9. Summitt, R. L., Jr., Stovall, T. G., Steege, J. F., and Lipscomb, G. H. "A Multicenter Randomized Comparison of Laparoscopically Assisted Vaginal Hysterectomy and Abdominal Hysterectomy in Abdominal Hysterectomy Candidates." *Journal of Obstetrics and Gynecology,* 1998, *92,* 321–326.

10. Summitt and others, "A Multicenter Randomized Comparison of Laparoscopically Assisted Vaginal Hysterectomy . . ."; Van Den Eeden, S. K., and others. "Quality of Life, Health Care Utilization, and Costs Among Women Undergoing Hysterectomy in a Managed-Care Setting." *American Journal of Obstetrics and Gynecology,* 1998, *178,* 91–100.

11. Cardoza, communication to the author.

12. McDermott, communication to the author.

13. Cardoza, communication to the author.

CHAPTER SIXTY

Improving Health and Reducing the Costs of Chronic Diseases

Robert E. Stone

Chronic diseases like diabetes, cardiac disease, and respiratory disease place a tremendous financial burden on the nation's health care system and society as a whole. Diabetes alone costs our country nearly $138 billion each year in direct and indirect health care costs, and the cost of cardiovascular disease and stroke is estimated to exceed $298.2 billion.[1]

The best way to reduce these costs is to improve the health of people with these diseases.

Seems simple enough, doesn't it? But the care provided to people with chronic conditions rarely supports this goal. For example, diabetes care rarely meets minimum national standards: fewer than 30 percent of individuals with diabetes receive treatment consistent with either the American Diabetes Association (ADA) Standards of Care or the measures supported by other national organizations.[2] Similar deficiencies can be found in the care of people with cardiac disease. For instance, beta blockers are frequently underused in the treatment of heart attacks, despite substantial evidence that they improve survival rates.[3]

A key reason that care for chronic diseases is not up to par is that health care delivery is fragmented and compartmentalized. Chronic diseases often affect and are affected by other health care conditions, frequently requiring different types of health care providers and multiple delivery sites. Successful treatment also requires the patient's commitment to self-management and, often, significant changes in lifestyle and personal health behaviors. But integrated supportive care is hard to find. A physician office visit, an outpatient test, and an inpatient hospital stay are all examples of the *components* found in a typical health care experience and in the subsequent billing and reimbursement. Even though each isolated component may serve patients well, the overall lack of integration and coordination of services ultimately fails to provide them with the care they need.

Managing the complex and multiple needs of patients with chronic diseases is challenging to all involved. For instance, a recent federally funded study found that primary care physicians lacked confidence in their ability to effectively treat diabetes and in their knowledge of accepted care management standards.[4]

A POPULATION MANAGEMENT APPROACH

Population management provides a solution to these problems. Population management, a comprehensive, total health care approach to disease management, is a way for health plans to improve the health of their members with chronic conditions while addressing the plan's need to reduce costs.

Although nearly 60 percent of managed care plans reported in 1997 that they had implemented at least one disease management program, and 78 percent planned to increase their budgets for these initiatives over the next year,[5] population management offers two improvements over traditional disease management. First, population management programs encompass the *entire* population of people who have a specific disease, regardless of the severity of their illness. This approach embraces the provision of preventive care for the less severely afflicted and at the same time manages the existing ailments of those who are high cost or who are at high risk for complications. In contrast, traditional disease management programs manage only members with the most severe forms of a disease and often only those who volunteer to participate. As a result, fewer members benefit from the additional services and early interventions. A typical asthma disease management program offers a good illustration of this shortcoming. Approximately 5 percent of a commercial HMO's members have asthma, but asthma programs interact with only 0.5 percent of the entire plan population, or 10 percent of all those with asthma. Therefore the plan generates savings only on 0.1 percent of the plan population, or 2 percent of all the members with asthma.[6] A population management program, in contrast, provides assistance for the needs of the entire 5 percent.

Total health care management is the second feature that distinguishes population management from disease management. Population management programs address all of a participant's health care needs, whatever the condition and wherever the care is delivered. Traditional disease management programs tend to manage only those conditions associated with the underlying disease state. For example, a traditional diabetes disease management program might focus only on improving metabolic management. In some instances, disease management programs do not engage in any type of meaningful care management but instead serve as an information clearinghouse, distributing treatment guidelines to physicians or educational materials to patients.

CARE ENHANCEMENT AND DIABETES

Population management can be applied to the management of any chronic condition. The diabetes care enhancement programs offered by American Healthways, Inc., provides good evidence of the success of this approach.

American Healthways[7] is a pioneer in developing population management programs for people with chronic conditions. Its programs are designed to provide the physician and patient with the support needed to improve health status and clinical outcomes while also addressing a managed care plan's need to achieve savings. Its diabetes programs are rooted in clinical evidence, such as the landmark Diabetes Control and Complications Trial (DCCT). (Nearly a decade ago, the DCCT confirmed that frequent and consistent interactions between the patient and a continuously available care team that provided support, education, proactive interventions, and continuous monitoring of clinical status could improve outcomes for people with diabetes.[8] The U.K. Prospective Diabetes Study has reported similar results.[9])

Like the DCCT protocol, American Healthways's programs employ a multidisciplinary team that interacts with both the patient and the physician to change and maintain desired behaviors. Supporting the patient and the physician are

- *Nurse care managers,* who coordinate and integrate all of the health care needs, including inpatient and outpatient resources
- *Patient support advocates,* who are a source of immediate support for the patient
- *Provider support coordinators,* who work with physicians and hospitals to determine needs and to assist them in providing better diabetes care

American Healthways's programs are designed to ensure the effective integration of services for people with diabetes, regardless of the source or site of the services. The ability to integrate services effectively relies heavily on information systems capable of collecting data, analyzing trends, and monitoring outcomes on an ongoing basis. American Healthways designed its electronic medical record (EMR) and PopulationWorx[SM] software to capture these data, which the company uses to provide physicians and patients with regular feedback on how treatment is progressing and to help physicians identify possible complications early.

American Healthways's EMR tracks and measures changes in specific laboratory values for members of the health plan, as well as changes in process measures of the specific clinical services that a given population should receive within a specific time frame. The laboratory values tracked include hemoglobin A1c levels. Research has demonstrated that A1c levels are closely linked to complications and costs.[10] The process measures for clinical services include whether or not a member has had a dilated retinal exam (DRE) and a foot exam. The EMR also houses information on utilization of clinical services that are potentially avoidable, such as hospitalizations and emergency room visits. Clinical information is segmented by primary care physician, type of member (for example, Medicare or commercial), and other categories.

Although all patients require a basic set of interventions all the time, not all patients need the same treatment at the same time. Therefore American Healthways's EMR captures not only patient data but also the data to tailor appropriate and timely individual interventions. EMR data serve as critical inputs for American Healthways's patient stratification model, which is derived from a variety of clinical, social, cost, and utilization inputs. This stratification model is dynamic and recategorizes patients as new data become available. Tracking each patient's stratification level and individual needs, the EMR prompts American Healthways staff to interact with patients and physicians when necessary. American Healthways's information technology also effectively integrates both the clinical and claims data for each patient in the population.

Evidence of Efficacy

American Healthways has submitted outcome results from its programs for a number of customer populations, both commercial and Medicare, for third-party validation, which has subsequently been published in peer-reviewed journals.[11] Unpublished enterprise-wide data for commercial diabetes and congestive heart failure (CHF) populations also show statistically significant improvements in adherence to standards of care measures, reduction of patient utilization, and reduction in total health care costs for the program populations (Table 60.1 summarizes the savings).

Year 1 Diabetes

- Members who have had one or more A1c tests increased 10.1 percent.
- Members who have had one or more DREs increased 12.7 percent.
- Hospital admissions per 1,000 members decreased 15.4 percent.
- Bed-days per 1,000 members decreased 16.3 percent.
- Total health care costs for commercial members with diabetes had an aggregated decrease of 14.8 percent (adjusted for nondisease trend).

Table 60.1. Aggregated Return on Program Investment.

	Diabetes		Congestive Heart Failure
	Year 1	Year 2	Year 1
Program members	57,498	34,945	1,328
Total gross savings	$42,515,906	$32,233,531	$9,112,415
Management fees	17,249,275	10,483,450	1,992,000
Total net savings	25,266,631	21,750,081	7,120,415
Return on investment	1.46	2.07	3.57

Year 2 Diabetes

- Members who have had one or more A1c tests increased 21.9 percent.
- Members who have had one or more DREs increased 43.4 percent.
- Hospital admissions per 1,000 members decreased 27.0 percent.
- Bed-days per 1,000 members decreased 25.7 percent.
- Total health care costs for commercial members with diabetes had an aggregated decrease of 20.5 percent (adjusted for nondisease trend).

Year 1 CHF

- Members who have had one or more LDL-C tests increased 68.6 percent.
- Members receiving ACE inhibitors increased 7.0 percent.
- Hospital admissions per 1,000 members decreased 26.8 percent.
- Bed-days per 1,000 members decreased 27.9 percent.
- Total health care costs for commercial members with diabetes and CHF had an aggregated decrease of 36.2 percent (adjusted for nondisease trend).

Societal Impact

American Healthways believes that approaches that coordinate, integrate, and manage the many different aspects of health care required by people with diabetes yield a positive societal impact. By continually improving the health status of these patients, the severity of complications is reduced and in some cases completely avoided. The resulting cost reductions compound over time. If American Healthways's first-year financial outcomes are extrapolated to the eleven million people diagnosed with diabetes, one could expect the company's population management approach to save society more than $6 billion. American Healthways's cost-savings model projects that savings will increase over time. After five years of program implementation, the model predicts approximately a 30 percent reduction in annual health care costs.

The impact of American Healthways's approach on work productivity and overall quality of life for society as a whole is difficult to quantify. However, as the health status of individuals with diabetes improves, society as a whole will benefit from fewer lost days from work and a reduction in premature deaths.

GREATER ACCEPTANCE OF CARE ENHANCEMENT

Different organizations take different approaches to disease management, and the resulting inability to accurately compare outcomes among programs has become a primary barrier to a wider acceptance of population management. Although other studies and outcomes reports have addressed standards of care compliance for diabetes, their findings are not comparable to the ones reported here, due to differences in sample size, evaluation time, program type, delivery model, and enrollment measurement method. For example, although the HEDIS measure for eye exams includes only health plan members over age thirty-one who have been continuously enrolled in the health plan, our outcomes are population based and reflect the entire population of members with diabetes regardless of their length of time in the health plan.

Publication of outcomes enables health care providers, consumers, and payers to make critical choices that affect the overall quality of care. The number of programs and organizations dedicated to this task is unprecedented—the Joint Commission on Accreditation of Healthcare Organizations (JCAHO), the National Committee for Quality Assurance (NCQA), and the Foundation for Accountability (FACCT)—to name a few. But for the health care sector to maximize the value of these studies, the measurements used should be consistent across all organizations.

CARE ENHANCEMENT AND CONSUMER-DRIVEN HEALTH CARE

Chronic diseases such as diabetes have no cure and affect all aspects of a person's life. Effective management of these diseases is challenging and complex, requiring a support team that not only understands physicians' needs but also recognizes and proactively addresses the unique needs of each patient.

Care enhancement provides the level of personal support and attention that many say is absent from today's health care system, and at the same time it improves health and reduces costs. If health plans and disease and population managers share their clinical outcomes with consumers, those consumers will come to understand and place a value on this type of initiative. Consumer-driven health care is a friend to care enhancement.

Notes

1. American Diabetes Association. "Diabetes Facts and Figures." [www.diabetes.org], Sept. 2003; American Heart Association. *1999 Heart and Stroke Statistical Update.* Dallas, Tex.: American Heart Association, 2000, p. 28.

2. National Committee for Quality Assurance (NCQA). *1997 Health Plan Employer Data and Information Set [HEDIS].* Washington, D.C.: NCQA, 1997; Martin, T. L., Selby, J. V., and Zang, D. "Physician and Patient Prevention Practices in NIDDM in a Large Urban Managed Care Organization." *Diabetes Care,* 1995, *18,* 1124–1132.

3. Gottlieb, S. S., McCarter, R. J., and Vogel, R. A. "Effect of Beta-Blockade on Mortality Among High-Risk and Low-Risk Patients After Myocardial Infarction." *New England Journal of Medicine,* 1998, *339,* 489–497.

4. Larme, A. C., and Pugh, J. A. "Attitudes of Primary Care Providers Toward Diabetes." *Diabetes Care,* 1998, *21,* 1392–1396.

5. InterStudy. *HMO Industry Report.* InterStudy Competitive Edge series, II. Modesto, Ca.: InterStudy, Oct. 1997; Rauber, C. "Disease Management Can Be Good for What Ails Patients and Insurers." *Modern Healthcare,* 1999, *29*(13), 48–54.

6. Al Lewis, executive director, Disease Management Purchasing Consortium, personal communication to the author.

7. For more than twenty years American Healthways has worked with hospitals, health plans, and physicians to improve patients' health, enhance the fundamental care experience, and reduce the cost of care. It is the nation's largest, most experienced disease and care management company, providing services to 465,000 health plan equivalent lives, and the nearly 100,000 physicians who care for them, in all fifty states, Puerto Rico, and the District of Columbia. It also provides comprehensive diabetes services to eighty hospitals nationwide. In 1996, the company launched its first disease management programs, helping HMOs and physicians coordinate the health care needs of people with diabetes. Today, American Healthways's care enhancement programs are offered by twenty-nine regional and national health plans to approximately 250,000 patients and the nearly 30,000 physicians responsible for their care. Building on its successful model for diabetes, the company is expanding its product line to include programs for cardiac and pulmonary disease.

8. The Diabetes Control and Complications Trial Research Group. "The Effect of Intensive Treatment on the Development and Progression of Long-Term Complications in Insulin-Dependent Diabetes Mellitus." *New England Journal of Medicine,* 1993, *329,* 977–986.

9. U.K. Prospective Diabetes Study (UKPDS) Group. "Intensive Blood Glucose Control with Sulphonylureas or Insulin Compared with Conventional Treatment and Risk of Complications in Patients with Type 2 Diabetes (UKPDS 33)." *Lancet,* 1998, *352,* 837–853.

10. Gilmer, T. P., O'Conner, P. J., Manning, W. G., and others. "The Cost to Health Plans of Poor Glycemic Control." *Diabetes Care,* 1997, *20,* 1847–1853.

11. Rubin, R. J., Dietrich, K. A., and Hawk, A. D. "Clinical and Economic Impact of Implementing a Comprehensive Diabetes Management Program in Managed Care." *Journal of Clinical Endocrinology and Metabolism,* 1998, *8,* 2635–2642; Hoffman, J. C. "Broad Disease Management Interventions: Reducing Healthcare Costs for Plan Members with Congestive Heart Failure." *Disease Management & Health Outcomes,* 2001, *9,* 527–529; Stone, R. "A Population-Based Approach to Diabetes Management." *Journal of Clinical Outcomes Management,* 2000, *7*(12), 49–51.

CHAPTER SIXTY-ONE

The Impact of Horizontal Integration in Hospitals

HCA Healthcare Corporation

Thomas F. Frist Jr.

Thirty years ago the hospital sector began an organizational transformation through the creation of horizontal networks similar to those that have been developed in other industries, such as the grocery, hotel, and restaurant sectors. The driving force in the early days of this reorganization was the need for access to capital to finance new hospitals, services, and technology to deal with infrastructure demands caused by population shifts from the rust-belt to the sun-belt states. But as a result of the Nixon era price and wage controls imposed on the health care industry, in 1972 serious efforts were also started to achieve the cost advantages inherent in a horizontally integrated hospital system.

Over the ensuing three decades, the horizontal integration phenomenon gained credence and momentum. In the mid-1970s and early 1980s, the dominant traditional not-for-profit hospital sector began to emulate it too. In its early stages the shift was fueled by a me-too defensive attitude among some not-for-profit leaders who said, in effect, "We can operate hospitals as well or better than the public for-profit companies such as American Medical International (AMI), Hospital Corporation of America (HCA), Humana, and National Medical Enterprises (NME)." Until the 1980s and early 1990s, much of the integration effort by the not-for-profits was effected through affiliation, management contracts, and purchasing consortia. In the 1990s, it was the increasing penetration of managed care, along with Medicare and Medicaid payment constraints, that gave a new boost to merger, acquisition, and consolidation activity in both the investor-owned and not-for-profit sectors.

Many of the advantages to be realized by horizontal merging of assets were obscured or never achieved in the nineties due to the simultaneous but conflicting phenomenon of vertical integration. That movement was stimulated by environmental changes that had created excess hospital capacity. At the same time, a changing public and private payment system accelerated the shift from inpatient to outpatient care and from more expensive acute inpatient care to less costly alternative caregivers—niche players, such as ambulatory surgery centers, skilled nursing facilities (SNFs), and home health care providers. This sea change was further enabled by new clinical technology. The results were devastating and life threatening to many freestanding hospitals. A decade later, industry graveyards are filled with the aborted efforts of vertically integrated hospitals to develop hospital-owned or -affiliated organizations to fill unused capacity or gain market share. The inscriptions on the tombstones read SNFs, home health care, disease niche providers, risk-taking products (HMOs), and physician practice management (PPM) groups.

CURRENT STATUS OF HORIZONTAL INTEGRATION

Why are an increasing number of hospitals looking to merge with a system? What is different now?

First, hospital providers are experiencing unprecedented, unabated pressures to decrease costs, pressures arising from state Medicaid payment changes, increased managed care, growing numbers of uninsured patients, and the sobering impact of the federal Balanced Budget Act on Medicare. These pressures have led hospitals to challenge the validity of their previous integration strategies. Second, the tools and technology now available enable hospitals to achieve savings and measure performance output as never before. We are moving into an information stage, where informed customers and third parties will demand ever-increasing accountability from providers. Last, the industry-wide government investigation into "fraud and abuse" has likewise caused vertically integrated providers to divest, close, or abandon many marginal activities that may place them in jeopardy of violating the law.

As we enter the twenty-first century the hospital sector is entering an era of *back to the basics.* Market leaders will find increasing pressures to consolidate to increase productivity and measurably improve quality.

For these reasons and others I believe we are just now entering the halcyon days of horizontal integration. The data support this view. The American Hospital Association (AHA) defines a *hospital system* as an organization that owns or manages multiple facilities (not including networks that coordinate care among institutions or alliances for managed care contracting). Given that definition, the AHA's 2001 annual survey reports that of the nation's 6,116 hospitals, 50 percent, or 3,074, belong to systems. That is an increase from 1,956, or 37 percent of 5,229 hospitals, in 1994.

Among these hospital systems there are almost as many distinguishing differences as there are common traits. They can be categorized by number of hospitals, number of beds, geography, and whether they are not-for-profit or investor-owned. The two most frequently mentioned categories are not-for-profit hospital systems and the investor-owned multihospital organizations. The former can be subdivided into religious-sponsored and nonreligious (501[c][3]) organizations. The latter may be either publicly listed or privately held companies. Both not-for-profit and investor-owned systems may be further distinguished as managed or owned, rural or urban, regional or national, and multiservice or specialty.

Over the past three decades numerous authors have debated the merits of not-for-profits versus for-profits in costs, charity care, teaching, research, and other important societal issues. That is not the purpose of this chapter. Rather, my aim is to present timely and meaningful information about the pros and cons of a horizontally integrated hospital system, through a case study of the largest system—Hospital Corporation of America (HCA), of which I am a cofounder, a former CEO, and now chairman emeritus. This study analyzes the system in light of today's environment, to which U.S. hospitals must learn to adapt so that they can continue to serve a public that has ever-higher expectations of them.

HOSPITAL CORPORATION OF AMERICA

At HCA horizontal integration has produced advantages in many areas: establishing quality assurance, providing shared services, developing and retaining human resources, purchasing, innovating, balancing risks and rewards, obtaining capital funding, designing and constructing new facilities, diversifying geographically, developing an information system, providing managed care, and maintaining support services.

Quality Assurance

Unquestionably, sound finances and cost-effective operations are essential in the competitive, market-driven health care system of 2002. Experience has shown, however, that a short-term focus on financial performance at the expense of the clinical programs and services will, over time, threaten the long-term ability of the institution to fulfill its mission. It is in the less frequently discussed and less frequently appreciated area of quality assurance that the benefits of a large, horizontally integrated multihospital system can be distinguished from those of a freestanding hospital or small multihospital system. The ability to share timely, accurate aggregated patient care data from a large group of hospitals and physicians can be immensely meaningful to the member hospitals and to the entire system. Added beneficiaries are government policymakers who all too often have been forced to use outdated or incomplete data for major state and national health care policy decisions.

HCA illustrates the scale of a large horizontally integrated system. In 2000, HCA's hospitals and affiliated physicians admitted 1,553,500 inpatients, registered 11,356,900 outpatients, and treated 4,534,400 emergency room visitors. The system housed 1,310,100 surgical procedures, including 23,061 open-heart surgeries, and HCA-owned hospitals delivered over 210,140 babies. These patient encounters represent approximately 6 percent of the hospital-based care delivered in the United States in 2000.

Shared Services

Another significant strategy that differentiates HCA and points to the value of a large system of hospitals with common ownership is its shared services initiative. This multiyear plan, expected to be fully implemented in 2004, is designed to remove certain local back-office functions, such as accounts receivable, payroll, billing and collecting, and supply management, from hospitals around the country and consolidate them into regional service centers. The supply chain portion of the initiative is developing centralized warehousing, electronic ordering and paying, and fleet management.

Although this strategy is not new to business, no hospital company has successfully implemented a similar approach. The advantages of doing so will go well beyond simple reduction of full-time equivalent (FTE) positions. Centralizing and specializing functions such as the processing of accounts receivable, improving relationships with major payers, and accelerating the information flow have already produced significant improvement in reducing accounts receivable days across the company, this with the project only about two-thirds completed. Perhaps most important, this strategy allows local hospital managers to give less attention to back-office functions and thus focus more attention on core clinical operations.

As has been demonstrated in other industries, quality measurement trend lines correlate directly with the financial performance of the institution. Through our information systems, management can monitor outcomes and related data in each hospital on a monthly basis. Additional quality measurement tools include employee, patient, and physician satisfaction surveys; for example, systemwide, the Gallup Organization conducts satisfaction surveys of over 100,000 patients per quarter, and every hospital must conduct at least one physician attitude survey and one employee attitude survey per year. The findings from these surveys, together with patient survey results, outcomes data, and Joint Commission on Accreditation of Healthcare Organizations (JCAHO) results, are used to construct a quality index. Senior managers at the hospitals have a significant portion of their variable compensation determined by the quality index.

Additional means for realizing the full potential for quality improvement in HCA hospitals are our national panels of physicians, each panel representing a field such as cardiology, orthopedics, oncology, emergency medicine, and so forth. These standing panels meet on a regular schedule throughout the year to provide physician input on all corporate-sponsored quality initiatives, to advise our purchasing department on contracts for physician-preferred supplies and equipment, and to provide a forum for discussion of other issues in each field.

Most important for HCA over the years has been its ability to identify and disseminate *best demonstrated practices* in the clinical specialties. Identified best demonstrated practices are used to establish new services at a hospital or to encourage and facilitate improvements in existing clinical programs. The power of our ability to share such data through interhospital networking is immense. This timely and accurate information enables local hospital medical staff and boards of directors to fulfill their governance roles far more effectively.

Human Resources

Unequivocally, the most important resource for HCA is its people. How well the hospitals fulfill their commitment to *putting the patient first* depends directly on how successfully the company attracts, motivates, and retains a highly qualified workforce. Although the local market determines the salaries, wages, and benefits for HCA hospitals, the HCA system has accretive advantages over an independent, freestanding hospital.

The ever-increasing mobility of the U.S. workforce over the past decades has created an unanticipated benefit for HCA employees and for the company itself. Whether a move is generated by a spouse's career-related relocation, a geographical preference, or a career advancement opportunity, thousands of HCA employees have moved from one HCA hospital to another over their careers without losing continuity of employment. HCA also presents attractive, challenging advancement opportunities for the aspiring health care executive that are simply not available in a freestanding institution. Within HCA the possibilities for positive career move changes are almost limitless: a master of health administration intern could rise from that position to assistant administrator to small hospital CEO to large hospital COO to large hospital CEO to multihospital division CEO to corporate senior management. Therefore a well-developed corporate recruiting, training, and tracking process for key talent is critical to the ultimate success of HCA hospitals.

Another benefit of size lies in employee benefits. The cost of benefit design and administration is inversely related to the size of the workforce, whether the benefit is health and life insurance, disability and workers' compensation insurance, or some other employer-provided product or service. A concrete example of this economy of scale is provided by the spin-offs of the LifePoint and Triad hospitals from HCA. After the spin-off the administrative cost of providing employee benefits for 5,500 employees at LifePoint's twenty-three hospitals and the 14,000 employees at Triad increased by 200 percent on a per employee basis.

Purchasing

The power of purchasing is the first and most frequently mentioned benefit of a horizontally integrated system. The value of aggregated purchasing of supplies, equipment, and services is directly related to size. As the committed volume and compliance to contract increases, the cost per unit decreases. A high level of adherence to contract is more easily achieved in a large system that owns all its facilities and has in place advanced processes, systems, and measurement tools that ensure compliance.

HCA, with strong operational support that has led to over 80 percent compliance with national contracts, now has a significant pricing advantage over other industry buying groups. With quality defined by the clinician or end-user as a constant, price is the primary measurement for value added, but for HCA an additional highly valued ingredient is the early availability of new technology and priority delivery in times of supply limitations. During its recent reorganization, HCA created the Healthtrust Purchasing Group to combine the purchasing power of its owned facilities with those of several other health care companies, including Triad and LifePoint. The total supply expense for hospitals using this purchasing group exceeds $5 billion annually, with supply costs as a percentage of net revenues ranging from 15.5 to 16.4 percent over the past year.

New Products and New Services

When HCA was founded in 1968, hospitals did not have coronary care units with sophisticated monitoring equipment. The technology era of medicine, with its advances in the diagnosis and treatment of patients, was just emerging. Over the last quarter century, every aspect of medicine has benefited from these remarkable developments. Many health care economists agree that the increased costs associated with the medical technology era have been more than offset by the improved outcomes.

Time after time, HCA, through its resources and affiliations, has been able to identify and gain access to new medical technology for its hospitals earlier than would have otherwise been possible. Frequently, this early access provides an enormous advantage for HCA hospitals over their competitors and, more important, delivers a tremendous benefit to medical staff and patients. The innate advantage of size brings at least two other notable advantages to HCA hospitals. First is the attractiveness of a large system such as HCA to developers and manufacturers of new medical technologies and services who wish to pilot their products. Second is the ability of the company to spread the risks and rewards of evaluating new, often expensive, medical technology among the hospitals.

Risks and Rewards

Our ability to balance the risk-reward equation when evaluating new services is as important as our early access to new technology. Examples of areas in which it was important to strike this balance are the development of psychiatric services and hospitals in the 1970s, the establishment of ambulatory service centers in the 1980s, and the creation of HMOs in the 1990s. In these efforts, along with numerous others such as vertical integration endeavors (SNFs, PPMs, and home health care, for instance), the company could evaluate each service without betting the family store as would a freestanding hospital.

Although the primary purpose of research and development of new services and products is to add value to the local hospital, a by-product has been the development of new lines of business that stand on their own. In many cases these business units have become more valuable as noncore strategic entities and have been spun off as freestanding companies. Some examples of this phenomenon are HCA International, HCA Health Care Indemnity (captive insurance), HCA Psychiatric Company, HMO/Equicor, and HCA Ambulatory Surgery. One recent spin-off is medtropolis.com, an Internet company in which HCA placed certain assets plus $50 million. Its primary focus will be to support our hospitals and the constituencies we serve. However, the potential for benefit to HCA is far greater if it is successful in executing its business plan. This latest Internet venture could not have been undertaken absent the aggregation of HCA's hospitals under one umbrella, networked together through a common information system. Through such spin-offs, billions of dollars have been generated from nonhospital patient revenue sources over the years. These dollars have provided a critical source of capital that gives HCA hospitals the added advantage of being able to maintain modern, up-to-date health care facilities to serve their communities.

Availability of Capital

The hospital sector has always been capital intensive. In 1968, Hospital Corporation of America built its first hospital, in Erin, Tennessee, at a cost of $16,000 per bed, or $30 per square foot. In 1995, HCA's MountainView Hospital, built in Las Vegas, cost $330,000 per bed and $183 per square foot. The latter is a full-service community hospital. It would not be unusual for a 300-bed, tertiary care teaching hospital to cost as much as $135 million, or $220 to $230 per square foot, in 1999 dollars.

Between 1997 and 2000, HCA spent an average of $1.1 billion per year to keep its approximately 220 hospitals modern and up to date—a level of spending equal to 110 percent of depreciation. Over the years since HCA's founding, as the company's size increased and its balance sheet strengthened, access to new capital sources expanded and its cost of capital decreased. Since 1997, HCA has accessed or had the ability to access domestic and foreign capital markets including public bond markets, commercial bank borrowing, commercial paper, equities, and foreign bank borrowing. Because of its large size and significant number of high-quality, geographically diverse hospitals, the company's cost of capital has been historically lower than the cost for most hospital companies. For HCA the lack of access to the tax-exempt market is partially offset by its access to multiple sources of capital and the equity markets.

Design and Construction

Over the last thirty years a corporate resource consistently highly valued by HCA hospitals has been the design and construction department. HCA has designed, built, and equipped over 150 hospitals and in excess of seven million square feet of medical office buildings. The emphasis has been on encouraging innovation and creativity while realizing significant cost savings during the construction phase. As a by-product of designing and building multiple hospitals, HCA can continually improve the operational efficiency of the final product through extensive postconstruction critiques.

One of the unanticipated but greatly appreciated benefits of the multihospital system with its corporate and sister hospital resources occurs in times of natural disasters, such as tornadoes, hurricanes, floods, and earthquakes. The company's human and physical resources enable its local hospitals to continue to function during these times, when nearby non-HCA facilities' capabilities are impaired. These same resources have on numerous occasions proven invaluable in enabling HCA's local hospitals to respond quickly and efficiently to mass tragedies such as train wrecks, plant explosions, or terrorist actions such as the bombing of the federal building in Oklahoma City in 1995 and the Littleton, Colorado, school shooting. In such instances, experience has demonstrated the value of being able to get nurses, physicians, chaplains, and psychologists from sister facilities on site within hours. This shared support has reduced the pain and suffering of the victims and their families and has frequently made the difference between life and death.

Geographical Diversification

Not infrequently, individual hospitals throughout the United States suffer from major detrimental events in the economic environment that are outside their control and unique to their geographical location. These threatening events include military base closings, factory closures, and business sector downturns. As part of a large, well-financed and well-dispersed system, an HCA hospital in this situation may well be able to survive or transition through the difficult period. One example of a local occurrence that will threaten numerous stand-alone hospitals is California's mandate that hospitals meet certain earthquake preparedness requirements. The current estimated capital expenditure for California hospitals to become compliant by 2008 is $12 billion. As a result some hospitals are already making plans to close or to merge facilities—to the detriment of the consumer.

Information Systems

The availability of accurate and timely clinical and financial information is absolutely critical to a well-run hospital. It has added importance for a publicly owned hospital system that must make frequent reports to shareholders. HCA has a state-of-the-art data-processing center in Nashville with branches in Anchorage, Phoenix, San Antonio, Fort Worth, Orlando, and Louisville. These are interconnected with each of the hospitals and physician's offices associated with the medical centers. Its build-or-buy philosophy has enabled HCA to continually improve its products and services while reducing costs. In 2000, information system costs represented less than 3 percent of net revenues, another example of HCA's ability to achieve economies of scale in both unit costs and professional talent when compared to individual hospitals or small hospital systems.

Of particular value to large systems is the ability to pilot new applications before deploying them systemwide. At HCA, information technology (IT) projects are carefully evaluated to ensure that personnel and financial resources support the business strategy and overall company goals of improving quality of care, efficiency, and outcomes while reducing costs. Over the years the ability to spread over many hospitals the research and development costs for the new products needed to deal with changes in regulations and reimbursement has provided distinct cost, quality, and timeliness advantages for HCA over the independent or small-system hospital. For example, HCA is currently addressing the complex issues related to the impending federal outpatient prospective payment system.

Managed Care

The growth of managed care has created significant business challenges for all health care providers. These challenges include price pressures, the costs of administering complex payer contracts, maintaining continued access to patient populations, and conducting interventions such as utilization review programs. HCA's philosophy toward managed care is that the provision of care is driven at the local level but is significantly enhanced by competitive advantages related to the overall hospital system. In short, the company provides invaluable processes, tools, and managed care expertise to support its local markets.

As a hospital system, HCA has more leverage than other providers in managed care contract negotiations. The pool of talented professionals available at the corporate and division levels is a resource that cannot be matched by an independent hospital. The managed care teams provide local markets with education and training, templates and guides, contracting support, internal consulting services, legal support, and information systems and reporting. Their resources include software applications, reference materials, and reporting tools delivered over HCA's intranet. This exchange of information and ideas contributes insight and leverage for addressing common problems, administrative requirements, and reimbursement issues with managed care payers.

Corporate Support Services

Overall, the cost of maintaining the corporate office support services, excluding information systems, is approximately 1 percent of net revenues. Using corporate departments for work in such areas as Medicare cost reports, internal audits, compliance, legal services, and corporate communications enables the company to provide higher-quality and more consistent service to its hospitals at a lower cost. We often question whether certain shared services should be built or bought. We do not always choose to build. For example, in biomedical engineering, the company achieves its desired end result by partnering with General Electric to provide services. We also partner where needed with McKesson for supply and pharmaceutical distribution and Marriott for food services.

SUMMARY

Health care expenditures in the United States have recently accounted for about 15 percent of GNP. The hospital sector, the largest cost component, recently represented 38 to 40 percent of all health expenditures. During the past three decades hospitals have emerged from their cottage industry roots and adopted many of the proven good business practices developed in other industries. But as the new millennium begins, hospital leadership cannot afford to accept the status quo. Even though the hospital sector has made much progress in improving cost and quality through the implementation of sound management and organizational principles, the environment in which hospitals operate has changed even faster. As freestanding hospital boards look to the future, they must seriously consider the benefits of a quality-oriented, financially sound horizontal integration.

CHAPTER SIXTY-TWO

An Innovative Approach to Population Health

Kaiser Permanente Southern California

Les Zendle

Kaiser Permanente[1] is a national medical care program made up of Kaiser Foundation Health Plan, Inc. (KFHP), the health services entity; Kaiser Foundation Hospital (KFH), the hospital entity; and nine Permanente Medical Groups, the provider entity. These three entities have a long history and culture of cooperation—they have worked together in an exclusive relationship for more than fifty-five years.

Kaiser Permanente is the largest nongovernmental health care provider in the world, serving over 8.2 million members in nine states and the District of Columbia. Programwide revenue in 2001 was nearly $17 billion. In Southern California, Kaiser Permanente (KFHP, KFH, and the Southern California Permanente Medical Group [SCPMG]) serves 3.1 million members, almost exclusively in eleven Kaiser Permanente major medical centers staffed by more than four thousand physicians. Each medical center contains executive leaders from all three arms who report to the KFHP-KFH CEO and the SCPMG medical director. Clinical regional coordination occurs through the SCPMG associate medical director (for clinical services), who facilitates the meetings held for the medical centers' chiefs of service by specialty. For example, all eleven chiefs of obstetrics and gynecology participate in a meeting every two months. In addition, there are regionwide physician coordinators for multispecialty issues such as elder care, HIV/AIDS, women's health, pain management, and perinatal services.

661

This chapter describes the *care management* approach used by Kaiser Permanente Southern California (KPSC) to reduce undesirable variability in care and to enhance health promotion and self-care among patient populations with chronic diseases or conditions. Through care management, KPSC, where I am associate medical director, has improved health outcomes (quality), increased member satisfaction (service), and better utilized limited health care resources (cost).

EVIDENCE OF THE NEED FOR CARE MANAGEMENT

Americans spend more than one trillion dollars a year on health care.[2] Where does all this money go? It is no secret that patients with chronic illnesses use a disproportionate amount of resources. About 20 percent of patients use an estimated 80 percent of health care resources.[3] Although sound evidence shows that certain tests and treatment strategies produce better outcomes and lower costs for patients with several chronic diseases,[4] in practice substantial variation in treatment exists.

Its organizational structure and culture make KPSC a natural setting for improving the management of chronic care. In the early 1990s, KPSC began to combine its long-standing integrated health care delivery system with an increased emphasis on evidenced-based medicine and population care management. It developed *models of care* for specific diseases and populations at risk, with the aid of various consultants, including David M. Eddy, MD, PhD, a KPSC senior consultant on health policy,[5] and Allen Bredt, MD, an Assistant to the Associate Medical Director (for Clinical Services). In 1997, KPSC began a formal region-wide care management program, led by Joel Hyatt, MD, another Assistant to the Associate Medical Director (for Clinical Services). In 1998, these efforts were combined with the rest of the Kaiser Permanente national program (and Group Health Cooperative of Puget Sound) to form Kaiser Permanente Care Management Institute (CMI).

KPSC POPULATION CARE MANAGEMENT MODEL

Although implementation of Kaiser's *population care management model* varies somewhat for each targeted disease or condition, each approach contains the following key elements:

- *Computerized information systems* linking electronic data from the pharmacy, laboratory, hospital, and outpatient systems to identify patients and improve care

- *Multidisciplinary teams* (with such members as primary care physicians, specialists, dietitians, social workers, and educators) to provide coordinated services

- *Clinical practice guidelines* (developed and approved by Permanente physicians) to identify the medical approaches that work best

- *Health education* (delivered one-on-one and through classes, groups, newsletters, videos, and so on) to help patients learn self-care strategies from professionals and from each other

- *Outreach* (friendly but firm phone calls and letters) to encourage patients and remind them of appointments and important activities

- *Inreach* (systematic electronic prompts, faxed reminders, and reports) to help physicians track the status of their patients

Results: Diabetes

KPSC has more than 120,000 members diagnosed with diabetes. In most cases patient education, early intervention, and appropriate medical treatment can prevent or delay the costly complications of diabetes.[6] The KPSC Diabetes Care Management Program combines the elements listed previously to produce an integrated, coordinated *systems* approach.

Is it working? Results show improvement in various measures of diabetes care between 1994 and 2000. Appropriate retinal eye examinations increased from 47 to 65 percent. Between the first quarter of 1999 and the third quarter of 2001, improvements have been noted in several additional measures: hemoglobin A1c testing (a blood test that measures glucose control) increased by 2 percent, from 79.8 to 81 percent; glycemic control (HgA1c < 8.0) increased 9 percent, from 52.5 to 57 percent; the lipid screening rate has increased by 18 percent, from 65.1 to 77 percent; and urine microalbumin screening (to detect early kidney disease) has increased by 83 percent, from 38.7 to 71 percent. These intermediate outcome measures were accompanied by more concrete outcome results—a decrease in myocardial infarctions from 14 to 11 per 1,000 diabetic members and in limb amputations from 5.1 to 2.9 per 1,000 diabetic members.

Results: End-Stage Renal Disease

By the end of 1998, KPSC's Renal Care Management Program was treating 2,969 active end-stage renal disease (ESRD) patients and over 5,000 pre-ESRD (predialysis) patients. The Renal Care Management Program includes all the key elements of the KPSC population care management model.

Results show decreased gross (crude, unadjusted) mortality rates (GMRs) for KPSC dialysis patients. The 1998 GMR of 15.04 percent compares to 16.53 percent in 1997 and a 19.9 percent GMR for all dialysis patients in Southern

California. The 1998 data also show increased use of fistulae in preference to grafts for vascular access (50 percent of all new accesses were fistulae compared to the previous year, in which 27 percent of new accesses were fistulae). This has resulted in a 1998 fistula prevalence rate of 31 percent, compared to the network average of 18 percent, and in a decreased rate of thrombosis (with KPSC experiencing 0.70 episodes per patient per year versus a national average of 0.80 episodes). KPSC's hospital utilization rate of 9.0 days per ESRD patient compares favorably with the national average of 11.3 in the 1996 U.S. Renal Data Service data.

In 1998, SCPMG also began a joint partnership venture (called Optimal Renal Care, LLC) with Fresenius, a national company that manages dialysis units, to export its expertise in renal care management.

Results: Heart Disease

Congestive heart failure (CHF) and coronary artery disease (CAD) are the two types of heart disease most suited to care management strategies. KPSC has developed and implemented comprehensive models of care for each.

CHF outcomes (such as inpatient, outpatient, and emergency room utilization) are currently being collected. Since the first quarter of 2000, there has been a 33 percent reduction in the inpatient discharge rate among members with congestive heart failure, from 0.91 to 0.61 percent. Improvements among members with CAD are demonstrated by a 12 percent increase in the rate of eligible patients receiving beta blocker treatment after myocardial infarction. The rate was 94 percent between 1996 and 1998, compared to 65 to 75 percent for all California health plans. In 2000, 88.5 percent of post–myocardial infarction patients were receiving short-term beta blocker treatment. In addition, lipid-lowering treatment in appropriate patients following myocardial infarction has improved from 29 percent in 1995 to 77.1 percent in 2000, an increase of 266 percent. Finally, the volume of cardiac surgery procedures has been shown to be related to superior outcomes. KPSC's Los Angeles Medical Center performed over 1,600 open-heart surgeries in 2000, compared to fewer than 300 at the average Southern California hospital performing heart surgery.

Results: HIV/AIDS

Kaiser Permanente may have been the first large health plan to develop an integrated approach to HIV and AIDS. Its programs have been recognized by both the government (it received a Leadership on HIV/AIDS award from the Centers for Disease Control and Prevention in 1997) and advocacy groups (such as Being Alive, in 1996) for their high-quality, compassionate care and excellent outcomes for patients with HIV and AIDS. As of 2000, approximately 4,600 members were receiving treatment for HIV. They are closely monitored to assure appropriate and early interventions to optimize health.

In addition to the usual elements of the population care management model, quality improvement programs have been developed to promote HIV antibody testing in pregnant patients and patients with symptoms of any sexually transmitted disease, timely T-cell and viral load testing in patients identified as HIV positive, and cervical cancer screening for female patients identified as HIV positive. The results are impressive. For example, between 1995 and 2000, the percentage of pregnant women with evidence of voluntary testing for HIV infection increased from 63 to 90 percent, far above the community rate for this population. The HIV screening rate among high-risk populations, 55 percent in 2000, is expected to increase significantly in 2001 and 2002 as a result of concerted efforts to remind providers and educate members.

Results: Asthma

The Asthma Care Management Program, the most recent of KPSC's care management programs, was initiated as part of a Kaiser Permanente nationwide effort. Over 98,000 KPSC members with asthma have been identified, and over 8,000 have been stratified as high risk. In August 1997, the Kaiser Permanente National Asthma Clinical Practice Guidelines were approved. In addition, national asthma outcome measures were created from tracking the following data across the entire Kaiser Permanente national program:

- Hospital and inpatient admissions, readmissions, and lengths of stay
- Ambulatory visits during regular hours, after regular hours, and to emergency departments
- Medication usage (especially the use of an inhaled anti-inflammatory)
- Continuity of care (prior outpatient visits by hospitalized patients and the number of primary care providers seen by asthma patients in one year)
- Findings of surveys assessing patient satisfaction and functional status

Results show that emergency room use among adult members with asthma was down by 66 percent from the first quarter of 1999 to the third quarter of 2001, from 9 percent to less than 3 percent. The percentage of adult high-risk members using inhaled anti-inflammatories had increased by 8 percent, from 78.4 to 85.0 percent.

SOURCES OF COMPETITIVE ADVANTAGE

Disease management strategies for chronic diseases are of course not new nor are they unique to Kaiser Permanente. But the Kaiser Permanente setting offers special characteristics that lead to the kind of excellent results I have presented here.

For one thing, a single multispecialty medical group cares for all KFHP members in a large geographical area. Because the entire medical group—not individual physicians—is capitated by the health plan, there are no incentives for individual physicians to withhold the care that can improve outcomes. In addition, Kaiser Permanente's data systems—which employ clinical information, not information from insurance claims as network-type health plans do—and management control systems allow consistent collection of data for the entire population. And in Kaiser Permanente, all clinical decisions and programs like population care management are directed by physicians and not by third-party intermediaries. Last, Kaiser Permanente's vertical integration (of multispecialty physician care, basic and advanced inpatient services, home health care, ambulatory care, laboratory services, radiology services, pharmacy services, and so forth) and horizontal integration of services (across the Southern California geographical area, for example) permit care to be managed in the most appropriate setting and patients to receive the most appropriate tests and treatments. Although individual departments have annual budgets, Permanente Medical Center, KFH, and KFHP senior managers are held jointly accountable for per-member per-month costs across an entire region or within a service area. This accountability frees up the movement of funds to ensure optimal quality and cost-effective initiatives.

BARRIERS TO DIFFUSION

There are three main barriers to the diffusion of this approach: financing, data systems, and implementation.

Efforts like Kaiser's require a substantial initial investment to set up programs and deliver services to at-risk patients who may have been underserved in the past. The returns on these investments are not rapid. Although the programs are generally cost effective, many months or even several years must pass before a return is realized. The information systems that accompany these programs also require a considerable investment, and the clinical systems needed to measure outcomes in a population are complex. Also, implementation is much harder than development.

At the same time, it is important not to underestimate the competitive advantage of Kaiser Permanente's integrated system and capacity to coordinate and measure clinical practices. The physicians who practice at Kaiser Permanente share a culture and a long history—a commitment to quality assessment, innovation, and improvement. They support evidence-based clinical practice guidelines and care management strategies.

CONSUMER-DRIVEN HEALTH CARE

One of the reasons we Americans react so negatively to the term *managed care* is that we do not like to be managed by others. People, especially those with chronic diseases, want to be involved in making decisions about their health. They want knowledgeable health care providers to support them in taking care of themselves. Kaiser Permanente's population care management programs provide them with the involvement and support they seek.

Consumers also want to have the data that will enable them to make choices about their health care. They want accurate and timely measurements that inform them about the ability of different health plans and providers to deliver the best results and outcomes. KPSC's population care management programs publicly report quality data that help consumers make informed choices. These data can be used by others, such as the Pacific Business Group on Health, which publishes a report comparing outcome results from all California health plans. In 2001, this report published results for perinatal care, women's health, diabetes, asthma, hypertension, heart disease, and mental illness.

Kaiser Permanente believes its population approach to improving the health outcomes of patients with chronic disease benefits not only its members but also society as a whole.

Notes

1. The history of Kaiser Permanente begins in 1933, when Sidney R. Garfield, M.D., completed his surgical residency and set up a twelve-bed hospital in the middle of the Southern California desert to provide medical care for workers on the metropolitan aqueduct that was to bring water from the Colorado River to Los Angeles. He arranged for the construction companies to pay him ten cents per day per man for both industrial and nonindustrial care. In 1938, Garfield was asked by Henry J. Kaiser to set up a similar plan in the State of Washington for the workers building the Grand Coulee Dam and their families. This arrangement helped Kaiser Industries attract skilled workers to its shipyards and steel mills in California and Oregon between 1940 and 1945. After World War II, Henry J. Kaiser established a nonprofit foundation to offer a health plan, based on Garfield's multispecialty group practice, to employees of other companies. The Permanente Medical Group in Northern California was formally established in 1949, and the Southern California Permanente Medical Group in 1953. In 1955, the current arrangement combining the Kaiser Foundation Health Plan, Kaiser Foundation Hospitals, and Permanente Medical Groups was established by The Tahoe Agreement, so named because it was drawn up at a meeting at Henry J. Kaiser's Lake Tahoe estate. At first, Kaiser Permanente existed only in California and Oregon. In 1973, however, the Nixon administration–sponsored HMO Act became law, and by 1985, the

Kaiser Permanente program had spread to seventeen other states and the District of Columbia. For more information, see Kay, R. *Historical Review of the Southern California Permanente Medical Group.* Pasadena, Ca.: Southern California Permanente Medical Group, 1979; Smillie, J. *Can Physicians Manage the Quality and Costs of Health Care?* New York: McGraw-Hill, 1991.

2. Smith, S., and others. "The Next Ten Years of Health Spending: What Does the Future Hold?" *Health Affairs,* 1998, *17*(5), 128–140.

3. Hoffman, C., Rice, D., and Sung, H. "Persons with Chronic Conditions: Their Prevalence and Costs." *Journal of the American Medical Association,* 1996, *276,* 1473–1479.

4. Wehrwein, P. "Disease Management Gains a Degree of Respectability." *Managed Care,* 1997, *6*(8), 39–46.

5. Eddy, D. *Clinical Decision-Making: From Theory to Practice.* Sudbury, Mass.: Jones and Bartlett, 1996.

6. Rubin, R., Dietrich, K., and Hawk, A. "Clinical and Economic Impact of Implementing a Comprehensive Diabetes Management Program in Managed Care." *Journal of Clinical Epidemiology,* 1998, *83,* 2635–2642.

CHAPTER SIXTY-THREE

The Right Care

Vanderbilt Medical Center

Harry R. Jacobson

Vanderbilt University Medical Center is one of 125 academic medical centers across the nation that train the next generations of physicians, conduct research into the causes and cures of human disease, and provide a full range of health care services from primary care to advanced tertiary care. Like most of those academic centers, Vanderbilt has subsidized its teaching and research missions with profits from its health care services enterprise. And also like most of those academic centers, it has watched the margins from its health care business shrink. Insurers, both commercial and governmental, have trimmed reimbursements and sought pricing on the margin in exchange for volume. Government payers have publicly questioned the payments for medical education that are embedded components of reimbursement strategies. The cuts in reimbursement are amplified by a renewed vigor on the part of government payers to remove reported fraud and abuse. Finally, the mushrooming costs of regulatory compliance and bureaucratic obstacles to timely payment for services rendered add to the financial stresses of academic health centers and, indeed, of all health care providers.

As the margins from health care shrink, the appetite for resources to meet the needs for training and discovery continues to grow. The pace of growth in scientific knowledge is exponential. The tools for assimilating and reducing that knowledge to distilled learning both for undergraduate and practicing physicians are stressed. Indeed, recent studies show that new standards of care move into practice at rates that are unacceptably slow.

Many believe that we stand at the brink of an era that will see unprecedented advances in our understanding of the basic rules of living organisms and an intimate understanding of how we operate as human beings and, importantly, how to fix us when we do not work properly. Obtaining that knowledge has proven to be an extraordinarily expensive operation. To understand the basics of human life we need to see and understand at a molecular level. We must comprehend a staggeringly large number of combinations and permutations of genes, and we must learn to manipulate them and to create molecules in replicable ways for the billions of individual cells that constitute us.

So academic centers face this challenging situation: their teaching and research missions require significant new investment. However, traditional sources of support, margins generated from providing health care services and government support for graduate medical educators, are eroding rapidly. What is an academic medical center to do?

The solution is staring us in the face. Academic medical centers must apply their strengths in research and education to innovate in health care delivery. They must perfect and export models for evidence-based medicine.

Here is the logic. There is significant waste in our health care system, created by wild variation in the kind and quality of care provided. Best practices are not routinely followed, and new standards are slow to be incorporated into practice. Reducing that variation by developing and implementing standards of care could represent a paradigm shift—leading to both better quality and cost savings.

This sea change in U.S. medicine can come about only if we can do the following: (1) design and continually refine our standards of care, (2) develop tools to assist providers in applying those standards and give them incentives to do so, and (3) develop systems that continually test for and correct variation. The discussion that follows outlines steps that Vanderbilt University Medical Center has taken to begin to address these issues. First, I examine the development of care pathways that harnessed evidence from multidisciplinary sources to control the cost of care, variation from standards, and quality of outcomes. Second, I look at an enabling information technology that ensures that care providers have the right information at the right time so the care they provide is effective and efficient.

ROLE OF PROVIDERS

An international working group has proposed that one of the five major ethical principles guiding health care providers should state: "All individuals and groups involved in health care, whether they provide access or services, have the continuing responsibility to help improve its quality."[1]

Improving the quality of health care requires providers to understand how *quality of care* is defined and measured. A multidimensional construct, the quality of health care can be evaluated on the dimensions of structure, process, and outcome. Thus quality of care needs to be examined in terms of the characteristics of the providers and facilities (structure); the care delivery between provider, facility, and patient (process); and the impact of the care on patient's health status (outcome). To improve quality, providers must examine each of these dimensions and the interaction among them.

Within each of these dimensions of quality, providers need to improve the effectiveness and efficiency of the care system while ensuring and improving its compassion toward patients. The effectiveness of care must be continually examined and improved, reducing the unexplained and system-determined variations in care and promoting the use of evidence-based care. Vanderbilt's case management system was implemented to reduce the total costs of care while maintaining or improving the effectiveness of care.

Providers should embrace clinical epidemiology and outcomes research as approaches that will assist in the determination of the most effective strategies of care. New structures and processes of care need to be developed to reduce excess variation and to ensure that the best practice of medicine is provided to each patient at each encounter. Real-time decision support for providers will be required as part of the solution. WIZ Order, an integrated order-entry and information retrieval system developed at Vanderbilt, is designed to be that decision support tool.

The Vanderbilt University Medical Center has embraced the concepts of clinical improvement. This chapter describes three medical center initiatives that address improving the effectiveness, efficiency, and compassion of the health care system. First, the case management initiative has created a program that has reduced the costs of care while maintaining effectiveness of care. Second, the Informatics Center has developed a computerized physician-order system (WIZ Order) that has the capacity to reduce unwanted variations in care. Third, the medical center has partnered with the Department of Veterans Affairs to implement a physician training program, the National Quality Scholars Program.

CASE MANAGEMENT SYSTEM

From its inception in 1994, case management at Vanderbilt has been viewed as a process and a system, not a role. The foundation of the Vanderbilt case management model is the case management triad, which consists of a nurse case manager, a social worker, and a utilization management (UM)/DRG specialist. These triad members work collaboratively with the health care team to ensure that cost and quality outcomes are met for their assigned patient population. Although triad members share some role functions, each discipline has a unique focus that brings specialized skills and expertise to the collaboration and to patient care.

Clinical Pathways

Vanderbilt University Medical Center began to develop and employ *clinical pathways* in 1990. Its early experience mirrored that of numerous other institutions nationwide in that the work was largely nursing, driven with little physician involvement and limited impact on patient outcomes.

One positive result from this early pathway effort was the development of a computerized documentation system, Pathways, that linked the clinical pathway and nursing flowsheet, electronically captured variance from pathway goals, and used a charting-by-exception (CBE) format. Pathways was well received by nursing staff at Vanderbilt, and time-motion studies revealed significant reductions in the time nurses spent charting activities compared to the time required by the previous charting method.[2] The early success of Pathways challenged Vanderbilt to design an enhanced, networked generation of the system, currently titled Pathworx. Pathworx has the potential to further transform patient care at Vanderbilt by knitting clinical pathways together with physician order entry and facilitating tracking and understanding of variances and costs of care. It can also ultimately be used as the basis for an acuity system that allows nurse staffing to be based on the clinical care requirements of patients.

The development and use of clinical pathways at Vanderbilt has matured with the case management model. Pathway work is now physician driven and has resulted in significant improvements in cost and quality outcomes.[3]

Results

The case management system has produced a number of substantial results.

Length of Stay. Case management efforts focused initially on care coordination and discharge planning. Vanderbilt University Medical Center (VUMC) experienced an accelerated decrease in length of stay (LOS) compared with the LOS of other academic medical centers and with other not-for-profit hospitals nationally. This decrease in LOS was particularly dramatic in fiscal year 1993–1994, when the case management program was established (see Figures 63.1 and 63.2).

Charges and Cost. In a comparison of average charges at Vanderbilt with those at other academic medical centers nationally and at local (nonacademic) hospitals in middle Tennessee, Vanderbilt fares favorably. The reductions are again

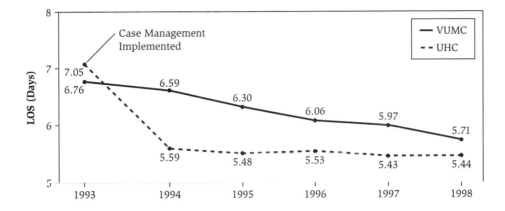

Figure 63.1. Average Length of Stay: VUMC Versus UHC Teaching Hospitals.

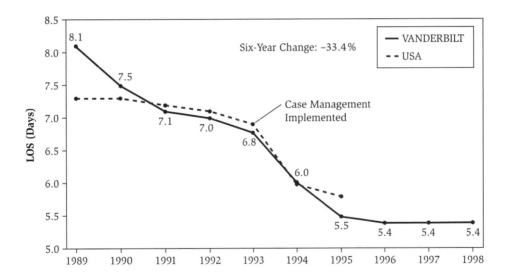

Figure 63.2. Average Length of Stay: VUMC Versus Not-for-Profit Hospitals Nationally.
Source: AHA.

most dramatic in the initial year of case management, 1993–1994 (see Figures 63.3 and 63.4).

Case Mix Index. A comprehensive analysis in 1995 indicated that the case mix index (CMI) at Vanderbilt was inappropriately low given the severity of illness among the patient population and the intensity of service provided. Incomplete physician documentation, which did not support accurate ICD-9 coding, was

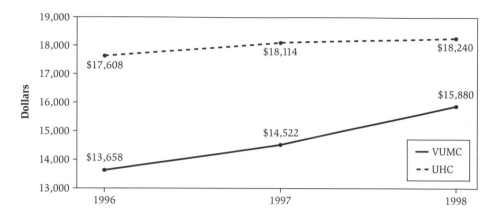

Figure 63.3. Average Charges: VUMC Versus UHC Teaching Hospitals.

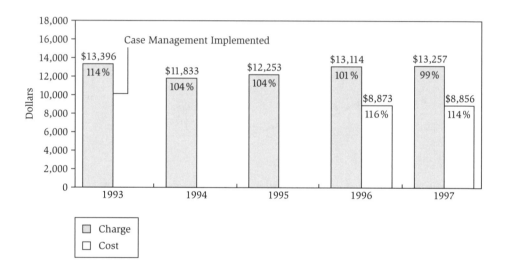

Figure 63.4. VUMC Clinically Adjusted Average Charges and Costs.

Note: Comparisons between Vanderbilt's charges and costs and other hospitals' charges and costs are expressed as percentages.

Source: The Delta Group Inc.

identified as the root cause. The redesigned UM/DRG specialist role provides concurrent chart review and physician prompting as needed to assure accurate and complete documentation. These efforts have resulted in an increase in the CMI to a more appropriate level for an academic medical center and have ensured the integrity of case type and severity data.

Reduction of Bad Debt. The UM/DRG specialist screens patients for admission appropriateness, completes authorization and certification processes, and appeals denied claims. In effect, Vanderbilt closed the loop by bringing front-end (authorization) and back-end (appeal and write-off) processes together, resulting in a significant reduction in dollars written off for claims the payer determined to be "not certified" or "not medically necessary," from 3.4 percent of total patient charges in 1995 to 0.29 percent in 1998.

A Population-Specific Result. The impact of case management on specific groups of patients is best illustrated by an example. The early work of Michael Koch, M.D., to use pathways and case management in the care of patients with radical prostatectomy was groundbreaking at the national level and an important model at Vanderbilt. It also marked the first physician-led effort at Vanderbilt to rationalize care for a specific patient type around cost and quality outcomes. Koch used evidence-based medicine (EBM) to challenge existing paradigms of care for patients with urological disorders. Results for the first one hundred consecutive radical prostatectomy patients showed

- A 47 percent decrease in charges
- An average LOS reduction from 6 to 2.9 days
- No increase in complications, readmissions, or other adverse events
- A high degree of patient satisfaction
- Improvement in key quality indicators, notably blood loss and allogenic blood transfusions[4]

This positive experience with prostatectomy led to the development and use of pathways for all adult and pediatric urology procedures. The entire service is now managed via an integrated pathway–case management model through which improvements in quality and cost are continuously achieved and disseminated into practice.

WIZ ORDER SYSTEM

Both people and machines have difficulty determining how to apply best practice and general medical knowledge to specific clinical cases.[5] There may be a wealth of information in a patient's medical record and a large body of medical literature containing facts pertinent to similar patient problems and guidelines for management. The crucial issue is how to quickly and efficiently reconcile one body of information with the other. Computers have been promoted and used as tools for the management of medical information.[6] Although recent trends may be changing, it is still the case that the majority of computer programs actually used in clinical practice offer only focused accounting, scheduling, patient monitoring, record-keeping, or bibliographical retrieval capabilities. In general, available commercial programs provide only one such service, rather than offering multiple capabilities in an integrated program.

The writing of orders is the final common pathway for actions in clinical medicine (aside from counseling and comforting patients and their families). Because patient care providers convert their decisions into actions at the time of order writing, interventions that provide patient-specific decision support are best implemented at this time. Direct care provider computerized order entry has, however, been a challenge for medical information experts.[7] Busy care providers, and particularly physicians, are reluctant to use systems that slow their work and fail to provide obvious direct benefits.[8] Changes in the workplace engendered by these systems can cause major stress and disruptions throughout an institution.[9] Preparing for these workplace stresses requires extensive planning and training.[10] At times the cost of such implementations can be prohibitive.[11] In institutions where comprehensive electronic medical record systems have been developed, direct care provider order entry has often been one of the last pieces to be implemented.[12]

Nevertheless, once implemented, direct care provider order entry, when linked with electronic medical record and decision support tools, has been shown to be beneficial in a number of domains. Tierney and colleagues showed in one study that presentation of previous test result values decreased the ordering of new tests of the same type by 13 percent[13] and in another study that displaying a computer-generated prediction of the likely test result (that is, the probability that it would be abnormal) decreased charges of ordered tests by 9 percent.[14] The same group also demonstrated that displaying the price of tests decreased the ordered tests by 14 percent[15] and that the use of physician order entry for inpatients reduced the charges per admission by 12 percent[16] when compared to manual order entry results. A system that displays comments about the orders being entered can help the care provider to follow medical guidelines, standard of care practices, and protocols.[17] When medical orders, and particularly orders for medications, are available in an electronic medical record, computerized decision support systems that generate alerts can be developed,[18] and have been shown to improve the management of digoxin therapy,[19] prophylactic perioperative antibiotic use,[20] therapeutic antibiotic use,[21] and blood transfusions[22] and to help in detecting adverse drug events[23] and nosocomial infections.[24] Computer-generated reminders have been shown to significantly increase physicians' response to clinical events that might need correction[25] and are more effective than delayed feedback.[26]

The Department of Biomedical Informatics at Vanderbilt has developed and implemented Horizon Expert Orders,[27] a software-user interface that makes relevant information readily available to the care provider as a by-product of the order-writing process. The provider may browse information in the patient's electronic record (notes and results together with active orders and prior changes), access information and decision support tools (local pathways or information via the intranet, general guidelines, or information resources available via the Internet), and make and record decisions. Horizon Expert Orders then translates those decisions into orders and passes them to the departments or systems that carry them out.

Horizon Expert Orders improves process quality. First, it resolves ambiguity at the source. Although the provider may record an order in clinical shorthand— for example, "Gen 80 IV q8H" for "Gentamicin sulfate 80 mg administered over 30 minutes every 8 hours starting now"—the system then displays its interpretation of that shorthand for verification and correction. Second, it repeatedly checks in the background for potential problems. For example with the gentamicin order, it will check the electronic record to see whether the dose is too high or low in relation to the patient's kidney function and to see whether this new drug may interact with another that the patient is taking.

Horizon Expert Orders guides the provider toward best practice as he or she makes individual decisions. First, the orders needed to care for a patient according to locally developed pathways for problems and procedures are packaged in *order outlines* that can be rapidly tailored to individual patients. Second, eligibility criteria for various clinical trials are available on-line. If a trial is selected for a patient, the system will step the provider through the orders needed to start the patient's workup and treatment. Third, policies are on-line together with tools to document compliance and generate related orders. For example, if a patient is to be placed in restraints, the provider is prompted for the indication and type, and the system generates orders that include the justification and instructions to the nurses.

Finally, Horizon Expert Orders encourages care that is sensitive to resource consumption and cost. If a provider wishes to order empiric antibiotics to treat an infection before the causative organism is known, the best choices in light of the patient's record are displayed, with the lowest cost of comparable choices listed first. Similarly, providers are prompted to convert from intravenous drugs to oral drugs that are less expensive when the record suggests the switch might be appropriate.

Horizon Expert Orders is now being used throughout the Vanderbilt University Hospital, with the exception of the Emergency Department. Ten thousand orders are generated through the decision support interface on an average day.

NATIONAL QUALITY SCHOLARS PROGRAM

Improvement in health care delivery will require leaders and providers who are equipped with the skills necessary to change and improve the system. The Vanderbilt University Medical Center has committed to creating programs that will train future leaders of health care who will be capable of improving the health care systems and the health of the populations they serve. The initial program, the National Quality Scholars Fellowship Program, is under way in partnership with the Department of Veterans Affairs and five other academic medical centers. The two-year program provides training to physicians who have completed their clinical training and who seek the knowledge, skills, and methods to design, introduce, implement, and evaluate improvement in health care systems. Through scholarly investigation, program fellows will advance the science and practice of health care improvement and shape the future of health care.

THE PRACTICE OF EVIDENCE-BASED MEDICINE

The practice of evidence-based medicine holds great promise. Simply following the best standard of care can predictably improve outcomes, reduce the severity and frequency of complications, and lead to a higher quality of life. Intuition says that following that standard of care will reduce costs—first, by eliminating variation and unnecessary expense and, second, by reducing the future demand for services.

Mechanisms that make the most recent standard of care available to all physicians could improve outcomes and reduce costs on a macro basis. Policymakers in Washington are desperately looking for ways to corral the cost of Medicare. With no other tools available to them, they have made unilateral, across-the-board cuts in reimbursement to providers through the Balanced Budget Act. Careful empirical formulation of standards of care and a system that makes just-in-time deliveries of those standards to physicians could begin to cut real health care expenses across the board and especially in Medicare and Medicaid, which serve the elderly and individuals with chronic disease.

Managed care held great promise for changing the existing U.S. medical system to a more efficient system that optimizes the health of a population. It has never fully lived up to that promise, focusing instead on managing cost and access rather than on managing health. A physician-driven movement to practice evidence-based medicine could help fulfill the promise.

Implementing evidence-based medicine will require several new tools. First, circulating new standards of care to the community of practicing physicians must happen more quickly than is possible through the current approach of peer-reviewed literature, presentation at national meetings, and traditional continuing medical education. The Internet could be a powerful new tool for distributing standards of care. Indeed, Vanderbilt, partnering with Duke University, Emory University, Washington University in St. Louis, Oregon Health and Science University, Mt. Sinai Hospital, and New York University, has developed evidence-based guidelines for over one hundred clinical disorders and has made them available over the Internet through IBM Solutions. Finally, order-entry systems like that at VUMC offer tools for real-time assembly of standards of care and immediate feedback to the physician.

Notes

1. Smith, R., Hiatt, H., and Berwick, D. "A Shared Statement of Ethical Principles for Those Who Shape and Give Health Care: A Working Draft from the Tavistock Group." *Annals of Internal Medicine,* 1999, *130,* 143–147.

2. Ashworth, G., and Erickson, S. "Enhancing an Outcome-Focused Collaborative Case Model with Charting by Exception." In L. Burke and J. Murphy (eds.), *Charting by Exception Applicators.* Albany, N.Y.: Delmar, 1994.

3. Price, B. J., Bernard, G. R., Drew, K., Foss, J., and others. "Impact of a Critical Care Pathway for Unstable Mechanically Ventilated Patients." *Critical Care Nursing Clinics of North America,* 1998, *10*(1), 75–85; Koch, M. O., and Smith, J. A. "Cost Containment in Urology." *Urology,* 1995, *46*(12), 14–25; Koch, M. O., and Smith, J. A. "Clinical Outcomes Associated with the Implementation of a Cost Efficient Program for Radical Retropubic Prostatectomy." *British Journal of Urology,* 1995, *76*(1), 1–6; Payne, J. L., McCorty, K. R., Chapman, W. C., Wright, J. K., and others. "Outcomes Analysis for 50 Liver Transplant Recipients: The Vanderbilt Experience." *American Surgeon,* 1996, *62,* 320–325; Geevarghese, S. K., Bradley, A. E., Wright, J. K., Chapman, W. C., and others. "Outcome Analysis in 100 Liver Transplantation Patients." *American Journal of Surgery,* 1998, *175,* 348–353; White, R. "Developing a Critical Pathway for Vascular Access Management." *ANNA Journal,* 1997, *24*(1), 70–77.

4. Koch and Smith, "Clinical Outcomes Associated with the Implementation of a Cost Efficient Program for Radical Retropubic Prostatectomy."

5. Osheroff, J. A., and others. "Physicians' Information Needs: Analysis of Questions Posed During Clinical Teaching." *Annals of Internal Medicine,* 1991, *114,* 576–581; Forsythe, D. E., Buchanan, B. G., Osheroff, J. A., and Miller, R. A. "Expanding the Concept of Medical Information: An Observational Study of Physicians' Information Needs." *Computers & Biomedical Research,* 1992, *25,* 181–200.

6. Bankowitz, R. A., and others. "A Computer-Assisted Medical Diagnostic Consultation Service: Implementation and Prospective Evaluation of a Prototype." *Annals of Internal Medicine,* 1989, *110,* 824–832; Miller, R. A. "Medical Diagnostic Decision Support Systems: Past, Present, and Future." *Journal of the American Medical Informatics Association,* 1994, *1,* 8–27.

7. Sittig, D. F., and Stead, W. W. "Computer-Based Physician Order Entry: The State of the Art." *Journal of the American Medical Informatics Association,* 1994, *1*(2), 108–123.

8. Dambro, M. R., Weiss, B. D., McClure, C. L., and Vuturo, A. F. "An Unsuccessful Experience with Computerized Medical Records in an Academic Medical Center." *Journal of Medical Education,* 1988, *63*(8), 617–623; Spillane, M. J., and others.

"Direct Physician Order Entry and Integration: Potential Pitfalls." In R. A. Miller (ed.), *Proceedings of the Fourteenth Annual Symposium on Computer Applications in Medical Care.* Los Alamitos, Calif.: IEEE Computer Society Press, 1990; Massaro, T. A. "Introducing Physician Order Entry at a Major Academic Medical Center: I. Impact on Organizational Culture and Behavior." *Academic Medicine,* 1993, *68*(1), 20–25; Massaro, T. A. "Introducing Physician Order Entry at a Major Academic Medical Center: II. Impact on Medical Education." *Academic Medicine,* 1993, *68*(1), 25–30; Williams, L. S. "Microchips Versus Stethoscopes: Calgary Hospital, MDs Face Off over Controversial Computer System." Comment. *Canadian Medical Association Journal,* 1992, *147,* 1534–1540, 1543–1544, 1547; McDonald, C. J., and others. "The Regenstrief Medical Record System: 20 Years of Experience in Hospitals, Clinics, and Neighborhood Health Centers." *MD Computing,* 1992, *9*(4), 206–217; Teich, J. M., Hurley, J. F., Beckley, R. F., and Aranow, M. "Design of an Easy-to-Use Physician Order Entry System with Support for Nursing and Ancillary Departments." In M. Frisse (ed.), *Proceedings of the Sixteenth Annual Symposium on Computer Applications in Medical Care.* New York: McGraw-Hill, 1992.

9. Massaro, "Introducing Physician Order Entry at a Major Academic Medical Center: I."

10. Massaro, "Introducing Physician Order Entry at a Major Academic Medical Center: II."

11. Dambro and others, "An Unsuccessful Experience with Computerized Medical Records . . ."; Spillane and others, "Direct Physician Order Entry and Integration."

12. Bankowitz and others, "A Computer-Assisted Medical Diagnostic Consultation Service"; Miller, "Medical Diagnostic Decision Support Systems."

13. Tierney, W. M., McDonald, C. J., Martin, D. K., and Rogers, M. P. "Computerized Display of Past Test Results: Effect on Outpatient Testing." *Annals of Internal Medicine,* 1987, *107,* 569–574.

14. Tierney, W. M., McDonald, C. J., Hui, S. L., and Martin, D. K. "Computer Predictions of Abnormal Test Results: Effects on Outpatient Testing." *Journal of the American Medical Association,* 1988, *259,* 1194–1198.

15. Tierney, W. M., Miller, M. E., and McDonald, C. J. "The Effect on Test Ordering of Informing Physicians of the Charges for Outpatient Diagnostic Tests." *New England Journal of Medicine,* 1990, *322,* 1499–1504.

16. Tierney, W. M., Miller, M. E, Overhage, J. M., and McDonald, C. J. "Physician Inpatient Order Writing on Microcomputer Workstations: Effects on Resource Utilization." *Journal of the American Medical Association,* 1993, *269,* 379–383.

17. Halpern, N. A., Thompson, R. E., and Greenstein, R. J. "A Computerized Intensive Care Unit Order-Writing Protocol." *Annals of Pharmacotherapy,* 1992, *26*(2), 251–254; McDonald, C. J., and Overhage, J. M. "Guidelines You Can Follow and Can Trust: An Ideal and an Example." *Journal of the American Medical Association,* 1994, *271,* 872–873.

18. Hales, J. W., Gardner, R. M., and Huff, S. M. "Integration of a Stand-Alone Expert System with a Hospital Information System." In M. Frisse (ed.), *Proceedings of the*

Sixteenth Annual Symposium on Computer Applications in Medical Care. New York: McGraw-Hill, 1992.

19. White, K. S., and others. "Application of a Computerized Medical Decision-Making Process to the Problem of Digoxin Intoxication." *Journal of the American College of Cardiology,* 1984, *4*(3), 571–576.

20. Larsen, R. A., and others. "Improved Perioperative Antibiotic Use and Reduced Surgical Wound Infections Through Use of Computer Decision Analysis." *Infection Control & Hospital Epidemiology,* 1989, *10,* 316–320; Classen, D. C., and others. "The Timing of Prophylactic Administration of Antibiotics and the Risk of Surgical-Wound Infection." *New England Journal of Medicine,* 1992, *326,* 281–286.

21. Evans, R. S., and others. "Computer Surveillance of Hospital-Acquired Infections and Antibiotic Use." *Journal of the American Medical Association,* 1986, *256,* 1007–1011; Pestotnik, S. L., and others. "Therapeutic Antibiotic Monitoring: Surveillance Using a Computerized Expert System." *American Journal of Medicine,* 1990, *88*(1), 43–48.

22. Gardner, R. M., and others. "Computer-Critiqued Blood Ordering Using the HELP System." *Computers & Biomedical Research,* 1990, *23*(6), 514–528; Lepage, E. F., Gardner, R. M., Laub, R. M., and Jacobson, J. T. "Assessing the Effectiveness of a Computerized Blood Order 'Consultation' System." In *Proceedings of the AMIA Annual Fall Symposium.* New York: McGraw-Hill, 1991, pp. 33–37; Gardner, R. M., and others. "Computerized Continuous Quality Improvement Methods Used to Optimize Blood Transfusions." In C. Safran (ed.), *Proceedings of the Seventeenth Annual Symposium on Computer Applications in Medical Care.* New York: McGraw-Hill, 1993.

23. Evans, R. S., and others. "Development of a Computerized Adverse Drug Event Monitor." In P. D. Clayton (ed.), *Proceedings of the Fifteenth Annual Symposium on Computer Applications in Medical Care.* New York: McGraw-Hill, 1991; Evans, R. S., and others. "Prevention of Adverse Drug Events Through Computerized Surveillance." In M. Frisse (ed.), *Proceedings of the Sixteenth Annual Symposium on Computer Applications in Medical Care.* New York: McGraw-Hill, 1992; Evans, R. S., and others. "Using a Hospital Information System to Assess the Effects of Adverse Drug Events." In C. Safran (ed.), *Proceedings of the Seventeenth Annual Symposium on Computer Applications in Medical Care.* New York: McGraw-Hill, 1993; Kuperman, G. J., and others. "A New Knowledge Structure for Drug-Drug Interactions." In J. G. Ozbolt (ed.), *Proceedings of the Eighteenth Annual Symposium on Computer Applications in Medical Care.* Philadelphia: Hanley & Belfus, 1994.

24. Kahn, M. G., Steib, S. A., Fraser, V. J., and Dunagan, W. C. "An Expert System for Culture-Based Infection Control Surveillance." In C. Safran (ed.), *Proceedings of the Seventeenth Annual Symposium on Computer Applications in Medical Care.* New York: McGraw-Hill, 1993; Rocha, B. H., and others. "Computerized Detection of Nosocomial Infections in Newborns." In J. G. Ozbolt (ed.), *Proceedings of the Eighteenth Annual Symposium on Computer Applications in Medical Care.* Philadelphia: Hanley & Belfus, 1994.

25. McDonald, C. J. "Protocol-Based Computer Reminders, the Quality of Care and the Non-Perfectibility of Man." *New England Journal of Medicine,* 1976, *295,*

1351–1355; McDonald, C. J., Wilson, G. A., and McCabe, G. P., Jr. "Physician Response to Computer Reminders." *Journal of the American Medical Association,* 1980, *244,* 1579–1581.

26. Tierney, W. M., Hui, S. L., and McDonald, C. J. "Delayed Feedback of Physician Performance Versus Immediate Reminders to Perform Preventive Care: Effects on Physician Compliance." *Medical Care,* 1986, *24*(8), 659–666.

27. Geissbuhler, A., and Miller, R. A. "A New Approach to the Implementation of Direct Care-Provider Order Entry." In J. J. Cimino (ed.), *Proceedings of the AMIA Annual Fall Symposium.* Philadelphia: Hanley & Belfus, 1996.

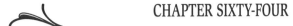

CHAPTER SIXTY-FOUR

Achieving Focus in Hospital Care

The Role of Relational Coordination

Jody Hoffer Gittell

Regina Herzlinger's book on market-driven health care draws on best practices in other industries to generate lessons for transforming health care.[1] One of Herzlinger's central recommendations is that health care organizations should organize their staff around areas of patient focus, rather than attempting to offer a wide range of diverse services. In making this argument, Herzlinger builds on a rich tradition of scholarship supporting the benefits of focus, starting with Wickham Skinner's classic work, "The Focused Factory."[2] When organizations create areas of focus, physical and human assets can be specifically tailored to accomplish a narrowly defined set of objectives, whether in manufacturing[3] or service settings.[4] However, evidence of the performance benefits of focus in health care have been largely anecdotal, drawing frequently on James Heskett's case study of Shouldice Hospital, the Canadian hospital whose delivery system is organized around repairing hernias, with 100 percent of staff time allocated to patients in need of hernia repair.[5] Herzlinger's book

I am grateful to Paul Adler, Richard Bohmer, Amy Edmondson, Regina Herzlinger, and anonymous reviewers for valuable input regarding the ideas in this chapter. I also thank Julian Wimbush for assistance with data collection and William Simpson of the Harvard Business School's Faculty Research Computing Center for advice regarding the statistical analyses presented in this chapter. I especially thank the health care providers and patients from the nine hospitals that participated in the study discussed here. Funding was provided by the Division of Research of the Harvard Business School.

expands the repertoire of evidence well beyond Shouldice but does not draw a statistical link between the degree of focus and health care performance.

In this chapter, drawing on a study I conducted across nine hospitals, I present statistical evidence for the performance quality and efficiency benefits of focus in health care service delivery. In addition, I present a novel argument about how focus works. Certainly asset specificity is likely to be part of the story, as it is in manufacturing settings. Facilities, equipment, and training programs can be designed more appropriately when they are used to accomplish a narrowly defined set of objectives. But I show that focus also helps to strengthen relationships among care providers working with a particular patient population, thereby enhancing the coordination of care for those patients by facilitating shared goals, shared knowledge, and mutual respect. Although the stakes are particularly high in health care, namely life or death, other industries can benefit similarly from the working relationships that are facilitated by focus.

COORDINATION

Leading management theorists have long viewed *coordination*—broadly defined as the management of interdependencies among tasks—as a critical organizational function.[6] Henri Fayol argued that coordination is one of the five tasks that successful organizations must accomplish, and Ronald Coase cited it as the fundamental reason that organizations exist.[7] Coordination is not only an executive function. It is carried out at every level, including the coordination of day-to-day tasks by workgroups within organizations that enables both higher quality outcomes and greater efficiency.[8] Researchers in multiple industry settings have shown that effective coordination can shift the production possibilities frontier outward, enabling organizations to achieve higher levels of productivity rather than simply negotiating trade-offs between the quality and the efficiency of service delivery.[9]

Because the delivery of health care services involves multiple providers with distinct areas of expertise and specialized knowledge, coordination is particularly difficult to achieve in this setting.[10] It is often left to patients to sort their way through the system, receiving diagnoses and treatments from a loosely connected set of providers. Even in the hospital setting, where resources are presumably brought together in one organization to improve the coordination of their deployment, coordination often falls to patients and their families. According to sociologist Anselm Strauss and his colleagues: "Coordination of care, for which personnel are constantly striving but know they are not often attaining, is something of a mirage except for the most standardized of trajectories. Its attainment is something of a miracle when it actually does occur."[11]

And yet the pressures for hospitals to achieve coordination in health care have risen dramatically. Some payers have reduced the number of days for which they will reimburse a hospital for any given episode of care, often by more than one-half, from twelve to five days for a hip replacement, for example. Hospitals that keep patients longer than the number of reimbursed days suffer a financial loss. Other payers provide a fixed fee to the hospital for a patient with a particular diagnosis, so that a hospital earns more money if the patient is discharged quickly and less if the patient stays longer. Shorter lengths of stay require coordination within the hospital setting to move patients quickly through testing and treatments to achieve their target dates of discharge.

Pressures to maintain quality have continued at the same time that pressures to reduce costs have increased. Hospitals compete for managed care contracts and referrals based not only on their costs but also on their quality of care as measured by the quality ratings of the Joint Commission for Accreditation of Healthcare Organizations (JCAHO), the National Committee for Quality Assurance (NCQA), and managed care organizations.[12]

Together, these cost and quality pressures have motivated new efforts to improve the coordination of patient care. One administrator said of her hospital's efforts: "As the screws have tightened, we've had to look at processes. We've moved from patients experiencing individuals as caregivers to experiencing systems as caregivers. Our length of stay is 4.9 or 5.0 days now, while it was 8.0 in the recent past. Because of the reduction in length of stay and downsizing, you have to substitute many more caregivers, and there's less time to build individual relationships with patients."[13]

Under these high-pressure conditions, coordination is increasingly necessary but also increasingly difficult to achieve. The consequences of failure are severe. Both the quality and the efficiency of patient care are reduced by poor coordination among providers.[14] For example, failure to coordinate can lead to devastating errors in medication and treatment.[15] Furthermore, recent work suggests that errors in patient care stemming from coordination failures are more likely than other errors to result in costly malpractice claims.[16] Poor coordination also results in scheduling problems, such as delays in testing or treatment, conflicting information given to patients and their families, and loss of confidence in the provider.[17] Confused, misinformed patients may not follow treatment advice due to lack of understanding, a particularly troublesome outcome now that much of the recovery period occurs outside the hospital and depends for its success on patient cooperation.

The era of consumer-driven health care will intensify these pressures. Many consumers will seek out focused teams for treatment of chronic diseases and disabilities and for services for currently underserved populations such as women and American Indians. Those focused provider teams that follow the

Buyers Health Care Action Group (BHCAG) model will need to price their services accurately and control them carefully so they can achieve satisfactory financial results. The increased accountability that accompanies consumer-driven health care will require these providers to achieve these financial results while they also attain exemplary quality ratings.

THE THEORY OF RELATIONAL COORDINATION

The theory of relational coordination argues that in highly interdependent task settings, such as health care, effective coordination is far more dependent than has previously been recognized upon the *relationships* that exist among participants, particularly relationships involving shared goals, shared knowledge, and mutual respect.[18] There is some precedent in organizational theory for this view. The *social capital* theorists, who have long conceived of communication and relationships among parties as forming a pattern of ties called *social networks,*[19] have begun to explore the possibility that relationships play an important role in coordination.[20] Other scholars have explored the impact of shared goals, shared knowledge, and mutual respect (or, more often, the lack thereof) on the effectiveness with which people work together.

Shared Goals

In their classic *Organizations,* James March and Herbert Simon[21] described the potentially disintegrative effects that occur when members of distinct functional areas in an organization pursue their own goals without reference to the overarching goals of the work process in which they are engaged. Other research suggests that participants with shared goals for the work process can more easily coordinate their work with each other.[22]

Shared Knowledge

Organizational scholar Deborah Dougherty[23] demonstrated that participants from different functional backgrounds often reside in different *thought worlds* due to differences in their training, socialization, and expertise. Because these thought worlds create obstacles to effective communication, they undermine the effective coordination of work processes. Karl Weick's *sense-making* theory suggests that collective mind, or shared understanding of the work process by those who are participants in it,[24] can link these distinct thought worlds and therefore enhance coordination.

Mutual Respect

John Van Maanen and Steve Barley's[25] groundbreaking work on occupational communities suggests that members of distinct communities who are divided by differences in status may bolster their own status by actively cultivating disrespect for the work performed by others. When members of these distinct occupational communities are engaged in a common work process, these divisive relationships can undermine coordination. Several scholars have suggested that respect for the competence of other participants in a work process may be fundamental to the effective coordination of work processes.[26]

Relational Coordination

The theory of relational coordination has been built from these insights.[27] The bottom line of this theory is that relationships of shared goals, shared knowledge, and mutual respect enable participants to coordinate more effectively the work processes in which they are engaged. Shared goals motivate participants to act with greater regard for the overall work process. Shared knowledge informs participants how their own tasks and those of others contribute to the overall work process, enabling them to act with greater regard for the overall work process. Respect for the work of others further reinforces the inclination to act in line with the overall work process. This web of relationships in turn reinforces frequency, timeliness, and problem solving in communication, enabling participants to coordinate effectively the work process in which they are engaged. Consistent with this theory, relational coordination has been shown to play a central role in achieving high levels of performance in the context of both flight departures and patient care.[28]

HOW FOCUS WORKS

Focus is expected to improve performance by supporting higher levels of coordination—operational flows are designed so they better support task interdependencies. The theory of relational coordination suggests a novel reason why focus may serve as a source of performance advantage for organizations. When everyone who is involved in a particular work is focused on that particular work process for most or all of their time, they interact more intensively and extensively about a particular set of issues and therefore have a greater likelihood of developing strong relationships of shared goals, shared knowledge, and mutual respect. Organizations that organize staff around particular areas of focus should therefore be particularly effective at generating high levels of relational coordination and achieving higher performance.

The positive impact of focus on relational coordination increases with the scale of the operation. In a small operation the benefits are smaller, because staff members tend to be familiar with what others are doing by virtue of the small scale. The scale of larger organizations, however, makes it difficult to coordinate a wide variety of activities. As scale increases, focus becomes particularly valuable for achieving the relational coordination that leads to higher levels of quality and efficiency performance.

THE STUDY

To examine these concepts, I studied nine hospitals. In each hospital, I surveyed the staff members responsible for providing care to joint replacement patients. These staff members represented five functional areas of specialization—physicians, nurses, physical therapists, social workers, and case managers—central to the care of joint replacement patients. I measured focus with a survey that asked each care provider what percentage of his or her time was spent working with joint replacement patients as opposed to other patient populations. Their answers were averaged within each of the nine patient groups to reveal the percentage of staff time allocated to joint replacement patients as opposed to other patient populations.

I used the same survey with each staff group to measure relational coordination, asking each care provider about his or her interactions with the other doctors, nurses, therapists, social workers, and case managers involved in caring for joint replacement patients. Seven questions (Exhibit 64.1) probed the frequency, timeliness, accuracy, and problem-solving tendency of the communication experienced with other group members and also the degree of shared goals, shared knowledge, and mutual respect experienced with them. Performance was measured along two dimensions—the quality of care and the efficiency with which care was delivered. Quality of care was assessed by patients in a survey they received after hospitalization. Patient-assessed quality of care has not traditionally been considered a relevant outcome in health care settings. However, "as the orientation to health care began shifting from scientific mandates and medical techniques to markets and the more human side of health care—a service delivery system, patient satisfaction has become an important dimension of the quality of care."[29] The discovery of the importance of patient satisfaction occurred through clinical work on patient-centered care,[30] and that satisfaction has continued to grow in importance as a dimension of health care quality.[31] The efficiency of care delivery was measured as the number of days spent in acute care. Control variables were included to factor out the effects of differences in patient age, health conditions, type of surgery (hip versus knee), psychological well-being, race, gender, marital status, and the volume of joint replacements performed by the group in the past six months on these measures of performance.

Patients rated their satisfaction with the quality of their care at 4.1 points out of 5 ("very good" but not "excellent") on average. Patient length of stay was 5.11 days on average. Multilevel regression analyses were conducted to test the model of focus, relational coordination, and performance described previously.

Exhibit 64.1. Relational Coordination Survey Items.

COMMUNICATION

Frequent communication	How frequently do you communicate with each of these [functions] about the status of joint replacement patients?
Timely communication	How timely is the communication you receive from these [functions] regarding the status of joint replacement patients?
Accurate communication	How accurate is the communication you receive from these [functions] regarding the status of joint replacement patients?
Problem-solving communication	When an error has been made regarding joint replacement patients, do the people in these [functions] try to solve the problem or blame others?

RELATIONSHIPS

Shared goals	To what extent do people in these [functions] share your goals with regard to the care of joint replacement patients?
Shared knowledge	How much do people in each of these [functions] know about the work you do with joint replacement patients?
Mutual respect	How much do people in these [functions] respect you and the work you do with joint replacement patients?

Note: Respondents were asked to answer each question with respect to each of the five functions involved in caring for joint replacement patients. Answers were measured on a 5-point Likert scale.

RESULTS

The nine care provider groups (hospitals) included in this study differed in the average percentage of their time focused on joint replacement patients, average level of relational coordination experienced by staff members, and quality of care and length of stay experienced by their patients. They also differed in the volume of joint replacements they performed annually and in the characteristics of their patients.

Across the sample, care providers working with joint replacement patients spent 68 percent of their time working with this patient population. Seventy percent of providers reported high or very high frequency of communication with their colleagues in other functional areas, 79 percent high or very high timeliness of communication from those colleagues, 80 percent high or very high accuracy of communication from their colleagues, and 66 percent high or very high focus on problem solving rather than on blaming communication from their colleagues when an error had been made. Seventy-one percent reported a high or very high level of shared knowledge with their colleagues, 83 percent high or very high levels of shared goals, and 71 percent high or very high levels of mutual respect. When these dimensions of relational coordination were combined into an equally weighted index, 77 percent of providers surveyed were found to have high or very high levels of relational coordination with their colleagues.

The model suggests that focus on a particular patient population fosters high levels of relational coordination among the providers who work with those patients. It also suggests that the larger the scale of the operation, the greater the effects of focus on relational coordination. Focus and the product of volume and focus are associated with significantly higher levels of relational coordination. Consistent with this model, focus and the product of focus and volume are significantly associated with improved quality of care and with shorter hospital stays. Finally, the model also suggests that the effects of focus on performance are transmitted at least in part *through* relational coordination. When relational coordination is added to the quality model, focus no longer has a significant effect on quality of care. When relational coordination is added to the efficiency equation, focus no longer predicts shorter hospital stays. These results indicate that the effects of focus on quality and efficiency performance are transmitted in part *through* the effect of focus on relational coordination. In other words the quality and efficiency benefits of focus exist at least in part due to the impact that focus has on relational coordination.

CONCLUSION

This study demonstrated four aspects of focus. First, focus does work in health care, consistent with Herzlinger's argument, as it has also been shown to work in manufacturing settings. Second, it provided insight about *how* focus works in health care settings. Focus improves both quality and efficiency performance by fostering higher levels of relational coordination among care providers. Groups whose members devote a higher percentage of their time to working with a particular patient population tend to develop stronger relationships (shared goals, shared knowledge, and mutual respect) and more effective patterns of interaction. Third, focus results in increased quality of care for the patient *and* reduced hospitalization costs for the payer. Organizations whose providers spend a high percentage of their time working with a particular patient population can achieve both quality and efficiency outcomes.

Last, focus requires a certain minimum scale. An organization can realistically create focus only around work processes that have sufficiently high volume to meet minimum economies of scale. Trying to create focus through dedicated staffing without the requisite scale results in underutilized staff,[32] a slack resource that can scarcely be afforded in the current health care environment. The groups in this study had relatively high volumes of procedures and as a result had the realistic option of dedicating staff and other resources to the care of joint replacement patients. (The groups included in this study had performed between 353 and 920 joint replacements in the six months preceding the study period, relative to a median volume of 256 joint replacement procedures per year for U.S. hospitals.[33]) However, even within these high volume operations, I found that the benefits of focus are greater the larger the scale of the operation.

Note that the entire organization need not be focused around serving a particular patient population. The key is achieving focus at the level of the workgroup. Indeed, a separate variable measuring the degree of organization-wide focus was included in all of the analyses, as an additional control variable. In none of the equations did organization-wide focus contribute positively to performance. Only at the level of the workgroup did focus make a difference for performance. This finding is consistent with earlier findings from manufacturing, suggesting that focus need not be organization-wide, but rather can be achieved at the level of the individual plant. In health care we see hospitals attempting to achieve focus at the level of service lines within the hospital. The present study suggests that to achieve performance benefits, staff members should be allocated to those service lines as exclusively as possible, to foster high levels of relational coordination with each other. With highly focused workgroups dedicated to delivering care to particular patients, the organization as a whole should be able to offer a broad range of services without sacrificing the quality or efficiency of care delivery.

Managers of organizations that have sufficient operational scale to achieve focus around particular patient populations can maximize the resulting benefits through supportive managerial practices, such as hiring and training for teamwork and allocating time and attention to resolving conflicts as they emerge. Executives of hospital organizations that lack sufficient operational scale to achieve focus around particular patient populations can create it by marketing key programs or by combining several similar programs (say, orthopedics patients as a whole) to create focus around several related patient populations. Even when staff members are pulled in many directions, providing care to multiple, fragmented patient populations, a degree of focus can be achieved through the efforts of case managers, who can serve as the central point for coordinating the care of particular patient populations.[34]

What are the implications of these hospital findings for executives in a consumer-driven health care system? Increasingly, health care is being delivered *outside* the walls of hospitals, across a wide array of settings such as physician offices, outpatient clinics, rehabilitation hospitals, skilled nursing facilities, and home care. As a result there is an increasing need to achieve coordination *across* settings. Focus can be a valuable tool for achieving coordination beyond hospital walls, by facilitating relationships across the range of settings in which providers are focused on delivering services to the same patient population. For example, organizations that provide disease management for patients with congestive heart failure can develop partnerships with complementary providers so that the full range of services needed by this patient population can be delivered efficiently and conveniently. The benefits of focus demonstrated by this study can therefore be extended from the in-patient setting as providers address the growing challenge of coordinating care in the broader consumer-driven health care system.

Notes

1. Herzlinger, R. E. *Market-Driven Health Care: Who Wins and Who Loses in the Transformation of America's Largest Service Industry.* Reading, Mass.: Addison-Wesley, 1997.

2. Skinner, W. "The Focused Factory." *Harvard Business Review,* May–June 1974, 113–121.

3. Brush, T., and Karnani, A. "Impact of Plant Size and Focus on Productivity: An Empirical Study." *Management Science,* 1996, *42,* 1065–1081; Hayes, R., Wheelwright, S., and Clark, K. *Dynamic Manufacturing: Creating the Learning Organization.* New York: Free Press, 1988.

4. Heskett, J. L., Hart, C., and Sasser, W. E. *Service Breakthroughs: Changing the Rules of the Game.* New York: Free Press, 1990; Heskett, J. L., Sasser, W. E., and Schlesinger, L. A. *The Service Profit Chain: How Leading Companies Link Profit and Growth to Loyalty, Satisfaction and Value.* New York: Free Press, 1997.

5. Heskett, J. L. *Shouldice Hospital.* Harvard Business School Case No. 683-068. Boston: Harvard Business School, 1989.

6. Malone, T., and Crowston, K. "The Interdisciplinary Study of Coordination." *Computing Surveys,* 1994, *26*(1), 87–119; Kogut, B., and Zander, U. "What Firms Do? Coordination, Identity, and Learning." *Organization Science,* 1996, *7*(5), 502–518; Van de Ven, A. "A Framework for Organization Assessment." *Academy of Management Review,* Jan. 1975, pp. 64–78; Thompson, J. D. *Organizations in Action: Social Science Bases of Administrative Theory.* New York: McGraw-Hill, 1967; Lawrence, P. R., and Lorsch, J. W. "Differentiation and Integration in Complex Organizations." *Administrative Science Quarterly,* 1967, *12,* 1–47; Galbraith, J. *Designing Complex Organizations.* Reading, Mass.: Addison-Wesley, 1973.

7. Fayol, H. *Industrial and General Administration.* Paris: Dunod, 1925; Coase, R. H. "The Nature of the Firm." *Economica,* 1937, *4,* 386–405.

8. Arrow, H., McGrath, J. E., and Berdahl, J. L. *Small Groups as Complex Systems: Formation, Coordination, Development and Adaptation.* Thousand Oaks, Calif.: Sage, 2000; Allen, T. *Managing the Flow of Technology.* Cambridge, Mass.: MIT Press, 1984; Ancona, D. G., and Caldwell, D. "Bridging the Boundary: External Activity and Performance in Organizational Teams." *Administrative Science Quarterly,* 1992, *37,* 634–665; Katz, R. "The Effects of Group Longevity on Project Communication and Performance." *Administrative Science Quarterly,* 1982, *27,* 81–104; Keller, R. T. "Technology-Information Processing Fit and the Performance of R&D Groups: A Test of Contingency Theory." *Academy of Management Journal,* 1994, *37*(1), 167–179.

9. Abernathy, F. H., Dunlop, J. T., Hammond, J. H., and Weil, D. *A Stitch in Time: Lean Retailing and the Transformation of Manufacturing: Lessons from the Apparel and Textile Industries.* New York: Oxford University Press, 1999; Womack, J. P., Jones, D. T., and Roos, D. *The Machine That Changed the World: The Story of Lean Production.* New York: Macmillan, 1990.

10. Gerteis, M., Edgman-Levitan, S., Daley, J., and Delbanco, T. *Through the Patient's Eyes: Understanding and Promoting Patient-Centered Care.* San Francisco: Jossey-Bass, 1993.

11. Strauss, A., Fagerhaugh, S., Suczek, B., and Wiener, C. *Social Organization of Medical Work.* Chicago: University of Chicago Press, 1985.

12. O'Leary. D. "What Will the JCAHO Do to Quantify Quality?" *Physician's Management,* 1988, *28*(8), 110–122; "NCQA Releases HEDIS 2.0 Standards: Quality Monitoring Group Prepares to Test Report Card Measures." *QRC Advisor,* 1994, *10*(3), 1–3.

13. Gittell, J. H., and Weiss, L. "Coordination Networks Within and Across Organizations: A Multi-Level Framework." *Journal of Management Studies,* 2004, *41*(1).

14. Argote, L. "Input Uncertainty and Organizational Coordination in Hospital Emergency Units." *Administrative Science Quarterly,* 1982, *27,* 420–434; Baggs, J. G., and others. "The Association Between Interdisciplinary Collaboration and Patient Outcomes in a Medical Intensive Care Unit." *Heart and Lung,* 1992, *21,* 18–24; Knaus, W. A., Draper, E. A., Wagner, D. P., and Zimmerman, J. E. "An Evaluation of Outcomes from Intensive Care in Major Medical Centers." *Annals of Internal Medicine,* 1986, *104,* 410–418; Shortell, S. M., and others. "The Performance of Intensive Care Units: Does Good Management Make a Difference?" *Medical Care,* 1994, *32,* 508–525; Young, G., and others. "Patterns of Coordination and Clinical Outcomes: A Study of Surgical Services." *Health Services Review,* 2000, *33,* 1211–1236.

15. Edmondson, A. "Learning from Mistakes Is Easier Said Than Done: Group and Organizational Influences on the Detection and Correction of Human Error." *Journal of Applied Behavioral Science,* 1996, *32*(1), 5–28.

16. Martin, P. B. "Review of Coordination of Care Issues in CRICO Claims." *Forum* (Risk Management Foundation of the Harvard Medical Institutions), 1996, *17*(4), 2–5.

17. Gerteis and others, *Through the Patient's Eyes.*

18. Gittell, J. H. "A Relational Theory of Coordination: Coordinating Work Through Relationships of Shared Goals, Shared Knowledge and Mutual Respect." Working

paper, 2002; Gittell, J. H. "Supervisory Span, Relational Coordination and Flight Departure Performance: Reassessing Post-Bureaucracy Theory." *Organization Science*, 2001, *12*(4), 467–482; Gittell, J. H. "Relationships Among Service Providers and Their Impact on Customers." *Journal of Service Research*, 2002, *4*(4), 299–311.

19. Granovetter, M. "Economic Action and Social Structure: The Problem of Embed-dedness." *American Journal of Sociology*, 1985, *91*, 481–510; Granovetter, M. "The Strength of Weak Ties." *American Journal of Sociology*, 1973, *78*, 1380–1390; Burt, R. S. "The Contingent Value of Social Capital." *Administrative Science Quarterly*, 1997, *42*, 338–365; Burt, R. S. "The Social Structure of Competition." In N. Nohria and R. Eccles (eds.), *Networks and Organizations: Structure, Form and Action.* Boston: Harvard Business School Press, 1992.

20. Leana, C., and Van Buren, H. J., III. "Organizational Social Capital and Employ-ment Practices." *Academy of Management Review*, 1999, *24*, 538–555.

21. March, J. G., and Simon, H. A. *Organizations.* New York: Wiley, 1958.

22. Saavedra, R., Earley, P. C., and Van Dyne, L. "Complex Interdependence in Task-Performing Groups." *Journal of Applied Psychology*, 1993, *78*(1), 61–72; Wageman, R. "Interdependence and Group Effectiveness." *Administrative Science Quarterly*, 1995, *40*, 145–180.

23. Dougherty, D. "Interpretive Barriers to Successful Product Innovation in Large Firms." *Organization Science*, 1992, *3*(2), 179–202.

24. Weick, K. "The Collapse of Sense-Making in Organizations: The Mann Gulch Disaster." *Administrative Science Quarterly*, 1993, *38*, 628–652; Weick, K., and Roberts, K. "Collective Mind in Organizations: Heedful Interrelating on Flight Decks." *Administrative Science Quarterly*, 1993, *38*, 357–381.

25. Van Maanen, J., and Barley, S. R. "Occupational Communities: Culture and Control in Organizations." In B. M Staw and L. L. Cummings (eds.), *Research in Organizational Behavior.* Vol. 6. Greenwich, Conn.: JAI Press, 1984.

26. Rubenstein, A. H., Barth, R. T., and Douds, C. F. "Ways to improve Communica-tions Between R&D Groups." *Research Management*, 1971, *14*, 49; Eisenberg, E. "Jamming: Transcendence Through Organizing." *Communication Research*, 1990, *17*, 139–164.

27. Gittell, J. H. "Relational Coordination: Coordination in the Context of Relation-ships." Working paper, 2002.

28. Gittell, "Relational Coordination"; Gittell, J. H., and others. "Impact of Relational Coordination on Quality of Care, Post-Operative Pain and Functioning, and the Length of Stay: A Nine-Hospital Study of Surgical Patients." *Medical Care*, 2000, *38*, 807–819.

29. Chilingerian, J. "Evaluating Quality Outcomes Against Best Practice: A New Frontier." In J. R. Kimberly and E. Minvielle (eds.), *The Quality Imperative: Mea-surement and Management of Quality in Health Care.* London: Imperial College Press, 2000.

30. Gerteis and others, *Through the Patient's Eyes.*

31. Gold, M., and Wooldridge, J. "Surveying Customer Satisfaction to Assess Managed Care Quality: Current Practices." *Health Care Financing Review,* 1995, *16*(4), 155–73; Berwick, D. "The Year of 'How': New Systems for Delivering Health Care." *Quality Connections,* 1996, *5*(1), 1–4.

32. Gittell, J. H. *Reading Rehabilitation Hospital: Implementing Patient-Focused Care.* Harvard Business School Case No. 898-172. Boston: Harvard Business School, 2000.

33. Jeffrey Neil Katz, M.D., Brigham and Women's Hospital, personal communication to the author.

34. Gittell, J. H. "Coordinating Mechanisms in Care Provider Groups: Relational Coordination as a Mediator and Input Uncertainty as a Moderator of Performance Effects." *Management Science,* 2002, *48*(11), 1408–1426.

CHAPTER SIXTY-FIVE

Consumer-Driven Health Care
Is a Message of Hope

James F. Rodgers

I have heard the story of consumer-driven health care delivered to physicians by a variety of speakers, and the response is invariably positive. Answering to patients, rather than a remote bureaucrat, is a message of hope in what many physicians argue is an otherwise gloomy medical practice environment.

Clinicians are trained in a vast and rapidly growing high-tech field to enable them to tailor the best care possible to each individual they see. The current system has erected a variety of barriers to the realization of that ideal. Physicians say those barriers are growing. An insurance clerk sits at a computer terminal and matches a doctor's order against some statistical description of efficient practice and overrules a clinical decision, irrespective of the consumer's interest or desires. A drug formulary fails to recognize the latest developments in the literature, and a patient is treated with a second-best drug, irrespective of cost considerations and without the patient's awareness of the choice that has been made. An insurer refuses to pay for a higher-cost treatment, in spite of the high nonmonetary cost to the patient, in pain and suffering or lengthened recovery time, of the lower-cost treatment.

After hearing physicians' favorable reception of a speech on consumer-driven health care, one health policy expert asked me if physicians really understand how profound the changes would be if consumers were put in the driver's seat. Do doctors really understand how demanding a consumer-driven market can be? Do they realize that the whole structure of medical practice may have

696

to change to accommodate patient convenience and efficiency? Do they realize how revolutionary the changes might be?

I suppose no one can truly know what changes would ensue, but I believe that part of the reason for physician enthusiasm about consumer-driven health care is the challenge of the wholesale changes that would be required as well as the promise of change away from the status quo. Practicing doctors do not have much of a stake in keeping things as they are, and they believe that they can fare well in a system that rewards serving patients. Many physicians realize that consumers would be a lot more cost conscious if they were spending their own funds for health care and consequently that successful medical practices would change significantly to accommodate such a new environment. I think physicians would appreciate the change to a consumer-driven marketplace—an environment in which they could be rewarded for serving their client in the way that client chooses.

Why is it that medical practice should expect radical change from such a marketplace?

The short answer is that the current system thwarts economizing behavior, causing relative prices to inadequately express consumers' collective judgment about relative values. For example, a patient tolerates the inconvenient gatekeeper visit before obtaining specialty care because insurance subsidization favors it. A physician allocates a small amount of time to patient communication (in person, over the phone, or on-line) because it is not compensated by insurance. A patient has little, if any, awareness of the relative cost of treatment options, because his or her outlays are unaffected by the choice.

We can gain some insight into how medical practices might change by examining how the existing marketplace undermines the power of competition among health plans and providers to drive allocation towards consumer preferences. A large segment of the employer-based population is overinsured, leading health plans to obtain large returns from focusing on nonprice rationing. In the individual and small-group markets, the greatest return to health plans often comes from selecting healthy patients. Responding to consumers by tailoring insurance or delivery packages is far down the list for plans when they are considering how to gain a competitive advantage.

In addition, providing patients with convenience and information may be undervalued relative to other attributes because of the potential for consumer abuse of such service qualities. However, they are also relatively undervalued because for many traditional services, insurance is so complete and cost sharing is so absent. I expect that a consumer-driven marketplace will move to right this imbalance.

Because physicians have shown themselves to be quite adaptable to managed care contracting, I expect they would adjust relatively quickly, though not painlessly, to the new order. In spite of the growth of practice size over the last several decades, most physicians practice in relatively small groups. Feedback from consumer-driven markets tends to be swift and sure for these small businesses. Physicians would tend to be much more adaptive than larger hospital and health plan organizations.

This favorable reaction of medicine to consumer-driven ideas, however, will not make such a marketplace happen. There are many impediments. Employer-based health insurance limits consumer choice. High-income families, on average, are too heavily subsidized. State-mandated benefits limit choice.

Yet physicians are not the only ones who need hope in today's environment. Who is satisfied with the health care system as it currently exists? Patients are not, and they have precipitated a political backlash against managed care because the current system is unresponsive to them. They are likely to get some relief via legislation. Employers are concerned about the potential for another cost explosion, as well as the possible loss of their shield against liability suits against self-funded health plans. Some kinds of health plans are having difficulties as well; maybe their competitors have excessive market power or maybe employers insufficiently value their service to patients.

The confluence of all these interests makes it possible that a political consensus favoring change could emerge and move us toward consumer-driven changes within a few years.

CHAPTER SIXTY-SIX

An Academic Health Center Perspective

Roger J. Bulger

What's in a name? *Consumer,* in the context of health care, could mean *patient* or *client,* or it could refer more broadly to a *payer* or to a *population* or *community* at large. If I were naming the model that this book is calling *consumer-driven health care,* I would prefer to call it *person-driven health care* or *person- and community-driven health care*—the implication would of course be that the new system should be driven by those whose health status the system is meant to address.

Having been asked to answer probing questions about consumer-driven health care from the perspective of an academic health center leader, I am pleased to do so, and I have endeavored to make clear when I am speaking from my personal point of view and when I am expressing the point of view of the academic community in so far as it is ascertainable as a broadly discussed and widely supported perspective. There are, for example, some general lessons that have recently been learned about academic health centers (such as that there is no single best organizational model or structure for the academic health center to use in coping with the new service delivery world); there are also some values and opinions about health care that most academic health center leaders share (for example, the membership of the Association of Academic Health Centers has been on record for more than a decade as favoring universal access to effective health care for all Americans).

The elements of the consumer-driven model that are most attractive are these: (1) that it offers universal access to health care, presumably through a variety of government supports to cover gaps in the market-based sector; and (2) that it offers choice of provider and care venue by the consumer, choices that will likely involve quality and cost evaluations.

Thus, from the academic health center perspective, consumer-driven care should give academic health center providers an excellent chance of recruiting patients who seek the highest-quality and most advanced treatments. Second, the provision of financial support to cover the previously uninsured will allow academic centers to sustain their commitment to caring disproportionately for those who currently cannot pay, as it also helps to reverse their declining financial status. Finally, it seems evident that the proposed new model tends to move individuals into the position of rationers of their own health care, a position doctors do not want, system managers do not covet, and the government has been avoiding. In summary, as presented, consumer-driven care (1) offers advances in reaching universal access, (2) stimulates data-driven quality efforts in order to evaluate clinical value, and (3) takes a big step toward solving the rationing dilemma.

Is all this too good to be true?

From the point of view of the academic health center sector, the consumer-driven health care model is attractive, credible, and feasible. If such a system comes fully into play, the academic sector will need to continue to develop and refine many of the changes that have already been initiated in many centers as they have confronted the challenges of market-driven health care over the past five or six years.

The Organization Study Committee of the Association of Academic Health Centers has just completed a two-year study of the overall impact of health care market evolution on the teaching, research, and community service activities of our nation's university-based academic health centers. In brief, that study shows

- The academic health centers of our country are responding with major adjustments in form and function, both to sustain their core functions and to lead the health sector in new approaches to deal with this volatile environment.

- The new financial realities require that research, education, clinical care, and community service be managed as though they were four separate businesses, each with its own business plan, goals, and performance guidelines: these changes in turn suggest that these four venues must be reintegrated at the school and campus level.

- Vast organizational and cultural changes are required in many academic health centers for faculty to operate successfully in this new environment. High degrees of individual faculty autonomy and the medieval fiefdom characteristics found in department- and specialty-oriented schools must yield to a more team-oriented, resource-constrained, supradepartmental approach.

- The backbone to these cultural changes will be built when medical schools and academic health centers make their fund flows and financial workings transparent. The black box within which many Merlin-like department chairs and deans have financed academic programs with cross-subsidizing legerdemain unintelligible to faculty and trustees must give way to a completely open process, allowing school departments and individual faculty to know whence come the funds to support their efforts and also allowing them and others to compare those investments with the outcomes and productivity they have generated.

- Tenure policies and obligated salary levels will be argued at those institutions where faculties enlarged over the past decade may no longer be affordable.

- Advances in education and research are already requiring new, flexible responses in deployment of faculty to achieve desired goals. New technologies may do more to alter traditional disciplinary and professional silos than most of us now appreciate; certainly cost cutting, efficiency, and value added will become much more prominent considerations in the conduct of both teaching and research programs.

In closing, let me speculate beyond the reach of the Organization Study Committee to suggest two things. First, the consumer-driven movement will be pushed forward by the evolution and miniaturization of the electronic medical record, giving patients control and possession of their records and creating an expanded network of acceptable providers.

Second, the twenty-first-century academic framework that is most worthy, in my personal vision, to replace that of the twentieth century teaching hospital, is a learning integrated delivery system (LIDS). In such a system the academic center would be a crucial piece of a network aimed at providing comprehensive services for individuals and able to address population-based community needs. In the new information and learning age, a LIDS would be a dramatic intersection of societal, professional, university, and business values (Figure 66.1). Society might reasonably expect these academic health centers to seek innovative workforce models or service arrangements to address, more effectively and efficiently, the expanding array of acute, chronic, and preventive care problems that will continue to confront our delivery systems. As the Internet becomes a more universal education tool, the academic health center and the university could (and in my view, should) take on the role of an honest and objective broker of health services and health promotion information. Thus our society's highest learning institutions can help individuals make their best choices as they pursue healthy lives.

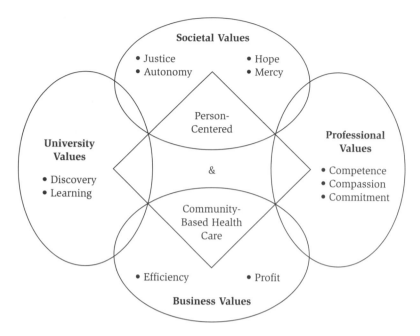

Figure 66.1. Twenty-First Century AHC-Based Learning System.

If we are to meet this expansive vision in the context of the consumer-driven health care model, we will also require universal access to health care, and that universal access will require government support. Finding appropriate and sustainable ways to provide this support will test all our resources and collective ingenuity. It is, however, in rising to such a challenge that America might finally get health care right!

References

Bulger, R. J. "Commentary: Health Plan Responsibilities for Medical Education and Research." In K. G. Gervais and others (eds.), *Ethical Challenges in Managed Care: A Casebook.* Washington, D.C.: Georgetown University Press, 1999.

Bulger, R. J. "What Will Health Care Look Like in the Future?" In E. J. Sullivan (ed.), *Creating Nursing's Future: Issues, Opportunities, and Challenges.* St. Louis: Mosby, 1999.

Bulger, R. J., Osterweis, M., and Rubin, E. R. (eds.). *Mission Management: A New Synthesis.* Vol. 1. Washington, D.C.: Association of Academic Health Centers, 1999.

Rubin, E. R. (ed.). *Mission Management: A New Synthesis.* Vol. 2. Washington, D.C.: Association of Academic Health Centers, 1999.

CHAPTER SIXTY-SEVEN

Consumer Choice in Consumer-Driven Health Care

François Maisonrouge

Consumer-driven health care will inevitably happen. The pace at which we get there is the question. And this pace may not necessarily be the same in all developed economies. After all, even though consumer-driven health care may facilitate the onset of universal access to care in the United States, other economies already ensure this access.

The thesis developed in this book provides the basis for a desirable health care model, but one that needs to overcome formidable obstacles before taking hold. The principal obstacles will come from two categories of participants in the health care sector: the physicians and the consumers themselves.

THE PHYSICIAN

Since Hippocrates, physicians have viewed themselves, and indeed have been regarded by the community, as charged with a mission imbued with a certain holiness. Recently, some physicians have had to spend some of their time filling in HMO forms, but on balance, physicians could continue to play God. The question to be asked is, With what docility will God punch in at the focused factory?

Of course, certain of these factories provide superb care and challenging professional circumstances. The examples of the Cleveland Clinic and the Texas

703

Heart Institute come to mind, but not all diseases can be neatly categorized. For all that one can imagine in terms of interventional cardiology or orthopedic surgery (high-throughput factories) or diabetes (chronic disease-oriented factories), health care spending is still largely devoted to the maintenance in some semblance of health of those whose variety of ailments do not fit a clear mold. Today many hospitals are not institutions; they are vast buildings, made of bricks and mortar, housing numerous cottages occupied by sole practitioners. This is why certain hospital mergers in Boston and New York that look logical on paper are experiencing such difficulties in taking hold.

These are psychological factors, but there are immediate economic ones as well: the existing infrastructure does not lend itself to the focused factory format. Closing down a multifunction hospital is like closing down an army base: the reaction tends to be that it may make sense on a national level, but not in my constituency! In fact pressures are great on national legislatures, by physicians' associations and by those legislators who are physicians themselves, to maintain the status quo.

THE CONSUMER

It is not uncommon today for patients to show up in their doctor's office with reams of printout detailing all the literature ever published on their particular disease. Other than the obvious comments relating to the expertise behind the diagnosis and the technology behind the diagnostics, certain observations seem relevant.

Although a substantial proportion of patients and caregivers to patients (1) have access to the Internet, (2) are well enough to use it, and (3) are interested enough to use it, a great percentage of the patient population still relies on the old model in which patients are more passive. True, the margin, and it can be a large proportion, will be an agent of change, but the old system will not starve quickly. Also, the intensity of patient activism tends to be very different depending on the country. The UK for instance, spends 7 percent of its GNP on health care, half of the U.S. percentage. This has been achieved not by rationalizing health care but by rationing it. Submit Americans to the UK's National Health Service, and the Capitol would be set afire by an angry mob in a week!

More important, individuals' interest in their health suddenly becomes acute when disease strikes. This is precisely not when the decision is made to choose a health plan. The devolution of choice to the consumer would be extremely powerful but for the fact that at the time of choice most consumers would be healthy and therefore predictably apathetic.

Two factors, therefore, that create impediments to the advent of consumer-driven health care are the attitudes of average physicians and the lack of ability or motivation among consumer themselves. To mitigate these factors of conservatism, the movement toward market-driven health care will require

- Enormous political will, to accept the unavoidable social consequences of the dismantling of a large part of the provider infrastructure
- Support systems for the consumer, to raise the interest level of the healthy in their health (a natural job for the hordes of people fired from HR jobs in corporations!)

The following issues will also influence the exercise of choice among consumers.

Who Is the Consumer?

The rise of consumer-driven health care will require health care providers and payers to think carefully about who their customer is. They will make a mistake if they assume that the patient is always the consumer. In many cases important health care decisions do not rest with the patient but with the caregiver. In the case of the elderly, who clearly will represent the bulk of health care demand, I believe the decision maker (the true customer) will often be a close relative.

Diagnostics

Diagnostics will have a dramatic impact on the practice of medicine. The first wave of the new research in genetics will be felt in diagnostics. Simple, rapid, and sensitive diagnostic and prognostic tests will dramatically alter the architecture of medicine: that is, the empirical diagnostic skill of a physician will in many cases become redundant. This will be accompanied by a rise in the use of paramedics (reducing costs and increasing accessibility) and expert-based computer systems. Medicine will become more mechanistic, driven by algorithms—this could see consumers' and physicians' being left with *less* room for qualitative choice.

DTC Advertising

Direct-to-consumer (DTC) advertising (so far mainly for drugs in the United States) will accelerate consumer demand for certain health care products and services. Some, though not all, pharmaceutical companies have awakened to the possibility of creating consumer pull for their products. I expect that use of DTC models will increase in the United States, particularly narrowcasting on the Internet. For example, use Yahoo to search for "coronary stent"—up pops an advert for a Johnson & Johnson stent and maybe the name of an expert center and, indeed, a physician. Broadcasting on TV will clearly broaden further in the United States. In Europe, however, the pace of such developments is likely to be much slower.

Interests of U.S. Versus European Consumers

There is clearly a huge gulf between the consumer in the United States and in Europe. Arguably, U.S. health care has historically enjoyed considerable drive from the consumer. With the traditional U.S. model having been powered by an ethos of open access to specialists and the fee-for-service profit motive, the U.S. health care system has been characterized by overutilization of goods and services. The advent of managed care providers has seen a more rational use of resources but has also led to what is perceived by the consumer as restrictive choice. The rapid growth in POS (point-of-service) plans appears to be releasing the pressure from this perception, largely through plan augmentations (for example, choice of surgeon) when disease intervention is needed; this augmentation is accompanied by a copay. This model has evolved rapidly in the marketplace and seems to point the way for most Americans.

Meanwhile in Europe the rise of consumer-driven health care will be perceived as creating more choices and will be warmly embraced. The focus in Europe will clearly not be on access (which remains firmly on the U.S. agenda) but rather on outcomes. European consumers will be driven by the realization that in some centers, regions, or countries their outcome for a given disease treatment may be markedly better or worse. A significant issue driving consumerism could therefore prove to be clinical audit information.

Regulation

Finally, regulation is also an important issue affecting consumer choice. Up to now a large part of the regulatory function in the United States has been filled by physicians, themselves self-regulated. As the physician loses some status, so will he or she lose some authority and ability to act as a regulator. The Financial Accounting Standards Board (FASB) and the Securities and Exchange Commission (SEC) regulate a huge but finite universe of companies and their financial disclosure. In the case of health care the explosion of transactions to be regulated is daunting. It is clear today, for example, that European authorities are incapable of enforcing their own laws regarding direct-to-consumer advertising of prescription pharmaceuticals: any European can access the Web site extolling the virtues of drug X. We smugly think that this is fine, and even morally right, because what is good for America is good for the rest of the world. But what will we think when a child in Peoria dies of a common disease because she was treated with the perfect remedy her mother found on a rain forest Web site?

The Internet has opened vast, daunting boulevards that circumvent present medical practice. I suspect that in good time, good information will drown out bad. In the meantime regulators will feel like the little Dutch boy facing a leaky dike.

CHAPTER SIXTY-EIGHT

Individual Genetic Profiles

The Empowerment of the Health Care Consumer

Tony L. White

The Internet allows consumers to research and purchase everything from concert tickets to mortgages from their living rooms. Using the Internet as a one-stop shop for information, services, and products, consumers are driving a revolution in many industries in how products are developed, marketed, and sold. As consumers have demanded better selection, lower prices, and ease of access to specialty goods, manufacturers and providers of goods and services have been forced to reexamine their business models. Most companies have come to understand that their survival in the twenty-first century will depend on their ability to react quickly to regional, seasonal, and trend-based consumer demand. In a growing number of industries, the consumer is king.

This transformation has yet to occur in the health care industry. Far from being king, the consumer of health care service and products is to a large extent a minor participant in the health care process. Insurance companies determine which doctors a consumer may visit and decide which treatments will be reimbursed. Physicians make the diagnosis and determine treatment regimens. Consumers have had little say in most of the decisions that affect their own health.

However, as we enter the twenty-first century, forces similar to those that have empowered the consumer in other industries will drive a revolution in the health care system. The power the consumer wields in purchasing everything from airline tickets to zebra-print suits will have significant impact on the way medicine is practiced, pharmaceuticals are developed, and health care services are provided. The central forces in the health care revolution are the rapid advancements in the genomic sciences, the tremendous computing power now available, and the integration of the Internet into our day-to-day lives.

Consumers have already been empowered in other industries as a result of their ability to obtain information on a wide range of subjects. They use this information to make rational, informed decisions about the products or services that best fit their need. The barrier to consumer empowerment in the health care system has been the paucity of medical information available to the consumer. However, the time when the consumer will have easy access to information on his or her own genetic risk factors and health issues will be here more rapidly than any of us could have imagined even a few years ago. Companies such as Applera, where I am chairman and CEO, are developing the tools and technologies to turn that vision into reality.

The availability of individual genetic profiles will have enormous impact not only on the consumer but on scientists, the pharmaceutical industry, physicians, and insurers as well. The three most significant changes in health care, all of which will be driven by genomic information, will be

1. The shift from diagnostic to prognostic disease management
2. The application of personalized, rather than statistically determined, treatment regimens
3. The transition from symptom-based medicine to condition-based medicine

In the current health care model the majority of illnesses are identified at the time when a patient presents to his or her physician with symptoms of disease. As a result of many factors, including limited access to health care, financial constraints, and the fast pace of our daily lives, many patients are not seen by a physician until their disease has progressed significantly. By the time a diagnosis is made, treatment may require invasive or complicated regimens such as surgery, hospitalization, or chronic medication. For certain diseases, such as cancer and some forms of heart disease, late diagnosis is synonymous with mortality.

PROGNOSTIC DISEASE MANAGEMENT

Although the diagnostic approach to identifying disease conditions is the model by which our generation has lived and died, a more prognostic approach is becoming standard practice and will be the model known by the generation being born today. The identification of genetic variations that increase the risk of certain diseases will enable patients to work with their doctors to best manage their health and avoid disease. Tests already are on the market to detect specific genes or genetic variants that increase risk for certain forms of breast, ovarian, and colon cancer and that determine how aggressive some forms of cancer are. Additionally, knowledge of a patient's genetic profile will enable physicians to select the most appropriate treatment regimen for diseases where genetic variation influences treatment efficacy.

PERSONALIZED MEDICINE

Selection of treatment regimens based on the genetic profile of the patient is known as *personalized medicine.* It is personal in the sense that it takes into account the underlying genetic cause of the illness, whether that is the human genetics or the genetics of an invading microorganism such as a virus or bacterium. It is also personal in the sense that it takes into account the effect of genetic variation on the individual's response to drugs.

To date almost all medications and therapies have been developed on a statistical basis—they have some therapeutic benefit for most people and are safe for and well tolerated by most people. Statistical medicine is not a bad approach, unless you are one of the unfortunate few who does not tolerate the drug well or for whom the therapy is not efficacious. As I discuss later, the ability to tailor therapy to fit the genetic makeup of the individual will have enormous benefit for all members of the health care community.

CONDITION-BASED MEDICINE

The third transforming principle will be a shift from symptom-based medicine to condition-based medicine. Today, most illnesses are not diagnosed until a patient presents to the physician with symptoms such as pain, nausea, loss of appetite, lack of energy, and so on. The doctor assesses these symptoms and uses available diagnostics to determine the cause of the symptoms and recommend treatment options. In very few cases will the doctor be able to determine the specific molecular condition that caused the disease. Moreover, with today's technology the doctor cannot determine that there is a problem until symptoms appear.

The completion of the multiple genome projects ongoing in the public and private sectors and at Celera Genomics, an Applera Corporation business, however, will provide the blueprint of the human body that will enable the health care system to predict, diagnose, and treat disease based on the condition, rather than the symptoms, of the patient. These treatments will respond to and will correct the specific molecular cause of disease. Assessing disease from actual conditions, rather than from a collection of symptoms, will lead to earlier and more accurate diagnoses and therapies that treat the underlying cause of disease rather than merely ameliorating the symptoms. Celera completed the sequence of the human genome in 2001 and is now embarking on identifying the individual variations that result in disease or affect response to various therapies.

OVERVIEW OF GENOMIC TECHNOLOGIES

Almost fifteen years ago the sequencing of the human genome was started in the academic community. From the beginning it was apparent that the sequence alone was only a piece in the much larger puzzle of how our genes make us who we are. The pharmaceutical industry, faced with declining profits and shrinking margins, realized that the human genome held the key to new and better products and improved approaches to developing drugs. Genome research has rapidly moved from the academic community into the pharmaceutical industry, speeding the discovery of novel genes and increasing our understanding of how these genes affect the development and progression of disease.

Once the human genome has been sequenced, the next step is to elucidate the intricate networks of biochemical pathways that regulate all life processes. This process, known as functional genomics, employs a wide variety of molecular biology and computer-based technologies. An understanding of how some proteins interact with one another to cause, for example, cell growth, cell death, increased blood pressure, or slower metabolic rates will enable us to manipulate these pathways for therapeutic benefit.

Yet even a complete map of the biochemical roadways that control every cell in our bodies is not sufficient information to transform the health care system completely. Even though the overall map will be the same for all human beings, the subtle, genetic variations that make each of us unique will regulate whether we develop certain diseases, how we will develop them if we do, and how we will respond to specific therapies. These variations are known as single nucleotide polymorphisms, or SNPs. It is knowledge of these SNPs that will allow the health care community to transform itself into a prognostic, condition-based system in which all members of the community work in partnership to maintain the health of every individual within it.

Applera Corporation is providing the systems that make this research possible. Our Application and Biosystems division has been the leader in developing automated and high-throughput systems that enable high-speed sequencing and genome analysis. Celera Genomics has completed the sequencing of the human genome and will serve as the portal for providing genomic information to all members of the health care community. Celera will then migrate into a diagnostic and drug development company using these new tools. We also are developing the next set of technologies that will be required to transform the health care system. These include DNA chips on which the complete genome of the individual can be analyzed, new computing technologies to analyze, store, and distribute these data, and ultra-high-throughput, automated systems that will speed the pace of genome research.

HOW WILL GENOMICS DO THIS?

The understanding of how SNPs affect health, disease, and drug response coupled with the knowledge of an individual's genetic profile will forever change the way all segments of the health care industry provide their products and services. The availability of this information will allow the consumer to take the lead in managing his or her health.

Payers

Health care costs continue to escalate at unprecedented rates as a result of the high cost of the newest pharmaceutical products, the frequent need for multiple, costly diagnostic tests, and the all too common trial-and-error approach to selecting treatment regimens. For insurance companies, predictive and personalized medicine should provide multiple mechanisms through which costs can be reduced. Pharmaceutical products will become less expensive due to increased efficiencies in the drug development process. When physicians select the right treatment the first time, insurance companies save money because they do not pay for medications that will not be beneficial. With better diagnostic tools in the hands of our medical professionals, insurance companies will pay for fewer tests. When a doctor intervenes early in a disease process, the insurance company saves money by avoiding the expensive treatments that are frequently necessary with later-stage, more complicated disease conditions. And when a doctor works with patients to prevent disease and maintain optimal health, we all benefit.

Additionally, the ability to track the relationship among genetic factors, treatment regimens, and clinical outcomes will enable a greater understanding of which treatments work best for each genetically defined patient population. The Internet will facilitate the sharing of information that will be necessary for these databases to become useful tools for providing the best care for all patients.

For the consumer this means improved care and lower insurance costs. Money that payers now use to fund ineffective treatments and uninformative tests can be shifted back to the consumer, focusing more on preventive medicine and resulting in consumer access to a larger number of services and service providers.

Providers

Genomics will also change pharmaceutical and physician practices.

Pharmaceutical Companies. The pharmaceutical industry has already accepted that the genomic revolution will be the key to its success in the future. Genomic information already is being used to select new and better drug targets, enabling the development of novel products that promise to have better efficacy and fewer side effects than existing drugs. The selection of better targets at the beginning of the development process should reduce the number of clinical failures, reducing the risks and costs associated with drug development today. Additionally, research in the field of pharmacogenomics will determine which genetic variants will respond favorably or unfavorably to a given compound and will allow the design of clinical trials that are more likely to succeed. Pharmacogenomics will not only increase the efficiency of the development process for new drugs but also give old drugs, which have failed due to toxicity or limited efficacy, new uses in a genetically defined patient population.

Moreover, the Internet is enabling various research groups within a pharmaceutical company to share information in real time. A chemist who identifies a compound that produces a desirable effect on one protein can promptly share that information with others who are working on related compounds or related proteins, speeding the research process of the entire organization.

As medicine becomes more personalized, the market place will likely demand more products that meet very specific patient needs, and these individualized and personalized products will have small markets. Those companies that continue to pursue blockbuster products such as Prozac or Viagra may find themselves losing ground to competitors who develop a series of products for smaller markets of individuals with a selected disease.

The ability to select highly qualified drug targets, design more clearly defined clinical trial protocols, and achieve statistical significance in smaller clinical trials should reduce the time and cost required to develop new drugs. In turn, this will make niche markets significantly more appealing and lucrative to the pharmaceutical and biopharmaceutical industries. Developing multiple products for one or a group of related indications should help to keep marketing costs from skyrocketing, as a single salesperson will be able to sell several drugs during each call. Moreover, product demand will depend less on physicians' preference and more on the disease state of individual patients.

For the consumer this revolution will result in better, less expensive drugs that address the underlying cause of their disease rather than just ameliorate their symptoms. Each patient will have access to drugs that have been designed for his or her individual genetic profile rather than for a statistically defined patient population. Consumers and physicians will be able to select drugs that provide the necessary therapeutic benefit without causing adverse side effects.

Physicians. The availability of individual genetic profiles will enable physicians to know almost instantaneously what the disease risk factors are for every one of their patients. With the ability to practice predictive medicine, physicians will be able to spend more time working with the consumer to design lifestyle modification programs that reduce those risks and prevent disease. Early diagnosis of disease will allow physicians to intervene at the start of the disease process, increasing cure rates and reducing the development of chronic conditions. Physicians will be able to select from a large number of genetically tailored therapies, enabling them to prescribe a treatment regimen that will be safe and efficacious for every individual patient. This is a significant advantage over the current approach in which multiple regimens may need to be evaluated until the right treatment is selected. When new products reach the market, physicians will be able to log into a database and determine, with just a click of the mouse, which of their patients will benefit from them.

Additionally, physicians will be able to share information with their colleagues over the Internet. Start-up companies are building their businesses by providing the latest clinical and medical information, continuing medical education credits, treatment outcome data, and resources for physicians over the Internet. Physicians who access these resources can easily remain on the cutting edge of their profession and will be better prepared to meet the changing needs of their patients.

For consumers, the availability of their own genetic profiles will enable them to develop relationships with health care providers that are partnerships geared toward maintaining the health of the individual. Moreover, their physicians will be up to date on the latest information and treatment options. Consumers will consult with their physicians before they are sick and will have more information, as described in the next section, about their own risk profiles and disease conditions.

Patients

One of the most significant changes in the status of the individual in the health care system is that the term *patient* is more and more frequently being replaced with *consumer* or *customer*. This signifies the increasing power and responsibility that has both been taken by and given to the individual.

As discussed earlier, traditionally patients have been only marginally involved in decisions about their health and have had limited access to, and little understanding of, their own medical data. The Internet will be the primary engine driving consumers to become more knowledgeable about and more involved in their long-term health and medical condition. A variety of *e-health* companies have come into existence to fill the information needs of both consumers and physicians. On-line support groups exist for diseases such as lupus, multiple sclerosis, Alzheimer's, and cancer. The availability of this information is empowering patients to become more involved in their own health care. Patients still visit their doctors, but these visits have become more consultative, with the patient asking questions based on information that is gathered in large part from on-line sources.

The vision my colleagues and I have for Celera is to provide genetic and medical information to consumers as well as to providers and payers. We are generating the data and will build the infrastructure that will enable us to provide the individual with a detailed picture of his or her own genetic profile. Along with the genetic data, the consumer will be able to access information on drugs that should be avoided due to safety or efficacy concerns arising from the consumer's individual genetic variation. The power of the Internet will allow the consumer to access information on diseases to which he or she is susceptible, including educational information, treatment outcome data, recommendations for moderating risk factors, and references for local physicians who have particular expertise in these diseases. From their own computer terminals, consumers will be able to access test results and know whether or not they might develop heart valve defects from taking a weight-loss drug or develop liver toxicity in response to certain diabetes medications or experience life-threatening allergic reactions in response to an antibiotic.

Consumers will consult with their physicians to gain additional insight into the information available over the Web, access diagnostic tests, obtain guidance on appropriate prophylactic and therapeutic regimens, and receive treatment. In the health care system of the twenty-first century, consumers will have the ability to control their health decisions in the same manner that they control decisions on investing, travel, and shopping. Additionally, consumers will benefit from lower insurance costs, less expensive pharmaceutical products, and safer and more effective treatment options. The system will at long last be centered on caring for the health of the consumer, rather than treating disease when it arises.

ISSUES TO CONSIDER

This transformation of the health care system is by no means trivial and raises important questions and concerns that will need to be addressed if the resulting system is to provide the benefit that we believe it can. The transformed health care playing field will require a new set of rules and novel configurations of teams and players. Many of the technologies and processes of the new system already are here, and the next generation of technologies already is under development. The issues that will accompany the transformation of the health care industry already exist and need to be addressed today. The health care system needs

- Ethics guidelines and laws to deal with potential privacy and discrimination issues

- Assessments of the extent to which patients want a large amount of genetic information and personal health responsibility and of the methods by which consumers can be educated about their own health

- Guidelines for determining the financial responsibilities, if any, of those patients who do not modify their behavior to avoid diseases for which they are at risk

- An evaluation of the informatics technologies that need to be developed to manage the vast amounts of data being produced and to use these data to their full potential—this includes a careful discussion of who should create these technologies and databases

- Insurance companies that focus more and spend more on preventive, predictive, and diagnostic medicine

- New curricula that train physicians to think about medicine in terms of patient-specific risks and treatments rather than in terms of statistics

- Pharmaceutical companies that accept the value of developing multiple products that will be used to treat smaller patient populations

- Dialogue among the FDA and other regulatory agencies to establish new trial protocols and approval criteria that take into account pharmacogenomics and patient stratification based on genetic profiles

- A time frame for integrating technologies, processes, and constituents into a single community focused on the health of the individual consumer

Although the complete transformation of the health care system to a model that is driven by the needs of the individual consumer will evolve over the next ten to twenty years, the first steps in this transformation already have been taken. The promise of the genomic revolution will be realized only through a transformation of the way we think about health care and related issues. Our dialogue about the ways genetic information is generated, stored, accessed, and used already lags behind the technology that makes these processes possible. The leaders of the insurance, pharmaceutical, and medical communities must come together today with consumer advocates to develop the legal and ethical infrastructure on which the new health care paradigm will be built so that we may all reap the benefits of the genomic revolution.

CHAPTER SIXTY-NINE

Delivering the Right Drug to the Right Patient

Mark Levin

Envision a time when there is no uncertainty in medicine. Patients are given precisely the drug they require—and that drug actually eradicates their disease. Although this scenario may seem futuristic, the biopharmaceutical industry is striving to make it reality. How can we succeed? By harnessing the information unleashed by the genomics revolution.

Most current diagnostics and therapeutics detect and treat only the symptoms of disease. Yet due to genetic variation, disease manifests itself slightly differently in each person. As the human genome is mapped, we at Millennium Pharmaceuticals, where I am chairperson and CEO, expect to be able to design diagnostics, therapeutics, and predictive medicine products that target the underlying molecular causes of disease. Thus, by analyzing an individual's genetic makeup, health care providers will be able to predict the types of diseases to which that person is genetically predisposed so that preventative measures such as diet and lifestyle adjustments may be taken. They will be able to accurately diagnose a disease—and prescribe therapeutics that both treat its specific genetic variant and are effective in that particular patient, eliminating side effects and months of trial and error. Ultimately, health care providers may be able to alter the genes themselves, curing disease at its source.

This type of personalized and precise medicine should dramatically reduce both direct health care costs and indirect costs to the overall economy. More important, it should significantly improve quality of life, especially for patients who suffer from chronic or fatal diseases.

THE TOOLS OF CHANGE: EXISTING SHORTCOMINGS AND NEW OPPORTUNITIES

Genomics allows researchers to establish which genes, in which cells or tissues, are mutated—turned on or off or up or down—under definitive conditions. We expect this increased knowledge to provide entirely new strategies for combating human disease, and new targets for drug development. Simultaneously, advances in technologies such as high-throughput compound screening, informatics, and robotics are enabling the rapid development of drugs precisely tailored to these specific, validated molecular targets.

These scientific innovations are the tools that enable change; they allow us to see the limitations of current medical practices and the potential we have to truly treat disease.

Current Diagnostics Are Imprecise and Current Therapeutics Palliative

Drawing on years of training and clinical experience, physicians diagnose disease on the basis of a combination of subjective observations and objective testing. Although they are overwhelmingly correct, the occasional misdiagnosis at best postpones effective treatment and at worst proves fatal. Likewise, current predictive medicine is largely based on family medical histories; although genetic background is a strong indicator of predisposition to disease, it is not absolute—nor does it enable presymptomatic diagnosis of diseases such as multiple sclerosis, for which predisposition requires a specific confluence of eight or more genes.

Health care providers know that what is good for most people is not good for everyone. Yet new therapeutics are vetted among broad populations who may or may not share genetic characteristics with a specific patient, which can cause frustrating delays in determining the optimal therapy for that patient. For example, a certain antidepressant may take a month to reach a potent level in the bloodstream—and may be effective in only 60 percent of patients. The 40 percent on whom it has no impact then have to try an alternative, again waiting to determine whether this new option works. More important, with the notable exception of antibiotics, drugs generally treat the symptoms of a disease, without attacking or changing its root cause. For example, arthritis drugs ameliorate phenotypic pain symptoms, but the disease state continues to progress unchecked. Using genomics, the biopharmaceutical industry is striving to eliminate these halfway technologies and palliative therapeutics, creating a more effective health care system.

Disease Is Expensive in Terms of Pain, Time, and Money

Diseases—from cancer to epilepsy—drain both financial and human resource capital. Direct treatment costs mount rapidly, especially for chronic diseases that are never cured. These expenditures are compounded by the indirect costs of disability insurance, lost work time (of both the patient and caregivers), and premature mortality; together they pose a staggering financial burden on the world economy. And this burden does not reflect the physical and emotional anguish endured by these patients. A quick statistical overview of three disease states forms a framework for considering the overall impact of disease on society:

- Each year, more than 51 million Americans are affected by one or more mental disorders[1]—worldwide that number jumps to 450 million.[2] Psychiatric disorders are the largest single reason for hospitalization in the United States. Annually, mental illness exacts $67 billion in direct treatment costs; that figure rises to approximately $150 billion when indirect costs are included.[3]

- An estimated 24.7 million Americans suffer from asthma, including more than 15 million children.[4] One study shows that the average amount spent by a family on medical treatment for children with asthma is 6.4 percent of total family income.[5] Overall, asthma annually costs the United States $12.7 billion; an estimated $8.1 billion is in direct medical costs.[6]

- Nearly 62 million Americans have one or more forms of cardiovascular disease (CVD). In 1999, CVD was listed as a primary or contributing cause of death on 60 percent of death certificates. The American Heart Association projects that the total cost of CVD in 2002 will be $329.2 billion; of this, $199.5 billion is in direct medical costs.[7]

By eradicating these and other diseases, society would be able to eliminate significant medical costs—and the tremendous personal costs of the disease burden.

Genomics Holds the Key to the Cure

It is not possible to create therapeutics that stop or slow disease without understanding—at a molecular level—how disease happens.

The human genome is composed of three billion base pairs (see the Glossary at the end of this chapter). Mutations in a single base pair can affect, or even destroy, a gene's function. Relative levels of expression between and among different genes at different times and under different environmental conditions can spell the difference between health and disease. An enormous amount of data is generated within a potentially infinite number of combinations and permutations. Our challenge is to convert this wealth of information into diagnostics, therapeutics, and predictive medicine products.

METHODS OF CHANGE: UNIQUE APPROACHES, A SINGLE GOAL

What pain reliever do you reach for when you have a headache? For some people aspirin is the answer, but in others aspirin produces terrible stomach pains and leaves the headache undiminished. Biopharmaceutical companies are discovering why.

All human deoxyribonucleic acid (DNA) sequences are 99.9 percent identical. The 0.1 percent that differs is responsible for most diseases—both common and rare—as well as most of the variability in drug responses from one person to the next; it is this 0.1 percent on which genomic research primarily focuses. The most common type of variation lies in the position of a single nucleotide, known as single nucleotide polymorphisms or SNPs. Essentially, if you know the entire genetic sequence of ten healthy people and compare it to the entire genetic sequence of ten people with diabetes, there will be certain SNPs in the diabetes group that are directly related to their disease. Additionally, patients who experience negative side effects from certain drugs may have an SNP that correlates to that reaction.

As our knowledge of the role genes play in disease initiation and progression increases, we will discover the variations that cause different illnesses in different groups of people; these SNPs will then become targets for diagnostic testing and therapeutic intervention. Through pharmacogenomics, the study of how response to a drug is affected by a person's genetic makeup, pharmaceutical companies will parlay this knowledge to design and implement cost-effective clinical trials—and to develop drugs tailored to the specific basis of a disease as it afflicts a particular, genetically characterized group of people. Ultimately, that means safer, more effective drugs.

Affymetrix Puts the Genome on a Chip

Someday soon, you may walk into the local pharmacy, hand over a card the size of your driver's license, and emerge with a drug precisely matched to your genetic profile. How? Your genotype will be stored—in its entirety—on the card. By scanning it, the pharmacist will know exactly which therapeutic will create the optimal response in your system.

This scenario may be possible due to the work occurring now at Affymetrix, Inc. A California-based company, Affymetrix is focused on gathering and analyzing the complex data increasingly available about the human genome. Integrating semiconductor wafer manufacturing, computer software, and biological research, the company has transformed the serial process used in conventional analysis into a massively parallel process in which thousands of reactions occur simultaneously. The process is both fast and simple, so it is cost effective and has vast potential for widespread use.

Affymetrix's current product, the GeneChip® system, includes disposable DNA probe arrays that contain selected gene sequences on a chip, instruments to process the arrays, and software to manage the information. This technology is designed to uncover fundamental information about genomics, including what the gene is (gene discovery), where it is on the genome (gene sequencing), how it reacts under various conditions (expression monitoring), and how it relates to human health (polymorphism screening).

As researchers continue to increase the amount of genetic information that can be analyzed on chips, this important enabling technology may greatly further our understanding of the complexities of DNA.

Genset Pioneers High-Resolution SNP Mapping

Before SNPs can be analyzed, they have to be discovered. Genset is a Paris-based genomics company that has harnessed large-scale genome mapping and sequencing operations to comb the genome for SNPs. The company is developing a high-resolution map of the human genome, comprising 60,000 uniformly spaced markers. Here, just as in printing, resolution refers to the level of detail; a high-resolution map should allow researchers to quickly identify mutations linked to disease or other traits. Although the gene sequences Genset maps initially do not necessarily correlate with any known disease states, the company believes that this broad coverage will enable it to apply a systematic genomewide approach to gene discovery and pharmacogenomics. When the map is complete, Genset will use it to analyze DNA samples from patients with specific diseases and from healthy individuals, seeking the markers for those disease states.

Millennium Targets Genes Related to Specific Disease States

Cambridge-based Millennium Pharmaceuticals, Inc., shares many goals with Affymetrix and Genset but has chosen a more targeted approach. Rather than mapping evenly spaced, random SNPs, the company establishes correlations between various genes and a disease state, then seeks those specific gene targets. Primary areas of interest are obesity, cardiovascular disease, cancer, respiratory diseases, infectious diseases, and diseases of the central nervous system. Millennium believes that this focused approach will more rapidly uncover those genetic differences that have an impact in clinical situations. To this end, Millennium has assembled a comprehensive, integrated drug discovery platform, encompassing the most powerful, innovative tools available. The company uses this proprietary platform literally to industrialize the process—identifying disease-related genes, elucidating the role of those genes in disease initiation and progression, validating drug targets, and then developing potential predictive medicine and therapeutic products.

Millennium also has pursued unique business approaches to further its impact. The company completed four mergers from 1997 to 2002 in order to build fully integrated capabilities at scale throughout the drug development value chain, from gene to patient. By means of these mergers as well as other innovative in-licensing agreements with drug discovery firms, Millennium has continued to advance a promising portfolio of drug candidates and products based on the company's genomics knowledge and in-depth understanding of disease. In addition, Millennium has established first-of-a-kind strategic alliances with major companies such as Abbott, Aventis, Bayer, and Monsanto designed to create transforming relationships that move the industry into a new era of biopharmaceuticals. Millennium's unique approach to business relationships is exemplary of the kind of innovative relationships that can harness the wealth of opportunities available in the genomics revolution.

THE IMPACT OF SUCCESS: COST SAVINGS, IMPROVED OUTCOMES, MARKET SHIFTS

Each of the approaches described here—along with those being pursued by dozens of other biopharmaceutical companies worldwide—has a single end goal: to attack disease at its root cause. Even though the cumulative impact on society is wholly speculative, it is easy to imagine.

As I illustrated earlier, disease imposes a tremendous economic burden on society. Even if products developed using genomics prove expensive, their cost, assuming they are effective, should be more than offset by the direct savings realized by eliminating long-term patient care. That cost-benefit ratio for third-party payers is augmented by the societal benefit of a healthier workforce—and the personal benefits to patients worldwide.

Of course these products may also completely change the face of medicine as we know it. They may not only reorder the way patients seek and receive care but are very likely to alter the function of the health care workforce. Just as the polio vaccine blessedly reduced the need for leg braces and rehabilitation centers, these products could affect everything from the manufacture of insulin pumps to the size and focus of hospitals. In the future, patients may receive most of their care at centers directly targeting the prevention or management of specific diseases; this trend is already being manifested in specialties ranging from cancer management to cataract removal. Ultimately, if we are successful, genomics-based medicine may achieve what people have been striving toward forever; after all, the whole idea of medicine is to put itself out of business.

BARRIERS TO DIFFUSION: ETHICAL ISSUES AND THERAPEUTIC SCARCITIES

Any innovation brings new concerns and poses new problems. Inevitably, some people will view these as reasons to forgo the advantages the innovation also brings. Indeed, they may fight to retain the status quo, preferring problems they are comfortable addressing. This is particularly true during the initial, formative stages of a revolutionary concept. Genomics-based medicine is no exception.

Could Absolute Knowledge Lead to Discrimination?

The prospect of personalized and precise medicine assumes a thorough molecular characterization of all patients. We will know each person's predisposition to developing a disease, precisely how sick he or she is, and his or her level of responsiveness to different therapeutic regimes. Some commentators view this knowledge as a future diary, which, were it to fall into the hands of those with interests inimical to the individual, could result in various forms of harm, including employment discrimination, insurance discrimination, and stigmatization.

Indeed, there exist documented examples of how people can fundamentally misunderstand and misuse genetic information. In 1949, Nobel laureate Linus Pauling discovered that a chemical abnormality in hemoglobin was responsible for sickle-cell anemia. Testing was introduced—and when the results became available, people who did not have the disease but were carriers of one copy of the gene were fired and denied health insurance. These people were truly wrongly discriminated against.[8]

The potential for discrimination leads some people to believe that technology and its uses should be significantly curtailed. However, Millennium and its fellow biopharmaceutical companies believe that proper controls can prevent these problems; we are actively advocating for legal measures that ensure confidentiality and offer protection against discrimination.

Diagnostics Have Little Value Without Corresponding Therapeutics

On a much more practical level, diagnostic or predictive products will not receive the necessary consumer push without an effective, economically accessible therapeutic or preventative medicine to treat the disease in question. The current situation with the BRCA 1 gene test illustrates this. The discovery of BRCA 1 was heralded by scientific journals and the lay press; the gene is thought to be responsible for slightly less than half of hereditary breast cancer. Yet there is no acceptable preventive treatment for breast cancer—consequentially, there is limited current demand for the diagnostic, whose only practical purpose is as an incentive for women to increase practices that lead to self-diagnosis. However, in the long term, market demand is likely to increase as a selection of drugs becomes available to treat individual genetic forms of breast cancer.[9] Indeed, a drug is now available for the treatment of patients with metastatic breast cancer whose tumors overexpress the HER 2 protein—and appropriate immunohistochemical testing can diagnose or predict this condition.[10] This is an optimal blending of the diagnostic and the therapeutic.

CONSUMER-DRIVEN HEALTH CARE: EDUCATION CREATES DEMAND

In theory, genomics-based medicine will eliminate all choice in health care, because for each condition in each person there is only one right answer. Yet, assuming this research is successful, from a consumer standpoint these predictive medicines, diagnostics, and therapeutics can only improve overall care. Parents will know that their child is susceptible to certain disorders and will take care to prevent them. Physicians will no longer have to guess at what is wrong. Drugs will no longer be over-, under-, or misprescribed.

Therefore, we believe that consumers who know the options will demand genomics-based solutions, and third-party payers will be forced to provide them. Some of that burden rests on the biopharmaceutical companies: our first job is to discover, develop, and deliver on the promise of genomics. Our second job is to educate consumers effectively. Together, we can deliver on the promise of personalized and precise medicine, delivering the right drug to the right patient at the right time.

GLOSSARY

Base pairs	In nature, the four building blocks of DNA are always found in pairs: adenine with thymine, guanine with cytosine. Thus the base sequence of each single strand can be deduced from that of its partner strand.
DNA (deoxyribonucleic acid)	The molecule that encodes information. Located in the nucleus of the cell, it determines the structure, function, and behavior of the cell.

Gene	The fundamental physical and functional unit of heredity; a DNA segment that codes for the manufacture of one protein. An estimated 100,000 to 150,000 genes make up the human genome.
Genetics	The study of the patterns of inheritance of specific traits.
Genetic map	A physical map of the human genome that describes its various regions. All twenty-four (twenty-two plus two sex chromosomes) of the human chromosomes have been mapped, but the degree of detail or resolution is still insufficient for these maps to be used as efficient tools for identifying gene mutations.
Genome	The human genome contains 23 chromosomes, 100,000 to 150,000 genes, and 3 billion nucleotides. These genes encompass the complete set of instructions needed to develop and build an organism.
Genomics	The study of all genetic material in the chromosomes of a particular organism, involving the identification of both the genes and their functions.
Mutation	An error in a gene resulting in a change in its sequence. Some mutations may be disease forming, and others harmless.
Nucleotide	The building block of DNA, composed of one of four bases linked to a sugar molecule and one phosphate group.
Pharmacogenomics	The study of how a patient's genetic makeup determines that patient's response to a therapeutic. Identification of the genetic markers that predict drug efficacy and toxicity should result in great strides forward: in theory, the risk and costs of clinical trials can be reduced; flawed drugs can be amended to address only responsive patients or to eliminate a side-effect problem; and new custom-made diagnostics and therapeutics can be created.

Single nucleotide polymorphism (SNP)

An alteration in a single nucleotide on a stretch of DNA. Some of these variations may be involved in a disease process, although the majority probably are not. These alterations are useful as unique signposts for researchers scanning the entire genome for abnormalities.

Notes

1. Continuing Medical Education, Inc. "Mental Health Information and Statistics." [www.mhsource.com/resource/mh.html], May 2002.

2. World Health Organization. "Mental Health." [www.who.int/mental_health/en], Sept. 2003.

3. Continuing Medical Education, "Mental Health Information and Statistics."

4. American Lung Association, Epidemiology and Statistics Unit. *Trends in Asthma Morbidity and Mortality.* New York: American Lung Association, Feb. 2002, pp. 5, 7, 15, 25.

5. National Institutes of Health (NIH), National Asthma Education and Prevention Program Task Force on the Cost Effectiveness, Quality of Care, and Financing of Asthma Care. NIH Publication No 55-807. Bethesda, Md.: NIH, 1996, p. 88.

6. American Lung Association, *Trends in Asthma Morbidity and Mortality.*

7. American Heart Association (AHA). *2002 Heart and Stroke Statistical Update.* Dallas, Tex.: AHA, 2001, pp. 4, 33.

8. Markel, H. "Scientific Advances and Social Risks: Historical Perspectives of Genetic Screening Programs for Sickle Cell disease, Tay-Sachs disease, Neural Tube Defects and Down's Syndrome, 1970–1997." Appendix 6. In N. A. Holtzman and M. S. Watson (eds.), *Promoting Safe and Effective Genetic Testing in the United States: Final Report of the Task Force on Genetic Testing.* Bethesda, Md.: National Human Genome Research Institute, 1997.

9. Murray, M. N., and Butler, C. A. "Myriad Genetics: Pronet Has Unrecognized Upside." New York: Lehman Brothers, 1998.

10. Genentech, Inc. "Herceptin." [www.gene.com/gene/products/information/oncology/herceptin], May 1999.

PART FIVE

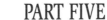

THE ROLE OF GOVERNMENT

The government's vast powers can help or hinder the consumer-driven health care movement. The twelve chapters in Part Five take a thoughtful look at the government's potential role in providing consumers with insurance, access, and information.

PROVIDING INSURANCE

Most of the authors of the first five chapters in Part Five believe that government will help the movement to marshal consumer-driven health care, in order to solve one of this great nation's most pressing needs—the lack of health insurance for more than forty million people.

Jon Gabel, vice president of health system studies at the Health Research and Educational Trust of the American Hospital Association (Chapter Seventy) (with thanks to the Schering-Plough Foundation for the $30,000 they donated to help Jon write this paper), and David Kendall, senior fellow for health policy at the Progressive Policy Institute (Chapter Seventy-One), espouse a tax credit to subsidize the individual purchase of health insurance.

The respondents on this topic are health insurance experts. In Chapter Seventy-Two, Eric Berger, director of planning and public policy at US Oncology; Carrie Gavora, a health care analyst and consultant; and Daniel Johnson, former president of the American Medical Association, and currently a visiting fellow in health policy at the Heritage Foundation, speculate on the proactive and reactive potentials for government action on consumer-driven health care. In Chapter Seventy-Three, Karen Ignagni, president and CEO of the AAHP-HIAA, argues for even-handed, contemplative regulation of the insurance sector, noting the sector's vast potential to do good. And in Chapter Seventy-Four, health insurance analyst and investor Ken Abramowitz describes how consumer-driven health care plans can encourage "adult," that is, mature, behavior in the consumption of health care.

PROVIDING ACCESS

But will the mere provision of insurance guarantee adequate health care access, especially among poor individuals and families who may lack the other resources needed to access health care–convenient transportation, baby-sitters, sometimes even telephones? The writers in the next three chapters in Part Five illustrate how the government can respond to these needs. The chairman and CEO of AmeriChoice Corporation, Anthony Welters, describes the cost effectiveness of the personalized care protocols that his entrepreneurial firm developed for the Medicaid recipients it serves (Chapter Seventy-Five). Drawing on her years of experience as the CEO of one of the nation's largest neighborhood health centers located in Chicago, Constance Jackson urges consumer-driven government policies that will improve access (Chapter Seventy-Six). As she illustrates, when poor individuals and families in Illinois were allowed a choice, health plans developed that were tailored to meet all their needs, including transportation and access for those who lacked phones. Consumer choice also drew a welcome number of new physicians into the community.

The respondent on the issue of providing access, Kevin Vigilante, a physician who treats inner-city patients in Providence, Rhode Island, and a clinical associate professor of medicine at Brown University School of Medicine, urges that government-subsidized low-income people can and should be treated as consumers and given as much choice and control as everybody else (Chapter Seventy-Seven).

PROVIDING INFORMATION

Arming consumers with sound information about preventive care, diseases, and conditions and about the quality of physicians and health plans will be critical to the success of consumer-driven medicine, as previous chapters in this book have emphasized. The government has a role to play here as well, as the next three chapters in Part Five illustrate. In Chapter Seventy-Eight, Regina Herzlinger, the lead author and editor of this volume, advocates the establishment of a health care public commission that will force public disclosure and broad dissemination of audited provider and insurer outcome data. She bases her model on the existing partnership between the public Securities and Exchange Commission and its private sector counterparts, organizations that fashion accounting principles and audit them. In Chapter Seventy-Nine, one respondent, former congressman and retired law firm partner Robert Shamansky, presciently warns cogently of the shortcomings of the SEC. In Chapter Eighty, a second respondent, market economist Rita Ricardo-Campbell, advocates total consumer-driven solutions, with government regulatory powers modeled on those used for banks.

ADDITIONAL ROLES FOR GOVERNMENT

Finally, in Chapter Eighty-One, health industry consultant Rich D'Amaro takes a novel and creative approach to additional roles for government, proposing regulations that would encourage public health and education and reward nonprofit hospitals for disposing of their excess capacity.

CHAPTER SEVENTY

The Uninsured

Understanding and Resolving an American Dilemma

Jon R. Gabel

In the midst of the strongest U.S. economy in thirty years, the Census Bureau reported that the number of Americans without health insurance rose to forty-one million in 1998, 17 percent of the nonelderly population.

You could almost hear Lyndon Johnson boasting, "You never had it so good!" So went the American economy of the 1990s. From 1992 to 2000, the economy added twenty-three million new jobs,[1] the gross domestic product grew 34 percent in constant dollars from 1992 to 2000,[2] and the Dow Jones Industrial Index soared from less than 3,000 in January 1991 to 11,800 in early 2000. *Newsweek* reported that between 1995 and 1998, the number of millionaires rose by one-third, and the number of billionaires increased by an estimated 32 percent from 1997 to 1998.[3]

But it was not till the eighth year of the economic expansion that the absolute number of uninsured declined. In 1987, the uninsured had constituted just 13.7 percent of the nonelderly population. Among the nonelderly the uninsured outnumber those with public insurance (Medicaid and Medicare) and those who buy their health coverage directly from an insurance company (coverage termed *individual insurance*).[4]

The United States is unique among the advanced economic nations of the world in having a substantial segment of its population without insurance coverage. In no other country in the industrialized world is serious illness closely associated with economic hardship.[5] And yet, a 1999 public opinion poll found that 60 percent of Americans believed that the uninsured do not have problems getting necessary health care. College-educated Americans more strongly hold those views.[6]

I am grateful for the financial support of the Schering-Plough Foundation that made this chapter possible. I thank Regina Herzlinger for inviting me to write the paper on which this chapter is based for the Consumer-Driven Health Care Conference and for arranging financial support. I thank Jeremy Pickreign and Samantha Hawkins for their research assistance and review comments. I appreciate the helpful suggestions of Deborah Bohr, Molly Collins, Thomas Rice, and Heidi Whitmore.

This chapter reexamines the uninsured in America. Following the humiliating defeat of President Clinton's Health Security Act in 1994, many observers predicted that the issue of the uninsured would not take center stage again for many years. Pollsters now report growing concern about health care among the American public; incremental legislation, such as the 2003 Medicare Prescription Drug Act, may extend coverage to more Americans in the near future.

The chapter begins with a brief review of health insurance coverage in America. It then discusses who the uninsured are and why their ranks are growing. It also looks at where the uninsured receive their medical care. Then it reviews the leading studies that link the lack of health insurance to reduced health status. Finally, it briefly outlines alternative approaches for covering the uninsured. In the spirit of the consumer-driven health care movement, it proposes a market-based initiative for achieving universal coverage that enhances consumer choice of health plans and providers.

HEALTH INSURANCE COVERAGE IN AMERICA

The American system of health coverage reflects the American character. It is pluralistic and entrepreneurial, with elements of the Wild West and political pragmatism. Other advanced Western nations, such as Canada, Germany, and the United Kingdom, trace the birth of their health insurance systems to a specific legislative act. In the United States, our primary source of health insurance coverage is the employer, with 152 million American workers and their dependents receiving their coverage through a place of employment today. One cannot point to any legislative act by our national government that created this employer-based system. Instead, it is an accidental system that grew out of rulings by the executive and judicial branches of government to overcome labor shortages during World War II. In 1942, federal officials ruled that increased health benefits were not subject to the limits of federal wage controls. In a 1943 ruling the Internal Revenue Service concurred with this decision, which in turn was later affirmed in judicial review.[7] Following these rulings, job-based health insurance grew dramatically. In 1940, only a few Americans received their health insurance through their employer. Enrollment in Blue Cross and Blue Shield plans alone increased from 1.4 million members before the war to 60 million in 1951.[8]

The Internal Revenue Service rulings stimulated dramatic growth in job-based insurance. Employer contributions for health insurance were tax exempt for workers and tax deductible for employers. Employer groups now purchased health insurance at substantially lower prices than individuals. This was due not only to the economies of mass purchasing but also to the special treatment the tax code afforded. Suppose the marginal tax rate of a worker was 40 percent, and also assume that the annual cost of a health policy was $1,000 a year and the employer paid for the entire cost of coverage. Then the worker's tax burden was reduced by $400, and the net cost of insurance was not $1,000 but $600. Not all employer groups, however, purchased insurance for their workers, and lower-income workers faced lower marginal tax rates than higher-income workers. Firms with many skilled and higher-income workers were and remain far more likely to offer coverage. Building a health insurance system from the tax exemption of employers' contributions redistributes income regressively. It resembles the Sheriff of Nottingham rather than Robin Hood. In 1998, the estimated value of the tax subsidy for job-based coverage was $111 billion dollars.[9] For those with family incomes greater than $100,000 per year, the subsidy averaged $2,357. For those with incomes of less than $15,000 per year, it averaged $71. The passage in 1965 of legislation launching Medicare coverage for the elderly and disabled and Medicaid coverage for the poor represents an effort to protect the most economically vulnerable members of our society. As the subsequent sections of this chapter discuss, many Americans, largely low-income workers and their families, continue to fall through the cracks.

WHO ARE THE UNINSURED? WHY DO THEIR NUMBERS GROW?

In the 1997 Hollywood blockbuster *As Good As It Gets,* Helen Hunt plays a waitress employed in a New York City restaurant. She is unable to obtain necessary medical care for her asthmatic son because her HMO refuses to cover the necessary therapy. Movie critics noted the sneering response of audiences to this denial of care. In reality, our New York waitress matches the profile of an uninsured American—an individual employed by a small business, most likely in the retail or service sector, and earning an income less than 200 percent of the poverty level.

Today, policymakers have substantial data on the uninsured. When the first count of the uninsured came from the 1977 National Medical Care Expenditure Survey, conducted by the then Department of Health, Education and Welfare, health care experts were surprised to learn that the uninsured were a near-poor working population. Conventional wisdom had been that the uninsured were unemployed individuals and their dependents. In a subsequent section I discuss changes in the composition of the uninsured over the twenty years since then, but I first will examine economic and demographic characteristics of today's uninsured.

Employment Status

If Americans view the disadvantaged as falling into two categories, the deserving and nondeserving (a welfare population that does not want to work), the uninsured fall into the deserving category. Eighty-four percent of the uninsured are in families where the head of the household held a job within the past year.

Fifty-two percent of the uninsured are in families where the head of household was employed full-time all year, and 32 percent are in families where the head of household worked either part time or had a spell of unemployment. Only 16 percent of the uninsured are in families where the head of household did not hold employment in the previous year.[10]

Income

No factor better predicts who will have job-based health insurance and who will be uninsured than income. As income rises, the likelihood that a family will have health insurance coverage from an employer increases, and the likelihood that the family will be uninsured decreases. For example, only 35 percent of individuals in families with annual incomes between $10,000 and $20,000 a year have job-based health insurance, and an equal percentage are uninsured. In contrast, more than 90 percent of those in families whose annual income is greater than $50,000 are covered by job-based health insurance, and less than 8 percent are uninsured. The one exception to this pattern is found in families earning less than $5,000 per year. The heads of household for these families are largely individuals who are not part of the workforce and receive their insurance coverage through Medicaid. Hence, only 18 percent of the poorest Americans are uninsured.[11]

More than 92 percent of Americans with private coverage receive their insurance through their employer (or their spouse's employer).[12] It is logical, therefore, that income and job-based coverage should be so highly correlated. If workers are paid roughly according to their productivity, every dollar contributed by an employer for health insurance coverage is a dollar that could have been used to increase wages. As previously discussed, due to the current exclusion of employer contributions for health insurance from taxation, this is not a one-to-one dollar substitution of health insurance payments for wages. Low-income workers, such as those earning minimum wage, may prefer income to health insurance. More likely, employers are unlikely to contribute $4,000 dollars a year for a minimum wage worker earning less than $11,000 per year.

Employer Size

Virtually all large employers offer health coverage to their workforce, whereas less than half of employers with ten or fewer workers do so.[13] Hence individuals working for small firms are far more likely to lack coverage than employees of large firms are. Roughly 34 percent of workers in firms with fewer than ten employees and 24 percent of self-employed workers lack coverage. In contrast, about 12 percent of employees in firms with five hundred or more workers lack coverage and about 8 percent of public employees do.

Wage rates largely explain the differences in coverage among large and small firms (small firms are those with fewer than 250 workers). Wages for workers in large firms (500 or more workers) average 32 percent higher than wages among smaller firms.[14] A second factor explaining the higher coverage rate among large firms is that administrative costs for insurance coverage, particularly marketing costs, are spread among many workers in large firms. Among the nation's small firms more than 30 percent of the premium dollar goes for the cost of administration (as opposed to medical claims expenses), whereas among the largest firms this figure is less than 10 percent.[15]

A third factor, beyond numbers of employers and wage rates, is a complex one. The inability to pool medical risks makes it more difficult for small employers to offer health benefits. Insurers have historically subjected small employers to rigorous medical underwriting as a means of rating the financial risk for insuring a group. This usually entails requiring employees to fill out questionnaires about their own and their dependents' medical history. If the small firm is already a client, the insurer will also review the medical claims experience of the past year and ascertain whether any employees have been diagnosed with a chronic condition that is likely to result in large medical expenses in the next year. Simple economics dictates that insurers estimate the medical risk for a small group. One very sick dependent, such as a dependent with terminal cancer, is likely to incur medical expenses of $50,000 within the next year. If there are only five employees in a firm, the premium income from that firm is likely to be about $20,000; hence if there is a very ill dependent, the insurer is certain to lose money on the small firm's account. In contrast, insurers can take advantage of the law of large numbers for large employers. They can spread the risk of catastrophic cost among tens of thousands of employees. For small employers (and for individuals) the inability to pool risks leads to a system in which the people who need the most protection against catastrophic costs cannot buy health insurance. In an attempt to remedy this situation, nearly forty states have passed legislation placing limits on insurers' ability to conduct medical underwriting.

The bottom line is that small employers must pay higher premiums to cover the greater risk of insuring a small group. In some states small employers with sick employees or sick dependents must pay higher premiums to buy coverage or, in some cases, are viewed as "uninsurable" by insurance companies.

Race and Ethnicity

Hispanics and African Americans are more likely to be uninsured than whites (Anglos). Thirty-six percent of Hispanics, 23 percent of African Americans, and 14 percent of whites are uninsured. These disparities reflect the decreasing likelihood that Hispanics and African Americans will be covered by job-based health insurance. Seventy-one percent of nonelderly whites are covered through job-based coverage as opposed to 42 percent of Hispanics and 51 percent of African Americans. Hispanics and African Americans are much more likely to work at low-wage jobs that don't offer health coverage, and this factor largely explains the higher rates of uninsurance.

Age

Young adults are the most likely age cohort to lack coverage, but for all cohorts more than 13 percent of individuals lack coverage. Nearly 34 percent of Americans aged twenty-one to twenty-four are uninsured, and 24 percent of Americans aged twenty-five to thirty-four are uninsured. Young workers have lower wages than older workers and are less likely to work for a firm that offers health insurance. Among the near elderly, those between fifty-five and sixty-four, one of every seven lacks insurance coverage. This is an age group in which chronic conditions are commonplace.

Education

Rates of uninsurance are much higher among Americans with less education. College graduates are far more likely to have job-based coverage than are high school graduates or school dropouts. Eighty percent of college graduates have employer-based coverage, compared to 63 percent of high school graduates and 34 percent of school dropouts.[16]

Demographic Changes

The percentage of nonelderly Americans without health insurance rose from 13.8 percent in 1977 to 19.7 percent in 1997. This increase was attributable to the decline of job-based health insurance, which covered roughly 70 percent of the population in 1977 but fell to less than 65 percent in 1997. In fact, if it had not been for expansions in Medicaid eligibility in the 1980s and early 1990s and the passage of the Child Health Insurance Program (CHIP) in 1997, the number of uninsured would have grown even more substantially.[17]

Over the past ten years, the ranks of the uninsured not only grew but changed composition also. More of the uninsured are workers, and fewer are children. Expansions in Medicaid and CHIP largely explain reductions in the percentage of the uninsured who are children.

A new wave of immigrants, many from Latin America and East Asia, has also changed the composition of the uninsured. Roughly one-quarter of the uninsured today are noncitizens, largely recent immigrants to the United States. An estimated 40 percent of the increase in the number of uninsured over the past ten years is attributable to the increase in immigrants from Latin America.[18]

Voluntary Versus Involuntary Uninsured

When asked in household surveys why they lack health insurance, nearly two-thirds of the uninsured respond that they cannot afford it. The second most common reason mentioned is that they are unemployed or that their firm does not provide coverage. Only 7 percent indicated that they were uninsured by choice or that they did not believe in health insurance.[19]

Among families where at least one worker is offered health coverage, 10 percent in 1996 declined health insurance altogether, up from 7 percent in 1987.[20] In all, about one of every three uninsured working families without health coverage had an opportunity to participate in an employer-based plan, and two out of every three had no such opportunity. As the subsequent section shows, the rising price of health insurance, particularly the employee's monthly contribution for coverage, has priced many workers out of the market.

Why the Number of Uninsured Is Growing

Two factors primarily explain the long-run increase in the number of uninsured Americans. First, the price of health insurance (and health care services), in constant dollars, is rising. From 1977 to 1998, in 1998 dollars, the cost of job-based insurance increased 2.5-fold and employees' contributions for coverage increased 2.5-fold.[21] Like other goods and services, health insurance at higher prices is affordable to fewer employers and employees.

Second, real wages for American workers without college degrees have fallen during the past twenty-five years. Since 1973, real wages for school dropouts have declined 18 percent; during these same years, college graduates have enjoyed a 17 percent increase in hourly wages.[22] Even during the remarkable economic expansion of the 1990s, median family income for high school dropouts declined 4 percent, whereas family income for college graduates increased 3 percent.[23] Hence low-income workers have fewer dollars in real wages to purchase health insurance. Moreover, real monthly contributions for workers were on average 3.5 times as great in 1998 as in 1977.

Other changes in the economy have contributed to the decline in job-based coverage and the consequent rise in the number of uninsured Americans. The goods industries—manufacturing, mining, and transportation and public utilities—now account for a diminished share of the nation's employment. These industries have traditionally been ones associated with high productivity and wages and offered their workers health insurance. Yet from 1977 to 1998, manufacturing's share of total employment declined from 24 to 15 percent of the workforce. The service industry has been a major source of job growth over more than two decades, as its share of employment rose from 19 to 29 percent of the nation's jobs.[24] Productivity and wages are lower in the service sector, and individual firms are smaller. Consequently, a smaller percentage of workers in the service sector have the option of buying job-based health insurance.

The nature of employment also has changed over the past twenty or so years. Today's workers are more likely to have part-time or temporary status at their jobs. They are also far more likely to be self-employed and independent contractors. In the 1970s, major corporations such as IBM and AT&T boasted of having never laid off workers. The same corporations today boast about downsizing efforts that have rendered their firms more efficient. Consequently, at any given time, more workers are in their probation period, waiting to reach eligibility for health benefits (as well as retirement benefits). Many of these aforementioned changes represent an effort to minimize labor expenses by reducing the percentage of workers covered by the firm's health insurance plan.

Underlying these factors—the decline in employment in the goods industry, falling real wages for less-skilled workers, and the restructuring of work—are two powerful economic forces—the information revolution and the globalization of the U.S. economy. Both of these forces produce greater wealth overall for society, but they reduce the demand for low-skilled U.S. workers, thereby driving down their wages. Globalization compels U.S. companies to seek lowest-cost production processes, and this can include moving plants from high-wage U.S. locations to third-world nations. The unskilled in America are competing with the unskilled of Indonesia for employment or contracts with multinational corporations.

We can see the differential effects of the twin forces of globalization and the information revolution in the divergent trends in job-based insurance according to educational status. In 1979, about 80 percent of the nonelderly in families where the head of household was a college graduate had job-based insurance. In 1997, that figure was still 80 percent. Among school dropouts the percentage of workers and their families with job-based health insurance fell from 54 percent in 1979 to 36 percent in 1997.[25]

WHERE DO THE UNINSURED OBTAIN THEIR CARE?

Three major groups of health care providers deliver services to the uninsured—hospitals, physicians, and community health care centers. Collectively, these providers dispensed an estimated $49.4 billion of uncompensated care, defined as charity care and bad debt, to the uninsured.[26] This represented slightly more than 5 percent of national health care spending. Uncompensated care is, however, concentrated among a minority of these providers. Emergency rooms and outpatient clinics have historically been the site of much charitable care in the United States. Major teaching hospitals provide nearly two-thirds of the uncompensated care in the largest metropolitan areas of the country.[27] Public hospitals accounted for 37 percent of hospital uncompensated care in 1994, up from 33 percent in 1994. For more than two-thirds of the nation's hospitals, uncompensated care constitutes less than 5 percent of total expenses. Nearly two-thirds of physicians report providing charity care, with the average physician estimating that he or she spends one-eighth of his or her time delivering charity care.[28]

Although the number of Americans without health insurance has grown substantially in recent years, the amount of uncompensated care provided by hospitals, in terms of inflation-adjusted dollars, has grown only slightly, from

$15.7 billion in 1985 to $16.8 billion in 1994. Data from the American Medical Association, based on self-reports of physicians, suggests a major increase in the volume of uncompensated care provided from 1990 to 1994. However, data from household surveys show no increase in the number of visits by the uninsured to physicians' offices; this self-reported increase in uncompensated care may reflect bad debts from insured patients more than free care to the uninsured.[29]

What explains why the number of uninsured is increasing while the amount of uncompensated care has risen only slightly? The most common explanation is the new medical marketplace. Managed care has emerged as the dominant form of private health insurance in the country. Under the old system of indemnity insurance, hospitals and physicians could subsidize care for the uninsured from their profits from indemnity insurance. Insurers largely paid physician and hospital charges and did not prospectively question the course of treatment. By negotiating discounts and by paying providers on a lump-sum basis (capitation), managed care organizations have placed financial pressure on hospitals and doctors to control their operating expenses. Uncompensated care is by definition the most unprofitable activity that providers are engaged in and, consequently, one of the primary activities to curtail when providers see their net incomes decline.

DOES LACK OF INSURANCE ENDANGER HEALTH?

One reason many Americans believe that uninsurance does not jeopardize health is that they do not see the uninsured dying in the street.[30] Yet a compelling group of studies demonstrate that lack of insurance has substantial effects on health status, from the ability to receive needed care to reducing life expectancy. This section highlights findings from these studies.

The Uninsured Have Greater Difficulty Obtaining Necessary Care and Suffer Greater Economic Hardships in Paying for Care

Many Americans hold views similar to the editorial writers of the *Wall Street Journal*. They see the uninsured receiving charity care through community hospitals and clinics as well as kindly physicians. In fact the uninsured do ultimately receive care at these institutions, but their experience in obtaining health care differs sharply from those with private and public insurance. According to household surveys, the uninsured report far greater problems than the insured in obtaining necessary care. One recent survey of 3,993 households found the uninsured four times as likely to report problems "getting necessary medical care in the last year" as the insured and three times as likely to report problems "paying medical bills in the past year."[31] Nearly half of the uninsured who reported problems in getting necessary care or paying medical bills had a serious medical condition. More than two-thirds of the uninsured report their problems in paying bills as serious, and 79 percent report their problems in obtaining care as serious. Medical care expenses remain one of the leading causes of bankruptcy in America, with states with higher numbers of uninsured having higher rates of bankruptcies.[32]

Difficulties in obtaining medical care result in lower use of services among the uninsured compared to the insured population. One-third of the uninsured report that they do not have a regular source of care, compared to 17 percent of the privately insured population.[33] Having a regular source of care is important for obtaining coordinated care and receiving preventive care services. When individuals in similar health are compared, the uninsured use roughly 60 percent of the ambulatory and 70 percent of the inpatient services that privately insured individuals use.[34] Furthermore, the disparity in use of services has grown. From 1986 to 1994, the number of annual physician visits for the uninsured fell from 3.1 to 3.0, whereas the number of annual physician visits for privately insured persons grew from 4.2 to 4.6. This has occurred even though the health status of the uninsured, defined as either self-described health status ("excellent," "very good," and so on) or the presence of chronic conditions, is lower than that of privately insured individuals. The percentage of individuals without a usual source of care, moreover, has risen from 28 to 36 percent for the uninsured and fallen from 15 to 11 percent among the privately insured.[35]

The Uninsured Are More Likely to Be Hospitalized for Avoidable Illnesses

Because the uninsured delay care, receive fewer preventive services, and are less likely to have a regular source of care, they are more likely to be hospitalized for medical conditions that do not require hospitalization among the insured. In a study of admissions to Massachusetts and Maryland hospitals, researchers from Harvard Medical School found that the odds of hospitalization for avoidable medical conditions were 26 to 182 percent higher for uninsured than for privately insured patients in three different age groups (under eighteen, eighteen to twenty-four, and twenty-five to sixty-four). For example, among patients with diabetes, the uninsured were 132 percent more likely to be hospitalized in Massachusetts and 182 percent more likely in Maryland than were the privately insured. Among patients with asthma, the uninsured were 84 percent more likely to be hospitalized in Massachusetts and 61 percent more likely in Maryland.[36]

The Uninsured Are Sicker Upon Hospital Arrival

Having delayed care, uninsured patients admitted to the hospital are in worse health than are privately insured admitted patients. In a study of ten million discharge abstracts from 1,200 hospitals, researchers at Georgetown University and

Johns Hopkins Medical School found that the state of health of uninsured patients was worse for thirteen of sixteen groups of patients defined by age, sex, and race (for example, one group was white females aged thirty-five to forty-nine). The abstracts included information on primary and secondary diagnoses. The researchers defined patients' state of health according to the likelihood of death in the hospital for patients in that condition.[37] For the median cohort, the probability of death for uninsured patients, given their medical condition upon arrival at the hospital, was about 60 percent greater than the probability for privately insured patients.

Researchers at Harvard Medical School conducted a similar study from the cancer registry of the State of New Jersey and hospital discharge abstracts from the state's hospitals. They examined the state of health and the likelihood of death of patients with breast cancer at the time of their admission to a hospital. The researchers concluded that the uninsured were 49 percent more likely to die, given their state of health at admission, than were privately insured patients.[38]

The Uninsured Receive Fewer Hospital Services and Are Discharged Earlier

Although the uninsured face more serious problems than privately insured patients upon admission to the hospital, they are less likely to receive discretionary procedures in the hospital. This is particularly true for procedures that involve considerable cost to the hospital. For example, according to research by Georgetown and Johns Hopkins Medical School researchers the uninsured are 74 percent less likely to have a total knee replacement and 44 percent less likely to have a colonoscopy.[39]

Even though the uninsured are in worse medical condition upon admission to a hospital, they are discharged sooner than privately insured patients. For five procedures where physicians have considerable discretion as to the course of care, the Georgetown and Johns Hopkins researchers found that uninsured patients stay 12 to 38 percent fewer days than privately insured patients with the same medical condition.[40]

The Uninsured Are More Likely to Die in the Hospital

Uninsured patients are far more likely to die in the hospital than are patients with private insurance coverage and with similar demographic characteristics (age, sex, and race). For example, a black male aged thirty-five to forty-nine without insurance is 3.2 times as likely to die after admission to a hospital than is a black male aged thirty-five to forty-nine with private insurance. An uninsured white male aged fifty to sixty-four is 23 percent more likely to die than is a white male aged fifty to sixty-four with private insurance.[41]

The Lack of Insurance Reduces Life Expectancy

Following a representative sample of the U.S. population from 1971 to 1987, researchers at the University of Rochester, Department of Family Medicine, examined the mortality rate among 5,161 Americans. In 1971, each respondent was asked about his or her source of health insurance as well as about such other sociodemographic characteristics as age, race, gender, education, income, employment status, exercise habits, smoking habits, obesity, and alcohol consumption. These individuals were then reinterviewed in 1982, 1984, 1986, and 1987. After controlling for other baseline characteristics, the researchers found that the uninsured had a 25 percent greater mortality rate than insured individuals.[42]

A CONSUMER-CHOICE PROGRAM TO ACHIEVE UNIVERSAL COVERAGE

This review of the literature has established that the uninsured are largely a low-income, working population disproportionately employed by small firms. As the percentage of Americans with job-based health insurance has declined, the number of uninsured Americans has risen, increasing from less than 14 percent to nearly 20 percent of the nonelderly population over the past twenty years. Two factors are behind the decline in the percentage of Americans covered by job-based health insurance: (1) a more than doubling of the real price of health insurance since 1977, and (2) declining real wages for non-college-educated workers. Decreasing real wages are attributable to declining demand for unskilled workers; this in turn is a consequence of the information revolution and the globalization of the U.S. economy. All these factors suggest that in the future, the number of uninsured will increase. A recession could lead to more than fifty million uninsured Americans. The primary mechanism for financing nonelderly health care—the exclusion from taxation of employer contributions for health benefits—exacerbates this erosion in coverage. This tax subsidy helps most those that need help least and helps least those that need help most—such as our waitress-mom, working for a small firm and earning only slightly more than the poverty threshold.

If the editorial writers of the *Wall Street Journal* and a majority of the American public were correct in their surmise that the uninsured could get care when they need it, then we would not have to worry that the uninsured are growing in number. The evidence, however, is to the contrary and is compelling. The uninsured are four times as likely as privately insured individuals to report difficulty obtaining care, and use 60 percent fewer medical care services than do other individuals in equivalent health with private insurance. They are three times as likely to report not having a regular source of care. The uninsured are much more likely to be hospitalized for avoidable medical conditions resulting from asthma or diabetes. When the uninsured are hospitalized, they arrive in poorer health, receive fewer discretionary, high-cost services such as knee replacements, have shorter hospital stays, and are far more likely to die in the hospital. Overall, uninsured individuals have a mortality rate that is 25 percent greater than that of privately insured individuals, after controlling for other economic and demographic factors.

So why has this nation not extended coverage to its uninsured citizens, who largely fall into the category of the deserving near-poor? Certainly an important factor is that the public and the press are not cognizant of the health hazards of uninsurance. Another explanation is that Americans are less compassionate and egalitarian than citizens from other Western nations. But public opinion polls indicate that Americans are in principle as egalitarian as citizens from nations with universal health care coverage.[43] I suspect a more important factor is the political impotence of the uninsured. Their demographics are the demographics of nonvoters. The uninsured do not contribute money to political candidates and do not play golf with the rich and powerful.

Perhaps the reason is that universal coverage is perceived as costing too much. Experts have estimated the expense of extending health insurance to the uninsured as costing as little as $20 billion per year, after netting out existing safety net programs for the uninsured.[44] My back-of-the-envelope calculation is $60 billion. Neither estimate is an overwhelming figure when one considers that this nation already spends more than one trillion dollars every year on health care. Other political factors have doomed previous political initiatives. The public's lack of understanding of the complexities of health care finance combined with the essential role that health care plays in our lives means opponents of health care initiatives can frighten the public with campaigns that play loose with the truth. The infamous advertisements featuring a married couple called Harry and Louise were highly effective in defeating President Clinton's Health Security Act. Similarly, the president and congressional Democrats were successful in frightening senior citizens about the 1995 Republican initiative to reform Medicare, even though the Republican plan used economic principles similar to those behind the Health Security Act. I infer that when political opponents can persuade a large number of people that those franchised under the current system will be made worse off by a proposed change in health care financing, the proposal stands little chance of passage.

Proponents of universal coverage have also long squabbled among themselves, seeking the perfect and ending with nothing. In 1993 and 1994, valuable energy and time was lost debating employer and individual mandates, managed competition versus single-payer plans, and the like. Policy analysts see health care reform as an opportunity to reorganize health care delivery, but politically this has often worked to the disadvantage of advocates of universal coverage.

Fortunately, the most workable political solution is consistent with the American political character. Americans distrust centralized political power (they also distrust big corporations and CEOs) and cherish the opportunity to make consumer decisions. A majority of Democrats are unlikely to support a single-payer solution, let alone Republicans and Independents.

So the question is, Should we take the route of shoring up our current employer-based system, or should we consider an individual-based system? An employer-based system has a number of strengths. It is a system workers are familiar with. An infrastructure is already established, including talented benefit managers among the largest employers. Human resource staffs serve as ombudsmen to workers and see that their consumer questions are answered and that workers enroll in the plans. Large groups serve as an efficient means of pooling risk. All these factors, however, do not diminish the fact that this system is breaking down and that ongoing economic forces dictate that it will erode further. The job-based system, moreover, is supported by a regressive tax subsidy. Universal coverage in the context of an employer-based system requires employer mandates, government-sponsored health insurance purchasing groups, and subsidies for low-income workers and small firms. The end result is a Rube Goldberg–like system.

Hence the best strategy is to promote a system in which individuals purchase their health insurance directly from private insurers and managed care organizations. An individual-based system will allow consumers greater choice of health plans. Such a strategy should slowly phase out job-based insurance. The phaseout should reflect employees' decision to purchase health insurance directly from insurers. These insurers should be subject to clearly defined rules of competition, just as the buying and selling of stock on the New York Stock Exchange is subject to the rules of the Securities and Exchange Commission (SEC) and the Financial Accounting and Standards Board (FASB).

The following outlines provide the objectives and principles and the basic design of such a system.

Objectives and Principles

1. Universal health care coverage is an objective that can be achieved through a system of individual choice. Employer-based coverage will not be immediately phased out but should wither as individual insurance proves more attractive to consumers.

2. The system permits diverse plans to match the diverse tastes of the American public.

3. Health plans compete on the basis of price, service, and quality, not by excluding sick individuals from coverage.

4. It is equally as profitable for health plans to treat sick as to treat the healthy.

5. The system does not attempt to achieve the impossible. The objective is for the formerly uninsured to obtain adequate coverage, not to have coverage equivalent to that purchased by those in the top 5 percent of the income distribution.

6. The government and its agents set and police the rules. Within these constraints the market sets prices and builds delivery systems.

Basic Design

1. The federal government provides progressive, refundable tax credits to individual families. For families whose incomes are below 175 percent of the poverty income level, credits are set at a level that allows purchase of single or family coverage without an additional monthly contribution by the family. That single or family policy is situated at the twenty-fifth percentile of premiums for employer-based health coverage.

2. Families that choose to purchase higher-priced plans pay the difference between the refundable credit and the premium in monthly contributions.

3. Medicaid is expanded to cover all individuals with income below the poverty level.

4. All Americans must purchase health insurance—either through an employer-based plan, Medicare, Medicaid, or individual insurance. Families must show proof of coverage when filing taxes. Using electronic information systems, federal and state governments work cooperatively to identify nonparticipants, and if necessary, randomly assign nonparticipants to a plan until each individual or family makes a choice.

5. States have the responsibility to serve as the sponsor, or administrator, of plans. They license plans that meet financial solvency and consumer protection requirements. They establish minimum benefit requirements set at the twenty-fifth percentile of the prevailing job-based coverage in the state.

6. States license all types of health plans—fee-for-service, preferred provider organizations, point-of-service plans, health maintenance organizations, and medical savings accounts. Medical savings accounts receive the same tax benefits as other plans do.

7. To minimize potentially explosive marketing costs, states provide citizens with consumer-friendly information on plan benefits, costs, member satisfaction, and performance.

8. The state sets geographical and standard age-sex categories for risk rating. Medical underwriting and preexisting condition clauses are not permitted.

9. The state reviews the marketing materials of health plans to see that plans are not discriminating against the sick.

10. Each plan contributes 5 percent of its monthly health revenues into an income-earning risk pool. Each year the state rates the risk of the member population of each health plan and redistributes pool revenues according to the comparative risk of each plan.

Certainly many insurers and managed care organizations will protest the rules embedded in these principles and in the design and term them "too regulatory." Critics from the left will consider them inadequate. Instituting the basic design will not be easy. But the chances of achieving universal coverage are greater with instituting an individual choice system than with salvaging a job-based one. "Compassionate conservatives" will find appeal in individual choice. Moderates and liberals now are willing to accept a system that is less than perfect if it leads to universal coverage or substantially reduces the number of uninsured Americans. Thus a system of individual choice is the best hope for remedying an American dilemma.

Notes

1. U.S. Bureau of Labor Statistics. [www.bls.gov].

2. U.S. Department of Commerce, Bureau of Economic Analysis. [www.bea.doc. gov/bea/newsrel/gdp199f.fhtm].

3. Brandt, M., and others. "They're Rich (and You're Not)." *Newsweek,* July 5, 1999, p. 38.

4. Fronstin, P. "Sources of Health Insurance and Characteristics of the Uninsured: Analysis of the March 1998 Current Population Survey." EBRI Issue Brief No. 204. Washington, D.C.: Employee Benefits Research Institute, Dec. 1998.

5. Reinhardt, U. "Employer-Based Health Insurance: R.I.P." In S. Altman, U. Reinhardt, and A. Shields (eds.), *The Future U.S. Health Care System: Who Will Care for the Uninsured?* Waltham, Mass.: Health Administration Press, 1998.

6. Blendon, R., Young, J., and Desrochez, C. "The Uninsured, the Working Uninsured, and the Public." *Health Affairs,* 1999, *18*(6), 206–207.

7. Employee Benefits Research Institute (EBRI). *Fundamentals of Employee Benefit Programs.* (5th ed.) Washington, D.C.: EBRI Education and Research Fund, 1996.

8. Law, S. *Blue Cross: What Went Wrong?* New Haven, Conn.: Yale University Press, 1974.

9. Shiels, J., and Hogan, P. "Cost of Tax-Exempt Health Benefits in 1998." *Health Affairs,* 1999, *18*(2), 176–181.

10. Fronstin, "Sources of Health Insurance and Characteristics of the Uninsured."

11. Fronstin, "Sources of Health Insurance and Characteristics of the Uninsured."

12. Fronstin, "Sources of Health Insurance and Characteristics of the Uninsured."

13. Gabel, J., and others. *Health Benefits of Small Employers in 1998.* Report prepared for the Henry J. Kaiser Foundation by KPMG, 1999, p. 5.

14. U.S. Bureau of the Census. "County Business Patterns." Washington, D.C.: U.S. Bureau of the Census, Nov. 1996.

15. Thorpe, K. "Inside the Black Box of Administrative Costs." *Health Affairs,* 1992, *11*(2), 41–55.

16. Unpublished data from 1998 Current Population Survey, Employee Benefits Research Institute, Washington, D.C.

17. Holahan, J. "The Changing Role of Medicaid." In S. Altman, U. Reinhardt, and A. Shields (eds.), *The Future U.S. Health Care System: Who Will Care for the Uninsured?* Waltham, Mass.: Health Administration Press, 1998.

18. Kenneth Thorpe, personal communication to the author.

19. Davis, K., Rowland, D., Collins, K., and Morris, C. "Health Insurance: The Size and Shape of the Problem." *Inquiry,* 1995, *32,* 196–203.

20. Cooper, P., and Schone, B. "More Offers, Fewer Takers for Employment-Based Health Insurance: 1987 and 1996." *Health Affairs,* 1997, *16*(6), 142–149.

21. Gabel, J. "Job-Based Health Insurance, 1977–1998: The Accidental System Under Scrutiny." *Health Affairs,* 1999, *18*(6), 62–74.

22. Bluestone, B. "The Inequality Express." *American Prospect,* Winter 1995, pp. 81–83.

23. U.S. Census Bureau. "Historic Income Tables—Households." [www.census. gov/hhes/income/histinc/h13.html].

24. U.S. Bureau of Labor Statistics. [data.bls.gov/CBT-bin/surveymost?ec].

25. U.S. Bureau of the Census, *Current Population Survey.* Washington, D.C.: U.S. Bureau of the Census.

26. Author's calculations based on Cunningham, P., and Tu, H. "A Changing Picture of Uncompensated Care." *Health Affairs,* 1997, *16*(4), 167–175.

27. Reuter, J., and Gaskin, D. "The Role of Academic Medical Centers and Teaching Hospitals in Providing Care to the Poor." In S. Altman, U. Reinhardt, and A. Shields (eds.), *The Future U.S. Health Care System: Who Will Care for the Uninsured?* Waltham, Mass.: Health Administration Press, 1998.

28. Readers should regard the physician figure for uncompensated care with caution. It is based on estimates of uncompensated care drawn from an American Medical Association survey of individual physician practices and not on audited financial statements.

29. Cunningham and Tu, "A Changing Picture of Uncompensated Care."

30. Altman, S., Reinhardt, U., and Shields, A. "Healthcare for the Poor and Uninsured: An Uncertain Future." In S. Altman, U. Reinhardt, and A. Shields (eds.), *The*

Future U.S. Health Care System: Who Will Care for the Uninsured? Waltham, Mass.: Health Administration Press, 1998.

31. Donelan, K., and others. "What Happened to the Health Insurance Crisis in the United States? Voices from a National Survey." *Journal of the American Medical Association,* 1996, *276,* 1346–1350.

32. Bleakley, F. "Personal-Bankruptcy Filings Are Soaring: High Debt, Downsizing and Medical Woes Are Cited for Four-Month Record." *Wall Street Journal,* May 8, 1996, p. A2.

33. Rowland, D., Feder, J., and Keenan, P. "Uninsured in America: The Causes and Consequences." In S. Altman, U. Reinhardt, and A. Shields (eds.), *The Future U.S. Health Care System: Who Will Care for the Uninsured?* Waltham, Mass.: Health Administration Press, 1998.

34. Long, S., and Marquis, S. "The Uninsured Access Gap and the Cost of Universal Coverage." *Health Affairs,* 1994, *13*(2, Supplement), 211–220.

35. Cunningham and Tu, "A Changing Picture of Uncompensated Care."

36. Weissman, J., Gatsonis, C., and Epstein, A. "Rates of Avoidable Hospitalization by Insurance Status in Massachusetts and Maryland." *Journal of the American Medical Association,* 1992, *268,* 2388–2394.

37. Hadley, J., Steinberg, E. P., and Feder, J. "Comparison of Uninsured and Privately Insured Hospital Patients: Condition on Admission, Resource Use, and Outcome." *Journal of the American Medical Association,* 1991, *265,* 374–379.

38. Ayanian, J., Kohler, B., Abe, T., and Epstein, A. "The Relation Between Health Insurance Coverage and Clinical Outcomes Among Women with Breast Cancer." *New England Journal of Medicine,* 1993, *329,* 326–331.

39. Hadley and others, "Comparison of Uninsured and Privately Insured Hospital Patients."

40. Hadley and others, "Comparison of Uninsured and Privately Insured Hospital Patients."

41. Hadley and others, "Comparison of Uninsured and Privately Insured Hospital Patients."

42. Franks, P., Clancey, C., and Gold, M. "Health Insurance and Mortality: Evidence from a National Cohort." *Journal of the American Medical Association,* 1993, *270,* 737–741.

43. Reinhardt, "Employer-Based Health Insurance."

44. Long and Marquis, "The Uninsured Access Gap."

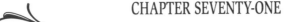

CHAPTER SEVENTY-ONE

A Health Insurance Tax Credit

The Key to More Coverage and Choice for Consumers

David B. Kendall

In the twentieth century no fewer than seven U.S. presidents, from Theodore Roosevelt to Bill Clinton, have attempted to achieve universal health care coverage.[1] Behind these repeated efforts has been the presumption that all Americans are entitled to health care coverage. But because most people today have coverage, they are not eager for reform, especially if it means they must give up something. The time has come to help the uninsured with a more practical political calculus. Rather than securing health care coverage for people who already have it, the nation's leaders should adopt a strategy that targets the uninsured but also benefits the insured. Specifically, this strategy should be aimed at the uninsured who cannot afford coverage and the insured who have no choice of coverage because they work for a company—typically a small firm—that offers only one plan.

The uninsured and insured have a common interest in expanding health care because health insurance markets work better when they are big and inclusive. For example, the nation's largest employer—the federal government—covers the great majority of its workers and offers more choices and better value than virtually all other employers.

The way to expand both coverage and choice is through a tax credit for individuals to purchase health insurance, through a job or on their own. A tax credit would offer lower- to middle-income workers the same kind of tax break that is used by most middle- to upper-income workers for job-based health insurance. It would increase competition and choice in the insurance markets for small employers and individual policies, where uninsured, lower-income workers are concentrated. In general, it would create a consumer-driven health insurance system that would both complement and compete against job-based health care.

In addition, the federal government should provide grants to the states for ensuring that tax credits are as useful and fair as possible.[2] Otherwise a federally designed tax credit risks being unsuitable for local markets and regulations.

This strategy will have to be pursued aggressively. After all, the additional cost of making health insurance more affordable will ultimately be borne by those with coverage. Most people with coverage are willing to pay something extra to ensure that others have coverage, but they are more likely to support change enthusiastically if they themselves receive something as well. Another problem is that the benefits of individual choice are not obvious to people who are used to letting their employers choose for them. But the lack of choice and control in health care is becoming more obvious as innovations give people choice and control in other services as diverse as pensions and electrical power.

This strategy can win support in both political parties because it uses both public financing that appeals to Democrats and private coverage that appeals to Republicans. It is a third way alternative to a government-run system or a fend-for-yourself marketplace. It will empower people with both coverage and choice.

THE LACK OF COVERAGE, CHOICE, AND OUTRAGE

More than forty million—one of every six Americans—were uninsured in 2003. That is an extraordinary number. Imagine if one of every six Americans lacked other basic goods like food or housing. The calls for action would be deafening.

Consider another disturbing statistic: at least one-third of workers and their families have no choice in their health care coverage because their employer chooses for them.[3] No one would tolerate employers controlling where people lived or shopped, as company towns once did in the nineteenth and early twentieth centuries. Why aren't elected officials rushing to help the uninsured and expand choice?

The lack of outrage over inadequate coverage and choice is partly a legacy of job-based health insurance. As a nation, we have come to expect that health insurance comes with a good job as a reward for hard work. Workers have generally been much more interested in getting and keeping a job with coverage than in having a choice of coverage. Workers without insurance have likely felt that coverage is either too expensive or a low priority. In other words, job-based health insurance makes it easy for people to excuse shortcomings, out of gratitude if they have coverage and as a matter of fate if they do not.

The story behind the statistics also helps to explain the lack of outrage. The survey that produced the statistic that one of every seven Americans is uninsured is meant to reveal the number of people uninsured for the whole year, but many researchers believe this number also includes people who are uninsured for less than a year, due to the way the survey questions are asked.[4] A more accurate but less frequently conducted survey shows that one in fifteen Americans were uninsured for at least a year in the mid-1990s (the latest time period for this survey).[5]

At the same time, this more accurate survey also shows that being uninsured is a relatively common experience. One of every five Americans went without coverage for at least one month in the mid-1990s.[6] Two-thirds of the people in this group were uninsured for less than a year. Such gaps in coverage are often related to losing a job or to going through a waiting period at a new job before benefits start.

People with higher incomes are more likely to have coverage, but many are uninsured nonetheless. Middle- to upper-income families (earning more than $40,000) make up a quarter of the uninsured and could be politically potent in the battle for reform. But they are also especially likely to be uninsured only in the short term. Families who are in the lower half of the income scale and are temporarily uninsured account for nearly half of all uninsured. Their sheer numbers could make this group important politically, but their own priority is much more likely to be securing a job or earning higher wages rather than getting health insurance. If it is not a personal priority, it is unlikely to become a political priority. Only about one-fourth of the uninsured are long-term uninsured, lower-income families, the group that is most likely to evoke public sympathy. Their problems are indeed significant, reflecting both the high cost of coverage and a lack of convenient access. Nonetheless, it is important to note that most of the neediest families (with incomes less than $20,000) do have coverage, in large part thanks to Medicaid.[7]

Although the plight of the uninsured periodically captures national attention, the cause of workers without a choice of coverage has never even registered on the radar screen. That is because most workers have a choice of what matters most to them: a choice of doctor. In spite of employers' widespread use of managed care plans that limit the choice of doctor, 95 percent of workers and their families can still choose their own doctor by going outside their plan's network of doctors at a cost similar to that for traditional fee-for-service coverage.[8]

THE RIGHT REASONS FOR REFORM

Given the sobering political realities behind the lack of choice and coverage, what hope is there for reform? The answer lies in the clear but poorly understood consequences of a lack of coverage and choice.

In general, the more participants in a market, the more choice and competition. A lack of health care coverage for some people therefore diminishes care choices for everyone. Moreover, in the health insurance market, the fact of large numbers of uninsured means that insurers feel forced to limit participants even further. That is, they have to compete almost as much on how well they can *exclude* people from coverage as they do on the value of their services. They must try to avoid people who wait until they become sick or injured to buy coverage, a problem known as *adverse selection*. Although this policy may sound inhumane, insurers explain it by pointing out that they cannot insure a burning house. However, if insurers did not have to market selectively, then they could offer everyone more choices, including better benefits, a greater range of products, and lower prices.

The lack of coverage is a public problem because as a matter of humanity, health care is often provided for free to those who cannot pay. As a result it may seem perfectly reasonable to some people to forgo insurance. Others, such as *yimbes* (young indestructible males), may not believe they are even at risk of needing expensive care. People who do not pay for coverage even though they could afford part or all of the cost are taking a free ride on everyone else when they become sick or injured and cannot pay for their health care.

The two markets where insurers are the most careful about whom they insure are the same markets where the uninsured are the most prevalent: small employers and individuals. Workers in very small firms (less than ten employees) are nearly three times more likely to be uninsured than are workers in large firms (more than one thousand employees).[9] Workers in very small firms are one-fourth as likely as their counterparts in large firms to have a choice of health plan.[10] Individually sold policies cover about sixteen million Americans. All of the thirty-nine million uninsured are potential participants in the individual market, although roughly one-fifth of the uninsured also have the opportunity to buy through a group policy but decline.[11] Individuals buying their own insurance are not, of course, constrained by their employer's choices, but they often find it difficult to shop for an individual policy. For example, they may face long delays in finding out whether an insurer will cover them and the price of that coverage. From the insurers' point of view, such delays make it less likely that they will insure "the burning house." Individual policies do, however, offer more choices in the selection of benefits (for example, a high versus a low deductible) than group policies do.

The lack of coverage is not the only reason for a lack of choice. Workers in small businesses are less likely than other workers to have a choice of coverage, in part due to the higher administrative costs of managing choices for small groups. In addition, government regulation of insurance premiums (that is, community rating laws) sometimes cause insurers to curtail their business or leave the insurance market altogether. Any strategy to increase coverage and choice must take these considerations into account.

The lack of coverage also, of course, hurts the uninsured themselves. When a devastating illness or accident occurs, the uninsured, whether lacking insurance long term or temporarily, can face a mountain of debt. Although many health care providers offer charity care, the amount of charity varies and its availability is inconsistent. Even those institutions that receive government funding for care of the uninsured regularly send bills to the patients who qualify for charitable care.[12] There are also health consequences from lack of coverage. The uninsured, who are more likely to delay obtaining preventive care or seeing a doctor for minor problems, can sometimes have costly and major problems down the road. In one study, the uninsured were found to be up to three times more likely than the insured with similar characteristics to die in the hospital.[13] In general, the uninsured are also about three times more likely to fail to receive needed care.[14] They face higher out-of-pocket costs than the insured, which deter access to care.

Those who lack choice but accept what is offered suffer less but still significantly. When all health plans were the same old flavor—fee-for-service indemnity—the choice of plan mattered little. But now that insurers give ever greater scrutiny to the bills they will pay, in order to reduce costs, their decisions have a big impact on patients' quality of life. For example, the limits on hospital stays and access to specialty care can have substantial impact on those less capable of caring for themselves at home and those with chronic conditions. Those without a choice of coverage cannot leave the plans that do not serve their individual needs. However, workers who lack choice are also less likely to have coverage. They are less likely to find a policy they can afford when an employer offers only one, relatively expensive, insurance plan. One study suggests that workers and their families who are offered only a non-HMO plan are three times more likely to decline coverage than those who have multiple choices including an HMO.[15] More choices let workers find the kind of coverage that suits their preferences and budgets.

The consequences of a lack of coverage and choice are not widely appreciated because they are not highly visible problems. The delays in health care that shorten the life spans of the uninsured or increase disability are hard to identify, track, and communicate. The costs of uncompensated care get absorbed into a complex web of provider charges to paying patients and support from government funding as well as charity. Frustration with impersonal treatment from managed care health plans has become absorbed in the drive for a patient bill of rights.

THE GROWING DEMAND FOR CHOICE AND COVERAGE

The consequences of a lack of choice and coverage will become more visible, however, as a result of the following societal and economic trends both inside and outside the health care system:

Rising health insurance prices will require employers and insurers to offer more choices so that individuals can make trade-offs between price and quality. After nearly a decade of lower medical inflation than before, thanks largely to the widespread adoption of managed care, double-digit premium increases are returning. No one knows, of course, whether the recent upward spike in prices will be short or long term, but either way it will demand a response. In the next round of the medical inflation fight, cost-saving techniques will have to become more customized because a one-size-fits-all approach has run its course. Moreover, by paying most of the premium regardless of an employee's choice of plan, employers continue to encourage employees to choose higher-priced plans. In fact, only 19 percent of employees who have a choice of plan are not subject to an outdated approach to health benefits.[16] A more customized approach would offer employees a range of choices and a basic, defined contribution that lets employees decide how much more money they want to spend on coverage. But without offering more choices, employers will not be able to encourage workers to be more price sensitive and yet remain satisfied with their benefits.

In the information age, when consumers have increasing control and choice over nearly all aspects of their lives, the health care system is looking increasingly archaic. The one-size-fits-all approach that dominates the health care sector stands in stark contrast to the trend toward mass customization in the rest of the economy. Made-to-order computers, movies on demand, customized local telephone service, and travel reservation systems that know your preferences are among the many examples of the systems that can efficiently deliver personalized service. The health care system lacks the convenience and reliability that consumers have come to expect from many other sectors of the economy.

The Internet and information technology are fueling consumer demand for control and choice in health care. One of the most common uses of the Internet is for health information. Informed people will be able to demand better service, higher quality, and lower costs from their doctor and health plan. The increasing use of information technology will enable more customized care. Online information about the health status of individuals can be collected anonymously and analyzed to reveal differences in how well their treatments, doctors, and health plans worked to make them healthy.

Rising health care costs and increased competition are straining the safety net for the uninsured. The drive for efficiency under managed care has already made it more difficult for doctors and hospitals to provide charity care. For example, doctors who are paid mostly by managed care plans provide 40 percent less charity care than doctors who receive little income from managed care plans.[17] That should not be a surprise because competitive markets can be expected to squeeze out providers' ability to provide charity care. As prices rise, higher-income insured Americans have the capacity and maybe even the desire to pay more to get more. The plight of the uninsured will become more prominent as the fragile safety net continues to fray.

WHERE TO START REFORM: TAX POLICY

The main reason for increasing subsidies to the uninsured for health insurance through a tax credit is that tax policy is already responsible for financing a good portion of most health insurance policies. Health benefits provided by employers, unlike wages, are excluded from all income and payroll taxes. This tax exclusion reduces the price of job-based health insurance by as much as 50 percent. Few people are even aware of this tax exclusion because, unlike a tax deduction, it is not claimed by individuals on their tax returns. Workers who pay for their own insurance get a deduction only if their total health care expenses exceed 7.5 percent of their adjusted gross income in any year, which rarely happens.

A historical accident, the tax exclusion for job-based health benefits grew out of wage and price controls during World War II. Unable to compete for scarce workers by increasing wages, companies greatly expanded health care benefits. In order to maintain the illusion that wage controls were working, the IRS simply deemed that health benefits were not wages and therefore not taxable. Congress subsequently codified the IRS ruling in 1953.[18]

From the 1940s to the 1960s, the expansion of job-based coverage made sense for most workers. They formed reliable, long-term relationships with big business and big labor. Since the 1970s, however, stiff global competition and corporate downsizing have eroded the workers' relationships with and confidence in big institutions. In today's economy one of every four workers does not hold a permanent, full-time job.[19] Only 13 percent of workers are unionized.[20]

Despite the increasingly strained connection between jobs and health insurance, the tax exclusion for job-based coverage has one very important virtue. It supports the public goal of covering people who might otherwise go without insurance. In effect, it encourages people to buy coverage before they get sick. It also benefits people who would buy coverage without the bribe because, as discussed earlier, it reduces the problem of adverse selection and thus makes health insurance markets more stable and competitive. In other words, as a form of charity, public financing for private health insurance can be very efficient.

A tax credit given to individuals directly instead of through the job would have the following advantages:

- A tax credit would give workers control over the tax subsidy, just as they have over tax breaks for home mortgages, charitable contributions, and pensions. Workers would not have to depend on employers to determine the amount of money to be spent on health insurance, the kind of benefits, the selection of health plans and doctors, and the information needed to make an informed choice. They would be free to join new and existing organizations that would compete on their ability to manage the competition for members' benefit.

- A tax credit would help workers who are between jobs. Few people take responsibility for these gaps because they are used to getting coverage through a job. Those who do go as far as pursuing coverage between jobs sometimes balk when they learn the high cost of paying for insurance themselves.

- A tax credit would be worth more to lower-income individuals. The value of the tax exclusion, just like all tax deductions, depends on one's tax bracket. Lower-income workers pay little or no income tax, which reduces the value of the tax break (that is, the exclusion from payroll taxes) to as little as 15 percent of the price of insurance. Put simply, workers who need the most help receive the least. The average value of the tax exclusion for families with incomes of more than $100,000 was roughly $2,600 in 2000. For families earning less than $15,000, the average value was about $80.[21]

- A tax credit could be capped at a fixed dollar amount to fight medical inflation. The existing tax exclusion is open ended: the more insurance coverage an employer buys, the bigger the tax break. That fuels medical inflation and makes health care even more unaffordable for the uninsured.

Why not replace the exclusion with a tax credit altogether? At roughly $125 billion in forgone tax revenues, the tax exclusion is worth just under half the cost of Medicare. Although it is well-intended, this strategy would be almost as far-reaching and just as controversial as President Clinton's 1994 proposed overhaul. It could be easily defeated by a coalition of employers, unions, and insurers who prefer the status quo with a slogan like, "Congress wants to tax your health benefits." The potential advantages of a new tax credit to individuals would quickly be lost amid the public's fear of losing their coverage altogether. Job-based coverage is far too deeply embedded in our society to be turned upside down in a frontal assault. It is instructive that the only successful government initiatives actually enacted for the uninsured have focused on non-workers: Medicare for retirees, Medicaid for welfare recipients, and the Children's Health Insurance Program (CHIP) for children. Reform must respect the fact that most people with job-based coverage are largely satisfied with it, even if there are probably better alternatives.

Rather than replacing the tax exclusion outright, a more practical approach would be to let individuals themselves choose between a new tax credit or the old tax exclusion.[22] This approach would create a new market that would simultaneously complement and compete with job-based coverage. It would demonstrate the benefits of individual control of health insurance and stimulate a broader movement toward a consumer-driven health care system. The immediate challenge in designing a tax credit is to create a new source of financing for uninsured workers without unnecessarily disrupting the job-based system.

DESIGNING A TAX CREDIT

The idea of a tax credit for health insurance is relatively easy to communicate, which helps make it politically feasible. The specific design of a tax credit, however, must confront some significant problems.

For starters, people have widely varying health care needs. Genetic, psychological, physiological, social, cultural, demographic, economic, and environmental factors all contribute to a wide variety of health conditions. As a result, each person sees the value of health care coverage differently. A fifty-year-old businesswoman living in New York City who has the gene that can lead to breast cancer has a view of health insurance very different from that of a twenty-one-year-old fast-food worker in the rural Southwest who drives a motorcycle without a helmet. From a social point of view as well, it makes little sense to treat each person the same, because each person's situation may, for a wide variety reasons, warrant more (or less) public support.

In the same way, the price of health insurance may vary for each person. Typically, an insurance company wants to charge a higher premium to individuals or groups that are more likely than others to need health care services given such risk factors as age, sex, geography, and health history. But it is unfair for people to pay more for health care conditions that are no fault of their own, especially when these people have low incomes. In response to this problem many state governments have enacted price regulations for health insurance, known as *community rating* laws, that lower the price of insurance for higher-risk, sicker people and raise the price for lower-risk, healthier people.

Community rating laws have three potential problems that can undermine their intent. First, instead of paying a higher premium, some healthier, low-risk people will simply drop coverage, thereby causing insurance premiums for sicker, higher-risk people to increase. Second, insurers will try to avoid covering higher-risk, sicker people or will skimp on their care in order to minimize losses. Third, because community rating laws treat the rich and poor in the same way, they create another inequity by forcing low-income people with low health risks to subsidize high-income people with high risks. One partial solution to the problems created by community rating is for employers or the government to adjust payments to insurers based on the age, sex, and health condition of people who sign up for that insurer. Medicare and larger employ-ers who offer a choice of plans currently use this process, known as *risk adjust-ment*. Risk adjustment helps prevent the problem of insurers who avoid selling coverage to older, sicker people or who skimp on such patients' care. It was a key aspect of the Jackson Hole Group's proposal for managed competition.[23]

Wharton School economist Mark Pauly and his colleagues have designed a customized tax credit that would offset the inequity of health insurance prices directly and avoid the need for community rating.[24] The Pauly tax credit would be worth the most to high-risk, low income people and worth the least (or noth-ing at all) to low-risk, high-income people. It would address the inequity of insurance pricing with highly targeted assistance instead of forcing everyone to pay the same price for something everyone values differently. The Pauly credit would be a fixed amount (as opposed to a percentage of the cost of insurance), calculated for each person so that it would not fuel medical inflation by encour-aging people to spend ever greater amounts beyond the cost of basic coverage. At the same time, the credit would provide the strongest possible inducement for everyone to get coverage because it would be dollar-for-dollar up to the fixed amount, thereby making coverage essentially free up to a given level. In con-trast, a tax credit based on a percentage of spending requires people to pay for the unmatched portion themselves, which would likely be insufficient to encour-age most people to buy coverage.[25]

Unfortunately, the sheer complexity of such a proposal has proven too daunt-ing for even the most ambitious legislator. No legislation has been introduced based on the Pauly tax credit proposal, despite many opportunities. Indeed, Mark Pauly himself has most recently proposed a simple flat-dollar tax credit as a starting point for reform.[26] Even with a more practical tax credit design, however, the need to reconcile the financing and pricing of health insurance remains important as a way to ensure that everyone has a chance to purchase coverage, and to build the biggest possible constituency in order to cover the currently uninsured.

TAX CREDITS AND STATE GRANTS

A practical approach to this problem is to divide responsibilities for solving it between the federal government and the states.[27] The federal government would provide a tax credit as a base level of financing coverage for the uninsured and give state governments funding to ensure, through supplemental subsidies, that everyone has an equal opportunity to purchase coverage.

The federal tax credit would be a fixed dollar amount (perhaps $1,500 for an individual and $3,750 for a family). It would decline in value for middle- to high-income families (above twice to three times the poverty level). It would be refundable, which means available to those who have not had to pay any income tax, and advanceable, which would give workers access to the credit at the time they had to pay insurance premiums. Finally, it would be available to the insured as well as the uninsured, so that workers who are struggling to afford coverage can remain covered.

The grants to the states would be performance based. The federal government would provide financing based on state improvements in coverage rates across demographic groups and other factors like access to care and health care quality. States could issue the supplemental subsidies either directly to individual insurance policyholders or through purchasing pools that are community rated. States could also use the grants to expand public programs like Medicaid and the State Children's Health Insurance Program (SCHIP).

Over time, as the states sorted out the best way to reconcile health insurance subsidies and insurance pricing, they would also gain insights on how to limit the federal tax subsidies in a fair way. If the customized subsidies prove effective, then the federal government could cap both the tax credit and tax exclusion accordingly. Similarly, if flat subsidies combined with a community rating system and risk adjustment proved better, then the federal government could use a flat cap on all tax subsidies while insisting that risk-adjustment systems be used widely. A mixed result—perhaps the most likely outcome—would require a flexible cap that allowed employers to choose a plan best suited for local markets and regulations.

ADDITIONAL MEASURES

Although tax credit and state grants are necessary parts of a successful strategy, other measures are also desirable, to expand coverage and choice for health care consumers.

Menus for Choice and Convenient Enrollment

Every state would provide a menu of health plan choices to everyone who lacks employer-sponsored coverage.[28] The menu of choices could be as formal as one offered by a purchasing group similar to the Federal Employees Health Benefits Program (FEHB) or as informal as a list of insurance products and prices compiled by the state insurance commissioner. Employers would still have a role, however, in distributing the menu and facilitating enrollment. All employees on their first day on the job and each year thereafter would receive an enrollment form for health insurance. The enrollment form would contain the menu of choices and permission for the employer to withhold payments for insurance. Employers would also enable employees to use their tax credit in advance by reducing tax withholdings by the amount of the tax credit.

Performance Information Disclosure

Good information for comparing health plans makes choice meaningful. Markets will always produce a certain amount of such information on their own (for example, *Consumer Reports* and Zagat's restaurant survey). But the health care sector produces a less than optimal amount of information, for several reasons: the need for scientifically sophisticated systems to measure and report health care outcomes and the lack of agreement over standards for reporting information and over the public benefit of measuring public health goals (for example, immunization rates). These problems warrant government action to require health plans and providers to report on their performance. As Harvard Business School professor Regina Herzlinger has argued, an agency like the Securities and Exchange Commission should be established for health care to ensure the production of a basic level of comparable performance information.[29]

Information Networks

Rapid access to the right information is important in health care for everything from saving lives to disseminating the latest scientific studies. Yet health care information systems are unconnected silos of data that have been constructed largely for submitting and paying claims instead of for caring for people. As a result, diagnostic tests are duplicated as people move among various health care providers, potentially dangerous drug interactions from multiple prescriptions are missed, and a patient's outcomes cannot be tracked over time and reported as part of the information that helps people choose health plans and providers. But linking these databases raises legitimate concerns about protecting people's privacy and ensuring that information is used by professionals confidentially. The government has important roles in both protecting privacy and catalyzing the creation of information networks that can share information, just as it did with the Internet.

Individual Mandate

Even with the most generous and well-designed tax credits and supplemental subsidies, some people will still choose to forgo coverage. They are essentially taking a free ride on the people with coverage, who would subsidize the payment of their bills if they needed costly care. A free-rider tax would be an appropriate penalty and an incentive to purchase coverage. Many health policy analysts have proposed an individual mandate as an upfront reform to prevent the problem of adverse selection.[30] But that approach is not practical until health care is made more affordable through tax credits and additional subsidies. In the area of children's coverage, the subsidy levels are nearing the point where the primary responsibility for coverage can and should be assumed by the families. If they do not arrange for their children to have coverage, then they should be required to forfeit the child tax credit and dependent deduction for federal income taxes.

SUCCESS THROUGH PRAGMATISM

A strategy based on tax credits and selective government interventions is not the only possible course for reform, but it is the one most likely to avoid gridlock. The traditional political posturing on health care has run its course, at least for now. A Canadian-style, single-payer system that puts the government in charge of most of the critical decisions over health care spending runs contrary to the U.S. belief in individual control and freedom. And conservatives cannot ignore a problem that continues to get worse even in the best economic times. Perpetual gridlock is becoming unappealing to both political parties. Republicans are moving beyond their just-say-no approach to health care reform that started with their successful opposition to President Clinton's plan and has continued throughout the debate about managed care abuses. Indeed, the GOP's enactment of a Medicare prescription drug benefit is a major political achievement, even if the policy itself leaves much to be desired. Democrats chastened by their own failures have become more pragmatic in the efforts to help the uninsured.

The United States will not enact universal coverage simply because other industrialized nations have done so or because the uninsured are deserving. To be successful in American politics, progressive action must bind together the interests of the middle class and the interests of those who are struggling to get into the middle class. A strategy to increase coverage among the uninsured and choice among the insured may offer a real chance for the nation to move steadily toward universal coverage.

Notes

1. The following U.S. presidents have proposed universal health care coverage: Theodore Roosevelt, Franklin D. Roosevelt, Harry S. Truman, Richard Nixon, Gerald Ford, Jimmy Carter, and Bill Clinton. See Starr, P. *The Social Transformation of American Medicine.* New York: Basic Books, 1982.

2 Lemieux, J., Kendall, D., and Levine, S. "A Progressive Path Toward Universal Health Coverage." Washington, D.C.: Progressive Policy Institute, Dec. 2000.

3. Trude, S. "Who Has a Choice of Health Plans?" Washington, D.C.: Center for Studying Health System Change, Feb. 2000.

4. Lewis, K., Ellwood, M., and Czajka, J. L. *Counting the Uninsured: A Review of the Literature.* Occasional Paper No. 8. Washington, D.C.: Urban Institute, July 1998.

5. Copeland, C. "Characteristics of the Nonelderly with Selected Sources of Health Insurance and Lengths of Uninsured Spells." Washington, D.C.: Employee Benefits

Research Institute, June, 1998. See also Bennefield, R. L. *Dynamics of Economic Well-Being: Health Insurance, 1992 to 1993.* U.S. Bureau of the Census, Current Population Reports. Washington, D.C.: U.S. Government Printing Office, 1996; Swartz, K., Marcotte, J., and McBride, T. D. "Spells Without Health Insurance: The Distribution of Durations When Left-Censored Spells Are Included." *Inquiry,* Spring 1993, *30,* 77–83.

6. Swartz and others, "Spells Without Health Insurance."

7. Copeland, "Characteristics of the Nonelderly," p. 7.

8. American Association of Health Plans. *Health Care Choices.* Washington, D.C.: American Association of Health Plans, Dec. 1997, p. 1.

9. Fronstin, P. *Sources of Health Insurance and Characteristics of the Uninsured: Analysis of the March 1999 Current Population Survey.* Washington, D.C.: Employee Benefits Research Institute, Jan. 2000, p. 10.

10. American Association of Health Plans, *Health Care Choices,* p. 3.

11. Cunningham, P., Schaefer, E., and Hogan, C. "Who Declines Employer-Sponsored Health Insurance and Is Uninsured?" Washington, D.C.: Center for Studying Health System Change, Oct. 1999.

12. Weissman, J. S., Dryfoos, P., and London, K. "Income Levels of Bad-Debt and Free-Care Patients in Massachusetts Hospitals." *Health Affairs,* 1999, *18*(4), 156–166.

13. Hadley, J., Steinberg, E. P., and Feder, J. "Comparison of Uninsured and Privately Insured Hospital Patients: Condition on Admission, Resource Use, and Outcome." *Journal of the American Medical Association,* 1991, *265,* 374–379.

14. Strunk, B., and Cunningham, P. *Treading Water: Americans' Access to Needed Medical Care, 1997–2001.* Washington, D.C.: Center for Studying Health System Change, Mar. 2001.

15. Cunningham, P. *Choosing to Be Uninsured: Determinants and Consequences of the Decision to Decline Employer-Sponsored Health Insurance.* Washington, D.C.: Center for Studying Health System Change, Mar. 2001.

16. Trude, S., and Ginsberg, P. *Are Defined Contributions a New Direction for Employer-Sponsored Coverage?* Washington, D.C.: Center for Studying Health System Change, Oct. 2000.

17. Cunningham, P. J., Gross, J. M., St. Peter, R. F., and Lesser, C. S. "Managed Care and Physicians' Provision of Charity Care." *Journal of the American Medical Association,* 1999, *281,* 1087–1092.

18. Helms, R. "The Tax Treatment of Health Insurance: Early History and Evidence, 1940–1970." In G. M. Arnet (ed.), *Empowering Health Care Consumers Through Tax Reform.* Ann Arbor: University of Michigan Press, 1999, p. 11.

19. Atkinson, R. D., and Court, R. H. *New Economy Index: Understanding America's Economic Transformation.* Progressive Policy Institute. [www.neweconomyindex.org], Nov. 1998.

20. Atkinson and Court, *New Economy Index.*

21. Sheils, J. "Health Insurance and Taxes: The Impact of Proposed Changes in Current Federal Policy." Washington, D.C.: National Coalition on Health Care, Oct. 18, 1997, p. 7.

22. Butler, S., and Kendall, D. B. "Expanding Access and Choice for Health Care Consumers Through Tax Reform." *Health Affairs,* 1999, *18*(6), 45–57.

23. Ellwood, P., Enthoven, A., and Etheredge, L. "The Jackson Hole Initiatives for a Twenty-First Century Health Care System." *Health Economics,* 1992, *1*(3), pp. 149–168.

24. Pauly, M., Danzon, P. M., Feldstein, P. J., and Hoff, J. *Responsible National Health Insurance.* Washington, D.C.: AEI Press, 1992.

25. Marquis, M. S., and Long, S. H. "Worker Demand for Health Insurance in the Non-Group Market." *Journal of Health Economics,* 1995, *14*(1), 47–63.

26. Pauly, M. "An Adaptive Credit Plan for Covering the Uninsured." In J. Meyer and E. Wicks (eds.), *Covering America: Real Remedies for the Uninsured.* Washington, D.C.: Economic and Social Research Institute, June 2001.

27. Kendall, D. B., Lemieux, J., and Levine, S. R. "A Performance-Based Approach to Universal Health Care." in J. A. Meyer and E. K. Wicks, eds., *Covering America.* Washington, D.C.: Economic and Social Research Institute, 2003.

28. Lemieux and others, "A Progressive Path Toward Universal Health Coverage," pp. 6–8.

29. For example, see Pauly, "An Adaptive Credit Plan for Covering the Uninsured."

30. Pauly, "An Adaptive Credit Plan for Covering the Uninsured."

CHAPTER SEVENTY-TWO

The Politics of Consumer-Driven Health Care

Eric S. Berger, Carrie Gavora, Daniel H. Johnson

As the chapters in this book establish, consumer-driven health care is a real and growing phenomenon in the American marketplace. Yet, as a market movement, it remains in its infancy, taking small but important steps in its quest to win over new converts. As such, it has long operated under government policymakers' radar screen. In fact, until very recently, consumerism in health care advanced without explicit guidance or policy direction from government. In light of a variety of forces, however, government is beginning to act to facilitate the growing demands for change in the nation's health care system. The convergence of double-digit premium inflation; consumer, provider, and payer dissatisfaction; and a tort system run amuck has initiated new pleas for Washington to "do something." The promise of government activism presents both challenges and opportunities for proponents of consumer-driven health care and gives rise to difficult questions: What role might government play in this emerging market, and will the government's presence advance or retard the market's potential to serve consumers better?

The advances being made by consumer-driven health care pioneers suggest that government may take on the role of market modifier, recognizing the potential benefits of patient-centered innovation and acting to facilitate their widespread availability. The federal government does not often take proactive stances, however, and the history of its efforts to do so has been decidedly mixed. The pressure to address rising costs and patient and provider dissatisfaction is already guiding government to provide relief to its frustrated constituencies by making those statutory and regulatory changes needed to advance the consumer-driven health care marketplace.

As this chapter documents, the history of government action in health care, the problems faced today, the rise of consumer-driven health care innovations, and how and why those innovations speak to people are important elements of a changing environment in Washington. Much remains uncertain as this story unfolds, but one thing seems increasingly likely: regardless of the impetus, government action will have a significant impact on the efforts of market innovators and their ability to reach and serve America's health care consumers and providers.

GOOD INTENTIONS GONE WRONG?
GOVERNMENT'S ROLE IN HEALTH CARE

Over the past half-century, the federal government has acted to advance market changes by providing the incentives and protections deemed necessary to support and strengthen them. Most frequently, however, these activities occurred in response to the demands of broad communities and narrow but intense special interests alike. In the case of proactive governance, a compelling illustration can be seen in the promotion of prepaid health care as a means of controlling costs. With respect to government's acting in response to pressure, federal tax policy favoring employer-purchased health insurance stands out. In each case the government's actions have had a deep and lasting impact—and serve as a useful lesson as lawmakers and observers consider the politics of consumer-driven health care.

The Health Maintenance Organization (HMO) Act of 1973 is an apt example of government's taking a proactive role in establishing the scope and design of health coverage in the private marketplace. Until 1995, federal law required employers with more than twenty-five employees to offer HMOs as a health insurance option, provided $375 million in subsidies to the HMOs, and preempted state laws that "prohibited physicians for receiving payments for not providing care."[1] To be sure, the HMO Act was a response to employer demands for less costly health coverage options. But lawmakers were largely given an empty slate on which to develop policy in this area, as employers did not offer any uniform concept of how their desire for cheaper coverage could be satisfied. The Nixon administration also asked Congress to develop an alternative to traditional indemnity insurance that would build on the initial advances in the field of prepaid health care.

Although some question the magnitude of the impact the HMO Act has had on health care, Nancy Dickey, past president of the American Medical Association (AMA), believes it has had long-term significance. Indeed, the act is often credited with (or blamed for, depending on the perspective of the observer) the rise of managed care in the 1980s and 1990s that in turn led to the patients' rights debate that continues today. As Dickey relates, "Managed care was only allowed to happen by the federal leg up the HMO Act offered. We have literally seen the health marketplace transformed."[2]

An equally monumental impact can be found in the 1943 Internal Revenue Service (IRS) ruling on the tax treatment of employer-provided health care. Constrained in attracting workers by the wage and price controls imposed during World War II, many employers responded by offering modest health insurance benefits. To protect their employees from the tax implications of this initiative, employers excluded the cost of these benefits from employees' wages. Although confident of the appropriateness of their action, employers sought clarification from the IRS to confirm that this practice was in fact legal. In response, an IRS rule clarified that employer expenditures for employee health care could be excluded from both income and payroll taxes. When the IRS reversed itself a decade later and issued a rule stating that employer expenditures for health benefits were part of employees' gross income and therefore subject to taxation, angry constituents, faced with sharply increased tax liabilities, forced the Congress to codify the original ruling in statute.[3] Today the health care tax exclusion is viewed as an integral element of health coverage in America because it has enabled employer-provided insurance to become the norm. Indeed, the exclusion is now one of the largest and most valued government subsidies provided to working Americans, accounting for an estimated $70 billion in avoided income taxes in 2002.[4]

It appears that the government's foray into health policy has produced a mixed bag of results. Seeking to foster lower-cost coverage options, the HMO Act made prepaid health care a reality and the dominant form of health coverage today. As the political debate of the last decade suggests, however, the act also helped to trigger a consumer- and provider-led backlash that translated into efforts to further regulate the insurance market. Likewise, the government's tax ruling on employer-provided health coverage made work-based coverage the norm. But even though this change worked well for industrial age workers, who often remained at the same firm for much if not all of their careers, it is less practical for today's entrepreneurial economy and more mobile workers. This has resulted in unintended *job lock* and workers' inability to retain the same health coverage if they do move from job to job.

CURRENT PROBLEMS, COMPOUNDING PRESSURES

Whether they view it positively or negatively, most observers seem to agree that the government's efforts to encourage employment-based health benefits and managed care have come at a cost. The restrictions placed on patients' choice of coverage and access to their providers, the both real and perceived trade-offs between cost and quality, and a dramatic increase in health care costs over the last decade have generated deep dissatisfaction and demands for change. For years, the government has responded with policies that tinker around the edges of the cost and access problems without addressing the source of the underlying frustration: consumers' lack of control over their health care resources and decision making.

One initiative to address consumers' needs was the creation of tax-favored medical savings accounts. MSAs enable employers and consumers to deposit funds into individual accounts where they grow tax free until used for medical expenses. Used in conjunction with insurance policies covering major medical expenses, MSAs allow consumers to seek the care they need, from the providers they want, at a cost they agree to, thereby empowering them to exercise greater control and choice. That is good news. The bad news is that the legislation passed in 1996 to make MSA use more widespread interfered with the very objective it sought to achieve. Following heated negotiations, lawmakers imposed several requirements on medical savings accounts, including a limitation on the number of policies that could be sold, an expiration date on those policies, a mandate establishing very high deductibles and onerous funding schedules, and a cap restricting firms exceeding a certain size from offering MSAs. As a result of these requirements, few insurance companies have actively marketed MSAs, and the number of policyholders remains low.

Meanwhile, efforts to address cost, control, and access issues have focused on regulatory solutions. Frustrated with denial of coverage for certain services, patients and providers have appealed to legislatures and the courts to place benefits mandates and legal risk on insurers. In the case of mandates this effort has had dramatic success: according to the Blue Cross Blue Shield Association, the number of laws with mandated benefits and those affecting providers reached 1,400 in 2001, an increase of more than 50 percent in just five years.[5] At the same time, the federal government has joined what has long been a state-level activity, and is now a key locus in the patients' rights debate, with its *body-part* mandates (mandates about care for specific body parts) as well as sweeping legislation achieving broad support. There is a growing awareness by lawmakers, however, that the regulatory approach has significant limitations. Consumer and provider discontent remains strong, and higher costs now confront employers and enrollees alike. As a result, political interest in mandates and statutory liability is on the wane, and lawmakers appear to be increasingly receptive to alternative strategies.

With respect to inflationary forces, the American Benefits Council projects that the premiums for health insurance benefits for an entry-level worker in

2007 will equal half that worker's salary.[6] With the Consumer Price Index growing only 3.04 percent for the twelve-month period ending February 2003,[7] this growth trajectory is not sustainable. Projected annual inflation rates for hospital care, prescription drugs, and other medical services also deviate sharply from the rate for the general consumer-driven economy.

At the same time, satisfaction surveys are finding that an ever-growing number of Americans are seriously concerned about health care today—dissatisfaction among those with coverage appears to be at an all-time high. And as surveys also indicate, employers share this sentiment. According to a Hewitt Associates analysis, for example, fully 99 percent of employers are "significantly or critically" concerned about health care cost inflation, and 75 percent agree with their employees' dissatisfaction with the health benefits those employees currently receive.[8]

For years, these trends imposed a notable degree of policy-making paralysis, as lawmakers sought to address both their constituents' dissatisfaction and to stem the growth of costs. As a result the search has turned to a different approach to meeting the health care system's many and complex needs.

THE RISE OF MARKET INNOVATORS

In light of the flaws of existing coverage models, a growing cadre of innovative companies is offering products that seek to address the cost, access, and control problems faced by employers, providers, and consumers alike. The innovators' objective is to capitalize on the pervasive discontent and capture a sizable slice of the nation's substantial health care market. But their impact may be even greater than that because their efforts appear to be forging a new path for government and the health care system as a whole.

The concept promoted by many of these innovators is often referred to as *defined contribution* or *consumer-driven health care*. They share a focus on enabling consumers to control their health care resources and therefore health care decision making. Just as important, these firms are pioneering new approaches that seek to combine the best features of employer-provided coverage—risk pooling and tax preferences—with incentives that reward consumers for prudent purchases of health care resources. Consider, for example, the products offered by Definity Health. Definity offers an MSA-type spending account (often referred to as a *personal care account*) combined with a high-deductible policy and the capability to roll over unused funds. Definity also offers full coverage of preventive health care services and well-patient doctor visits to encourage preventive care among enrollees and often includes an annual checkup at no cost to the enrollee. A similar firm provides a personal care account for enrollees that covers annual costs up to a preset limit (such as $2,000), establishes a deductible over that amount (such as the costs between $2,000 and $3,000), places responsibility for covering the deductible on the enrollee, and typically covers all costs above the deductible. Both companies make detailed medical information available to enable their enrollees to make informed choices. Both companies' products are thus designed to encourage active self-management by the enrollee, thereby increasing his or her control.

Other innovative companies focus on the supplemental benefits not typically covered by insurance. For example, HealthAllies offers its members access to discounted prices for vision, dental, and similar services. Vivius has developed a system that allows individuals to create their own *provider panel* of physicians and ties their premium costs directly to the decisions they make. And Pinnacle Choice offers health care cards that enable members to obtain medical goods and services at discounts of up to 80 percent off the customary price.

Although their approaches to consumer-driven health care differ, all these firms share a common and critical incentive for enrollees: they provide greatly improved choice and quality that enable enrollees to manage their own health status and health care resources effectively and efficiently.

To be successful these market innovators must now move their consumer-driven offerings from the secondary to the primary health care market. Although once considered a long shot at best, such a transformation appears to be taking place, due to the growing popularity (and media coverage) of innovations such as those described here. Just as telling, large managed care insurers are making forays into the consumer-driven market. If this trend continues, patient-empowering innovations may become a necessary element of any competitive insurer's menu of product offerings.

Perhaps the most significant sign that consumer-driven health care is here to stay, however, is the changing dynamic in the health care market's demand side. Not long ago, paternalism characterized the employment-based health benefits system. Many employers believed they were in the best position to make coverage and resource allocation decisions for their employees. This perspective, although by no means entirely gone, is certainly on the wane. Faced with a choice between centralized control, rising costs, and dissatisfied employees on the one hand and decentralized control, contained costs, and empowered employees on the other, a steadily growing number of employers are making or seriously considering making the switch, something that was taboo even two or three years ago.

Finally, even what some believe is the last vestige of prepaid health care may be disappearing. For years, consumers accepted limited control and restricted choice as the prices to be paid for low copayments and deductibles. In recent years, however, they have experienced a sharp rise in the costs from which low copays and deductibles had once insulated them. As a result the trade-off no longer works for many enrollees, and the appeal of consumer-driven alternatives is growing.

These changes have taken place with little attention paid by the federal government. This benign neglect may be due in part to the fact that Washington has traditionally focused elsewhere, with some lawmakers holding to the notion that regulatory measures, such as the Patients' Bill of Rights legislation, may solve the health system's ills. But their almost singular focus on regulatory solutions has raised concerns about the potential impact of such regulations on market efficiency and consumer satisfaction. Meanwhile, the public's anti-HMO fervor is being cooled by a growing concern over costs, access, and the sustainability of the coverage people already have. As a result, sweeping patients' rights legislation has stalled in Congress, and lawmakers have begun to look elsewhere.

A NEW ROLE FOR GOVERNMENT

Following the demise of regulatory-oriented legislation, government has turned its attention to patient-empowering alternatives. Although the market for consumer-driven health care serves an ever-growing segment of the American population, it is still in its nascent stage. As a result, little clamor has been heard for governmental action that could expedite its development and adoption. Nevertheless, health policy experts who favor consumer-driven health care have been hard at work building a consensus that, like the tax exclusion and HMO Act, could reshape the nation's health care system. Their efforts have already resulted in a series of specific statutory and regulatory proposals. Although many of these changes may appear innocuous at first blush, they could have a profound impact on the widespread adoption of consumer-driven health plans and they now enjoy an active and growing constituency.

The evolving role of government is perhaps best demonstrated by the late 2003 legislation authorizing Health Savings Accounts (HSAs). Included in the Medicare "Prescription Drug, Improvement, and Modernization Act," the HSA provision was hailed by free-market advocates as an unusual and bold step to empower health care consumers. In essence, the HSA legislation creates an improved MSA, which, in conjunction with a basic insurance policy, is free from taxation, may be invested to earn tax-free interest, and is used to pay for allowable health care services (non-health care uses of HSA funds result in tax and penalty obligations). Deviating from the MSA restrictions, HSAs are available to the nearly 250 million Americans not enrolled in Medicare. As a result, the vast majority of America's working population now has access to a health account that is fully portable and directed by them for their own health care needs.

HSAs could have a significant impact on the nation's health care system—and the future direction of health care policy. Americans with insurance coverage will likely find the ability to fully deduct HSA deposits, especially because the tax-free benefit is not limited solely to those who itemize their taxes. Those who lose their jobs will be able to retain health care coverage if they have built up HSA reserves. Meanwhile, employers are expected to find HSAs attractive because it offers the ability to shift funds from premiums to tax-free contributions while enabling employees to also deposit funds into their HSA, thereby allowing for tax-free, out-of-pocket payments. Finally, providers may applaud the efficiencies made possible by the HSA legislation because it will enable many of them to operate on a cash payment basis and, thus, allow them to reduce their prices and attract more patients without the administrative costs often associated with insurance coverage. Even better, the empowerment made possible by HSAs will enable patients to be more mobile in selecting the providers they want to see, ensuring that the promise of a competitive market becomes a reality in health care.

The advances in cost, efficiency, and competition that HSAs may achieve could have profound implications beyond market dynamics, however. If HSAs fulfill their promise, elected representatives will not fail to notice the lesson: efforts to facilitate consumer-driven health care can generate electoral benefits, and efforts to legislate or regulate away consumer empowerment could lead to political peril. Whether this connection is made depends in large part on the market's response to the HSA legislation—and on the role that advocates play in guiding government to additional needed reforms, such as allowing Section 125 health account balances to roll over into the new HSAs, removing state regulations and mandates that may interfere with the use of HSAs, and bringing the favorable dynamics enjoyed by the government's FEHBP system to market-based buying groups.

Either way, the first decade of the Twenty-First Century already has produced some very interesting political markers. Whereas some of the efforts already achieved or underway focus on changes needed to remove obstacles that have been created by government, others seek to reduce the number of uninsured through effective tax policy, to assist in educated decision making through expanded access to information, and to ameliorate unsustainable trends in liability through tort reform. Regardless of their specific nature, these initiatives indicate a growing and often bipartisan desire to forge new paths to address the health care system's woes—a desire that may bode well as market and political support for consumer-driven health care expands.

CONSUMER-DRIVEN POLITICS

The problems plaguing this nation's health care system, like the system itself, are large and therefore difficult to characterize accurately at a glance. But this storm cloud may carry an unusual silver lining: political pressure arising from widespread frustration has compelled government to take action, and that action may foster the consumer-driven marketplace that will best address the system's flaws.

The reader will be forgiven for greeting the prospect of government activism with a shudder. After all, the history of government's health policy role—both proactive and reactive—cannot be viewed as a story of resounding successes. The government can, however, be recognized as a force that may foster patient empowerment *if* it is subjected to the politics of consumer-driven health care. In this vocal society, discontent is not kept quiet long—and in that reality rests hope that the frustrations of patients, providers, employers, and even lawmakers will be translated into free market-oriented action.

What might the politics of consumer-driven health care mean for this market's future? As discontent with the status quo continues to rise, government action that could nip this promising flower in the bud (such as expanded market regulation) will come under increasing scrutiny. Likewise, when today's discontented constituencies become tomorrow's active advocates for change and for the innovative products developed by market pioneers, lawmakers will find political gain in fostering patient empowerment through such measures as those discussed here. In this manner consumer-driven politics for consumer-driven health care can help ensure that government action—whether undertaken to modify, or more likely to react to, the market—will be designed to meet the growing needs of the new and multifaceted consumer-driven health care constituency.

To be sure, the politics of consumer-driven health care are only now beginning to be felt. Nevertheless, one conclusion may already be made: the genie has left the bottle, and she's not going to be easily restrained again. As consumers experience products that reveal what a patient-centered, consumer-driven, provider-friendly health care system can be, consumers and caregivers alike are unlikely to allow that promise to go unfulfilled. Rather, they can be expected to play an increasingly active role in supporting, protecting, and furthering market innovations. And as the politics of consumer-driven health care grow, so too will the likelihood that the federal government will take even more action supportive of consumer-driven health care.

Notes

1. Brase, T. "Blame Congress for HMOs." Citizens Council on Health Care. [www.cchconline.org/privacy/hmoast.php3], Sept. 2003.

2. Mitka, M. "A Quarter Century of Health Maintenance." *Journal of the American Medical Association,* 1998, *280,* 2059.

3. Helms, R. "The Tax Treatment of Health Insurance: Early History and Evidence, 1940–1970." In G.-M. Arnett (ed.), *Empowering Health Care Consumers Through Tax Reform.* Ann Arbor: University of Michigan Press, 1999, p. 11.

4. Joint Committee on Taxation. *Estimates of Federal Tax Expenditures for Fiscal Years 2002–2006*. JCS-1-02. Washington, D.C.: U.S. Government Printing Office, Jan. 17, 2002.

5. Laudicina, S., Losleben, B., and Walker, N. "State Legislative Health Care and Insurance Issues: 2001 Survey of Plans." Washington, D.C.: Blue Cross Blue Shield Association, Dec. 2001.

6. American Benefits Council. "Health Premiums Predicted to Cost Nearly Half of Entry-Level Salaries by 2007: Employers May Be Forced to Choose Between Coverage and New Workers." News Release. Washington, D.C.: American Benefits Council, May 15, 2002.

7. Federal Reserve Bank of St. Louis. [www.research.stlouisfed.org/fred2/data]. Sept. 2003.

8. Hewitt Associates. *Health Care Expectations: Future Strategy and Direction, 2001*. Lincolnshire, Ill.: Hewitt Associates, 2002.

CHAPTER SEVENTY-THREE

Health Care

What Role for Regulation?

Karen Ignagni

When a marketplace is in transition, how should it be regulated? When regulation is dispersed among state and federal agencies, where should the locus of authority lie? When controversies arise, how can regulators distinguish between genuinely protecting consumers and protecting established interests against the challenges of change? What should be the test for government intervention? In an arena that arouses intense emotions, is it possible to design and maintain a regulatory model guided more by data than by anecdotes?

To some these questions may sound abstract or academic. They certainly have not been getting much attention in the nation's capital, where for the past half-dozen years the health care debate has rarely risen above the level of a partisan point-scoring contest. Indeed, hopes for holding any kind of substantive discussion soon are slim. But this simply points up the need to begin laying the groundwork for that discussion now.

Many if not most thoughtful Americans would actively welcome the substitution of a genuine discussion of health care regulation for today's thinly disguised mud-wrestling bouts. Recent polls show that voters by large margins believe politicians are using health care controversies to advance their own careers rather than trying to find ways to protect their constituents. This is an encouraging sign that voters are ready to move on—and up. People now realize that health care, like it or not, simply had to change—that the old system desperately needed an overhaul. They recognize that the inefficiencies and lack of accountability in the old system led to vast amounts of inappropriate care.

They see the connection between the rising cost of coverage and the high numbers of uninsured Americans, particularly children. Anxious for their parents or thinking about their own retirement, they realize that Medicare is on borrowed time unless efficiencies and incentives are put in place to make care both more affordable and more accountable. And despite being besieged by health plan horror stories, they appreciate what health plans offer and pronounce themselves well satisfied with the plan in which they participate.

This last is a very important point. By and large, consumers are putting aside the kinds of blind prejudices that can stymie efforts to reshape the health care debate. They may worry about receiving quality care or getting a coverage dispute resolved promptly, but surveys show that they are also suspicious of self-serving rhetoric aimed at dividing the world, Hollywood-style, into black hats and white hats, with HMOs routinely typecast as the heavies and all critics of HMOs assumed to be without blemish. They are suspicious too of panaceas such as the notion that turning back the clock or replacing the marketplace with a centrally controlled system would somehow resolve all our problems. In short, the public, increasingly sophisticated in health care policy matters and resentful of being manipulated by politicians and commentators, may be more ready for a substantive debate than the political spinmeisters realize.

If this hypothesis holds, then it is incumbent upon academics and corporate leaders to do the hard work of laying a foundation for this next level of the health care debate. That requires addressing and answering the kinds of questions outlined at the beginning of this chapter.

To help us shape this process, some core assumptions may be useful:

- Our goal should be to protect the public—period. The present regulatory system, coupled with the present superheated political climate, is a dangerously combustible mixture that lends itself all too readily to the purposes of those who have more to gain from pouring fuel on flames than from extinguishing them. As a fire-prevention measure, we should subject every regulatory proposal to a careful test of whom it is really intended to protect: consumers or those behind the proposal? When the principal effect of a proposed regulation would be to allow various interests to go on with business as usual, or as it used to be, that proposal should be set aside. Our focus should be on taking only those steps that meet the test of consumer protection—such as providing external review of coverage disputes, an approach that can remove barriers to care without undermining the principle of care management.

- Reducing the number of uninsured Americans should be of primary importance. At a time when more than forty-three million Americans lack health insurance, proposals that would increase health care costs and put coverage even further out of reach are irresponsible. More than twenty-seven cents out of every new health care dollar spent is expended on dealing with lawsuits or coping with government red tape or is spent to no effect (systemwide waste). Our goal should be to cut the current waste out of the system and be vigilant in resisting additional waste in order to make health insurance an affordable reality for more Americans.

- We should be moving toward a unified philosophy of regulation. The present hodgepodge of state, federal, quasi-governmental, and non-governmental regulation of health plans begs for reform. Growing without benefit of blueprints, it satisfies no one. Health plans find it burdensome in the extreme; purchasers and consumers of care find it unresponsive to their needs and expectations. Politicians, meanwhile, compound the problem by stuffing additional regulatory requirements into the matrix without regard to their overall impact. An accumulation of mandates, body part by body part, does not add up to a coherent regulatory theory. If the Hippocratic maxim—"first, do no harm"—were to be applied to the regulatory sphere, we might well opt for a moratorium on new requirements pending the evolution of a dynamic, responsive, marketplace-sensitive regulatory philosophy that balances the need for broad oversight against the impetus toward multilayered micromanagement. To create such a model, we may need to look beyond the limitations of the present system in order to build an evidence-driven, public-private regulatory process that responds to consumers' needs.

- Across-the-board consistency should be of paramount concern. At its present stage, the health care regulatory debate is a one-sided affair, largely focused on the perceived flaws of managed care rather than on systematically raising the bar for the health care system in its entirety. As a result the level of accountability required of health plans, and their burden of compliance, far exceeds that required of the fee-for-service sector. Leaving aside issues of fairness and systemwide quality improvement, this perpetuates a vicious cycle in which consumers, hearing only of the alleged failures of one part of the system, demand redress, and at the same time operate under the misimpression that no aspect of the old system needs equivalent attention.

- Performance standards are preferable to central control. As a practical matter, there is no way to put a regulator in every examining room or at the elbow of every decision maker at every health plan (and even if this approach were feasible, Americans would forcefully reject it). Regulatory efforts should be more focused on identifying and addressing anomalies rather than compounding the number of requirements that health plans must meet as a condition of being allowed to operate.

- Generally, we should encourage rather than punish. The still-evolving health care marketplace should be allowed to measure up to its highest potential—and to demonstrate its progress—rather than being distorted and held back by the imposition of complex, overlapping, micromanaging regulations that are, among other things, inherently inconsistent with the national goal of keeping health care affordable.

- The test for regulatory intervention in health care should be as strictly objective as possible. As in other fields, regulators should be more concerned with identifying and addressing patterns of substandard performance than with reacting to anecdotal accusations. This is a difficult area for regulators and their political overseers. To illustrate, the wrong way to make health care practices more transparent is to broaden the field of malpractice litigation, which among other things creates compelling reasons for practitioners to conceal their failures. The better way is to assiduously collect and scrutinize data on practice patterns and outcomes in order to identify outliers and encourage the broadest possible adherence to best practices.

The present health care debate has been limited by its size—too big or too small. From the Clinton health care proposal we learned, or should have learned, that sweeping efforts to rapidly transform the entire health care system are unlikely to meet with public approval. At the other extreme the legislative debacles of the more recent past should teach us that incrementally micromanaging one part of the health care system, ostensibly in the name of patient protection, simply leaves the ills of the old system unaddressed while undermining public support for change.

We can do better. Without for a moment underestimating the complexity of the regulatory challenge, we should be guided by the public's common sense—that is, our collective ability to set reasonable objectives designed to meet reasonable expectations—and by the need to develop a regulatory framework consistent with the basic goal of delivering accountable care at affordable cost.

Although few topics are more emotional than health care, there is at the same time a deepening public understanding of the perfectibility of the system within which care is organized, delivered, and managed to maximize effectiveness. Indeed, a demonstrable commitment to perfectibility is at the heart of true consumer protection. An approach to regulation based on this commitment—geared to identifying opportunities for improvement and to encouraging rather than limiting innovations aimed at continually raising the bar—will be worthy of public support.

There are of course those who simply do not believe that a marketplace economy can simultaneously serve the goals of corporate stockholders and consumers. Acting on that belief, they argue for regulating with a heavy, all-encompassing hand. But the heavier the hand, the more the belief that the marketplace will fail to deliver becomes a self-fulfilling prophecy. For those who believe, conversely, that a healthy marketplace offers the most promising antidote to the debilitating disease of overregulation and micromanagement, it has become an urgent matter to design—and communicate—a coherent and comprehensible regulatory approach that attracts support by clearly addressing public concerns and expectations.

That in broad strokes is the challenge we face now. When we meet it, the health care debate will rise to the level that the public expects—and is ready for.

CHAPTER SEVENTY-FOUR

Adult Health Insurance

Ken Abramowitz

Defined benefit programs are evil, because they treat beneficiaries as children. They will be replaced by defined contribution programs, because they treat beneficiaries as adults.

Two major forms of consumerism exist in the health care system today: *adult* consumerism and *infantile* consumerism. By far, infantile consumerism predominates, as it is a natural by-product of defined benefit health insurance purchased either by employers or by the government. Under this system, consumers buy highly subsidized insurance and are largely ignorant of the total costs involved as well as the financial ramifications of any particular service used. In turn, consumers demand unlimited amounts of service and freedom, and they become indignant when they do not receive instant service. Adult consumerism is displayed by the 10 percent of the working population who pay for health care insurance as individual consumers, unaffiliated with corporate buyers, as they are spending their own money. These consumers have a chance of behaving like adults because they are spending their own money and can make their own informed trade-offs among levels of deductibles and copayments and levels of freedom of provider choice.

As happened when corporations converted pension funds from defined benefit plans into defined contribution plans (401[k]s), a major opportunity exists for both corporate America and the government (the Medicare and Medicaid programs and the Department of Veterans Affairs) to move to *managed* defined contribution health plans. In this new system, employers would simply gross up the salaries of their employees and then allocate vouchers of $5,000 to $7,000 per family and $1,500 to $2,000 per single employee, so that employees could purchase a variety of family health plans for $7,000 to $12,000, depending on the benefits desired. Through such cafeteria-like benefit structures, the employees could make trade-offs among the freedoms desired and the expenses involved. The employer would still play a major role in employee education and health plan negotiation. The insurance carriers would continue to play a major role in provider network creation, provider payment negotiation, medical management, and disease management.

A less-managed alternative model could be employed for the nearly 15 percent of the total population (close to 25 percent of the working population) who are uninsured. By enacting a modest defined contribution health insurance mandate, subsidized by tax credits or deductions (depending on income level), the government could require 100 percent of these people to buy at least catastrophic health insurance, stripped of traditional insurance mandates. In turn, this population segment (and only this segment) should be authorized to establish MSAs. Through this mechanism these people would be empowered to become adult consumers.

If this experiment were successful, some might suggest that this model for the uninsured be expanded to those insured by corporate America or the government. However, there is a pitfall here. Individual consumers, acting alone and without help of corporate America, are likely to pay far higher prices and receive lower-quality care than that provided by the best-managed care plans. After all, the consumers who choose to spend $5.00 for Tylenol's $0.25 of acetaminophen will quickly run out of money. Consequently, we should maintain distinct policies and rules for the insured population and the uninsured population, as these segments have very different problems to overcome. The insured segment has a cost problem, and the uninsured segment has an access problem. Both problems can and must be solved separately.

CHAPTER SEVENTY-FIVE

AmeriChoice Corporation

The Personal Care Model

Anthony Welters

meriChoice Corporation is a diversified health care company that owns and operates health plans in New York, New Jersey, and Pennsylvania. AmeriChoice concentrates on the public sector market—Medicare, Medicaid, and government programs for children and the uninsured. The people AmeriChoice serves are those among us with the greatest needs, both medical and socioeconomic. (United Health Group bought AmeriChoice on June 18, 2002, for $560 million.)

THE PERSONAL CARE MODEL

In the late 1990s, AmeriChoice reevaluated its approach to delivering health care. The company, of which I am a founder and also chairman and CEO, historically has been committed to working with community-based organizations to improve the health and social infrastructures of the communities it serves. AmeriChoice, for example, was among the first health plans to develop school-based health clinics and to seed local physician practices in underserved areas. After nearly a decade, however, the company decided to build upon this community-based approach by shifting the focus to the individual member.

The AmeriChoice Personal Care Model™ (PCM) provides holistic and ongoing care planning and management to AmeriChoice members with chronic and catastrophic health needs. This approach addresses all the factors—medical, social, and environmental—that affect the individual's health status. In trying to maintain or improve health status, the PCM draws not only on medical resources but on social and economic resources as well. For example, a pregnant teen is linked not only with an obstetrician for prenatal care but with volunteers from a local women's association, who visit with the young woman through her baby's birth and after, offering advice and helping her learn parenting skills.

The Personal Care Model differs from traditional case management in two important ways:

- It emphasizes face-to-face contact with the member and the development of an ongoing relationship. In contrast, traditional case management is carried out by telephone, is targeted toward the provider, and stresses management of acute episodes.

- It recognizes that medical needs cannot be separated from an individual's social environment. Personal Care Unit care managers look not only for medical remedies but for practical, everyday solutions to maintain or improve health status.

The PCM is designed to control the cost of care provided by AmeriChoice plans. It does so by making care more effective through increased plan and provider accountability to the members served.

NEEDS STATEMENT

It is an unfortunate but well-documented fact that the medically underserved, low-income population experiences greater morbidity than the population at large. The costs of treating the most needy members of society, at more than $180 billion each year for Medicaid alone, are huge, consuming significant portions of federal and state budgets. Managed care was embraced by the states in the early 1990s as a means of controlling the costs of care for the Medicaid population. So too has Congress expanded managed care under the Medicare program in recent years as a means of controlling the costs of that program.

Traditional managed care models cannot meet the needs of the medically underserved population. Housing, transportation, and even access to simple forms of communication, such as a telephone in the home, are likely to be problems faced by the underserved. These challenges of daily living are exacerbated when the individual also faces a health problem, and may be insurmountable when the individual suffers from a chronic health condition that requires compliance with a complex medical regimen.

Disease management as practiced by health plans serving an employed, commercial membership will not suffice for the medically underserved. These persons require a more hands-on method of assistance in dealing with the health and life challenges they face. AmeriChoice's Personal Care Model embodies that hands-on approach.

SIZE OF MARKET

In determining which members to target in the initial phase of applying the Personal Care Model, AmeriChoice identified those chronic conditions for which there are proven interventions that can prevent or delay complications:

Diabetes

Congestive heart failure

Asthma and other pulmonary disease

HIV/AIDS and other chronic infections

High-risk pregnancies, including teen pregnancies

Complex and catastrophic cases (such as ventilator dependency)

Sickle cell disease

These are conditions found disproportionately among medically underserved, low-income populations. AmeriChoice estimates, for example, that as many as 10 to 15 percent of its Medicaid members have one or more of these conditions. Extrapolating that figure to the Medicaid population nationwide means that at least five million persons could benefit from the PCM approach. Its significance for the Medicare population is even greater, as the incidence of some of these targeted conditions increases with age.

PCM OPERATION

The Personal Care Model involves a number of interrelated steps, beginning with early identification of members at risk; continuing with evaluation of at-risk members' health status and living conditions; and culminating with the development, implementation, and refinement of the care plan. The model requires the active participation of all who come into contact with the member, including health plan representatives, providers, lay caregivers, family, friends, and community groups.

A health risk assessment is performed with each AmeriChoice member within the first month of the individual's enrollment in the health plan. The assessment surveys the member's health status, permitting early identification of chronic conditions or other special needs. The results of the assessment are forwarded to the member's primary care physician (PCP) and to the member's care manager within the AmeriChoice health plan. PCM candidates are also identified through health plan data, such as a record of frequent hospitalizations. They are also identified through referrals from PCPs and community-based organizations.

Personal care managers, a nurse and social worker team, visit with members who have been identified through the health risk assessment, plan data, or referrals as candidates for the PCM. They complete a broad-based assessment of the individual's status, including medical, emotional, and socioeconomic factors. Input from family members, friends, and caregivers is sought in order to obtain as complete an understanding as possible of the individual's situation. Finally, physicians who have been involved in the individual's care meet with the personal care managers to develop a comprehensive plan of care for the individual.

The care plan is implemented through a working partnership between the PCM member's primary care physician and an AmeriChoice personal care manager. The plan might call for a number of environmental interventions, such as making physical changes to the individual's living space, identifying alternative housing, or arranging for transportation services and home-delivered meals, in addition to strictly medical interventions. The plan might also involve community resources—churches, fraternal organizations, social service agencies—in the individual's care. The focus of the plan is to keep the individual well and in the community and to provide him or her with the resources needed to maintain the highest functional status possible.

The personal care manager coordinates care and monitors implementation of the care plan through home visits and contacts with the PCP and other providers of services. The personal care manager troubleshoots as problems arise and, working with the member and the PCP, suggests necessary revisions to the care plan as circumstances warrant or as the individual's condition changes. (Three illustrative case studies of the AmeriChoice Personal Care Model in action can be found at the end of this chapter.)

The tenets of the Personal Care Model are diffused throughout all areas of operation of the AmeriChoice health plans. The customer service representatives, for example, who staff the AmeriChoice twenty-four-hours-a-day, seven-days-a-week customer call center are schooled in the model and trained to be alert for needs that members may express that go beyond the medical. Providers are encouraged to subscribe to the Personal Care Model, and those who do receive priority handling. And all employee orientation and periodic in-service training includes sections on the PCM. It is AmeriChoice's intent to imbue every aspect of its operations with the Personal Care Model mission, enabling members to obtain the highest possible levels of health and social function.

EFFICACY AND COST EFFECTIVENESS

An immediate, measurable goal of the PCM is to reduce the number of hospitalizations experienced by AmeriChoice members with chronic conditions. Inpatient hospital stays consume more than one-half of Medicaid and Medicare dollars. Reducing their number results in immediate cost savings. The PCM also seeks to ameliorate the severity of a condition or disease and prevent its adverse consequences. Improving the dietary and medical compliance of persons with diabetes, for example, can forestall or prevent entirely complications typically associated with that condition, such as amputation and blindness.

The methods used under the Personal Care Model to obtain these results require some expenditure. The PCM entails intensive staffing not found in traditional care management models. It can also involve expenditures for housing, transportation, and other social supports that are not typically paid for by health plans. These staffing and other expenditures are generally more than offset by the reduction in medical costs that results from improved member compliance with a medical regimen.

Analysis of our data reveals a 47 percent reduction in inpatient days and a 47 percent reduction in inpatient costs for a cohort of 145 AmeriChoice members with severe asthma during a thirteen-month period in which they received PCM services, compared to their utilization and costs during a similar period without PCM services. Even more impressive was a study we conducted of 98 AmeriChoice members with diabetes, half of whom were covered by the PCM and half not covered, over a twenty-two month period. The report showed that inpatient admissions were cut by 51 percent and inpatient costs were a tremendous 65 percent lower when the members were in the PCM.

BARRIERS TO DIFFUSION

The effectiveness of the Personal Care Model depends on the organization's commitment to devoting the resources necessary to solving members' problems. The model will not prove effective unless everyone in the company is committed to doing what is necessary to ensure success. The PCM is not health care as usual. It requires care managers and providers to innovate on a daily basis in order to find creative solutions to members' problems. It requires dedication and perseverance to work through the many and varied life challenges faced by AmeriChoice's members.

These intangible requirements are perhaps the biggest barrier to the widespread adoption of the Personal Care Model by the health care system. The Personal Care Model is not easy; it exacts a toll on staff who are used to a more well defined and comfortable workload. For many physicians the Personal Care

Model demands a far greater involvement in a patient's care and living situation than they are accustomed to providing. And it is not easy for members either. Although the PCM provides the tools they need to better manage their disease and their lives, it will not work unless the members are prepared to partner with the health plan and assume responsibility for following their care plan.

EFFECT OF CONSUMER-DRIVEN HEALTH CARE

The Personal Care Model is consistent with and supportive of the movement in the states and the federal government to empower consumers of health care. The PCM attempts to give individuals the support and tools they need to lead healthier lives. It must be recognized that it is far simpler to empower the middle-class consumer through legislation than it is to afford the same rights to low-income persons. Having the "right" to go out of network for certain services is a wonderful right if there are doctors who are ready and willing to treat you. It is far less meaningful to those who live in an area where medical services are limited and who lack the means to travel outside that neighborhood. The Ameri-Choice Personal Care Model represents a means of empowering these health care consumers through the coordinated efforts of the consumer and his or her caregivers.

CONCLUSION

The AmeriChoice Personal Care Model establishes a new paradigm for health care delivery to the medically underserved. The PCM expands the focus of care for those with chronic conditions, looking beyond the disease or condition to the total environment in which the individual lives. The PCM changes the role of the health plan from mere payer to an active participant in the lives of its most vulnerable members. The following case studies show the AmeriChoice Personal Care Model in action.

V.C. is forty-five years old, single, and lives with her daughter, who has been diagnosed with schizophrenia, and her ten-year-old grandson.

V.C. suffers from congestive heart failure and diabetes. She is insulin dependent. She just moved to a new apartment about one month ago. She and her family pay $375 per month for their small apartment. They frequently run out of food because their total household income of $730 per month just covers rent and utilities.

The Personal Care Unit received a referral from the plan's Member Services Department. One of the social workers from the unit made a home visit to V.C. and her family. She noted the roach-infested conditions. There was no furniture—
V.C. and her daughter and grandson slept on dirty pieces of foam on the floor. The

grandson had never slept in a bed. V.C. injected her insulin herself twice a day without checking her blood sugar—she had no glucometer.

The personal care manager arranged to have furniture donated to the family by a charity, a St. Vincent De Paul store. Volunteers from the AmeriChoice health plan, using the AmeriChoice van, delivered the furniture. The family now has two full beds, a sofa, and a dinette set. They have also been connected with various food pantries in the area. The plan's Home Care Department sent out a glucometer and scale the day following the social worker's assessment. This was followed by a skilled nursing visit and instruction on use of the instrument. The personal care manager maintains contact with the family and V.C.'s PCP to continue coordinating their care.

D.H. is a twenty-three-year-old African American female who lives with sickle cell disease. AmeriChoice records indicate repeated hospital admissions to facilities throughout the plan's service area. Sometimes she had as many as three hospitalizations in one week. Because of this history, she was identified as a potential PCM member.

The first time a personal care manager met with D.H. she was a hospital inpatient. She was found to be a bright young woman who reported that her sister had died in the previous year of sickle cell complications. D.H. lives with her aunt but frequently stays with other relatives. She has never seen her PCP, who does not specialize in sickle cell disease. When D.H. has pain, she becomes frightened, and the relatives she is visiting at that time take her to the nearest hospital. This explains the hospital hopping.

With D.H.'s permission, her personal care manager changed her PCP to a physician with a large sickle cell practice. The timing was fortunate. While the personal care manager was making a home visit, D.H. complained of leg pain and was able to be immediately evaluated by the doctor. She was admitted to the hospital with deep vein thrombosis and immediately began treatment with her new PCP.

Transportation was also a problem for D.H., making it difficult for her to keep doctor's appointments. With the help of the health plan, an application for an area transportation program was initiated. The plan will also provide a cab voucher if necessary.

D.H. developed a fever after discharge from the hospital. She was visiting her grandfather, and he immediately took her to the nearest hospital—but not the one with which D.H.'s new PCP was affiliated. Subsequently, a member of the plan's inpatient case management team was able to assist in her transfer to her PCP's facility for IV antibiotics once her condition was stable. This promoted continuity of care. The Home Care Department was involved when she was discharged from the hospital, following up with skilled nursing visits.

The current plan is to provide D.H. with a level of comfort by maintaining frequent contact with her and encouraging her frequent contact with her PCP and compliance with the PCP's advice. With the help of her physician and the many resources of the AmeriChoice departments, we hope to provide D.H. with a better understanding of her disease, thereby giving her the knowledge to help direct her own care. This will have the impact of reducing her medical costs and, more important, will improve her quality of life by allowing her to maintain healthy functioning as an outpatient.

D.M. lives alone and recently broke her clavicle and could not perform activities of daily living (ADLs). This AmeriChoice member is legally blind, suffers from hypertension and chronic obstructive pulmonary disease, and was malnourished, weighing eighty-three pounds at five feet three inches in height. She also had a history of heart surgery dating to December 1998.

The personal care manager developed a plan of action for this member. This plan included a referral to the Association for the Blind and a referral to Elderly Waiver Services. D.M. was also encouraged to make an appointment for an orthopedic follow-up, and an appointment was subsequently confirmed. In addition, D.M.'s case manager called her PCP to request a home health agency skilled nursing visit to assess her nutritional status; homemaker services were begun as a result of this intervention. Finally, a social worker from the plan visited D.M. in her home to assess safety and psychosocial needs.

This member appreciated the interventions that helped her remain in her residence. Her quality of life was significantly improved.

CHAPTER SEVENTY-SIX

The Uninsured and Access

Constance G. Jackson

Truly transformative changes in the U.S. health care system must result in two outcomes: increased health insurance coverage that is as close to universal as possible and increased access to health care services. Consumer-driven health care provides better solutions to the issue of health insurance coverage but a significant government role is required to increase access.

UNIVERSAL HEALTH COVERAGE

Health insurance coverage is fast becoming a luxury. The number of uninsured in the United States—after reaching a high of forty-three million, or 16 percent of the population, in 1997 and then declining significantly in 1999 and 2000—began rising again in 2001 as unemployment levels rose. This phenomenon, which started during one of the strongest economic booms of the post–World War II period, signals increases of historic proportions in those without health coverage over the current economic downturn. With most of the current job growth coming from small businesses—many of which cannot afford health insurance coverage or are unwilling to shift resources away from profit-generating activities to provide it—the role of employers in health insurance purchasing will be decreasing, and that will be a significant opening for forging a consumer-driven health care system.

The current employer-driven system has resulted in an increasing number of people who work and yet are uninsured. They are unable to afford health insurance, but they are not poor and therefore they do not qualify for Medicaid, the federal health insurance program for the indigent. In addition, this system is also resulting in increasing numbers of uninsured children because, even when there is employer-provided coverage for the employee, many employees cannot afford to purchase dependent coverage. The health needs of the working uninsured and their families are increasingly straining the safety net system of public hospitals (often through inappropriate use of hospital emergency rooms), community health centers, and free clinics designed to treat the indigent uninsured. (The number of the poor who are uninsured has remained relatively constant at about nine million people, or 29.5 percent of those considered poor under federal poverty guidelines.) Lacking insurance, the working uninsured often avoid seeking primary and preventive care. When care is sought, a complicated calculus begins: "Can I do without the lab tests?" "Will half of the prescription be enough or can we use the leftover antibiotics from last year?" When the decision becomes, "Let's get one of little David's prescriptions and split it among the other kids," the end result can be one or more trips to a hospital emergency room. The longer-term consequence is to rob children of the most important ingredient in attaining a healthy life: a sense of entitlement. The child who learns to associate seeking health care with humiliation and anxiety is likely to become an adult who avoids seeking care except in the most extreme circumstances, thus creating another generation that loses the numerous benefits of preventive care.

The new uninsured are the young, those who are self-employed or employed by small businesses (according to the Census Bureau, 52 percent of the increase in those lacking health coverage in 2000 had annual household incomes in excess of $75,000), illegal immigrants, and those making the often rocky transition from welfare to work.

A consumer-driven health care system should move us closer to universal coverage. How rapidly this change occurs will depend on what forms of tax incentives and penalties are introduced and how quickly they take effect. If incentives are phased in at a dilatory pace over several years, consumers will make incremental changes and exploit any market inefficiencies in the transition. If incentives are immediate, consumers will make rapid adaptations where they perceive the benefit is substantial and within their short-term time horizon.

Any system based on tax incentives, whether in the form of a defined contribution account using pretax dollars or in the form of a tax credit, will be effective in motivating the behavior of the vast majority of consumers. However, the working poor—with household income around twice the federal poverty level (about $25,000 for a family of three)—may not be motivated. They are often too "rich" to qualify for most forms of government assistance, including Medicaid, and they already receive refunds of a substantial portion of their withheld taxes from the earned income tax credit. For these families the financial equation is often rounded to the nearest penny and the loss of one pretax dollar can drastically upset that balance. In this case, incentives and penalties for employers, who need productive employees, may be necessary.

Although coverage against catastrophic events would protect families from financial ruin in the event of serious disease, it could also be a factor that contributes to illness because it does not provide coverage for routine physical exams. Any mandated health coverage must make some provision for age-adjusted primary care, such as an annual physical exam or mammogram, to encourage preventive care and early detection of potentially serious illnesses. Without such coverage, many will forgo any routine care until they are in pain or unable to work. Often, by the time a condition is symptomatic, it is much more difficult and costly to treat.

ACCESS TO HEALTH CARE

The issue of access presents challenges that a consumer-driven system may not be able to fully answer. Those with little or no access to health care typically fall into two categories. They are either residents of rural or urban communities with no health providers within a reasonable distance or they are residents of poor or urban communities with health providers who do not provide accessible or culturally competent care. In the former case, the communities tend to be poor and isolated, both geographically and economically. Without government assistance, such as programs that forgive the medical school loans of physicians who practice in these areas for a stated number of years, these communities have little chance of attracting health care providers, even if all their residents are insured. In the latter case, although the communities have health care providers, those providers are either not willing or not able to provide care suited to community needs. For example, providers may not accept Medicaid insurance because of the low reimbursement rates, the slow payment, and the additional documentation required. Some restrict Medicaid patients to certain days and times, not wanting them to mix with their private insurance patients, resulting in long waits for visits.

Severely economically disadvantaged clients usually require supportive services such as transportation and child care if they are to access the health care system. In addition, they may require social services, either through referral to services like family counseling or through direct intervention such as negotiation with a landlord to increase the apartment temperature for an asthmatic child. These services are subsidized by government funding but are not usually reimbursed by private insurance. These needs, if unmet, coupled with racial and cultural differences and language barriers, can make interaction with the health care system an unpleasant and negative experience for those who may most need its care.

Increasing Medicaid rates so that they achieve at least parity with most private insurers' rates (or pay a premium to those physicians who provide supportive services) and streamlining the reimbursement process are the most effective ways to increase access.

Throughout the mid- to late 1990s, many state governments received permission from the federal government to compel their Medicaid patients to enroll in managed care plans. In most cases patients had to choose a plan or be randomly assigned to one. In Illinois the introduction of Medicaid managed care initially resulted in competition among hospitals, community providers, and traditional managed care companies to enroll the state's 1.3 million Medicaid patients in their plans before the mandatory assignment period began. The intense competition precipitated the development of health plans specifically geared to the needs of the Medicaid market, offering features such as free transportation services and free voice mail for enrollees without telephones. Door-to-door marketing and advertising on urban and foreign-language radio stations was conducted to reach potential enrollees, and a major campaign to contract with a diverse group of physicians, including traditional Medicaid providers, ensued. With capitated payments for Medicaid that offered consistent cash flow, and falling private insurance reimbursement rates, new physicians began to be drawn into the market, increasing access.

After the passage of the Balanced Budget Act of 1997, the federal government mandated additional financial responsibilities to the states for their portion of the Medicaid program and phased out the guarantee of 100 percent reimbursement to states for certain groups of physicians and health care providers. In Illinois the result was that payment rates were reduced. With state coffers overflowing from surplus tax revenues, overall health care costs rising at rates only slightly above inflation, and political pressure mounting from community groups against mandatory assignment of all Medicaid recipients, the mandatory Medicaid enrollment plan was abandoned. Without mandatory enrollment the health plans did not have enough members to spread their risk and make a profit. By May 1999, the result was low enrollment—with only 10 to 15 percent of eligible patients enrolled—and an exodus of the majority of the commercial health plans from the market. Around the same time, a major expansion of coverage of near-poor children had occurred, made possible by the federal legislation that created the State Children's Health Insurance Program (SCHIP).

Without the imposed discipline of managed care, Illinois, like other states, began to see a major reversal of fortune as costs soared from increased utilization and rising prescription drug prices and tax revenues began to decline as the economy slowed. By the end of 2001, facing a $1 billion budget deficit, Governor

George Ryan began a series of cuts to hospitals, Medicaid managed care companies, and pharmacies that have threatened to tear apart the nearly forty-year-old Medicaid safety net. The speed with which this expansion and subsequent contraction took place, a period of less than five years, illustrates how quickly the market can adjust to the demands of the consumer.

If there is one truth that can be distilled from the past period of escalating health care costs, it is that costs can never be controlled if the focus is only treating illness. Resources must be allocated to prevention and early detection, with incentives and penalties that motivate health care providers to keep patients healthy and promote consumers' participation in their own well-being. And these resources must be universally available and accessible.

CHAPTER SEVENTY-SEVEN

Consumer-Driven Health Care for the Uninsured

Kevin Vigilante

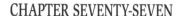

It has been said that the poor will be greatly disadvantaged when making choices about health care. I think this is condescending and patronizing. After years of working with inner-city and addicted populations, it is clear to me that the poor know just as acutely as the wealthy whether they are being treated with respect. Respect is probably one of the most important indicators of the quality of physician care. In my experience, physicians who treat all patients with equal respect, regardless of the patients' socioeconomic status, are generally the best and most committed.

No one should be forced to accept care from a physician who does not treat him or her with dignity. The consumer-choice model, properly administered, can provide choice and resources to the disadvantaged so they will not have to settle for second-rate care and callous attitudes.

Unfortunately, the consumer model has been tainted with the negative perceptions of managed care and the drumbeat for a state-based, single-payer system is once again quickening. Even some physicians who formerly opposed total state control are beginning to view it as preferable to the current managed care environment. But the consumer model is not predicated on the current managed care–employer structure. Consumers have little choice in the current system, making them feel more like hostages to managed care companies than real consumers with multiple options. Using tax credits to loosen the ties to an employer-based system of health insurance will help maximize choice and overcome some of the current restrictions of the managed care–employer monolith.

Medical savings accounts (MSAs), when properly constructed and not the anemic versions that have been tried thus far, also hold promise for overcoming the limitations of managed care. MSAs enable the individual to pay in cash for less expensive health care purchases and have generous coverage for more costly events. In either case consumers' choices and doctors' decisions are less likely to be limited by the dictates of a managed care CPA.

Information is fundamental to a consumer-based system. Choice is meaningless if it is reduced to throwing darts at a menu of health care options. Informed choice is what drives continual improvement in a competitive environment. Information barriers are high in health care, but they are no lower in a state-run system. In years past the English limited access to dialysis simply by failing to inform the elderly that it was a medical option. However, the marketplace holds great promise for lowering information barriers. New information technologies will change the way health and medical information are disseminated. No longer will information be limited to hushed discussions among physicians in hospital hallways nor will it be shrouded in the arcane language of medical jargon. As we learn to provide and use information on the Internet, medical information will become democratized; it will become increasingly accessible and understandable. When it is not, the consumer will quickly look for another provider who can make it understandable. An emerging cadre of sites will enable you to determine whether, for example, you are getting state-of-the-art treatment for HIV or acute myelogenous leukemia, and if not, where you should go to get it.

The consumer model will flourish under such conditions. Of course not all consumers will be able or motivated to do this kind of research, but as with cars and computers, those who do will help raise the standard of excellence for everyone. I have personally observed this phenomenon in HIV care. Only substandard physicians should feel threatened by the democratization of medical information. The rest need to embrace these changes and harness them. Some studies suggest that only between 10 to 20 percent of consumers need to be active information seekers to make a market competitive.[1]

Medicine is an art, a science, and now a big business. (It used to be many small businesses, run by physicians.) But medicine is first and foremost an ethical endeavor. Physicians must be the custodians of that ethic. We must commit ourselves to constructing a system that strives for excellence in the care of each patient and provides equal access for all patients, while realizing that efficiency is an ethical imperative in a system with limited resources. Excellence, equity, and efficiency can be opposing forces. By placing physicians at the center of these sometimes divergent vectors, we subject them to great tensions. However, physicians must be prepared to take leadership roles. To the extent that physicians effectively balance these forces, they will honor the ethic of medicine and do the greatest good for the greatest number.

Note

1. Thorelli, H., and Engledow, J. "Information Seekers and Information Systems: A Policy Perspective." *Journal of Marketing,* Jan. 1980, *44,* 9–26; Feick, L. F., and Price, L. L. "The Market Maven: A Diffuser of Marketplace Information." *Journal of Marketing,* Jan. 1987, *51,* 83–97.

CHAPTER SEVENTY-EIGHT

A Health Care SEC

*The Truth, the Whole Truth,
and Nothing But the Truth*

Regina E. Herzlinger

Americans are mad as hell at managed care.[1] My analysis of health care consumers caused me, long ago, to predict a managed care backlash;[2] but now that everybody knows that managed care is in trouble, I am not only proven a prophet, at least in this case, but also, and much more important, our elected representatives are rushing to the rescue. Their bills for patient protection often contain a shopping bag full of mandated benefits such as easy access to specialists and hospitals. The consumer activists who induced these mandates have presented perfectly reasonable evidence for each.[3] Take Mary Jo Sadosky's complaint when, exhausted and in pain, she was asked to leave a hospital twelve hours after giving birth to twins. Small wonder she fought for a ban against "drive-through deliveries."[4] Well intentioned? Sure. But away from the glow of C-Span cameras, reality strikes: regulation is no surefire problem solver.

Although one cannot argue with individual complaints, a one-size-fits-all medical care strategy is unlikely to prove effective. Mother Nature designed us in infinite variety—we sustain injuries and heal in many different ways. Worse yet, mandated benefits may suppress the innovations that offer the best hope for improving health care cost effectiveness. For example, a fifteen-year study

A prior version of this chapter appeared in Regina E. Herzlinger, "The 'Truth' About Managed Care," *Journal of Health Politics, Policy and Law,* 1999, *24*(5). See also Regina E. Herzlinger, *Protection of the Health Care Consumer* (Washington, D.C.: Progressive Policy Institute, Mar. 1999).

found that a program of frequent, at-home nurse visits lowered the rates of sub-stance abuse and welfare dependency among low-income mothers and reduced the incidence of child abuse.[5] Home visitation has also improved pregnancy out-comes and reduced injury rates.[6] Will a health insurer forced to follow a one-size-fits-all hospital maternity stay mandate also reimburse innovative home visit programs? Do not count on it.

Consider how innovation helped Dick Fosbury, the 1968 Olympic gold medal-ist in the running high jump. Unlike other jumpers, who faced the bar, Fosbury backed into it and flopped seven feet and four and one-quarter inches over it. His innovation promptly spread, and the *Fosbury flop* is now routinely used by other athletes. But imagine the result if well-intended Olympic officials had mandated forward-facing high jumps because backward jumps increase the chances of injury or are aesthetically unpleasing or fail to measure up to any other seemingly plausible reason. There would be no Fosbury flopping, no innovation. As Robert Waller, former CEO of the Mayo Foundation, has said, "Regulations put a stake in the ground that says, 'You have to meet that stan-dard.' But what's quality on Monday is not what's quality on Tuesday."[7]

BACK TO BASICS

If current public policy initiatives carry deadly consequences, we must go back to basics: *What lies at the core of consumers' complaints about managed care?*

To my mind, the answer is clear. Today's well-educated, assertive consumers want choice and control. The rest of the U.S. economy understands these desires. As one retailer comments, consumers say, "I want it the way I want it and when I want it."[8] But managed care takes choice and control away from them: for example, all the top-rated responses in one consumer survey favored overturning managed care's powers to select providers, require permission, and approve specialist care.[9]

The Internet vividly illustrates the consumer's power. The intermediary, on-line markets, such as Amazon.com, that enable consumers to obtain conve-nient, intelligent, comparative information succeed because of their "allegiance to buyers rather than products."[10] Their focus on the customer has helped to propel the rise in Internet retail revenues, and health care purchases are already among the leading-edge Internet purchases.[11] Today's consumers control even items once considered the province of experts. For example, although most pen-sion assets were once controlled by employers in defined contribution plans, currently up to 80 percent are controlled by individuals.[12] Consumers are so self-confident that individual trading on the New York Stock Exchange and the NASDAQ has grown 31 percent annually from 1994.[13]

Yet despite health care consumers' manifest desires for the choice and con-trol they find elsewhere, some argue that these wishes should be ignored. As one Beltway consultant observed: "The approach of trying to give people the power to operate in the current insurance market assumes too much about individual purchasing abilities."[14] Such sentiments erroneously assume that every market participant must be equally adept. But the fundamental lesson of Economics 101 is that price is determined by marginal participants, not the average ones. The importance of marginal consumers is illustrated by the success of markets for complex goods, such as computers, automobiles, and securities. Further, the sentiments are misplaced: the acclaimed, consumer-controlled Federal Employees Health Benefits Program (FEHB) (see the description in Chapter Seventeen in this volume) and the Buyers Health Care Action Group (BHCAG) (see Chapter Nineteen) provide early examples of the savviness of health care purchasers.[15]

Even if these opinions were more persuasive, they would still ignore the awesome power of the American people to shape the public policy they want. For example, in 1988, the Medicare Catastrophic Coverage Act was hailed as a Beltway star. The act's expanded benefits, protection against catastrophic medical expenses, and modest incremental costs pleased Democrats and Republicans alike. But the solons neglected to consult consumers. The elderly failed to join the lovefest. Angered with extra costs for unwanted benefits, they forced Congress to repeal this vastly unpopular legislation.[16] This debacle demonstrates that Beltway mavens cannot persuade the public to accept health care it does not want. And it wants choice and control.

WHAT WORKS: INFORMATION DISCLOSURE

Fundamentally, consumers complain that in managed care they cannot control what they buy. One reason is their limited choice. Currently, only 15 percent of employees in small firms and 50 percent of those in firms with 500 to 999 employees have more than one option.[17] With so little competition, health insurers can allegedly offer too little health care for the money. They can also spend too much on salaries (compensation for Oxford Health Care's CEO topped $29 million in 1996[18] as Oxford's providers languished for lack of payment,[19] for example), spend too little for customer service,[20] return too much to investors,[21] and paradoxically, return too little to capital (for example, New York's mammoth $7 billion Empire Blue Cross Blue Shield had an inadequate $39 million capital balance in 1992[22]).

Theoretically, greater consumer choice in the purchase of health insurance would better line up the interests of the buyers and insurers.[23] Consumers could then reward insurers that give them good value for the money and punish those that do not. Both Democrats and Republicans agree with this reasoning. A plethora of bills in Congress offer to expand consumers' choice, from proposals to enlarge people's choice of Medicare plans to approaches that would use the tax code to subsidize individual purchase of health plans.

When they have good information and freedom to choose health care plans and providers, consumers optimize in classic Economics 101 fashion. For example, when the satisfaction data collected by a Twin Cities employer coalition, the Buyers Health Care Action Group, were released, the information contributed to a nearly 20 percent drop in the membership of high-cost, low-satisfaction plans and a 50 percent increase in the membership of low-cost, high-satisfaction plans.[24] Information exerts powerful effects even in the absence of consumer control. When the State of New York provided standardized measures of the open-heart surgery performance of hospitals and surgeons, for instance, statewide death rates dropped.[25] Low-performance providers exited and others improved. Market share growth was inversely related to the mortality statistics.[26]

The trouble is, much of the needed information does not currently exist. Despite exemplary organizations such as the Foundation for Accountability, the Picker Institute, CalPERS (the California Public Employees' Retirement System), the federal government's own Office of Personnel Management, and the National Committee for Quality Assurance,[27] consumers presently lack the consistent, comprehensive, relevant, timely, and comparable information about providers and insurers that they need to reshape the health care market. Indeed, there is widespread agreement that health care quality measurement is in its infancy.[28] What to measure, how to measure and disseminate it, how to adjust for individual characteristics—these are but a few of the unresolved issues.[29] Small wonder then that most consumers simply ignore presently available data. They suspect its validity, questioning its statistical reliability and data integrity.[30] They may find some data irrelevant: for example, measures that pool us all into a vast sea neglect the significant differences among us,[31] and quality measures that focus exclusively on clinical dimensions ignore the busy U.S. consumer's overwhelming interest in courtesy and convenience.[32] Moreover, consumers want specific, timely information so they can readily identify the health professionals who can best treat them or a sick loved one. They are much more interested in the outcomes of specific providers who treat breast cancer than in the percentage of enrollees in a health plan who receive mammograms.

The paucity of such information prevents an effective response to the managed care backlash.

The securities market demonstrates the impact of information on performance. In this market the prices of publicly traded securities are fair in the sense that they fully reflect the impact of the ample publicly available information.[33] The information reflected in these prices effectively redirects capital from ineffective firms to effective ones. (This is not to say that the market is always right but rather that it reflects all the information publicly available at that time.) If health care markets resembled this *efficient* securities market, consumers would have a large quantity of reliable information available and could use it to reward effective health care insurers and providers.

There goes the backlash.

Efficient Markets and How They Got That Way

How can securities prices reflect the impact of all the complex publicly available information about the performance of each listed firm when many individual owners of securities cannot fully evaluate this information?

There are at least two possible explanations.[34] First, a group's consensus estimate is generally better than the average level of knowledge of the individuals within the group; as one example, the consensus forecast for the outcomes of football games consistently beats the estimates of individual forecasters.[35] Additionally, expert analysts help investors evaluate prices, through information freely available in the mass media and to clients of brokerage houses. The experts are also rated. The *Wall Street Journal,* for example, publishes its "All-Star Analysts" list. Mutual fund investors can compare annual evaluations of these funds in publications such as *Forbes, Money,* and *Consumer Reports,* or they can turn to mutual fund newsletters such as those produced by Morningstar and Value Line for quarterly updates. Investors use these assessments to reward recent good performers by allocating more money to them.[36] The growth in information retrieval services—especially in their electronic component—supports the market's continued efficiency.

The SEC: The Truth Agency

Many knowledgeable observers contend that the Securities and Exchange Commission (SEC) is a critical element of the efficiency of the securities markets.[37] As I discussed in Chapter Seven, the SEC was created in 1934 by President Franklin Delano Roosevelt to protect small investors. The regulation of securities was nothing new. As early as 1285, King Edward I required licensure of London brokers.[38] But FDR's SEC differed from traditional regulation, which relied on authorities to evaluate the worthiness of a security. He opted for sunlight, arguing that the "Federal Government cannot and should not take any action that might be construed as approving or guaranteeing that . . . securities are sound." Rather, his SEC was "The Truth Agency" ensuring full disclosure of all material facts. In his words, "It puts the burden of telling the truth on the seller."[39]

As in health care, there was plenty of truth waiting to be told. Requirements for listing securities on the stock exchange were minimal, there was no source of generally accepted accounting principles, and in 1923, only 25 percent of the firms traded on the New York Stock Exchange provided shareholder reports.[40] To put teeth in its mission, the SEC was given the power to enforce "truth in securities" and to regulate the trading of securities in markets through brokers and exchanges.

Private Sector Sources of Information

Surprisingly, much of the information that lies at the heart of the efficiency of the securities markets wells not from the SEC but from three private sector groups: the corporations themselves,[41] the FASB (Financial Accounting Standards Board), and the accounting profession. Much of the publicly available information emanates from each corporation itself and reflects the findings of the specific measurement approaches promulgated by the FASB and its predecessors. The SEC has legal authority to specify these accounting standards but it generally relies on the FASB, with the SEC's active oversight, to do so. Managers must hire an independent accounting firm to audit the financial statements. If the auditor cannot issue a clean opinion, the SEC may well bar the firm from access to the capital markets.[41] As a private nonprofit organization, the FASB must earn sufficient revenues to cover its expenses and the respect of its constituency. Two predecessor organizations collapsed in part because they could not reach a consensus on specific accounting standards acceptable to business, the accounting community, and the SEC. To fulfill its mandate the FASB must be politically aware and able to build consensus. Its structure and its process for issuing an accounting standard are designed to elicit broad-based, thoughtful involvement.[42]

The interaction among these groups promotes fuller consideration of diverse points of view. The process is completely public, and repeated rounds of drafts encourage wide participation. These characteristics are crucial to the FASB's success because in accounting, as in health care measurement, there is no widely accepted conceptual basis for the methods used. Despite a long history of accounting techniques—they were first codified in 1494—a conceptual foundation on which we can clearly adjudicate all accounting disputes does not exist. Despite the existence of the Elements of Financial Statements, consisting of six conceptual outlines, in practice, debates about fundamental accounting issues such as current versus historical costs value and capitalization versus expensing continue to roil the profession. As the FASB's first chairman noted, "Accounting . . . is an art whose rules are not susceptible to . . . tests of validity . . . accounting is rather a convention supported by general acceptance, consensus."[43] Unlike a government agency, they do not sing out of one hymnal. And being private sector organizations and individuals, they require the political and financial backing of supporters for their continued existence.[44]

Initially, in abdicating some of its authority to set accounting standards for the private sector, the SEC recognized the following advantages:[45] (1) practicing accountants were close to the firms that were subject to SEC regulations and thus could identify emerging issues more accurately than the SEC could, (2) private sector involvement encouraged greater compliance than government mandates could, and (3) the SEC could more objectively audit the work of the private sector information disclosers than its own work, thus resolving a conflict of interest. But the accounting abuses that emerged in 2001–2003 caused a shift in this stance. It appeared that the financial statements of massive firms such as Enron and Global Crossing did not accurately reveal their underlying economic status, despite audits by leading accounting firms and reviews by the audit committees of the firms' boards of directors.[46] In Enron's case, for example, much of the company's debt was lodged in special-purpose entities that were not consolidated in the financial statements.

Many blamed the structure of the accounting firms for these debacles. They had simultaneously offered lucrative consulting and low-profit auditing services to their clients, thereby setting up conflicts of interest with financial consequences. Past SEC attempts to bar accountants from offering consulting contracts had been stymied by the Congress. This time around, the SEC relied on its internal rule-making authority to reclaim some of its powers. In 2002, it introduced rules to prompt faster, more complete disclosure and to create a new entity to oversee the accounting professionals.[47] Similarly, the rule-making Financial Accounting Standards Board hoped to simplify and streamline its occasionally complex rules.[48]

TRANSLATING THE LESSONS OF THE SEC TO MANAGED CARE

The U.S. securities markets have precisely the characteristics that managed care consumers want: (1) prices are fair in the sense that they reflect all publicly available information, (2) buyers use this information to reward effective organizations and penalize ineffective ones, and (3) information and competition continually reduce transaction costs. The presence of these characteristics in the health insurance market would achieve an important social goal: *it would divert capital from health insurers and providers that offer a bad buy to those that offer a good one.* Poor-value-for-the-money insurers and providers would shrink or improve. Good-value-for-the-money insurers and providers would flourish.

Impact on Insurers

Currently, the magnitude of health insurance transaction costs is unclear. One broker has estimated that for a forty-person company these costs range from 2 percent to 2.5 percent. When pressed for more specific data, he said, "Asking about this . . . is like asking the military for their nuclear weapons plans. The information is not top secret—or it should not be—but it is treated that way."[49] Any attempt to compare health insurance prices is also a major research undertaking. Contrast this mysteriousness with the clarity of the transaction costs of brokers and the prices of securities. When Web sites such as Motley Fool openly compare the transaction costs of different brokers, investors can easily evaluate their services relative to their costs. This information has enabled low-price discount brokers to flourish and has forced full-price brokers to offer their customers more "free" services, such as proprietary research.[50]

Purchasers of health insurance armed with comparable transaction cost and price information will benefit from similar competition. Some brokers will offer low prices and others will provide extensive additional services to justify their fuller price. Public disclosure of these analyses would likely eventually lead to a list of "All-Star Health Insurance Analysts" in the *Wall Street Journal.*

Impact on Providers

Similarly, health care consumers have little information about the quality of their providers. Currently they have better quality information about the jar of tomato sauce they buy than about the surgeon who will operate on their breast or prostate cancer. Publication of data about the quality of individual providers, as measured by generally accepted health care outcome principles and audited by certified, independent appraisers of such information, will ameliorate this problem. Eventually, independent analysts will use this information to compile readily accessible ratings of providers, just as Morningstar does with its excellent system for classifying and rating mutual funds.

How to Make It Happen

The key to achieving these desirable characteristics in the health insurance market is legislation that replicates these essential elements of the SEC model:

1. *Registration.* The SEC requires firms that trade their securities in interstate markets and all such market makers to register with the agency. A corresponding health care agency would oversee the integrity of and require the public disclosure of information about health insurers, the policies they issue, and the interstate markets in which such insurance policies are sold. It would be armed with powerful penalties for undercapitalized and unethical market participants.

2. *Private sector disclosure and auditing.* The SEC relies heavily on private sector organizations. The new health care agency would delegate the power to derive the principles used to measure the performance of insurers and providers to an independent, private nonprofit organization that, like the FASB, represents a broad constituency. The agency would require auditing of the information by independent professionals, who would render an opinion of the information and bear legal liability for failure.

3. *Private sector analysis.* The securities evaluation process is conducted primarily by private sector analysts, who disseminate their frequently

divergent ratings. To encourage similar private sector health care analysts, the new agency would require public dissemination of all health insurance prices, related transaction costs, and the characteristics of the policies and providers, such as clinical measures of quality and customer satisfaction. To protect against the conflicts of interest that arise when analysts are employed by brokers, the agency may require separation of these two functions.

How Not to Make It Happen

Unfortunately, many of the well-intended patient protection proposals undermine one or more of these essential characteristics. All too often they require that health care regulators evaluate and micromanage health insurers and the markets in which they operate.[51] One well-intended proposal, for example, blurs the distinctions between information and evaluation, between oversight and micromanagement: its FASB analogue evaluates quality and its SEC analogue evaluates health care benefits and coverage problems. But the real FASB does not assess the quality of the output produced by corporations, nor does the real SEC evaluate whether the markets for the products that corporations sell yield effective, efficient outputs.[52] Instead, they ensure the provision of reliable, useful information that investors can use to perform their own analyses.[53]

The likely result of these proposals? Lack of innovation.

Wave good-bye to the health care Dick Fosburys.

The much-abused U.S. health care consumer needs, and wants, government protection.[54] We know that the SEC model works. We just need to take advantage of it.

Notes

1. See, for example, Tokarski, C. "HMOs Get Thumbs-Down in Hit Movie." *American Medical News,* Mar. 23–30, 1998, p. 9.

2. Herzlinger, R. E. "Healthy Competition." *The Atlantic,* August 1991, 69–81; Herzlinger, R. E. "The Quiet Health Care Revolution." *The Public Interest,* Spring 1994, pp. 72–90.

3. Annas, G. J. "Women and Children First." *New England Journal of Medicine,* 1995, *3,* 1647–1651.

4. Miller, J. "Mother and Newborn: How Long in the Hospital." *New York Times,* Aug. 20, 1995, sec. 13CN, p. 1.

5. Kitzman, H., Olds, D. L., Henderson, C. R., Hanks, C., and others. "Effect of Prenatal and Infancy Home Visitation by Nurses on Pregnancy Outcomes, Childhood Injuries, and Repeated Childbearing." *Journal of the American Medical Association,* 1997, *278,* 644–652.

6. Olds, D. L., Eckenrode, J., Henderson, C. R., Kitzman, H., and others. "Long Term Effect of Home Visitation on Maternal Life Course and Child Abuse and Neglect." *Journal of the American Medical Association,* 1997, *278,* 637–643.

7. Aston, G. "Congress at Odds Over Managed Care." *American Medical News,* Mar. 23–30, 1998, p. 12.

8. Lorie, E. "Retailers Provide Instant Furniture." *New York Times,* Aug. 4, 1994, p. C2.

9. Gorman, C. "Playing the HMO Game." *Time,* July 13, 1998, p. 32.

10. Hof, R. D. "The Buyer Always Wins." *Business Week,* Mar. 22, 1999, pp. EB26–28.

11. Forrester Reports. *Retail's Growth Spiral.* Cambridge, Mass.: Forrester Research Inc., Nov. 1998.

12. Shoven, J. B., and Wise, D. A. "Extending the Consumption-Tax Treatment of Personal Savings." *The American Economic Review,* May 1998, *88,* 197; Poterba, J. M., Venti, S. F., and Wise, D. A. "401(k) Plans and Future Patterns of Retirement Saving." *The American Economic Review,* May 1998, *88,* 179–184.

13. Franco, S. C., and Klein, T. M. *On Line Brokerage.* Minneapolis: Piper Jaffrey, Oct. 1998, p. 4.

14. New York Business Group on Health Care (NYBGHC). *The Nation's Health Insurance System.* Conference Proceedings. New York: NYBGHC, 1992, p. 61.

15. See Herzlinger, R. E. *Market-Driven Health Care: Who Wins, Who Loses in the Transformation of America's Largest Service Industry.* Reading, Mass.: Addison-Wesley, 1997, pp. 264–268.

16. Dahl, D. "Catastrophic Coverage: Lawmaking Gone Awry." *St. Petersburg Times,* Dec. 17, 1989, p. 3D.

17. "Managed Care Helped Employers Hold the Line on Costs." *On Managed Care,* Dec. 1998, p. 3.

18. Pollack, R., and Slass, L. *Premium Pay: Corporate Compensation in America's HMOs.* Washington, D.C.: Families USA Foundation, Apr. 1998, p. 24.

19. Frudenheim, M. "Shake-Up at a Health Giant: The Reaction." *New York Times,* Feb. 25, 1998, p. D3.

20. Rundle, R. "Under Attack, HMOs Address Patients' Gripes." *Wall Street Journal,* Nov. 27, 1998, p. B1; Woolhandler, S., and Himmelstein, D. "The Deteriorating Administrative Efficiency of the U.S. Health Care System." *New England Journal of Medicine,* 1991, *324,* 1253–1258.

21. McKinsey & Company. *1995 Health Care Annual.* New York: McKinsey & Company, 1995, pp. 270–273.

22. Hilgenkamp, R., and Herzlinger, R. E. *Empire Blue Cross and Blue Shield (A).* Harvard Business School Case No. 195-216. Boston, Mass.: Harvard Business School, Aug. 1995.

23. Kendall, D. B. "Better Luck Next Time: Moving Beyond Partisan Posturing over Patients' Rights." Washington, D.C.: Progressive Policy Institute, Oct. 1998.

24. Wetzell, S. Slide presented at a meeting of the American Medical Association, Palm Beach, Fla., Feb. 1999.

25. Chassin, M. R., and Galvin, R. W. "The Urgent Need to Improve Health Care Quality." *Journal of the American Medical Association,* 1998, *280,* 1003.

26. Mukamel, D., and Mushlin, A. I. "Quality of Care Information Makes a Difference." *Medical Care,* 1998, *36*(7), 945–954.

27. Herzlinger, R. E., and Burroughs, A. *Note on Health Care Accountability.* Harvard Business School Case No. 198-065. Boston: Harvard Business School, Mar. 1998. For evidence that profiling does not force New York's high-risk cases to seek care elsewhere, see Peterson, E. D., and others, "The Effects of New York's Bypass Surgery Provider Profiling on Access to Care and Patient Outcomes in the Elderly." *Journal of the American College of Cardiology,* 1998, *32,* 993–999.

28. Chassin and Galvin, "The Urgent Need to Improve Health Care Quality," p. 1000.

29. See, for example, Isaacs, S. "Consumers' Information Needs: Results of a National Survey." *Health Affairs,* Winter 1996, *15,* 31–41.

30. Edgman-Levitan, S., and Cleary, P. "What Information Do Consumers Want and Need?" *Health Affairs,* Winter 1996, *15,* 45.

31. Tumlinson, A., and others. "Choosing a Health Plan: What Information Will Consumers Use?" *Health Affairs,* May–June 1997, *16,* 229–238.

32. See Herzlinger, *Market-Driven Health Care,* chaps. 1–4, for descriptions of busy and intelligent health care consumers; see Edgman-Levitan and Cleary, "What Information Do Consumers Want and Need?" pp. 45, 52–53, for consumers' information interests.

33. In statistical terms, the efficient market hypothesis assumes that investment returns are serially independent and that their probability distributions are constant through time. The interpretation of the efficient market hypothesis has evolved to mean that if a market is efficient with respect to information, an investor is playing a fair game, meaning that prices behave as though everyone had access to the same information. See Fama, E. "Efficient Capital Markets: A Review of Theory and Empirical Work." *Journal of Finance,* 1970, *25*(1), 383–417; Beaver, W. H. *Financial Reporting: An Accounting Revolution.* Upper Saddle River, N.J.: Prentice Hall, 1989, pp. 130–152; Malkiel, B. *A Random Walk Down Wall Street: Including a Life-Cycle Guide to Personal Investing.* New York: Norton, 1996, p. 3.

34. Eugene Fama first proposed three definitions or standards to test the efficient market hypothesis: weak, semi-strong, and strong. The strongest form of the efficient market hypothesis asserts that all information known by market participants is fully reflected in market prices so it is impossible for insiders who trade on private information to earn abnormal profits. See Fama, "Efficient Capital Markets"; Joy, M. A. "Hunting the Stock Market Snarks." *Sloan Management Review,* Spring 1987, *3,* 22. Although it is not impossible for insiders to profit from private information, for the most part the stock market comes very close to meeting the strongest standard for efficiency. See Joy, "Hunting the Stock Market Snarks."

See also, for example, Jensen, M. "Risk, the Pricing of Capital Assets, and the Evaluation of Investment Portfolios." *Journal of Business,* Apr. 1969, *42,* 167–247.

35. Beaver, *Financial Reporting,* p. 150.

36. Ippolito, R. A. "Consumer Reactions to Measures of Poor Quality: Evidence from the Mutual Fund Industry." *Journal of Law and Economics,* 1972, *35*(1), 45–70; Malkiel, *A Random Walk Down Wall Street,* pp. 443–444.

37. See, for example, Seligman, J. *The Transformation of Wall Street.* Boston: Northeastern University Press, 1995, 561–568. However, see also Stigler, G. J. "Public Regulation of the Securities Market." *Journal of Business,* Apr. 1964, pp. 117–142; reprinted in Previts, G. J. *The Development of SEC Accounting.* Reading, Mass.: Addison-Wesley, 1981. In this classic article, the great economist George Stigler determined that government regulation of information disclosure is not essential to the efficiency of markets. In this view, if information is beneficial to the firm, its managers will advertise it; if it is detrimental, the firm's competitors will trumpet it; and if it exists, whether good or bad, analysts will ferret it out. No need for government.

As is usual with works of such significance, Stigler's analysis and similar research were widely criticized. (For similar research, see Benston, G. "Required Disclosure and the Stock Market: An Evaluation of the Securities and Exchange Act of 1934." *American Economic Review,* Mar. 1973, *63,* 132–155. For critiques, see, for example, Dopuch, N. "The Capital Market, The Market for Information, and External Accounting." *Journal of Finance,* 1976, *31*(2) 611–630; Deakin, E. "Accounting Reports, Policy Interventions, and the Behavior of Securities Returns." *Accounting Review,* 1976, *51*(3), 590–603.) Yet despite the abundant, intelligent research on the question of whether government action is needed to ensure an efficient market, the debate cannot be settled solely by empirical analyses.

There are two theoretical bases for government's presence in the information market. First, information disclosure conceived as a public good from the government's point of view enables free riders from the discloser's point of view. Because disclosers cannot charge these users for the benefits the users derive, they lack incentives for full disclosure. (See, for example, Stiglitz, J. E., Jaramillo-Vallejo, J., and Park, Y. C. "The Role of the State in Financial Markets." *World Bank Research Observer,* 1993, pp. 16–61; Dutt, J. "Unlikely Adversaries: Top Regulators in Dispute over Plan to Change Accounting Rule on Derivatives." *Washington Post,* Aug. 24, 1997, p. H1.) Absent government regulation, the quantity of publicly available information will likely be undersupplied. Second, disclosure may be made selectively, favoring some recipients and excluding others. (Eventually, of course, all investors would share the same information, but some would have a temporal advantage because they learned special information earlier than others did.) Such selective discrimination, however temporary, violates our national notions of equity. Regulations that penalize insider activity and require simultaneous dissemination of information level the playing field. There is also a third frequently voiced justification for government action, but it is less convincing to my mind. Some argue that government disclosure of public information may cost less than the sum of the costs of many private disclosures of the same information. But if the economies of collective action are so powerful, an industry group could attain them as well as a government organization. (See, for example, Beaver, *Financial Reporting,* p. 191.)

38. Skousen, F. *An Introduction to the SEC.* Cincinnati, Ohio: South-Western, 1991, p. 118.

39. Seligman, *The Transformation of Wall Street,* pp. 54–55.

40. Seligman, *The Transformation of Wall Street,* pp. 43–48.

41. Miller, P. W., Redding, R. J., and Bahnson, P. R. *The FASB: The People, the Process, and the Politics.* Burr Ridge, Ill.: Irwin, 1994, pp. 20–21.

42. Previts, G. J., and Marino, B. D. *A History of Accounting in America.* New York: Wiley, 1979; Armstrong, M. S. "The Politics of Establishing Accounting Standards." *Government Accountants Journal,* 1976, *25*(2), 8–13; Miller and others, *The FASB.* Miller and others, *The FASB,* pp. 30–58; Financial Accounting Foundation. *Guide Star: Financial Report.* Washington, D.C.: Philanthropic Research Inc., 1998; Financial Accounting Foundation (FAF). *Annual Report 1997.* Norwalk, Conn.: 1998, p. 24; McEnroe, J. E., and Martens, S. C. "An Analysis of the FASB's Independence." *Journal of Applied Business Research,* Winter 1996–1997, *13,* 129–132.

43. Reither, C. L. "How the FASB Approaches a Standard-Setting Issue." *Accounting Horizons,* Dec. 1997, *11,* 91–104. Armstrong, "The Politics of Establishing Accounting Standards," p. 10.

44. The independent accountants who audit the financial statements are usually professionals who must pass examinations and fulfill stringent educational requirements. Many work in the large accounting firms that audit nearly 80 percent of the publicly traded firms. Accounting firms may be held legally liable for negligence, fraud, and breach of contract. One firm was required to pay up to $145 million to the creditors of the bankrupt DeLorean Motor Company for negligent auditing (Phillips, D. "Jury Gives DeLorean Creditors Millions." *Detroit News,* Mar. 6, 1998, p. B1). Accountants have also been found criminally liable (Skousen, *An Introduction to the SEC,* p. 128).

45. Baker, R. E. "Accounting Rule-Making: Still at the Crossroads." *Business Horizons,* Oct. 1976, *19,* 66.

46. Pearlstein, S. "The Whole Story?" *Washington Post,* May 12, 2002, p. H01.

47. "SEC Seeks Reform in Financial Disclosure and Auditor Oversight." *Chemical Market Reporter,* Mar. 4, 2002, p. 18.

48. "FASB: Rewriting the Book on Bookkeeping." *Business Week,* May 20, 2002, p. 123.

49. Transcript of interview, conducted by Bea Bezmalinovic, with an insurance broker who prefers to remain anonymous, summer 1998.

50. Moore, W. K., and Scott, D. L. "Deregulation That Worked." *Akron Business and Economic Review,* Fall 1986, *17,* 109–120.

51. See, for example, "Bush Is Said to Be Set to Back Patients' Bill." *New York Times,* June 7, 2002, p. A16.

52. Etheredge, L. "Promarket Regulation." *Health Affairs,* Dec. 1997, *16,* 22–25.

53. Herzlinger, R. E. "Can Public Trust in Nonprofits and Governments Be Restored?" *Harvard Business Review,* Mar.–Apr. 1996, *74,* 97–107.

54. Stemberg, S. "Finding the Health Care System Unfit, Many Americans Fear the Care Won't Be There." *USA Today,* Nov. 23, 1998, p. 1D.

CHAPTER SEVENTY-NINE

Keep 'Em Honest

The Health Care SEC

Robert N. Shamansky

Information is vital for anyone who has to make decisions affecting his or her health care. What are some good ways of getting that information? Regina Herzlinger, Nancy R. McPherson Professor of Business Administration at the Harvard Business School, has proposed[1] the creation of an agency that would do for the purchasers of health care what the U.S. Securities and Exchange Commission (SEC) does for purchasers of securities. An issuer of stocks and bonds that wants to sell in the national market—as distinguished from selling within one state only—registers with the SEC specific information regarding the issuer and the nature of the securities being offered for sale. The SEC does not recommend or prescribe what particular security an investor should put his or her money into. Its function is to provide an investor with information that is reliable, so that the investor can make an informed decision. To that end, the SEC issues rules and regulations implementing the federal statutes governing the securities industry in the United States.

Likewise, we would require those who propose to sell health care to register with a similar agency (which I will call the *Health Care SEC*) and provide in their registrations information needed by a purchaser to make a reasonable decision.

THE HEALTH CARE SEC MUST BE UNDER CONSTANT SCRUTINY

The government agency created to regulate even a limited informational approach to health care, à la the SEC, will still be a bureaucracy, and bureaucracies—whether

811

in the public or private sector—need constant scrutiny and effective means for the public to correct the abuses perpetrated or ignored by the bureaucracy.

The SEC does a good job in regulating the securities sold in an economy measured in trillions of dollars. It does this with a staff of only 3,000 or so, which is small given its task. But if the SEC is the model for creating a government regulator of the health care industry, it is absolutely necessary to remind ourselves of the following immortal thoughts:

"The condition upon which God hath given liberty to man is eternal vigilance."[2]

"Power tends to corrupts. Absolute power corrupts absolutely."[3]

The regulator captured by the regulated.[4]

Let us assume a new government agency is going to be created. There must be built into the structure of this entity procedures and practices whereby those affected by the entity can view and obtain the maximum information about its decision-making processes. The expression enjoying popularity these days is that there must be as much *transparency* as possible.

It is safe to assume that any large economic interests affected by the new entity will have a full array of lobbyists, lawyers, and public relations operatives scurrying about Washington legitimately representing those economic interests. But what if you are not one of those interests but an individual who believes he has a legitimate gripe affecting not only himself but many others who may be similarly situated?

LEARNING FROM THE SEC

Most owners of securities are not particularly aware of the securities transfer industry, which provides the securities industry with the services needed to keep track of the many millions of owners of securities. These services include delivering dividends and interest, recording transfers of ownership when securities are bought and sold, and turning over to the fifty states as *unclaimed property* securities whose owners have been "lost" for various—depending on the state—periods of time. (Ohio's period is generally five years.)[5]

It took an investigation,[6] started by then representative and now senator Ron Wyden (D-OR), articles in various national publications,[7] and the interest of former SEC commissioner Steven Wallman to convince the SEC[8] to order the securities transfer industry to use current computer databases of national credit rating agencies to obtain good addresses for securities owners who were classified as lost after checks mailed to them had been returned to the transfer agent as undeliverable. The reluctance with which the SEC apparently took this very simple step can be seen by what the SEC *did not* do with respect to lost securities owners, even though the SEC was aware that these owners were affected in the following situations:

- The SEC applied the database search requirement only to securities owners lost *after* December 8, 1997, and not to the three million securities owners lost *before* that date, who were owed an estimated $450 million.[9]

- The SEC failed in 1997 to require the names of the lost securities owners to be posted on the Internet, even though it had considered such a step in 1996.[10] Contrast that failure with these actions: (1) a majority of states post the unclaimed property names for their state on the Internet and have published such lists of names in newspapers for decades[11] and (2) the U.S. government and the world Jewish community shamed the members of the Swiss Bankers Association into listing on the Internet their banks' Holocaust-era unclaimed accounts, which for the preceding fifty years the Swiss bankers had denied having.[12]

- The SEC ignored the fact that undelivered dividends and interest are held in accounts that do not earn the owners of the undelivered funds a single cent, and in effect it rewarded the holder of those funds for not delivering those dividends and interest, because the holder keeps the interest earned by the undelivered dividends and interest.

- The SEC failed to require the so-called heir finders, that is, the locators of, or searchers for, lost securities owners to bid openly for the privilege of locating lost securities owners.[13] Although the SEC acknowledged that "the charges of such firms can cost a securityholder a significant portion of his or her assets,"[14] it did nothing to protect lost securities owners from being exploited by heir finders, which typically charge from 25 to 50 percent of the value of the recovered assets.[15]

Bureaucracies are necessary. We are not going to function without them. However, that does not mean nothing can be done to shed the vital light of publicity and public inquiry on their workings, an exposure that bureaucrats by their very nature are loath to undergo. The new Health Care SEC must

- Put as much information as possible on the Internet.

- Collect, collate, and tabulate data regarding the various types of concerns that people direct to the Health Care SEC. For example, if increasing numbers of people are having a particular type of problem, that finding should be available to the public and the press on the Health Care SEC's Web site. The Health Care SEC should have a Web site with chat rooms, where concerned persons can exchange information and views on those problems. (The new SEC might well learn something from the exchanges.)

- Staff an e-mail operation to answer inquiries received via the Health Care SEC's Web site or e-mail, as the Internal Revenue Service is now doing.

- Have a real-time, live human being–type ombudsman, so that a bureau-crat in the middle rank can get a concern to the Health Care SEC's CEO via the ombudsman (rather than commit bureaucratic suicide by com-plaining to his or her immediate boss about that boss's or higher-up bosses' shortcomings, because every seasoned bureaucrat, whether in the public or private sector, knows intuitively that he or she may be punished for "not being a team player" or for "rocking the boat" or for "whistle blowing"[16]).

The real-time ombudsman must also be paralleled by a cyberombudsman at the agency's Web site for the benefit of the public and the press. The home com-puter, the Internet, and the exponential proliferation of computer users must be marshaled to create a constant dialogue via cyberspace about the processes and procedures employed by the Health Care SEC and about their outcomes. The objective should be to provide a forum that permits public discussion of peo-ple's problems with the agency's workings or failures to work and that sheds the glare of publicity on those who work for or are regulated by the agency. (In this vein the State of Ohio is a harbinger of things to come in the Internet era.[17])

It was a quantum leap for the securities transfer industry to go from doing nothing but remailing checks and notices to addresses already proven bad to using current databases to find good addresses for the remailing of checks and notices. It will be another quantum leap when a new federal regulatory agency is created and the enabling legislation requires access to that agency, scrutiny of it, and active discussion about it via the Internet.

The full effects of the technological change in telecommunications are incal-culable, but what is certain is that this technology is going to change signifi-cantly the way people get information and then act on that information. With respect to the Health Care SEC, close scrutiny of its workings by the public can be only for the better.

Notes

1. Herzlinger, R. E. *Protection of the Health Care Consumer: The "Truth" Agency.* Washington, D.C.: Progressive Policy Institute, Mar. 1999.

2. John Philpot Curran, "Speech Upon the Right of Election of the Lord Mayor of Dublin," July 10, 1790. See Bartlett, J. *Familiar Quotations.* (16th ed.) Boston: Little, Brown, 1992, p. 351.

3. "Letter From Lord Acton to Bishop Mandell Crichton," Apr. 5, 1887. See Bartlett, J. *Familiar Quotations.* (16th ed.) Boston: Little, Brown, 1992, p. 521.

4. Think of the now-defunct Interstate Commerce Commission during the heyday of the railroads.

5. *Ohio Revised Code,* §169.02(E) (Anderson, 1999).

6. Sub-Committee On Regulation, Business Opportunities, and Technology of the Committee on Small Business, 103rd Cong. "Return to Sender: Tens of Thousands of 'Undeliverable' Dividend Payments in Limbo: Individual Investors Lose Billions of Dollars of Shareholder Assets Because of Lax Transfer Rules, Indifference by Public Companies and Government Regulators: A Payday for Public Companies and States?" July 28, 1993.

7. See, for example, Lalli, F. "Playing Lost and Found with Your Money." *Money,* Jan. 1994, p. 7; Asinoff, L. "Lost and Found: How You Can Recover Your Family's Long-Forgotten Nest Egg." *Wall Street Journal,* June 14, 1996, p. C1; Vickers, M. "In Search of Lost Shareholders." *New York Times,* Sept. 3, 1996, p. 6; Caplin, J. "Have You Claimed All the Money Belonging to You?" *Money,* Dec. 1997, pp. 106–109.

8. Quinn, J. B. "Call All—Some? 'Lost' Securities Owners." *Washington Post,* June 28, 1998, p. H2.

9. *Federal Register,* 62, §§52229, 52235 (Oct. 7, 1997).

10. *Federal Register,* 61, §§44249, 44254, notes 29–31 (Aug. 28, 1996).

11. For instance, the Ohio Department of Commerce, Division of Unclaimed Funds, maintains the following Web sites to assist individuals in obtaining unclaimed funds:

    [www.com.state.oh.us./unfd/scripts/thqry.htm] and [www.com.state.oh.us/unfd/scripts/theresults.asp]. The National Association of Unclaimed Property Administrators also maintains a Web site: [www.unclaimed.org].

12. Sanger, D. E. "Swiss Banks Turn Up 4,000 More Holocaust-Era Accounts." *New York Times,* Oct. 14, 1997, p. A12.

13. National Association of Unclaimed Property Administrators (NAUPA). "Comments on Proposed Rules 17Ac2-2 and Related Form TA-2 and Rescind Rule 17a-24." New York: NAUPA, pp. 4–5, May 17, 1999.

14. National Association of Unclaimed Property Administrators, "Comments on Proposed Rules . . ."

15. Lyman, L. *The New SEC Lost Securityholder Rules: An Analysis.* Boston, Mass.: State Street Bank & Trust Company, Aug. 1998.

16. "Helping Whistle-Blowers Survive." *New York Times,* May 1, 1999, p. A14.

17. Doyle, T. "Legislation Provides Greater Public Input in State Agency Rule-Making Process." *Columbus, Ohio, Daily Reporter,* May 7, 1999. Both the House and Senate in Ohio passed without opposition a bill to reform the approval process for agency regulations. The bill creates *The Register of Ohio,* an electronic central register accessible via the Internet. From this on-line register, anyone can obtain information about hearings of the Ohio legislature's Joint Committee on Agency Rule Review. This new bill also requires that new agency rules can be enacted only after the public is given the opportunity to voice opinions at an open committee hearing.

CHAPTER EIGHTY

The U.S. Needs a Consumer-Driven Medical Care System

Rita Ricardo-Campbell

The United States needs a market-driven medical system of medical care, even though most of the payments for care are made by third parties, not directly by the consumer. For this market to evolve, consumers need information. Twenty years ago I advocated wider "dissemination of information through advertising" and through "directories of physicians by specialties, and of hospitals with representative charges, staffs, and tertiary specialists." I also suggested "that public libraries purchase the national directories of physicians by specialties and the *Physicians' Desk Reference* (PDR), which contains manufacturers' descriptions (FDA approved) of prescription drugs." And I pointed to the "need for new compilations about HMOs, PPOs, nursing homes, health insurance benefits." I argued that "unless consumers are knowledgeable about what they buy, the market cannot approach a competitive market."[1]

Over the last two decades the media have made a tremendous response to the public's interest in information about health. Individuals can take advantage of widely available information about prevention to maintain good health, magazine articles that rate hospitals and physicians, employer newsletters that describe the different health care delivery systems that the employer offers, and many similar offerings. There are books on prescription drugs and Internet sites that describe in lay terms recent health news, clinical trials, health insurance alternatives, and specific serious diseases from diagnosis to treatment. Major universities such as Harvard, the University of California-Berkeley, and Johns Hopkins mail well-researched newsletters to subscribers.

Despite the current enormous flow of information on matters of health, consumers believe they are still uninformed about quality factors in the delivery of care. For example, if they know that some HMOs give primary care physicians bonuses for keeping the average per capita cost of the physician's patient load below a given dollar amount, they may ask, Does my HMO do this? How big is the bonus? Am I restricted in seeing a specialist who is part of an HMO because of this? Patients know that if they are in a PPO plan, they must pay, say, 50 percent of an out-of-plan physician's bill rather than the 20 percent they pay in the plan, but they usually know little of the internal plan restrictions. However, public debate over the twenty-four-hour in-hospital stay for a mother after her baby is born did blow the lid off this common HMO restriction. The twenty-four-hour limit was pronounced unconscionable.

During the Reagan years I pushed for getting more information to consumers (in fact, my 1982 book was an informal guide to the Reagan administration's policies on health), especially in respect to hospitals. For several years, from 1984 on, health outcomes were published for specific operations performed in hospitals. These data were criticized when some elite hospitals argued that they got the worst cases and that therefore their above average death rates were due at least partly to their high caseloads of poorer risks, not their poorer procedures. The data did make it easier, however, for consumers to select more wisely where to go for particular surgical procedures. The Clinton administration ended this information flow in the early 1990s.

In response to these and other restrictions on medical care and medical information by for-profits and nonprofits alike, some have proposed new federal oversight by a health agency modeled on the Securities and Exchange Commission (SEC), with a private, advisory enforcer run along the lines of the Financial Accounting Standards Board (FASB). But the SEC and FASB are designed to protect the shareholders of private corporations, not the consumers of these corporations' products.

The regulatory approach more closely related to the protection of the consumers of health care involves the truth-in-lending laws in the banking system and the regularly scheduled bank examiners' visits. Such an oversight program for health care seems needed because the private, nonprofit National Committee for Quality Assurance, which accredits HMOs, has not routinely released information to all consumers and its data have not been publicized. A government-sponsored approach similar to the truth-in-lending regulations could overcome this drawback. The SEC, established in 1934, was designed to protect shareholders. To me, a truth-in-lending model under which examiners check on the accuracy of providers' and insurers' self-reported data is preferable.[2]

As useful as this reform may be, it will not improve the number of choices from which individuals can select their health care financing, even though it may improve their quality. KPMG has estimated that among employers with two hundred or more employees only 57 percent provide two or more health plans. Fewer smaller employers offer even this degree of choice, and many offer no health care insurance coverage at all.

Can the range of choices be improved? For over twenty-five years economists across the political spectrum have agreed that the basic problem lies in the seemingly benign offer, during World War II, of employer-paid health insurance benefits, in an effort to enlarge the labor pool that federal wage rate controls had helped to dry up. The federal government acquiesced by making employers' costs of health insurance for employees tax exempt. For others, government action for a tax cut could help level this playing field.

The discussion to determine the best federal government policy is being pushed by large employers who are developing their own options. IBM has redesigned its retiree health plan so that employees accumulate funds in an "account balance retiree health plan" and, when they retire, use these funds to purchase health care. This is close to a medical savings account. The 2003 Medicare Prescription Drug Act creates similar "health savings accounts." It favors defined contributions over defined benefits. The cashing-out of retirement health benefits to supplement Medicare benefits is also being put into practice and appeals to business firms that in the past have promised health benefits to retirees only to see total costs rising rapidly as the retirees live longer than expected and costs of new technologies and prescription drugs continue to rise.

In addition, support for legislation that would allow patients to sue HMOs for decisions they make that affect care continues to grow. Medical care consumers need to be informed about probable alternative medical outcomes stemming in part from their choices. Opportunities to pool employees of small businesses for the purpose of buying health insurance also need more attention.

Free markets do a better job than polls of revealing what consumers need and want. A competitive market accommodates billions of individual actions and, worldwide, has shown that it automatically works for the most efficient allocation of scarce resources. Medical care is expensive but "too expensive" is a relative term. Consider that *Newsweek* has reported that low- to middle-income individuals are willing to go into debt to pay for plastic surgery to improve their self-perceived looks. For example, a twenty-four-year-old Chicago waitress used $500 in tips as a down payment on a $4,425 laser resurfacing and took out a $178 per month loan for the rest.[3] The phrase "too expensive" involves value judgments. Although many may believe that six months of health insurance is the best use of a certain sum of their money, others may believe that it would be better to spend that sum on liposuction that might give them a better figure and a better job. The plastic surgery market for which there is no health insurance coverage is booming.

Beyond the issue of improving health care delivery for those with health insurance coverage, a more difficult problem is how to extend health insurance coverage to the forty-million-plus without it. Questions needing answers are: How many of these uninsured are children of workers who do not wish to pay a monthly fee to insure the health of their children? But to address such questions would take another book.

Notes

1. Ricardo-Campbell, R. *The Economics and Politics of Health.* Chapel Hill: University of North Carolina Press, 1982, p. 337.

2. Meredith, T. P., and Mishkin, B. S. "Truth in Lending 2001." *Business Lawyer,* *57*(3), May 2002, pp. 1163–1174.

3. "Our Quest to Be Perfect." *Newsweek,* Aug. 9, 1999, p. 56.

CHAPTER EIGHTY-ONE

Government's New Roles in the Era of Consumer-Driven Health Care

Richard A. D'Amaro

Those in government and other policymakers have long yearned for individuals to accept responsibility for their own health care. Widespread consumerism is the movement that could fulfill this long-sought promise. People who were passive and disengaged only a few years ago now enter their physicians' offices with articles, Web page printouts, and treatment plans. Once derided as sheep in the shepherding care of "providers," they are increasingly knowledgeable and assertive. The most common reason Americans now use the Internet is to seek health care information.[1] Nontraditional remedies, in addition to or instead of traditional ones, are being purchased at record levels. Consumerism is the assertion of economic and psychological self-interest and personal accountability: just what the policy doctors ordered.

Along the path of progress to this welcome destination, government, and particularly the federal government, played two central roles. One was a traditional role: setting policy. Through laws, regulations, the tax code, investments in basic research, and other policy instruments, government helped shape health delivery and payment systems. Government's other role has been as a buyer of health care. (It might be more technically accurate to say *payer,* but either word describes its role in health care.) In fulfilling this role the U.S. government adopted an approach different from that of the governments of other industrialized nations. Those nations selected socialized or nationalized systems that directly provide care. In the United States the government's Medicare and Medicaid programs became a conduit through which tax receipts pass to hundreds of thousands of certified private enterprises that are selected by consumers. Of the nearly $1.3 trillion spent in the United States on health care in 2000[2] (an amount exceeding the GDP of the United Kingdom[3]) the private sector distributed about half (54.8 percent), and the government, at all levels, distributed about half (45.2 percent).[4]

This testifies to a remarkable interdependence of public and private activity, perfectly adaptable to the wave of consumerism washing over health care. That wave will not eliminate government's roles but will instead allow government to concentrate on *health* rather than *health care.* This different emphasis will require changes in the nature, but not the structure, of the public-private interdependence. Government's conventional policy tools and purchasing power can be used to respond to and accelerate consumer influence. Among the useful actions that government can take, given these new market conditions, are these five:

- Require standardized data to be collected and disclosed
- Abandon minimum pricing and establish minimum benefits
- Increase support for public health
- Increase support for education
- Allow frozen charitable assets to thaw

REQUIRE STANDARDIZED DATA TO BE COLLECTED AND DISCLOSED

The Human Genome Project is an international research effort to map the human genome, among other things. Scientists are creating one of history's most complicated maps. But this database will likely be completed long before we have a map of another important and complicated source of data: the hundreds of millions of health care claims filed each year in the United States. The data contained in these claims describe in unimaginable detail the services performed by providers. They account for the makeup of our delivery system. Yet they remain completely unavailable to consumers and largely unavailable to researchers and entrepreneurs who could extract meaning from them and make it available to consumers.

True, the Centers for Medicare and Medicaid Services (CMS) has made Medicare data available, and a few intrepid souls have explored it. *The Dartmouth Atlas of Health Care* uses Medicare data to illuminate variability across the nation in medical costs and practice patterns.[5] Solucient[6] and Caredata.com[7] are two examples of private companies refining government data for resale. Generally missing from this data bank are claims processed by private insurance companies and third-party administrators for self-insured employers. This information remains proprietary and may or may not be used to analyze use patterns, demand rates, clinical variability, economic variability, or other activity or price measures. It remains lost to analysts and yet is certain to be important for a complete understanding of delivery system activity and costs. After all, the Medicare population's profile is different from the profile for commercial populations.

Consumers of course do not need or want raw data. They want meaningful, useful, practical information prepared by thoughtful and qualified people. Government should not prepare this information but should instead use its policy and purchasing pulpits to ensure that the raw data are available to the private enterprises that can convert it into something useful. Consumers want a J. D. Power report or a *Consumer Reports* magazine for health care. The market depends on information. Without it, consumerism will suffocate.

Government, using its policy and its purchasing powers, should intervene to require a freer flow of raw data out of the health care industry. The data could be submitted to a central clearinghouse, to which CMS could add data regarding its own purchasing activity, and be made publicly available, without charge, to anyone who wanted it. Downloaders would eagerly analyze the raw data and distill them into information for consumers, professionals, and corporate buyers. Data recasters would be permitted to make commercial, proprietary, or public databases. A health care information industry would be launched and consumerism's fire stoked.

What data should be available? None that imperil personal privacy or patient confidentiality. The urgent need is for information that describes the utilization patterns and costs of health care resources; the ultimate need is for cost-adjusted outcome data. Leaders in such fields as insurance, epidemiology, medicine, academia, and public health are most qualified to identify the useful information latent in the vast reserves of data collected over the past quarter-century. Government should convene these leaders and ask them to

- Identify a minimum, standard, required data set (MSRDS) to be collected and reported for every clinical encounter
- Select a historical date after which all available MSRDS data need to be supplied
- Specify the precautions necessary to protect confidentiality
- Establish technical protocols that make MSRDS data readily available

Requiring and assembling these data need not be onerous or expensive. Indeed most, if not all, of the MSRDS should be information that has been collected on claim forms for years.

The MSRDS would create a much-needed, standard industry data collection protocol. The health care industry, composed of dissimilar sectors, would benefit from government's across-the-board nudge compelling such a conversation and its timely conclusion. In the end this will be less costly than developing incompatible standards, competing standards, or no standards. As noted, it is not enough to collect data in the future. Raw data have been collected for years, some since the inception of Medicare. Such data should be mined to enable retrospective analyses.

Initially, the data will have shortcomings. For instance, very few outcome data are available today, let alone latent in existing data. Yet in time, outcome data will be crucial and are sure to be added to the standard MSRDS as our understanding of outcomes matures. Without compulsory and standard data collection, however, discovering the correlates of action and result seems a game of utter chance. Only a clearinghouse, perhaps privately sponsored by a consortium of trade organizations or foundations, that collects data from different populations, regions, ethnicities, and employers and from people of different education, incomes, and backgrounds will be of use. Understandably there will be profound concerns that the data will be put to Orwellian use. Strict and enforceable safeguards against such a malignancy are as essential as the data themselves, but these concerns cannot be an excuse for retaining the status quo.

ABANDON MINIMUM PRICING AND ESTABLISH MINIMUM BENEFITS

Medicare is the world's largest purchaser of health care.[8] Like the pricing practices of most large purchasers, its pricing has transcendent influence. Non-Medicare buyers set their prices as percentages of Medicare prices: they offer rates of 105 percent of Medicare or 98 percent of Medicare, for example. The federal price controls thereby produce private price controls. In an industry replete with troublesome price distortions, this adds yet another.

In an era of consumerism, price controls have no place. They will keep prices artificially high or artificially low, neither of which is good. A more fitting role for government than price control is defining the minimum insurance benefits that should be available to the public—particularly, but not necessarily only, government program beneficiaries. That is, rather than establish the prices for health care transactions, or for any level of insurance coverage, government should specify the safety nets of minimum allowable insurance coverage. This need not (should not) be a single, monoform safety net. Another fuel for consumerism is variety and choice, so there should be several acceptable safety nets. Some might emphasize primary care coverage while others might emphasize catastrophic care or formerly excluded or negligibly covered services, such as mental health. Only a few designs of minimum allowable coverage need be created.

Then, as health care buyers, Medicare and Medicaid should establish defined contributions to be paid through government toward the premium costs of their beneficiaries. With this defined contribution, a consumer would be able to select managed care or commercial insurance coverage and select coverage for office visits or coverage for pharmacy benefits. Consumers who see additional value in additional coverage could buy more coverage, but such additional coverage would be elective and would not deny others their minimum coverage. This approach locates decision-making nearer to the consumer. It also allows consumers to select a level of protection or risk that suits their circumstances.

In the policy arena the reforms that created health insurance portability and flexibility should be continued. The post–World War II triangular relationship among employee, employer, and insurer is archaic in an economy of high employee mobility. Employers should be encouraged to replace their current health insurance coverage models with defined contribution models that empower employees to go shopping for the plan and coverage that suits their needs—plans that may or may not be offered through the employer. Again, employees could augment the coverage at their own election and expense. This will tend to shift the insurance premium cost to employees, because it is likely that the defined contribution will be more static than premium prices. In the absence of increased value, consumers will resist these out-of-pocket increases and be a countervailing force against increases in premium prices.

The freedom of more choices cannot be separated from the cost of those choices. The United States has already endured a health care system in which consumers were shielded from the costs of their choices: the long-gone, cost-plus indemnity model. From 1960 to 1990, this model yielded 11 percent average annual growth in health care spending, growth consistently higher than overall economic growth.[9] The shift to defined premium contributions by employers should be coupled with a ten-year phase-out of the tax deductibility of employer-paid health insurance. This will gradually increase the cost of health insurance to the employee by at least the amount of his or her marginal tax rate.

Increasing this price burden will provides an enormous tank of gas to fuel the long consumerism journey. After all, consumerism is about getting value. The more a consumer has to pay, the more value the consumer will want, from both insurers and providers. Delivering more and more value will become an axiom for them. Subsidies, including tax-effect subsidies, distort the value equation and insulate sellers from the buyers' true demands.

INCREASE SUPPORT FOR PUBLIC HEALTH

Public health is like national defense: it requires two components to be effective—an elaborate infrastructure and individual commitment to the cause. The infrastructure is familiar and well-placed. It includes clean, fluoridated water, medicines that immunize against dread diseases, and the basic research that precedes the discovery of such medicines. It also includes food inspection, building codes that protect life and safety, health education, and dozens of other activities taken for granted—and often incorrectly omitted from the health care equation. Government's past investment in this infrastructure has been invaluable.

Individual commitment to the cause of consumerism holds the promise of improved public health. Consumerism can recruit more people to serve in the battle against perilous personal risks. Every year 658,530 Americans perish through murder, suicide, and accident, including automobile accidents.[10] The health care system is powerless to cure this carnage. People, acting individually, must buckle a seat belt, stop smoking, stop excessive drinking, stop drinking and driving, avoid addictive drugs, and avoid dangerous sex. The cumulative economic and social impact on morbidity and mortality of these personal choices is staggering. Some argue that consumerism's dark side is selfish self-interest, yet self-interest is the prescription for avoiding these risky behaviors.

The costs of successful public health innovations are usually discrete. The benefits are not. They are benefits that are measured for their effect on populations, not individuals. All the same, they can have a very real and beneficial effect for individuals. Government is the logical catalyst for these efforts.

INCREASE SUPPORT FOR EDUCATION

In the context of health care consumerism, education has two dimensions. First, implicit in the notion of an effective consumerism movement is an educated population. It is not possible to have an ignorant public and an effective consumerism movement. Second, and perhaps more important, study after study correlates health and well-being on one hand and education and income on the other. Former secretary of Health, Education and Welfare Joseph Califano reminds us that "[p]overty is the most persistent and pernicious companion of poor health. Individuals with family incomes under $9,000 a year have a death rate more than triple [that of] those with incomes above $25,000."[11] High school dropouts over age twenty-five have a median annual income of about $22,000, compared to nearly $36,000 for high school graduates and $70,000 for college graduates.[12] This underscores education's contribution to public health.

A government role that is directed toward health, not health care, ensures that literate youngsters graduate from high school, enter a growing economy that provides good jobs, and allows the bonds of unemployment and its inevitable poverty to be permanently broken. Whether support for this comes from local, state, or federal levels is a separate discussion; however, the link is undeniable, and the investment worthy for the long term.

ALLOW FROZEN CHARITABLE ASSETS TO THAW

This nation's hospital system was built with charitable dollars. Communities, philanthropists, and religious groups built thousands of hospitals. In 1946, Congress enacted the Hospital Survey and Construction Act, sponsored by Senators Lister Hill and Harold Burton and thus popularly called the Hill-Burton Act (Public Law 79-725). It enabled hospitals to be built and imposed requirements to provide free care. Over $4.6 billion in Hill-Burton grant funds and $1.5 billion in loans have been distributed to 6,800 health care facilities in more than 4,000 communities since 1946.[13] Investor-owned hospitals arose to supplement those owned by communities and religious organizations.

The hospital system today has excess capacity. Since the 1983 inception of Medicare's prospective payment system, the number of hospital admissions has fallen by about 12 percent.[14] The overall U.S. hospital occupancy rate continues to hover around 64 percent.[15] For a variety of reasons, substantial assets are frozen in their current form as hospitals though they might be more productive in other forms. Pure economic theory and market conditions ordain that this excess capacity will eventually evaporate. Some will go bankrupt; some have been, and more will be, bought and closed. But others will struggle to remain open, underwritten by taxpayers or sustained by charities—factors not considered in "pure" conditions. Meanwhile, government, as a health care buyer, and consumers pay some premium for this excess capacity. The excess capacity persists for a simple reason: there is no efficient way to convert a hospital's asset base to another use. Suppose a hospital board decides that the hospital's assets, if converted to cash and invested in a trust fund, would generate earnings sufficient to pay for the community's childhood immunizations forever. To sell the hospital does not rid the system of capacity. To shutter the hospital extracts no value from the assets and fails a test of fiduciary duty. To reinvest in, rebuild, or replace the hospital may be a last-gasp attempt to regain market share in a double-or-nothing investment gambit. Hospital administrators lack motivation to acquire and close a competitor because they believe they can defeat the competitor in a less costly war of attrition. Local businesses do not want to buy the capacity and remove it. How are consumers served by a long, painful struggle that squanders assets owned not by the hospital but by the community as a whole?

Again, government is in a unique position to set policy, though the policy course is not clear. One option is a kind of reverse Hill-Burton program, designed to eliminate rather than create hospitals. And just as Hill-Burton imposed a quid pro quo so might Hill-Burton II: permanent closure and perpetual charitable, civic, and health-promoting use of the proceeds. A hospital's decision to exit would have to be local, voluntary, and irrevocable. The period of time during which such an option might be exercised and the number of hospitals to be "bought" would have to be limited.

Georgia considered a similar idea. Public rural hospitals, in exchange for surrendering some licensed bed capacity to a statewide *bed bank*, would have received state grants.[16] This innovative policy was eliminated from the enacted legislation (Georgia Senate Bill 195) but had merit, even though it probably would not have reduced costs. Presumably the variable costs were already removed, and this proposal did nothing to reduce the ongoing fixed costs or liberate the assets for other uses. The most useful solutions will permanently remove capacity and thaw the assets for other charitable purposes.

SUMMARY AND CONCLUSION

Government, as an instrument of the people's will through policy and as a buyer of health services, has an unmistakable stake, opportunity, and obligation in the health care consumerism trend. The most important functions it can perform are those that the private sector cannot: require data to be available to others so that it can be manufactured into useful, widely disseminated information; effect policies that protect the citizens by establishing minimum coverages but let people make their own choices using defined contributions; encourage employers to use defined contributions, and slowly but steadily remove the masks that hide the real cost of health care from consumers, because doing so will, perhaps painfully, reduce prices and increase quality and value; aggressively fund public health, one result of which will be a more educated and employed populace; and finally, allow the hospital industry to invent methods that move assets to consumer-demanded uses.

Notes

1. Leschley, J. (then-CEO, SmithKline Beecham). Remark made at the *Wall Street Journal* Health Care Summit 99, Washington, D.C., May 5, 1999.

2. Centers for Medicare and Medicaid Services. "National Health Expenditures, 1996–2001." [www.cms.gov/statistics/nhe/historical/t3.asp], Sept. 2003.

3. U.S. Census Bureau. *Statistical Abstract of the United States, 1998.* Washington, D.C.: U.S. Government Printing Office, Oct. 13, 1998, table 1355 ("Gross Domestic Product, by Country: 1980 to 1997").

4. Health Care Financing Administration, *National Health Expenditures* . . .

5. Dartmouth Medical School, The Center for the Evaluative Clinical Sciences. *The Dartmouth Atlas of Health Care.* (J. Wennberg and others, eds.) Chicago: American Hospital Publishing, 1998. Additional information is available at [www.dartmouthatlas.org/pdffiles/ATLAST08.PDF].

6. Solucient is a health care information company based in Evanston, Illinois, that maintains a health care database. Additional information is available at [www.solucient.com].

7. In April 2001, J. D. Power and Associates formed this health care division, with the acquisition of Caredata Reports. Additional information is available at [www.jdpw.com/presspass/pr.pressrelrase.asq?ID111].

8. Centers for Medicare and Medicaid Services. *National Health Expenditures, Aggregate and Per Capita Amounts, Percent Distribution, and Average Annual Percent Growth, by Source of Funds: Selected Calendar Years 1980–2001.* [www.cms.hhs.gov/statistics/nhe/historical/t1.asp]. At over $500 billion per year, Medicare alone equates to half the GDP of the United Kingdom.

9. Health Care Financing Administration. *National Health Expenditures Aggregate and Per Capita Amounts, Percent Distribution, and Average Annual Percent Growth, by Source of Funds: Selected Calendar Years 1960–97.* Bethesda, Md.: Health Care Financing Administration, Oct. 1998.

10. Calculated from figures published by the U.S. Census Bureau. See *2001 Statistical Abstract of the United States.* Washington, D.C.: U.S. Government Printing Office, 2002.

11. Califano, J. A., Jr. *Radical Surgery.* New York: Times Books, 1994, p. 69.

12. U.S. Bureau of the Census. *Money and Income in the United States.* Current Population Reports P-60-209. Washington, D.C.: U.S. Government Printing Office, 1999.

13. U.S. Department of Health and Human Services, Health Resources and Services Administration, Office of Special Programs. [www.hrsa.dhhs.gov/osp/dfcr/about/aboutdiv.htm].

14. Calculated from figures published by the American Hospital Association. See "Fast Facts on U.S. Hospitals from Hospital Statistics." [www.aha.org/resource/ "newpage.asp], 2000.

15. American Hospital Association, Trend Analysis Group. *National Hospital Panel Survey Reports.* Chicago: American Hospital Association, June 1998.

16. Georgia State Health Planning Agency. Minutes of the Rural Health and Hospital Technical Advisory Committee, Oct. 20, 1998. Atlanta: Georgia State Health Planning Agency, 1998; Interview with Karen Decker, division director, planning and data management, Georgia State Health Planning Agency.

THE EDITOR

Regina E. Herzlinger is the Nancy R. McPherson Professor of Business Administration at the Harvard Business School. She is a prolific, iconoclastic, and acclaimed writer on the topic of health care. Her 2002 article on consumer-driven health care in the *Harvard Business Review* became an Amazon ebook best-seller.

In her previous book, *Market-Driven Health Care,* Professor Herzlinger predicted the problems that managed care plans and vertically integrated health care systems subsequently encountered, and introduced the concepts of "health care–focused factories" and "consumer-driven health care" to wider audiences. The book won the James Hamilton Book of the Year Award from the American College of Healthcare Executives. In 2003, she was elected one of health care's 100 most important people and awarded the HFMA's Board of Directors' award.

PARTICIPANTS IN THE CONSUMER-DRIVEN HEALTH CARE CONFERENCE, HARVARD BUSINESS SCHOOL, NOVEMBER 1999

E. Ratcliffe Anderson Jr.
G. Lawrence Atkins
James E. Austin
Pamela G. Bailey
Steve Bailey
Roger Battistella
Thomas R. Beauregard
Regina M. Benjamin
Eric S. Berger
Richard Bohmer
Sarah B. Bua
Amy S. Burroughs
Leonard Camarda
Thomas A. Cameron
James R. Castle
Becky J. Cherney
Jon A. Chilingerian
Dean Clancy
Kim B. Clark
Robert Coburn
Meryl Comer
Marcia Comstock

Judy Toran Cousin
Richard A. D'Amato
Corbette S. Doyle
Mary Jane England
John C. Erb
Matthew Eyring
Roger Feldman
Bernard T. Ferrari
James F. Fries
Thomas F. Frist Jr.
Jon Gabel
Robert S. Galvin
James S. Garrison
Lawrence N. Gelb
William W. George
John C. Goodman
Jessie C. Gruman
Edmund F. Haislmaier
Katherine M. Harris
John T. W. Hawkins
James L. Heskett
Jesse S. Hixson

Bruno L. Holthof
Steven S. Hyde
Lisa I. Iezzoni
Karen Ignagni
Constance G. Jackson
Harry R. Jacobson
Robert W. Jamplis
Daniel H. Johnson Jr.
Donald W. Kemper
David B. Kendall
Bradford J. Kimler
Amy Kroninger
Thomas J. Kuhlman
David J. Lansky
Louis Lasagna
Stacey Lauren
S. Robert Levine
Alfred B. Lewis
Ronald L. Lindsey
Mark E. Litow
Ron Loeppke
William H. Longfield
Stuart Lovett
François Maisonrouge
Brian J. Marcotte
Alfred Martin
Shaun Matisonn
Frank McArdle
Steven McGeady
Dwight McNeill
Scott F. Meadow
Mark Michel
Arnold Milstein
Ryan A. Moore
James W. Morrison Jr.
Stacey Muller
John G. Nackel
Thomas J. Nagle
Steven W. Naifeh
Chris O'Connell
Alan O'Dell
Dean Ornish

Mark A. Pearl
Diane C. Pinakiewicz
Gary P. Pisano
Thomas D. Policelli
Stephen Pollard
J. D. Power III
Wilfried Prewo
Richard L. Reece
Sharon Wildstein Reich
Rita Ricardo-Campbell
Russell J. Ricci
Ann Robinow
James F. Rodgers
Denise Hamilton Ross
John C. Rother
Alvaro Salas-Chaves
Bernard Salick
Greg Scandlen
Jennifer S. Schultz
Robert N. Shamansky
Steven J. Shulman
Warner V. Slack
Gregory White Smith
Danville D. Spiller
Charlie Stein
Robert E. Stone
Ellen Stovall
Cornelia K. Tilney
Jennifer Ulin
Daryl Urquhart
Kevin Vigilante
Robert R. Waller
Scott Walton
Albert S. Waxman
Alan Weinstein
Leon S. White
John A. Whittemore
Bonnie B. Whyte
Vicki M. Wilson
Ron Winslow
Seth M. Yellin
Les Zendle

THE CONTRIBUTORS

Ken Abramowitz, M.B.A., is managing director of The Carlyle Group, based in New York City. He currently focuses on health care buyouts, after having spent twenty-three years as a health care analyst at Sanford C. Bernstein & Co.

John W. Adams Jr., M.S., is president and chief executive officer of Cardio-Vascular Care Providers, Inc., and Global Healthcare Alliance, Inc., in Houston, Texas.

Laura L. Adams is principal at Laura Adams Consulting and a member of the faculty of the Institute for Healthcare Improvement in Boston.

Nancy E. Adler, Ph.D., is professor of psychology in the Departments of Psychiatry and Pediatrics at the University of California-San Francisco and also vice chair of the Department of Psychiatry and director of the Center for Health & Community.

Paul Belien lives in Antwerp, Belgium; he holds a degree in law from Ghent University (Belgium). From 1982 to 1995, he worked as a journalist. From 1995 to 2000, he was research director at the Centre for the New Europe (CNE), a Brussels-based think tank.

Eric S. Berger is vice president of planning and public policy at US Oncology, in Houston, Texas. He previously served as health policy analyst for the House Commerce Committee and as the State of Virginia's legislative and policy director for health and human resources.

Richard Bohmer, M.D., M.P.H., is assistant professor at the Harvard Business School in Boston.

Jeanne A. Brown, B.S.E., J.D., is the former general counsel of the Evergreen Freedom Foundation, based in Olympia, Washington, which works to advance individual liberty, free enterprise, and responsible government.

Roger J. Bulger, M.D., is president and chief executive officer of the Association of Academic Health Centers, based in Washington, D.C.

Becky J. Cherney is president and chief executive officer of Central Florida Health Care Coalition, based in Orlando.

Jon A. Chilingerian, Ph.D., former assistant health commissioner at Boston City Hospital, is a tenured professor of organizational behavior and health care management at Brandeis University, Waltham, MA.

Jon Christianson, Ph.D., is the James A. Hamilton Chair in Health Policy and professor of management at the Carlson School of Management, University of Minnesota at Minneapolis. He directs the Center for the Study of Healthcare Management in the Department of Healthcare Management at the Carlson School.

Graydon M. Clouse, M.B.A., is a freelance consultant in San Francisco and the author of a number of teaching case studies on the health care industry, focusing on innovations in software and services.

Robert W. Coburn is a principal in William M. Mercer Human Resource Consulting, in Baltimore.

Denton A. Cooley, M.D., is president and surgeon-in-chief of the Texas Heart Institute in Houston.

Richard A. D'Amaro is president of NuTec Health Systems, based in Atlanta, Georgia. He has been an active advocate for our health care system for over twenty-five years as an industry consultant.

Corbette S. Doyle is managing director at AON Financial Institution Alliance, in Franklin, Tennessee. She currently sits on the boards of Definity Healthcare and Sterling Life Insurance Company.

Amy C. Edmondson, Ph.D., is associate professor at the Harvard Business School, Boston, specializing in organizational behavior.

John C. Erb, M.H.A., is a senior manager and consultant with Deloitte & Touche, specializing in employer-sponsored health benefits programs.

Roger Feldman, Ph.D., is Blue Cross Professor of Health Insurance, Division of Health Services Research and Policy, School of Public Health, at the University of Minnesota in Minneapolis.

Bernard T. Ferrari, M.D., J.D., is head of the North American Corporate Finance and Strategy Practice at McKinsey & Company.

James F. Fries, M.D., is professor of medicine at Stanford University School of Medicine, in Palo Alto, California.

Thomas F. Frist Jr., M.D., is chairman emeritus of Hospital Corporation of America (HCA), Nashville, Tennessee. He cofounded HCA in 1968, along with his father, Thomas F. Frist Sr., M.D., and Jack C. Massey.

Jon R. Gabel, Ph.D., is vice president, health system studies, of the Health Research and Educational Trust, American Hospital Association, in Washington, D.C.

Carrie Gavora was a member of the professional health staff of the House Commerce Committee and the health care analyst for the Heritage Foundation, a public policy think tank.

Lawrence N. Gelb, M.B.A., D.M.H., is president and chief executive officer of CareCounsel, LLC, in San Rafael, California.

William W. George, M.B.A., was chief executive officer of Medtronic, Inc., from 1991 to 2001, after serving as an executive at Honeywell and Litton Industries for over twenty years.

Cynthia M. Gibson, M.S.W., is a program officer at Carnegie Corporation of New York, working in the program titled Strengthening U.S. Democracy and overseeing the subprograms Strengthening the Nonprofit and Philanthropic Sector and Youth Civic Engagement. She is a doctoral candidate in social policy at Rutgers University.

Jody Hoffer Gittell, Ph.D., is assistant professor of management at the Heller School for Social Policy and Management, Brandeis University, in Waltham, Massachusetts.

John C. Goodman, Ph.D., is president of the National Center for Policy Analysis, based in Dallas, Texas.

Jessie C. Gruman, Ph.D., is president and executive director of the Center for the Advancement of Health in Washington, D.C.

Jenny M. Hamilton, M.S.G., is executive policy advisor, Governor's Executive Policy Office, in Olympia, Washington.

Katherine M. Harris, Ph.D., is a full economist in the Health Program at the RAND Corporation, in Arlington, Virginia.

Eugene D. Hill III, M.B.A., is a general partner at Schroder Ventures Life Sciences, based in Boston, where he focuses on health care service and health care information technology investments.

David J. Hines is president and founder of Consumer's Medical Resources, Inc., based in Duxbury, Massachusetts.

Jesse S. Hixson, Ph.D., was principal economist for health policy at the American Medical Association.

Bruno Holthof, M.D., M.B.A, is a partner with McKinsey & Company, working in the New Jersey and Brussels offices.

Stephen S. Hyde, M.B.A., is managing partner of Clear Creek Resources, LLP, a business advisory firm based in Colorado Springs. He was also the founder and chief executive officer of Peak Health Care, Inc.

Lisa I. Iezzoni, M.D., M.Sc., is professor of medicine at Harvard Medical School in Boston.

Karen Ignagni is president and chief executive officer of the AAHP-HIAA (American Association of Health Plan–Health Insurance Association of America), based in Washington, D.C.

Constance G. Jackson, M.B.A., is president and chief executive officer, Urban Health Consulting, in London.

Harry R. Jacobson, M.D., is vice chancellor for health affairs at Vanderbilt University, in Nashville, Tennessee.

Daniel H. Johnson, M.D., is a former president of the American Medical Association and currently a visiting fellow in health policy at the Heritage Foundation.

Donald W. Kemper is chairman and chief executive officer of HealthWise, Inc., in Boise, Idaho, and founding chairman of the Center for Information Therapy.

David B. Kendall is senior fellow for health policy at the Progressive Policy Institute, in Washington, D.C.

Charles H. Klippel, J.D., is deputy general counsel at Aetna Inc., Hartford, Connecticut.

David Lansky, Ph.D., is president of the Foundation for Accountability (FACCT), in Portland, Oregon.

Mark Levin is chairperson of the board of directors and chief executive officer of Millennium Pharmaceuticals, Inc., based in Cambridge, Massachusetts.

S. Robert Levine, M.D., is chairman of the Juvenile Diabetes Research Foundation (JDRF), a mission-driven nonprofit organization seeking a cure for diabetes and its complications through the support of research.

Al Lewis, J.D., is executive director of the Disease Management Purchasing Consortium, based in Wellesley, Massachusetts, and founder of the Disease Management Association of America.

Stuart Lovett, M.D., is director of Perinatal Services at the Alta Bates Summit Medical Center in Berkeley, California; chief of service, Obstetrics and Gynecology, for Hill Physicians Medical Group of San Ramon, California; and medical director of East Bay Perinatal Medical Associates, based in Oakland, California.

François Maisonrouge is co-head of the Global Health Care-Life Sciences Group at Credit Suisse/First Boston, in England.

Brian J. Marcotte is vice president, compensation and benefits, at Honeywell International, Morristown, New Jersey.

Shaun Matisonn is head of risk management at Discovery Health, in Sandton, South Africa.

Molly Mettler is senior vice president of HealthWise, Inc., in Boise, Idaho, and chair of the National Council on the Aging.

Michael L. Millenson is the Mervin Shalowitz, M.D. Visiting Scholar at the Health Industry Management Program of the J. L. Kellogg School of Management at Northwestern University, Evanston, Illinois, and the author of *Demanding Medical Excellence: Doctors and Accountability in the Information Age.*

Arnold Milstein, M.D., M.P.H., is the National Health Care Thought Leader at Mercer Human Resource Consulting and medical director at the Pacific Business Group on Health.

James W. Morrison Jr. is president of Morrison Associates, in Scottsdale, Arizona, which provides strategic business advice on legislative and regulatory issues affecting health care and employee benefits. He is a former administrator of the Federal Employees Health Benefits Program.

Colleen M. Murphy is president and chief executive officer of Asparity Decision Solutions, in Durham, North Carolina.

Steven W. Naifeh, J.D., is the president of Woodward/White, Inc., in Aiken, South Carolina. He is the best-selling author of several books, including *Jackson Pollock: An American Saga,* which won the Pulitzer Prize and was a finalist for the National Book Award in 1990. He has been editor of *The Best Lawyers in America* since 1981. He was chairman of Best Doctors from 1997 until 2000.

Alan O'Dell is managing director of Shouldice Hospital, in Ontario, Canada.

Dean Ornish, M.D., is founder and president of the Preventive Medicine Research Institute and clinical professor of medicine at the University of California-San Francisco.

Mark A. Pearl, M.D., M.B.A., is a managing member at Henderson Capital Management, based in Wellesley, Massachusetts, where he works with entrepreneurial health care companies. He was a cofounder of CareAgents, which eventually became WebMD.

Gary P. Pisano, Ph.D., is Harry E. Figgie Jr. Professor of Business Administration at the Harvard Business School, Technology and Operations Management unit.

J. D. Power III is chairman and chief executive officer of J. D. Power and Associates, based in Westlake Village, California.

Rita Ricardo-Campbell, Ph.D., is a senior fellow at the Hoover Institution, Stanford University, Stanford, California.

Russell J. Ricci, M.D., is chief medical and strategy officer, HealthSTAR Communications, Woodbridge, New Jersey. He formerly was general manager of IBM Global Healthcare, based in Waltham, Massachusetts.

Ann L. Robinow is president and chief executive officer of Patient Choice Healthcare, Inc., in St. Louis Park, Minnesota.

James F. Rodgers, Ph.D., is vice president, health policy, of the American Medical Association.

John Rother is director of policy and strategy for the American Association of Retired Persons (AARP), based in Washington, D.C.

Alvaro Salas-Chaves, M.D., M.P.H., M.P.A., was the minister of social security, Costa Rica, now retired.

Bernard Salick, M.D., is chairman and chief executive officer of Bentley Health Care, Inc., in Beverly Hills, California. As founder of Salick Health Care, Inc., in 1983, he pioneered the concept of a twenty-four-hours-a-day, seven-days-a-week, consumer-driven, outpatient diagnostic and treatment center.

Leonard D. Schaeffer, Ph.D., is chairman and chief executive officer of WellPoint Health Networks, Inc., based in Thousand Oaks, California.

Jennifer S. Schultz, Ph.D., is a health services researcher in the Economic and Outcomes Research Department of IngeniX, Inc., in Minneapolis.

Robert N. Shamansky, J.D., is a former U.S. Congressman and retired partner at Benesch Friedlander Coplan & Arnoff in Columbus, Ohio.

Warner V. Slack, M.D., is a professor at the Harvard Medical School and president of the Center for Clinical Computing at the Beth Israel Deaconess Medical Center in Boston. His classic book, *Cybermedicine,* was republished in an expanded edition by Jossey-Bass in 2001.

Cynthia A. Smith, R.N., J.D., is a principal in William Mercer Human Resources Consulting.

Gregory White Smith, J.D., is vice president of Woodward/White, Inc., in Aiken, South Carolina. With partner Steve Naifeh he founded Best Doctors, Inc., in 1992.

Robert E. Stone, Ph.D., is executive vice president of American Healthways, in Nashville, Tennessee.

Joseph P. Tallman is president and founder of Access Health Group/McKesson, in Boulder, Colorado.

Lynn M. Taussig, M.D., is president and chief executive officer of National Jewish Medical and Research Center, in Denver, Colorado.

David Tinkelman, M.D., is vice president of health initiatives at National Jewish Medical and Research Center, in Denver, Colorado.

Daryl J. B. Urquhart is director of marketing of Shouldice Hospital in Ontario, Canada.

Mary K. Uyeda, Ph.D., is the senior health analyst for the Washington State Health Care Authority, in Olympia, Washington.

Kevin Vigilante, M.D., M.P.H., is clinical associate professor of medicine at the Brown University School of Medicine, Rumford, Rhode Island.

Anthony Welters, J.D., is chairman and chief executive officer of AmeriChoice Corporation, based in Vienna, Virginia.

Tony L. White is chairman and chief executive officer of Applera Corporation, based in Atlanta, Georgia.

Bonnie Whyte, C.F.C.I., C.A.E., is chief executive officer of the Employers Council on Flexible Compensation, based in Washington, D.C.

Vicki M. Wilson, Ph.D., is project director of the State Planning Grant on Access to Health Insurance, Governor's Executive Policy Office, in Olympia, Washington.

Seth M. Yellin, M.B.A., is an associate director in the mergers and acquisitions group at UBS Warburg in New York.

Les Zendle, M.D., was associate medical director of Kaiser Permanente Southern California, based in Pasadena, California.

NAME INDEX

A

Abe, T., 741
Abernathy, F. H., 684
Achman, L., 31
Adamache, K. W., 247
Advertising Age, 442
Aetna Press Release, 60
Akerlof, G., 475, 477
Aldana, S. G., 528
Alexander, G. C., 32
Allen, H., 105, 119
Allen, T., 684
Alter, D. A., 181
Altman, S., 736, 738, 739
American Benefits Council, 768
American Cancer Society, 596
American Child Health Association, 551
American Diabetes Association, 119, 120, 121, 555, 643
American Healthways, 645
American Heart Association, 718
American Hospital Association, 115, 826
American Hospital Publishing, 605
American Lung Association, 619, 620, 718
American Medical Association, 158, 738
American Medical News, 32, 115
Ancona, D. G., 684

Anderson, D., 106
Anderson, D. R., 119
Anderson, G. F., 35, 342
Anderson Consulting, 342
Andrews, F., 107
Andrews, M., 135
Annas, G. J., 797
Antonius, D., 168
Aon Consulting Inc., 18
Appleby, J., 17
Aranow, M., 676
Archives of Internal Medicine, 433
Argote, L., 685
Arista Associates, 108
Armstrong, D., 461, 802
Arnett, G. M., 766
Arnold, M., 344
Aron, D. C., 186
Arregui, M. E., 629, 632
Arrow, H., 684
Arrumada, B., 348
Asch, S. M., 106, 120
Ash, A. S., 170, 244
Ashton, C. M., 552
Ashworth, G., 672
Asinoff, L., 812
Aston, G., 798

Atkinson, R. D., 755
Atlas, 469
Audit Bureau of Circulations, 139
Austin, B., 565
Austin, B. T., 564
Auto Affordability Index, 14
Aventis Risk Report, 175
Ayanian, J., 741
Ayanian, J. Z., 39, 254

B

Baggs, J. G., 685
Bahnson, P. R., 802
Baigriie, R. J., 580
Bailey, S., 118
Baillie, J., 580
Baker, D. W., 44
Baker, R. E., 802
Banaszak, 431, 432
Bankowitz, R. A., 675, 676
Banthin, J. S., 378
Barley, S. R., 581, 686
Barnes, J., 105, 119
Barnes, V., 166
Barondess, J. A., 550
Barr, S., 159
Barrand, N. L., 299
Barrett, M. J., 105
Barringer, F., 164
Barth, R. T., 687
Bartlett, J., 812
Basinski, A. S. H., 181
Basler Zeitung, 323
Bates, D. W., 167, 254
Baumol, W. J., 104
Beach, W. W., 289
Beaver, W. H., 800, 801
Becher, E. C., 183
Becker, S., 597
Beckley, R. F., 676
Beddingfield, K. T., 246
Beine, K., 445
Benk, L. B., 85
Benko, L., 28
Benko, L. B., 157
Benner, P., 447
Benson, J. M., 58, 110
Benston, G., 801
Bentley, J. M., 168, 183
Berdahl, J. L., 684
Berger, M., 120

Bering-Jensen, H., 345
Berk, M. L., 119
Bernard, G. R., 672
Bernstein, N., 624
Bertko, J., 255
Berwick, D., 446, 670
Bezmalinobic, B., 803
BHCAG, 168
Bianco, A., 235
Biermannn, J. S., 583
Billings, J., 517
Black, F., 7
Bleakley, F., 740
Bledsoe, T., 538
Blendon, R., 347, 731
Blendon, R. J., 58, 110
Block, S., 7
Blue Cross of California, 22, 84
Bluestone, B., 737
Blumberg, L. J., 35
Blumenthal, D., 50
Blyskal, J., 174
Bodenheimer, T., 36
Boehm, E. W., 434
Boehm, J., 94, 102
Bogardus, S. T., 246
Bogle, John, 20
Bohmer, R. M. J., 574, 583
Bokser, S., 167
Bond, M. T., 230
Bonnard, J., 326
Borden, S., 105, 119
Boston Globe, 60
Bourna, C., 114
Bowen, W. G., 104
Bowlin, S. J., 248
Boyd, C. J., 181
Bradley, A. E., 672
Bradley, Bruce, 424
Branch, M. S., 580
Brandt, M., 731
Brase, T., 765
Brenner, B., 5, 21
Brinkley, J., 256
Brocato, F. ., 105
Brocato, F. M., 119
Brodie, M., 16
Brody, H., 345, 554
Brook, R. H., 76, 102, 106, 447
Brooke, J., 180
Brown, B. W., 526

Brown, E. R., 40
Brown, J. B., 120
Brown, L. D., 165
Brown, M. S., 602
Brown, R., 253
Brown, S. E., 517
Brush, T., 683
Buchanan, B. G., 675
Buchanan, R., 128
Buchmueller, T. C., 77
Budetti, P. P., 106
Buettner, R., 140
Bulllman, W. R., 563
Buntin, M. J. B., 255
Burda, D., 163
Burke, L., 672
Burroughs, A., 583, 800
Burstin, H., 254
Burt, R. S., 686
Business Week, 7, 9, 11, 47, 161, 802
Busquin, P., 345
Butler, C. A., 723
Butler, S., 757
Butler, S. M., 141
Byrd, J. C., 166

C
Caggiano, C., 7
Caldwell, D., 684
Califano, J. A., 825
Call, K., 480
Canadian Institute of Health Information, 628
Caplin, J., 812
Cardoza, D., 639, 641, 642
Caredata Reports, 820
Carey, C., 527
Carey, J., 169
Carey, M. A., 141
Casalino, L., 108
Castle, J., 461
Center for the Advancement of Health, 565
Centers for Disease Control and Prevention, 38
Centers for Medicare and Medicaid Services, 820, 823
Central Florida Health Care Coalition, 467
Chaines, A., 445
Chan, J. K., 106
Chang, Y., 50

Changes in Health Care Financing and Organization, 169, 183
Chapman, L. S., 528
Chapman, W. C., 672
Chassin, M. R., 167, 168, 183, 247, 454, 800
Chatfield, . A. M., 169
Chemical Market Reporter, 802
Chernew, M., 479
Chiang, Y. P., 253
Chicago American Bar Association, 112
Chicago Planlinx, Inc., 491
Chicago Tribune, 554
Chilingerian, J. A., 444, 445, 448, 449, 688
Chin, T., 140
Chorus, A. M. J., 354
Christensen, C. M., 444
Christianson, J., 89, 477, 480, 483
Churchill, N. C., 168
CiGNA, 22
Cimino, J. J., 676
Clancey, C., 742
Clancy, C. M., 345
Clark, K. B., 573, 683
Clark, N. M., 564
Classen, D. C., 676
Clayton, P. D., 676
Cleary, P. D., 447, 800
Clemson University, 538
Cleofe Molina, C., 363
Coase, R. H., 684
Coburn, R., 87
Codman, E. A.., 551
Coffman, G., 170
Cohen, M., 429, 430, 431, 432
Coile, R. C., 307
Colby, C. J., 120
Cole, R. E., 128
Colen, A., 342
Collins, C., 166
Collins, K., 736
Committee on Quality of Health Care in America, 552
Committee on Small Business, 812
Commonwealth Fund, 39, 40, 41, 44, 139, 179
Conlin, M., 102
Connelly, J., 461
Consumer Assessment of Health Plans, 473
Consumer Reports, 9, 13

Consumers Union, 31
Continuing Medical Education Inc., 718
Cooley, D., 143
Cooper, P., 737
Cooper, R. A., 582
Copeland, C., 751
Corey, E. R., 175
Coronel, S. A., 31
Costantino, G. N., 582
Coulam, R., 477
Court, R. H., 755
Cowan, C. A., 22, 34, 42, 142, 146, 160
Cox, J., 8
Coye, M. J., 108
Coyne, C., 248
Coyne, K. P., 14
Crane, D., 116
Crane, S. D., 20
Creedon, 293
Croasdale, M., 45
Crowston, K., 684
Cull, C. A., 106
Cummings, L. L., 686
Cummins, D. S., 45
Cunningham, P., 738, 739, 740, 753
Cunningham, P. J., 166, 431, 754
Cunningham, R., 106
Cunninham, P., 752
Curran, J. P., 812
Cutler, D. M., 110
Cyber Dialogue, 16
Czajka, J. L., 751

D

Dahl, D., 799
Daley, J., 557, 684
Daly, R., 180
Damato, K., 5, 155
Dambro, M. R., 676
Danzon, P. M., 35, 345, 758
Dartmouth Medical School, The Center
   for the Evaluative Clinical Sciences,
   114, 315, 605, 608, 820
Datastream International, 135
Davis, K., 736
Davis, M., 342
Deakin, E., 801
Deardon, J., 172
DeBare, I., 499
DeBuono, B. A., 247
Defeever, C., 463
Definity Health, 132

Delbanco, T. L., 445, 446, 447, 448,
   557, 684
De Morgen, 353
Denk, C., 166
Dennis, W. ., 159
Desrochez, C., 731
Detwiler, M. L., 291
DeVito, C. A., 253
DeVlin, B. H., 628
Diabetes Control and Complications Trial
   Research Group, 120, 645
Dickey, N. W., 45
Dietrich, C. L., 582
Dietrich, K., 663
Dietrich, K. A., 646
DiSalvo, T. G., 579
Dixon, R., 108
Dobbs, K., 114
Dolliver, B. K., 431
Donabedian, A., 445, 448, 449, 608
Donelan, K., 181, 739
Dooley, D., M. D., 115
Dopuch, N., 801
Douds, C. F., 687
Dougherty, D., 686
Dowd, B., 476, 477
Doyle, C., 196
Doyle, J. C., 551
Doyle, T., 814
Dranove, D., 183
Draper, E. A., 685
Drew, K., 672
Dreyfus, T., 244
Driest, P., 326
Drury, P., 483
Druss, B., 32, 35
Druss, B. G., 39, 105
Dryfoos, P., 753
Dubois, R. W., 246
Dubuono, B. A., 168
Duchon, L., 37
Duchow, L., 102, 157, 159, 162
Dunagan, W. C., 676
Duncan, J. ., 614, 615
Dunlop, J. T., 684
Dunn, D. L., 170, 255
Dunn, S. M., 622
Dutch Federation of Patients and
   Consumers Organizations, 345
Dutt, J., 801
Dutton, G., 29, 155
Dziuban, S. W., 183

E

Earley, P. C., 686
Eccles, R., 686
Eckenrode, J., 798
Eddy, D., 445, 662
EDGAR, 164
Edgman-Levitan, S., 557, 684, 800
Edlin, M., 120
Edmonds, C. H., 613, 614
Edmondson, A., 685
Edmondson, A. C., 574, 583
Eichenwald, K., 21
Eisenberg, E., 687
Eisenberg, J. M., 243, 449, 553
Eisenkop, S. M., 639
Ellis, R. P., 254, 299
Ellwood, M., 751
Ellwood, P., 758
Elrod, T., 476
Elsens, V. D., 538
Employee Benefit Plan Review, 21, 30
Employee Benefits Research Institute,
    9, 29, 34, 43, 148, 178, 179, 288, 386,
    732, 736
Employers Council on Flexible Compen-
    sation, 286, 287, 289
Engledow, J., 795
Enthoven, A., 95, 231, 758
Epstein, A., 741
Epstein, A. M., 455, 740
Erdem, T., 476
Erickson, S., 672
Esposito, A., 253
Estrada, C., 166
Ethan Allen Institute, 79
Etheredge, L., 758, 804
Evans, R. S., 676
Everett, D., 562
Ewigman, B. C., 639

F

Faas, A., 232
Fabrikant, G., 164
Fagerhaugh, S., 684
Fagerlin, A., 32
Fama, E., 800, 801
Fayol, H., 684
Feder, J., 740, 741, 753
Federal Agency for Health Care Policy
    and Research., 303
Federal Employees' Health Benefits Act of
    1959, 291

Federal News Service, 165
Federal Register, 813
Federal Reserve Bank of St. Louis, 768
Feldman, R., 476, 477, 480, 483
Feldstein, P. J., 77, 758
Fenley, L., 142
Ferris, T. G., 50
Fidel, S., 431
Fidelity Investments, 18, 19, 28
Figluilo, M. L., 107
Financial Times, 353
Fireman, B. H., 175
Flanigan, J., 46
Flexner, A., 607
Florence, C. S., 135
Floyd, M., 445
Food and Drug Administration, 580
Forbes, 12, 107, 162
Foreman, J., 554
Forrester Research Inc., 16, 434, 798
Forsyth, B., 477
Forsyth, D. E., 675
Fortune, 21
Foss, J., 672
Foundation for Accountability, 424
Fowles, J., 478
Fowles, J. B., 247, 255, 315
Fox, S., 16
Francis, W., 94
Franco, S. C., 798
Frankfurter Allgemeine Zeitung
    Infomation Services, 347
Frankl, V. F., 602, 608
Franks, P., 742
Fraser, V. J., 676
Frayling, L., 286, 287, 288
Freeman, J. L., 244
Freidson,, E., 551
Freudenheim, M., 40, 157, 582
Fries, J. F., 32, 527, 528
Fries, S. T., 527
Frisse, M., 676
Frogue, J., 180
Fronstin, P., 42, 160, 731, 734, 752
Frudenheim, M., 799
Fuchs, V. R., 96, 110
Fulcrum Analytics, 431

G

Gabel, J., 28, 178, 734, 737
Gabel, J. R., 49, 155, 166
Galbraith, J., 684

Galewitz, P., 582
Galloway, A. C., 574
Galvin, R., 606
Galvin, R. W., 454, 800
Garber, Alan, 549
Gardner, E., 106
Gardner, J., 163
Gardner, R. ., 676
Gardner, R. M., 676
Garnick, D. W., 575
Gaskin, D., 738
Gatsonis, C., 740
Gauthier, A. K., 255, 299
Gawande, A. W., 167
Geevarghese, S. K., 672
Geissbuhler, A., 676
Geldstein, M. S., 102
Gelick, E., 605
Genbank, 607
Genentech, Inc., 723
Gentry, C., 80, 86
Georgia State Health Planning Agency, 827
Gerteis, M., 557, 684, 685, 688
Giacomini, M., 299
Gibbs, D., 477
Gifford, D. L., 285, 286
Gillette, B., 28
Gillies, R., 106
Gilmer, T., 244
Gilmer, T. P., 646
Ginsberg, P. B., 47, 754
Ginsberg, P. R., 49
Gittell, J. H., 685, 686, 687, 691
Gladstone, M., 9
Glauber, H. S., 120
Glazer, J., 255
Glower, D. D., 574
Gokhale, J., 102
Golaszewski, T. J., 526
Gold, M., 31, 446, 688, 742
Gold, M. R., 175
Goldberg, S., 116
Goldberg, S. T., 5
Goldfield, N., 246
Goldmann, L., 582
Goldstein, B. D., 455
Goldstein, J. L., 602
Goldwasser, R., 143, 144
Golov, D., 168, 183
Goodman, J. C., 170, 225, 226, 230, 233,
    238, 341, 354

Goodman, M. J., 247
Goodwin, E. J., 246
Gorin, E. J., 628
Gorman, C., 798
Gottlieb, S. S., 643
Gould, K. L., 518
Gourville, J. T., 97
Govindarajan, V., 168
Grahm, P., 377
Granovetter, M., 686
Green, J., 247, 583
Greenfield, S., 243, 248, 496
Greenhouse, L., 43
Greenlick, M., 537
Greenstein, R. J., 676
Greenwald, J., 157
Greenwald, L. M., 253, 254
Greenwalk, J., 32, 85
Greer, A. L., 571
Grensburg, C. R., 43
Grey, B., 135
Griffiths, J., 60
Grimaldi, J. V., 21
Groome, P. A., 181
Grossman, J., 108
Grossman, J. M., 177, 754
Gruenberg, L., 247
Grumbach, K., 323
Gulati, R., 107
Guralnik, J., 562

H
Haburchak, D., 597
Hadley, J., 741, 753
Hagland, M., 43
Haines, A., 558
Hakim, D., 5
Hales, J. W., 676
Hallman, G. L., 613, 614
Halm, E. A., 167
Halpern, N. A., 676
Hamilton, J. M., 299
Hammond, J. C., 629, 632
Hammond, J. T., 684
Handbook of American Business, 158
Handelszeitung, 328
Hanks, C., 798
Hannan, E. L., 183, 244, 247
Hannen, E. L., 168
Hargraves, J. L., 57
Harper, D., 169, 183

Harper, D. L., 186
Harrington, C., 38
Harrington, H., 527
Harris, J. E., 449
Harris, K., 482
Harris Inereactive Poll, 432, 557
Hart, C., 683
Hart, J., 518
Harvard Business School Bulletin, 19
Harvard University School of Public
   Health, 117, 492
Hatcher, C. S., 170
Havighurst, C. C., 43
Hawk, A. D., 646, 663
Hawkins, S., 28
Hayes, R., 683
HayGroup, 769, 771
Health Affairs, 355
Health Care Choices, 751
Health Care Financing Administration,
   820, 824
Health Insurance Association of America,
   462
Health Systems Trust, 330
Healthwise, 538
Heffler, S., 255
Heinonen, O. P., 639
Hellinger, F. J., 255
Helman, R., 42
Helms, R., 755, 766
Helms, R. B., 345
Hemenway, D., 445
Hen, P. de, 325
Henderson, B. D., 172
Henderson, C. R., 798
Henderson, R. M., 573
Henikoff, L., M. D., 80
Henry Ford Museum, 29
Hensler, D. R., 43
Hernandez,R., 140
Herring, B., 38
Herschman, R., 29
Herzlinger, R. E., 84, 88, 89, 104, 105,
   107, 138, 144, 167, 184, 232, 235, 362,
   389, 445, 448, 487, 534, 582, 583, 632,
   683, 797, 799, 800, 804, 811
Heskett, J. L., 446, 683
Hewitt, M., 167, 596
Hewitt Associates, 43, 217, 286, 491, 492,
   768
Hiatt, H., 670

Hibbard, J., 537
Hibbard, J. H., 365, 455
Hilgenkamp, R., 799
Hill, S. C., 253
Himmelstein, D., 799
Himmelstein, D. U., 177, 179
HMO Disease Management Initiatives, 556
Hof, R. D., 798
Hofer, T. P., 167, 185
Hoff, J., 758
Hoffman, C., 562, 563, 595, 662
Hoffman, J. C., 646
Hofmann, M. A., 177
Hogan, C., 49, 50, 752
Hogan, P., 733
Holahan, J., 40, 736
Hollman, R. R., 106
Holmer, M., 482
Holmes, B. J., 182
Holtzman, N. A., 722
Hornbrook, M. C., 247
Horst, K. M., 166
Houdart, P., 325
Howatt, G., 102, 162
Hubbard, J. H., 166
Huff, S. M., 676
Hui, S. L., 676
Hulsey, T. C., 639
Hunt, D. L., 164
Hunt, K. A., 166
Hunt, S., 255
Hupfer, M. A., 615
Hurley, J. F., 676
Hurley, R., 108, 175
Hurley, R. E., 177
Hurst, Jeremy W., 355
Hussery, P. S., 342
Hwang, W., 35
Hyde, Stephen, 78
Hynes, A. K., 431

I

Iezzoni, L. I., 170, 243, 245, 247, 254, 299
Iglehart, J. K., 255
Ingber, M. J., 253
InSights Consulting, 538
Institute of Medicine, 104
Institute of Medicine, Health Sciences
   Policy Program, 606
Institutional Investor, 4, 8, 20
Internal Revenue Code, 105, 106., 276

Internal Revenue Code, 3121, 3306, 3401., 272

Internal Revenue Code. U.S. Code, Title 26 106 (2000), 271

Internal Revenue Code of Federal Regulations. Title 26, 1.106-1., 271

Internal Revenue Service., 288

Internal Revenue Service. *Medical Expenses.,* 287

Interstate Commerce Commission, 812

Interstudy, 556

InteStudy, 644

Ippolito, R. A., 801

Ireys, H., 35

Isaacs, S., 800

Iyengar, S. S., 97

J

Jacob, J. A., 37

Jacobius, A., 155

Jacobson, J. T., 676

Jaedke, K., 164

Jaklevic, M. C., 10, 50

Jamieson, G. G., 580

Janis, I. L., 455

Jaramillo, I., 363

Jaramillo-Vallejo, J., 801

Jensen, G. A., 233

Jensen, M., 801

Jernstadt, L., 462

Jewett, J., 166, 365

Jewett, J. J., 455

Johnson, B. C., 11, 101

Johnson, R. E., 286

Joint Committee on Taxation, 766

Jones, D. T., 684

Jones, R., 558

Jossi, F., 424

Jost, T. S., 250

Journal of Accountancy, 42

Jowell, P. S., 580

Joy, M. A., 801

Joyeaux, A., 32

Juniper, E. F., 622

Jupiter Media Metrix, 428, 429, 430

K

Kaga, 607

Kaganova, E., 247

Kahn, M. G., 676

Kahneman, D., 455

Kaiser Family Foundation, 117, 430, 492

Kaiser Family Foundation and Agency for Health Care Research and Quality, 42, 43, 44, 132, 423

Kaiser Family Foundation and Health Research Educational Trust, 41, 76

Kallner, H., 332

Kalmer, H., 526

Kamberg, C. J., 102

Kaplan, S., 496

Kaplan, S. E., 168

Karjalainen, O., 639

Karnani, A., 683

Katz, J. N., 248, 552, 691

Katz, R., 684

Kay, R., 661

Keane, M., 476, 482

Kearny, A. T., 434

Keenan, P., 740

Keenan, P. S., 255

Kefalides, P. T., 248

Keller, R. T., 684

Kelley, G., 444

Kemper, D. W., 535, 538

Kendall, D., 147, 609, 750

Kendall, D. B., 757, 758, 799

Kennedy, J., 461

Kerwin, K., 13

Kessler, D., 183

Khandker, R. K., 247

Kim, J., 40

Kim, M., 110

Kimball, R., 640

Kimberly, J. R., 688

King, R. T., 570, 584

Kitzman, H., 798

Klein, T. M., 798

Klein, W. M., 455

Kleinke, J. D., 110, 323

Knaus, W. A., 251, 685

Knepper, 431, 432

Knickman, J., 482

Knox, R. A., 47

Knutson, D., 170, 255

Koch, M. O., 672, 675

Kochaniek, J. W., 139

Kogut, B., 684

Kohler, B., 741

Kolb, K., 455

Kopacz, D. J., 571, 580

Kornberg, A., 606

Kotlikoff, L. J., 102
Kovar, M., 562
Kowalczyk, L., 47
KPMG, 76, 139
Kraines, R. G., 526
Kranish, M., 148
Krantz, D. S., 4
Krasner, M., 583
Kravitz, R. L., 248
Kronick, R., 95, 244
Kumar, D., 183
Kuperman, G. J., 676

L
LaCroix, A., 562
Lake, T., 108, 175
Lalli, F., 812
Lamphere, J. A., 299
Landers, S. J., 39, 168
Landon, B. E., 166
Lang, F., 445
Lankford, K., 46
Lansky, David, 608, 609
Larme, A. C., 644
Larson, D. E., 139
Larson, P., 537, 538, 539
Larson, R. A., 676
Laschober, M. A., 255
Laub, R. M., 676
Laud, P., 582
Laudicina, S., 767
Lavern, E., 184
Law, S., 732
Lawrence, P. R., 684
Lazenby, H. C., 142, 146
Leana, C., 686
Leape, L. L., 579
Leatherman, S., 76
Lee, C., 167
Lee, L., 244
Legnini, M. W., 167
Legorretta, A. P., 582
Le Grand, J., 345
Lemieux, J., 147, 750, 758, 759
Lemov, P., 345
Lepage, E. F., 676
Lepper, M. R., 97
Leschley, J., 820
Lesser, C. S., 47
Levin, M., 144
Levine, S., 750

Levine, S. R., 147, 609, 758
Levit, K., 34, 35
Levit, K. R., 22, 34, 160, 225
Levitan, S. E., 448
Levitt, B., 573
Levitt, L., 28
Levy, J. M., 253
Lewis, A., 644
Lewis, K., 751
Lewis, W. W., 11, 59
Lichtenberg, F. R., 110
Licking, E., 47
Lieberman, A., 527
Linde, K., 85
Lipscomb, G. H., 640, 641
Litsky, F., 111, 112
Lloyd-Jones, D., 579
Lohr, K. N., 102
London, K., 753
Long, S., 740, 743
Long, S. H., 758
Looney, W., 345
Lorie, E., 798
Lorig, K., 526, 538, 564
Lorsch, J. W., 684
Los Angeles Times, 140, 155
Lo Sasso, A. T., 155, 177
Losleben, B., 767
Lubalin, J., 477
Lucas, L., 18
Luft, H., 50, 575
Luft, H. S., 250, 299
Lux, H., 86
Lyall, S., 180
Lyles, A., 89
Lyman, L., 813

M
Maassen, B. M., 346
MacFarlan, M., 342
MacKillop, W. J., 181
Malflict, T., 341
Malkiel, B. A., 800, 801
Malmsheimer, R., 550
Malone, T., 684
Malye, F., 325
Managed Care, 155, 170, 388
Mandel, M. J., 23
Mangione-Smith, R., 554
Mango, P. D., 107
Manin, M. B., 286, 287, 288

Manning, J., 115
Manning, W. G., 228, 646
March, J. G., 573, 686
Marcus, S. C., 32, 105
Marin Independent Journal, 17
Mark, D. H., 575
Markel, H., 722
Marks, G. B., 622
Marmot, M., 181
Marquardt, C., 538
Marquis, M., 740, 743
Marquis, M. S., 228, 758
Marquis, S., 482
Marsa, L., 85
Marshall, M. N., 76
Martens, S. C., 802
Martin, A. B., 142, 146
Martin, D. K., 676
Martin, P. B., 685
Martinez, B., 47, 49, 94, 158
Martino, A., 342, 348
Martino, B. D., 802
Marwick, C., 120
Massaro, T. A., 676
Matisonn, S., 231, 332
Matthews, M., 230, 231, 238
Mattli, W., 184
Maurstad, H. L., 95
Mauss, D. W., 132
Mazzolini, J., 252
McCabe, G. P. Jr, 676
McCall, N., 482
McCarter, R. J., 643
McClellan, M., 110, 183
McClure, C. L., 676
McCormick, D. H., 107
McCormick, J., 7
McCorty, K. R., 672
McDermott, S., 638, 641
McDonald, C. J., 676
McDonnell, P. A., 22, 34, 160
McEnery, R., 168, 183
McEnroe, J. E., 802
McGeehan, P., 5
McGinley, L., 43
McGlynn, E. A., 106, 447, 552
McGrath, J. E., 684
McGuire, T. G., 255
McKeever, W., 431
McKenna, R., 414
McKibbon, A., 164

McKinnon, J. D., 461
McKinsey & Company, 324, 799
Mclaughlin, C. G., 28
Mclean, B., 21, 184
McManamin, P., 45
McMurty, D., 23, 160
McPhee, S. J., 575
McShane, D. J., 527, 528
Mechanic, D., 129
Medecine & Health, 252
MEDecision, 473
Medical Benefits, 46
Medical Post, 16
Medicare Payment Advisory Commission, 34, 50, 253
Meier, B., 43
Melloan, G., 347
Menard, M. K., 639
Menon, K., 168
Mercer Human Resource Consulting, 42
Meredith, T. P., 817
Mettler, M. K., 535, 538
Meyer, H., 235
Midwest Business Group on Health, 454
Millenson, M., 478, 557
Millenson, M. L., 551, 555
Miller, J., 797
Miller, M. H., 6, 7
Miller, P. W., 802
Miller, R. A., 675, 676
Miller, R. H., 50
Miller, T. E., 16, 94, 139
Milliyet, 463
Mills, R. J., 38
Mills, R. T., 4, 38
Milstein, A., 446
Minvielle, E., 688
Mitka, M., 766
Modern Healthcare, 15, 107, 175
Moeller, J. F., 378
Moffit, R., 135
Moffit, R. E., 94, 289
Moffitt, R. E., 34
Mokdad, A. H., 119
Monheit, A. C., 119
Monoson, R., M. D., 45
Montgomery, E. B., 527
Moody's Investor Service, 108
Moore, B., 114
Moore, D., 136
Moore, R.K, 597

Moore, S., 349
Moore, W. K., 803
Moran, G., 388
Morgan, J. P., 46
Morgan, R. O., 253
Morrisey, M. A., 233
Morrow, M., 554
Morton, F. M. S., 9
Moses, S., 34
Moskowitz, M. A., 170, 247
Moyers, B., 517
Moynihan, R., 582
Muhlhausen, I., 120
Mukamel, D., 800
Mullins, C. D., 110
Mumford, L. M., 313
Murphy, J., 672
Murray, E. K., 37
Murray, M. N., 723
Murray, S., 134, 135
Musgrave, G. L., 225, 233, 238, 341, 354
Mushlin, A. I., 800
Myers, L. P., 246
Myerson, A. R., 143

N
Naifeh, S. W., 137
Nangle, M., 614, 615
Nash, D. B., 168, 183, 246
Nasser, J., 14
Nastas, G., 551
National Association of Unclaimed
    Property Administrators, 813
National Committee for Quality
    Assurance, 491, 554, 643
National Economic Research Associates,
    348, 350
National Health Information, 106
National Institute for Health Statistics, 118
National Institute of Health, 606, 610, 718
National Public Radio, 117
National Underwriter, 21
Nation Center for Health Statistics, 142
Navarro, F., 79
Naylor, C. D., 180, 181
Neal, J. M., 571, 580
Ness, D., 84
Neuman, P., 253
Newacheck, P., 619
New England Journal of Medicine, 120
Newhouse, J. P., 171, 185, 244, 255

Newman, R. B., 639
News and Progress, 134, 168, 170
Newsweek, 819
New York Business Group on Health,
    15, 799
New York Daily News, 140
New York Times, 19, 20, 155, 160, 161,
    165, 180, 344, 351, 804, 814
New York Times Magazine, 236
Nichols, B., 142
Nichols, G. A., 120
Nichols, L. M., 35
Noble, H. B., 437
Nohria, N., 107, 686
Norris, F., 4, 7, 8
Nurss, J. R., 44

O
O'Conner, P. J., 646
Ohio Department of Commerce, 813
Ohio Revised Code, 812
Old Mutual Actuaries and Consultants,
    330
Olds, D. L., 798
O'Leary, D., 685
Olsfsonh, M., 32, 105
On Managed Care, 799
Ontario Health Insurance Plan, 631
Ontario Ministry of Health, 632
Oppel, R. A., 20
Oregon Health Sciences University, 537
O'Reilly, B., 87
Organization for Economic Cooperation
    and Development, 341, 342, 350
Ornish, D. M., 517, 518
Osheroff, J. A., 675
Overhage, J. M., 676
Oxley, H., 342
Ozbolt, J. G., 676
Ozminkowski,, R. J., 528

P
Pacific Business Group on Health, 166
PaineWebber, 135
Palmade, V., 11, 59
Palumbo, F. B., 110
Pan American Health Organization, 363
Parcell, C. L., 527
Park, Y. C., 801
Parker, R. M., 44
Paroa-Parsi, R., 89

Parrish, M., 181
Partners Health Initiative, 538
Passaro, V., 346
Patge, M., 9
Paul, S. D., 579
Pauly, M., 170, 758, 759
Pauly, M. V., 35, 38, 226, 238
Pauly, P., 141
Payne, J. L., 672
Pear, R., 42, 46, 50, 58
Pearlstein, S., 802
Pearson, S. D., 50
Pelletier, K. R., 528
Penn, M. J., 29, 31, 179, 182
Pensions & Investments, 9, 10, 11, 155
Percy, A., 38
Perenboom, R. J. M., 354
Perry, M. J., 167
Persily, N. A., 253
Pestotnik, S. L., 676
Petersen, E. D., 168, 183, 800
Phillips, D., 802
Phillips, E. H., 629
Phillips, K. A., 110
Pinches, G. E., 6
Pisano, G. P., 574, 583
Pockell, D. G., 37
Podolsky, D., 246
Pollack, R., 799
Pollitz, K., 37
Pollock, J. E., 571, 580
Ponka, J. L., 628
Pope, B. C., 247, 254
Pope, G. C., 254, 299
Porter, M., 95
Porter, P. K., 170, 226
Pozen, R., 20, 185
President's Advisory Commission on
  Consumer Protection, 552
Previts, G. J., 801, 802
Price, B. J., 672
PricewaterhouseCoopers, 16, 117
Priest, L., 463
Princeton Survey Research Associates, 166
Professional Target Marketing, 628
Puchalski, P. J., 299
Pugh, J. A., 644

Q
Quesenberry, C. P. Jr., 323
Quinn, J. B., 813

R
Rabkin, S. W., 120
Rainie, L., 16
Rainwater, J. A., 168, 250
Ramsey, R., 9
RAND Corporation, 481
Ray, G. T., 120
Ray, N. F., 106
Redding, R. J., 802
Redelmeier, D. A., 455
Reed, M. C., 32
Reekie, W. D., 344
Reents, S., 16, 139, 140
Regout, B., 11, 59
Rehfeld, B., 9
Reinhardt, U., 731, 736, 738, 739, 743
Reinhardt, U. E., 342
Reither, C. L., 802
Research!America, 606
Reuter, J., 738
Reuters Medical News, 47
Revenue Ruling 57-33. 1957-1 *Cumulative
  Bulletin 303.*, 272
Revenue Ruling 61-146., 272, 273
Revenue Ruling 61-146. 1961-2 *Cumulative
  Bulletin*, 25., 271
Revenue Ruling 2002-41, 276
Ricardo-Campbell, R., 816
Rice, D., 562, 563, 595, 662
Rice, N., 244
Rice, T., 28, 129, 155, 482
Richardson, N., 526
Ridley, M., 145
Riley, G., 253
Rind, D., 378
Robbins, A. W., 628
Robert, L., 169
Roberts, K., 686
Robertson, N. J., 167
Robert Wood Johnson Foundation, 105,
  106, 166
Robinow, A., 88, 478
Robinson, J., 108
Robinson, J. C., 48, 106, 158, 299, 478
Robitaille, S., 108
Rocha, B. H., 676
Rodriguez, T., 446
Rogal, D. L., 255
Rogers, M. P., 676
Rogers, P. G., 563
Rogers, W. H., 248

Romano, P. S., 168, 249, 250
Roos, D., 684
Rosenberg, L. E., 167
Rosenberg, R., 144
Rosenheck, R. A., 39
Rosenthal, G. E., 186
Rothman, M., 255
Rottenberg. S., 225
Rowland, D., 736, 740
Royal College of Surgeons of England, 628
Rozin, P., 455
Rubenstein, A. H., 687
Rubenstein, E. S., 342, 345
Rubin, R. J., 646, 663
Rundle, R., 799
Russ, C. S., 429, 430, 431, 432
Rutkow, I. M., 628

S

Saari-Kemppainen, A., 639
Saavedra, R., 686
Safran, C., 676
Sage, W. M., 43
Salas, A., 363
Salas-Chavas, A., 363
SalomonSmithBarney, 135, 157
Samuelson, R. J., 342
Samwick, A. A., 8, 17
Sanders, D., 94
San Francisco Chronicle, 43
Sanger, D. E., 813
Sangl, J., 482
Sasser, W. E., 446, 683
Satterthwaite, M., 183
Scalise, D., 17
Scanlon, D., 479
Scavini, M., 120
Schaapveld, K., 354
Schade, D. S., 120
Schaefer, E., 752
Schanier, J., 477
Schauffler, H. H., 446
Schellevis, F. G., 232
Scherwitz, L. W., 517
Schlesinger, L. A., 446, 683
Schmittdiel, J., 323
Schneider, E. C., 455
Schone, B., 737
Schroeder, S., 563
Schultz, J., 480
Schurz, J. W., 629

Schuster, M. A., 552
Schuster, M. S., 106
Schwarzschild, B., 169
Schwenditman, C. J., 6
Sciandra, F. G., 286, 287, 288
Scott, D. L., 803
Seby, J. V., 323
Segal Company, 288
Selby, J., 120
Selden, T. M., 378
Seligman, J., 169, 184, 801
Sell, S., 164
Seltz, C. A., 285, 286
Shakelle, P. G., 76
Shaw, G. B., 376
Sheils, J., 756
Sheldon, T., 341
Shelton, P., 445
Shemin, R. J., 574
Shepardson, L. B., 186
Sherlock, D., 50
Sherlock Company, 141
Sherman, H. D., 445, 448
Sherman, M., 138
Sherman, W., 140
Shields, A., 736, 738, 739
Shiels, J., 733
Shinkman, R., 499
Shore, A. D., 89
Shortell, S., 106
Shortell, S. M., 685
Shouldice, E. E., 627
Shoven, J. B., 798
Sidiropoulos, E., 330
Silber, J. H., 582
Silow-Carroll, S., 102, 157, 159, 162
Silva-Risso, J., 9
Silvestri, S., 603
Simborg, D. W., 246
Simon, H. A., 455, 686
Simone, J., 596
Simonson, D. C., 106
Sinclair, J. L., 32
Sinclair, M., 166
Sing, M., 253
Singh, G., 527
Singh, H., 107
Sinisi, M., 246
Sirio, C. A., 169, 183
Sittig, D. F., 676
Siu, A. L., 183

Skinner, W., 8, 17, 105, 683
Skousen, F., 801, 802
Slack, W. V., 376, 377, 378
Slass, L., 799
Slatalla, M., 140
Slater, R., 5, 19, 20
Sledge, W. H., 39
Smillie, J., 661
Smith, C. A., 299
Smith,, G. W., 137
Smith, J. A., 672, 675
Smith, M. D., 37
Smith, P. C., 244
Smith, R., 670
Smith, S., 662
Smoley, S. R., 249, 250
Snyderman, R., M. D., 46, 109
Sofaer, S., 455
Solucient, 820
Soman, D., 97
Soumerai, S.B., 607
Sox, H. C., 110
Spence, M., 478
Spillane, M. J., 676
Spragins, E., 589
Spranca, M., 479
Spring 2000, 147
Stafford, R. S., 579
Starfield, B. H., 313
Statistical Abstract of the United States, 8
Staw, B. M., 686
Stead, W. W., 676
Steege, J. F., 640, 641
Steen, P. M., 247
Steib, S. A., 676
Steinberg, E. P., 741, 753
Steiner, C. A., 582
Steinwachs, D. M., 313
Stephens Inc., 135
Stephenson, J., 35
Sternberg, L., 538
Sternberg, S., 804
Stevens, C., 614
Stigler, G. J., 182, 801
Stiglitz, J. E., 801
Stipp, D., 144
Stires, D., 161
Stoline, A. M., 550
Stone, R., 646
Stovall, T. G., 640, 641
Stratton, I. M., 106

Strauss, A., 684
Struebing, L., 447
Strunk, B., 753
Strunk, B. C., 177, 431
Stuart, B., 110
Studdert, D. M., 43
Suczek, B., 684
Sullivan, L. M., 248
Sullivan, L. W., 246
Sullivan, R., 517
Summitt, R. L. Jr., 640, 641
Sung, H. Y., 562, 563, 595, 662
Swiss Week in Review, 350
Switzerland. Federal Statistical Office., 350
Swope, C., 148

T
Tanielian, T., 32, 105
Tanne, J., 461
Taylor, M., 184
Taylor, W., 619
Teich, J. M., 676
Teleki, S., 40
Tengs, T. O., 229, 606
Ter Meulen, R. H. J., 87
Teske, R., 34
Testa, M. A., 106
Tetik, C., 629
Thamer, M., 106
The Business Roundtable, 555
The Economist, 103, 108, 180, 345, 387
Thomas, J., 255
Thompson, J. D., 684
Thompson, R., 388
Thompson, R. E., 676
Thorelli, H., 795
Thorpe, K., 735, 736
Thorpe, K. E., 135
Tierney, M., 29, 83, 158, 174
Tierney, W. M., 676
Toffler, A., 413
Tokarski, C., 797
Tollen, L., 255
Topol, E. J., 252
Toran, M. W., 43
Treasury Notice, 276
Trotter, C., 60
Trude, S., 32, 161, 750, 754
Tu, H., 738, 739, 740
Tudor, C., 253
Tumlinson, A., 800

Turner, G., 101
Turner, R. C., 106
Tversky, A., 455
Tweed, V., 351
Tye, L., 583

U
Ubel, P. A., 32
U.K. Prospective Diabetes Study Group, 645
Ulmer, M., 59
Ulrich, B., 143, 144
United Kingdom. HM Treasury., 328
Urquhart, D. J. B., 628, 632
U.S. Accounting Office, Health, Education, and Human Services Division, 246
U.S. Banker, 20
U.S. Bureau of Labor Statistics, 117, 155, 353, 731, 737
U.S. Census Bureau, 8, 15, 34, 38, 40, 41, 42, 49, 102, 128, 141, 160, 287, 288, 589, 735, 737, 738, 820, 825
U.S. Congressional Research Service, 94
U.S. Department of Commerce, 429, 430, 731
U.S. Department of Health and Human Services, 254, 597, 614, 826
U.S. Department of Labor, Bureau of Labor Statistics., 287
U.S. General Accounting Office., 178, 289
U.S. House of Representatives, 293
USA Today, 15, 16

V
Van Buren, H. J. III, 686
Van de Ven, A., 684
VanDorsten, J. P., 639
Van Dyne L., 686
Van Eijk, J. T., 232
Van Geest, J. B., 45
Van Maanen, J., 686
Van Overtveldt, J., 342, 345
Varmus, H., 607
Vatter, H. G., 128
Vaughn, D., 583
Vergara, F., 355
Versweyveld, L., 435
Vickers, M., 812
Vickery, D. M., 526
Vincent, J., 325
Vinicor, F., 621

Virnig, B. A., 253
Vise, D., 9
Vladeck, B. C., 244, 246
Vogel, R. A., 252, 643
Vogeli, C., 50
Von Korff, M., 564, 565
Von Stillfried, D., 344
Vuekovic, N., 39
Vuturo, A. F., 676

W
Wachter, R. M., 582
Wade, R., 115
Wageman, R., 686
Waggoner, J., 6
Wagner, D. P., 685
Wagner, E. H., 564, 565
Wagner, L., 34
Walker, J. F., 128
Walker, N., 767
Wall St. Journal, 8, 11, 128, 161, 171, 183, 184, 186
Wall St. Journal Europe, 342, 346, 348, 351
Walsh, E. G., 247
Walsh, J., 9
Walters, J., 9
Wang, J., 110
Wantz, G. E., 629
Ward's Reports, 13
Ware, J. E., 496
Warshawsky, M. J., 102
Washington State Health Care Authority, 299
Wasley, T., 345
Watson, D. I., 580
Watson, M. S., 722
Watson Wyatt Worldwide, 10, 176, 184, 491
Webb, A. B., 11, 59
Wechsler, J., 85
Wee, C. C., 44
Weekers, S., 326
Wehrwien, P., 662
Weick, K., 686
Weil, D. A., 684
Weinberger, M., 303
Weiner, J., 483
Weiner, J. P., 89, 313, 550
Weinstein, N. D., 455
Weiss, B. D., 248, 676
Weiss, L., 685

Weissman, J., 740
Weissman, J. S., 753
Weller, W., 35
Wellpoint Health Networks, 84
Wells, C., 583
Welters, A., 146
Wennberg, J. E., 552
Werdegar, D., 249, 250
Werner, R. M., 32
Western Journal of Medicine, 434
Wetzell, S., 800
Wheeler, D. J., 557
Wheelwright, S., 683
White, K. S., 676
White, R., 672
Whitford, D., 6, 129
Wiener, C., 684
Wiener, D., 7
Wilensky, G. R., 246
Wilkens, S., 79
Williams, D. D., 168
Williams, F., 5
Williams, L. S., 676
Williams, M. V., 44
Willliam M. Mercer, Inc., 556
Willliams, L. P., 553
Willoughby, J., 9
Wilson, G. A., 676
Wilson, I. B., 45
Wilson, P., 249, 250
Wilson, V. M., 255, 299
Winslow, A., 583
Wintfield, N., 247, 583
Wise, D. A., 798
Witter, J. W., 14

Wolfe, S., 461
Womack, J. P., 684
Wong, M.D., 102
Woody, T., 430
Woolcock, A. J., 622
Wooldridge, J., 446, 688
Woolhandler, S., 799
Woolhandler, S. J., 177, 179
World Bank, 363
World Health Organization, 256, 350, 718
Wright, E. C., 526
Wright, J. K., 672
www.faa.gov, 164
www.nhtsa.gov, 164
Wyn, R., 40
Wynia, M. K., 45

Y
Yegian, J. M., 37, 38
Ylostalo, P., 639
Young, G., 685
Young, J., 731

Z
Zabinski, E., 378
Zach, A. P., 250
Zaheer, A., 107
Zander, U., 684
Zettelmeyer, F., 9
Zezza, M. A., 22, 34, 160
Zhang, D., 120
Zhang-Salomons, J., 181
Zimmerman, J. E., 685
Zuger, A., 581
Zweifel, P., 350, 354

SUBJECT INDEX

A

AAPCC (adjusted average per capita cost), 253

Academic medical centers, 670, 699–702, 738

Academy of Medicine, 250

Access Health Group (AH), 501–508, 503–507

Access issues, 79
    accessibility of doctors, 431–432
    to cardiac surgery for women, 517
    denial of coverage/access to Medicare, 520
    of doctors through referral services, 461–462
    European, 354
    to evidence-based information, 535
    incentives for (BHCAG), 314
    to information, 429, 816–817
    limited access problems, 162–163, 791–793
    for poor/nearly poor people, 791–793
    universal access to knowledge, 609
    of universal health care systems, 180–181

Accountability, 182, 183–184, 263, 419–427, 608, 776

ACGs (adjusted clinical groups), 313

Activism/activists, 145–146

AcuMatch, 459–460

Acute care/disease management, 205–206, 503–505, 567

Acute Physiology and Chronic Health Evaluation (APACHE), 251

Adjusted average per capita cost (AAPCC), 253

Adjusted clinical groups (ACGs), 313

Administrative data, 245–246

Administrative services only (ASO) funding, 592–593

Adults, 311, 779–780

Advance selection networks, 90

Adverse selection concept, 591, 752

Advertising, direct-to-consumer, 431

Advisory Commission on Consumer Protection and Quality, 552

Advocacy, 377, 411, 493, 645

Aetna, 21, 47–49, 58, 59–60, 158, 281, 292

Affymetrix, 719–721

Agency for Health Care Policy and Research (AHCPR), 488, 553–557

Agent effects, 9

AHA (American Hospital Association), 115, 652

AH (Access Health Group), 501–508, 503–507
AHCPR (Agency for Health Care Policy and Research), 488, 553–557
AIDS, 556. *See also* HIV/AIDS
Aisner, James, 10
AlliedSignal (Honeywell), 213–218
Allocations, 76–77, 395, 524–525
Alternative caregivers, 652
Alternatives to managed care, 322–328
AMA (American Medical Association), 139–140
American Accreditation Health Care Commission (URAC), 141
American Association of Health Plans, White Paper on plan risk management, 79
American Child Health Study, 551
American Diabetes Association, 120–121
American Healthways, 645–648
American Hospital Association (AHA), 115, 652
American Medical Association (AMA), 139–140
AmeriChoice Corporation, 146, 781–788
Analyses, 476–480, 481–482
APACHE (Acute Physiology and Chronic Health Evaluation), 251
Applera Corporation, 708–711
Approaches to care
    care management at Honeywell, 216–217
    Consumer Assessment of Health Plans study (CAHPS), 303–304
    Federal Employees Health Benefits Program (FEHB), 293
    meeting need for information, 424–425
    to plan offerings for, 265
    right care approach, 204–205, 210
    of Washington State Health Care Authority (HCA), 298–299, 303–304
Archer, Bill, 279
Archer medical savings accounts (MSAs), 281–282
Architectural innovations, 573, 584
As Good as It Gets (film), 733
ASO (administrative services only) funding, 592–593
Asparity Decision Solutions, 487–489

Assessment
    of care, 420, 459–460, 688–689
    Consumer Assessment of Health Plans study (CAHPS), 303–304, 473–474
    of health plans, 302–305, 306
    of risk, 299–300, 327, 783–784
Association of Academic Health Centers, 700–701
Asthma management, 644
    Asthma Care Management Program (KPSC), 665
    barriers to success of DMP:Asthma program, 624–625
    Lung Facts, 621
    LUNG LINE, 620–621
    Managed Care Consult Line, 621
    by National Jewish Medical and Research Center, 621–625
    numbers of sufferers, 718
    Physician Line, 621
    quality of life results, 622–624
    statistics on, 619–620
Athletes, 111–112
Atlas system, 469–471
Audits, 555, 706, 804
Austria, Freedom Party (FPOE), 343
Automated systems, CareCounsel, 496–498
Automotive industry examples, 410–418, 477–478
Autonomy of consumers, 524–525

B
Balanced Budget Act (1997), 248, 792
Bank of America study, 527
Bankruptcies, 369, 740
Barriers/obstacles
    to accountability, 608
    to change, by providers, 550–552
    to choose, by chronically ill, 594
    consumers as, 704–706
    decision-making, removing, 307
    to diffusion
        of AmeriChoice plan, 785–786
        CareCounsel, 499–500
        genomics-based medicine, 722–723
        HCA, 305–306
        Healthtrac, 529–530
    of information, 425–426
    Kaiser, 666

to implementation, 314–315, 567–568
information, 795
to international consumer-driven
    health care, 365
to mandating standard system of risk
    adjustment, 266
to outcomes comparisons, 324
overcoming, 385–387
physicians as, 703–704
sense of entitlement of consumers as,
    389–390
to solutions, 818
to success of DMP:Asthma program,
    624–625
to use of managed care organizations,
    509
of vision/models of consumer-driven
    health care, 383–387
Base networks, 222
Base pairs, 723
Bed bank (Georgia), 827
Belgium, 36, 339–340, 343
Belien, Paul, 36
Benchmarking, 424, 551
Benefits
    of consumer-driven model, 378–379,
        382–383, 699–700
    defined benefit (DB) funds, 5, 8–9, 11,
        17, 33–37, 74–75, 210
    design of, 90
    for employers, 498–499
    establishment of minimum, 823–824
    expansion of, during World War II, 755
    of ideal health insurance, 237–239
    market context of, 492
    redesigned options, 220
    trading unwanted, 31–32
    types offered, 75
Benign uterine disease, 640–641
Bentley Health Care, Inc., 595–601
Best Doctors, 136–137, 458–465
Best practices, 218, 491, 655, 670
Beta (risk measurement), 6–7
BHCAG. See Buyers Health Care Action
    Group (BHCAG)
Bid rates, health plan, 300–301
Billionaires, 164
Black lists of doctors, 461
Blue Cross Blue Shield, 50, 233, 235, 519,
    767

Blue Cross of California, 160
Bogle, John, 5–6
Bradley, Bill, 147–148
BRCA 1 gene test, 722–723
Breakfast insurance metaphor, 57, 79
    choice and control in, 69–70
    consumer-driven, 68–69
    defined benefit (Phase One), 63–64
    human resource managed star
        (Bruce), 65–67
    managed breakfasts (Phase Two),
        64–65
    pricing, 70–73
    problems of, 67–68
Broomfield Care Center sorting
    method, 505
Budgets
    Balanced Budget Act (1997), 248, 251,
        253, 422–423, 792
    health care systems based on, 327–328
    Netherlands, PGB (persoonsgebonden
        budget), 326
Bundled services, 46, 80
Bureaucracies, 812–814
Business-to-business e-commerce,
    434–435
Buyers Health Care Action Group
    (BHCAG)
    background, 475–476, 476–480
    barriers to implementation, 314–315
    care systems, results of, 310–312
    competition for patients, 310
    data source for analyzing, 480
    enrollment patterns, 310, 312
    incentives for access/care by, 314
    mentioned, 87–89, 93–94, 104,
        134–135, 686, 799, 800
    provider reimbursement/risk
        adjustment, 312
    results, 481–482
    risk-adjusted payments, 314
    variation in illness burdens, 313
Buying-blind situation, 406–407

C
C. Everett Koop National Health Awards
    for Healthtrac, 528
CAD (coronary artery disease), 664
Cafeteria plans, 285, 286, 288, 392–393,
    780

CAHPS (Consumer Assessment of Health Plans study), 303–304, 473–474
Califano, Joseph, 825
California
    California Association of Hospitals and Health Systems, 249
    California Hospital Outcomes Project case study, 248–250
    California Public Employees Retirement System (CalPERS), 767–768
    FlexScape program (BC of California), 160
    Kaiser Permanente Plan, 184, 377
    Kaiser Permanente Southern California (KPSC), 661–667
    Public Employees Retirement System (PERS) study, 526–527
    ratings of hospitals, 113–114
    WellPoint plan, 317–321
Canada, 345, 628, 631–632
Cancer
    catastrophic care model for, 595, 597
    lung, 244–245
    per-member per-month (PMPM) basis for treatment, 600
    of reproductive tract, 639–640
    treatment of, 597–598, 640
Capital, availability of, 657–658
Capitalization, 351–352, 352–354
Capitation, 108, 252–256, 315, 599–600, 756, 792
Captive insurance (HCA Health Care Indemnity), 657
Cardiac care
    acute myocardial infarction (AMI) death rates, 250
    care management strategies for, 664
    congestive heart failure (CHF), 108–109, 211–212
    coronary artery bypass graft (CABG) surgery, 244, 247
    formation of cardiovascular care providers, 613–614
    Heart Hospital of Milwaukee, 114–115
    lifestyle changes for, 516–521
    MedCath Corporation, 113–116
    minimally invasive cardiac surgery, 572–576
    open heart surgery, 142–143
    risk-adjusted mortality rates, 168
    Texas Heart Institute, 142–143
CardioVascular Care Providers (CVCP), 613–618

Cardiovascular disease (CVD), 718
CareCounsel, 17, 491–492, 492–498, 499–500
Caredata.com, 821–822
Care enhancement program, 645–649
Caregivers, 622–623, 652
Care management approach (Kaiser Permanente), 662–667
Care managers (Personal Care Model), 782
Care systems. See Health care systems
Case management, 671–675, 782
Case mix index (CMI), 673–674
Case studies/examples
    Access Health Group (AH), 501–503
    adjustment of capititated payments (Medicare), 252–256
    AmeriChoice Personal Care Model, 786–788
    California Hospital Outcomes Project, 248–250
    Cleveland Health Quality Choice Program (CHQC), 250–252
    congestive heart failure (CHF), 211–212
    Consumer's Medical Resource (CMR), 512–515
    cost effectiveness, 512–515
    Hershey Foods, 248
    quality of care, 512–515
Casualty insurance model, 232–233
Catalogues, health plan, 90
Catastrophic care model, 595–601
Catastrophic insurance, 195, 220
CBE (charting-by-exception) format, 672
CDV (Customer-Delivered Value), 416–417
Celera Genomics, 709–710, 710–711
Center for the Advancement of Health, 564–565
Centers for Medicare and Medicaid Services (CMS), 530, 590, 821–822
Centers of excellence, 235–236
Central Florida Health Care Coalition, 467–474
Centralized functions, non medical, 654–655
Challenges
    of Best Doctors referral services, 463–464
    of consumer-driven health care, 186–187, 368–370
    to managed care businesses, 659–660
    to medical professionals, 636–637
    overcoming resistance, 398

Chamber of Commerce, 21
Changes
    in consumer reporting, 304
    consumer resistance to, 388
    consumers as engines of, 608–609
    demographic, in uninsured
        consumers, 736
    doctors' awareness of, 697
    in fee schedules, 312
    government (U.S.) as overseers of, 196
    guidelines for, 196–197
    industry, in future, 403–404, 407–409
    information as key to, 468–469
    insurers as engines of, 196
    methods of, 719–721
    organizational/cultural, 700–701
    patient behavior affecting, 444
    in provider orientation, 371
    providers as engines of, 196
    resistance to, 539
    in roles of insurers/providers, 381
Charitable assets, thawing of, 826–827
Charity care, 738
Charter Communications, 488
Charting-by-exception (CBE) format, 672
CHEC (Consumer Health Education
    Council), 178–179
CHF (congestive heart failure), 108–109,
    211–212, 647, 664
Childbirth length of stay laws, 180
Children
    American Child Health Study, 551
    Children's Health Insurance Program
        (CHIP), 756, 759
    Children's Health Insurance Program
        (SCHIP), 792
    Twin Cities Metro Area, 311
Chile, 365
Choice Plus, 478–479
Choices. See also Decision making
    advocacy for, 377
    among competing products, 295–296
    among insurance plans, 487–489
    benefits of consumer, 799–800
    of care systems by variable, 481–482,
        483
    choice cooperatives, 374
    consumer choice program for universal
        coverage, 742–746
    consumers', 703–706
    decision types, 423–424
    in defined contribution retirement
        plans, 28–29, 216

demand for, 753–755
    dissatisfaction with lack of, 323
    effects of, 97–98
    for elderly, 394–396
    enabling competition for, 195
    of Federal Employees Health Benefits
        Program (FEHB), 94
    government support for consumer-
        based, 263
    of health plans, 12
    for insurance plans, 75–76
    lack of, as problem, 60–61, 753
    Limited Access story, 162–163
    menus for choice/enrollment, 759
    methods of providing, 266–268
    need for information for, 422–423
    portability of pension plans, 18
    promoting, 133
    reducing/expanding, 374
    restrictions on, 766–768
    by size of employer, 752
    between tax credits or tax exclusions,
        756–757
CHQC (Cleveland Health Quality Choice
    Program), 169, 183, 250–252
Chronic diseases. See also Disease
    management
    behavior as factor of, 563
    care enhancement program (diabetes),
        645–649
    choices for care, 396
    costs of, 643
    focused factories for, 105, 590–593
    HMOs for, 589–590
    integration of care for, 45–46
    management of, 207–208, 554–555,
        561–568, 644–645
    outcomes measures for, 593
    out-of-pocket expenses for, 35
    reasons for focusing on, 562–564
    uninsured people with, 39
Claims, 86, 312, 315, 323–324
Clancy, Dean, 148
Class Warfare story, 161–162
Cleveland Health Quality Choice Program
    (CHQC), 169, 183, 250–252
Cleveland Tomorrow, 250
Clinical moments of truth, 446
Clinical outcomes, 216–219
Clinical pathways, 672
Clinical trials, 605
Clinton administration, 552, 743, 761, 777
Closed-panel HMOs, 318

CMI (case mix index), 673–674
CMR (Consumer's Medical Resource), 16, 139, 217–218, 220, 510–515
CMS (Centers for Medicare and Medicaid Services), 530, 590, 821–822
Coaching, 495–496
Coalitions, 250–251, 467–474
Coburn, Robert, 86
Codman, Ernest A., 608
Collaboration with consumers, 602–610
Collaborative management model, 561–562, 568
Commerce, health care Web sites, 434–435
Commonwealth Fund, 179
Communication, FACCT model of, 421
Communities
    community rating systems, 267, 757
    Healthwise community channel, 536–537
    occupational, 686–687
    online, 432–433
    resources of, 784
Comorbidity, 106, 116
Comparisons
    of average hospital charges, 672–674
    capitation versus linkage of payment to data submission, 315
    competition of non-HMOs versus HMOs, 157–159
    consumer-driven services versus managed competition, 95–96
    differences among purchasers in risk adjustment mechanisms, 301
    of health care systems, 343–351
    health care versus automotive industry, 410–418, 477–478
    health care versus other markets, 164–166
    individual versus group markets, 177–178
    information on comparative physician quality, 461–462
    insurance industry versus other businesses, 132
    of international systems, 354–355
    of models, 319
    multipurpose versus focused factory hospitals, 113
    outcomes, 324
    PCPs in South Africa versus United States, 332

performance, 456
pressure for comparative information in France, 325
quality of care, 455–456
self-insurance versus third-party administrators (TPAs), 228–230
of systems, 311
voluntary versus involuntary uninsured consumers, 736–737
Competition
    competitive bidding, 476–477
    competitive markets, 13–14
    consumer-led, 131–134
    foreign, 353
    health insurance product competition, 141–142
    managed, 95–96, 758
    non-HMOs versus HMOs, 157–159
    with other industries, 417
    of providers, 214–215, 219, 310, 372
    quality-focused, 425
    in services, 474
    sources of competitive advantage (KPSC), 665–666
Compliance industry, 373
Component innovations, 573
Components of health care experiences, 643
Comprehensive Sickle Cell Center, 106
Computer use. See also Internet
    for decision making, 487–489
    information systems, 662
    medical care, 378
    PopulationWorx software, 645–646
    WIZ Order system, 671, 675–677
Condition-based medicine, 709–710
Confidentiality, 378, 592–593
Congestive heart failure (CHF), 108–109, 211–212, 647, 664
Connectivity
    provider, 436
    between specialists/patients, 210
    technology for, 208–209
    via Internet, 433–434
Consortiums, 434, 593. See also Foundation for Accountability (FACCT)
Consumer Assessment of Health Plans (CAHPS), 473–474
Consumer Assessment of Health Plans study (CAHPS), 303–304, 473–474
Consumer Health Education Council (CHEC), 178–179

Consumer Price Index (CPI), 768
Consumers/consumerism. *See also*
  Patients
    adult versus infantile consumerism,
      779
    assessment of health plans by,
      302–305, 306
    autonomy of consumers, 524–525
    average consumers, 12, 14–17
    awareness of new technologies by, 584
    with chronic conditions, needs of,
      564–565
    collaborating with, 602–610
    consequences, attachment of weight
      to, 455
    Consumer Assessment of Health Plans
      study (CAHPS), 473–474
    consumer choice program for universal
      coverage, 742–746
    consumer-focused products, 318–321
    consumers' choices, 703–706
    core of complaints by, 798–799
    data use by, 822
    demands of, 414–415
    direct–to–consumer (DTC) advertising,
      705
    emergence of new, 403–404
    as engines for change, 608–609
    health organizations' responses to, 444
    Healthwise approach of, 532–533
    identification of consumers, 705
    implications of new technologies for,
      582–584
    interests of U.S. versus European, 706
    Internet use by, 414–415, 435–437
    marginalized consumers, 408
    needs of consumers
      changing, 421
      with chronic conditions, 564–565
      different-prices-for-different-needs
        formula, 72
      evidence of, 291, 299, 302–303,
        422–423
      in free markets, 818–819
      Healthwise consumers', 533
      for information, 816
      meeting information needs,
        424–425
      reduction of, 523–525
    new consumers, 405–407, 416, 534
    perception of health care differences
      by, 481–482

practice improvement, consumer-
  driven, 607–609
purchasing power, 364
resistance to change of, 398
resource use by, 537–538
rights of consumers, 346, 376–379,
  410–411
satisfaction of consumers, 57–58
  assessment of care by patients,
    688–689
  with Best Doctors, 462
  collection of information on, 479
  dissatisfaction, 323, 369, 510–511
  European, 322–323
  with FEHB, 293
  NCQA Member Satisfaction Survey,
    305
  patient ratings of, 169, 446–447
  studies on, 473–474
  ways of accomplishing, 447–448
Consumer's Medical Resource (CMR), 16,
  139, 217–218, 220, 510–515
Contributions to plans. *See also* Defined
  contributions (DC) plans
  average, 332
  defined, 4
  by employees (Europe), 341
  by employers, 76–77, 392, 824
  pretax, 18, 84–85
  spending account contributions, 267
    (*See also* Medical savings accounts
    (MSAs))
Control issues
  consumer control of health care, 45,
    798–799
  control of spending on health care
    needs, 12
  employee/employer, 195
  meeting needs of employees/employers
    for, 319
  over tax subsidy, 755–756
  payers' discretion for services, 377
  third-party payment, 229–230
Convenience of care, 448
Cooley, Denton, 142–143
Cooper Clinic (Dallas), 225
Coordination of care, 683–692, 784
Coordinators, provider support, 645
Copayments, 350, 431
Core Center for Infectious Diseases, 79–80
Coronary artery disease (CAD), 664
Corporate activism, 554–555

Corporate support services, 660
Cost effectiveness
    at Access Health Group (AH), 506
    of American Healthways approach,
        647–648
    better care for, 314
    bidding strategies for, 476–477
    case examples, 512–515
    cost–benefit ratio for third-party
        payers, 721
    cost–containment pressures, 369, 375
    disease prevention, 721
    escalation of costs, 510
    evidence, 424
    future choices for, 442
    genomics and, 710
    Healthwise approach, 537–539
    long-term savings for cardiac care
        patients, 519
    National Jewish asthma program,
        623–624
    need for cost control, 317–318
    reducing post–surgical infections, 632
    savings claims of managed care
        organizations, 323–324
Cost–plus indemnity model, 824
Costs. See also Expenses/expenditures;
  Financial issues; Prices/pricing
    affordability of right care, 210, 216
    asthma–associated, 619–620
    of chronic disorders, 562–563, 643
    comparison of average charges,
        672–674
    computer, 429–430
    controlling, 119
    cost–reducing impact of consumer-
        driven health care, 102
    of coverage, 737
    diagnosis and treatment, 596
    of disease, 717–718
    distribution, 369
    employer-based coverage, 42–43
    of employer liability, 43
    escalation of, 711
    evidence of cost effectiveness, 424
    of group plans to employers, 732–733
    hospital charges, 672–674
    improving outcomes for high-cost
        conditions, 216–219
    innovations for lowering, 104–110
    insulation of providers from, 214
    of insurance pools, 227

    lowered, through new technologies,
        209
    major medical insurance, 37
    managing expenditures, 327–328
    Merrill Lynch's, 86
    out–of–pocket medical expenses,
        31–32, 75
    and productivity, implications of, 382
    reasons for rising, 117–118
    self–funded health care, 77
    of universal coverage, 743
    unpredictability of, 600
    ways of controlling, 103
Coverage. See also Insurance coverage
    American system of, 732–733 (See also
        Health care systems)
    employment-based, 539–540
    exemptions for, 41
    individual-based coverage system,
        744–746
    mandated, 266, 760, 767
    media, 555–556, 582–583, 816
    prescription, 331–332, 397–398
Covered lives, 203
CPI (Consumer Price Index), 768
Credibility, 461
Credits, 387. See also Tax credits under
    tax issues
Criteria for catastrophic care, 596–597
Criticisms
    by consumers about managed care,
        798–799
    Federal Employees Health Benefits
        Program (FEHB), 294–295
    of Kaiser and Health Insurance Plan
        groups, 377
    MedCath, 115
    of MSAs, 334, 378
    of pharmaceuticals industry, 117–118
    of risk adjustment, 256–257
Cross–cultural attitudes toward health,
    248, 448
Crossing the Quality Chasm (Harvard
    Business Review), 104
Cross–subsidization, 116
Cure, path to, 604–605
Customer–Delivered Value (CDV),
    416–417
Customization, mass individual, 435–436
CVCP (CardioVascular Care Providers),
    613–618
CVD (cardiovascular disease), 718

D

D. S. Howard & Associates, 491
Danger control agents, 455
Dartmouth Atlas of Health Care
   (Wennberg), 552, 607–608, 821
Data/databases. *See also* Information;
   Medical records
   administrative, 245–246
   Affymetrix, 719–721
   availability of, 169–170, 324–325, 508
   Best Doctors, 136, 458–465
   CABG mortality data, 247
   collection costs, 167
   confidentiality of, 592–593
   on consumer decision making, 488
   converting of, into diagnostics, 718
   data analysis, 95
   on efficacy of Personal Care Model, 785
   empirical data, 471
   Health Plan Employer Data and
      Information Set (HEDIS), 166
   information networks, 760
   Kaiser data systems, 666
   major sources of data, 245
   minimum, standard, required data set
      (MSRDS), 822–823
   objective data, 76
   on outpatient quality, 473
   Paediatric Asthma Caregivers Quality
      of Life Questionnaire, 622–623
   on performance, 185, 800
   privacy of, 590–591
   protection from loss, 300
   reporting rules for, 456
   sources, 480–482
   standardized, 821–823
   supplying consumer-friendly data,
      218–219
   synopsis of consumer data, 491–492
   universal access to knowledge, 609
DB (defined benefit) funds, 5, 8–9, 11, 17,
   33–37, 74–75, 210
DCCT (Diabetes Control and Complications Trial), 645–648
DC (defined contribution plans). *See*
   Defined contributions (DC) plans
Deaths/mortality rates, 116, 574, 663–664,
   824–825
   acute myocardial infarction (AMI)
      death rates, 250
   annual report on death rates, 243–244
   CABG mortality data, 247

from coronary artery disease, 519
   risk–adjusted, 168
   severity–adjusted, 247
   of uninsured consumers in hospitals,
      741
Debt, 341–343, 675, 753, 819. *See also*
   Bankruptcies
Decision making. *See also* Choices
   among insurance plans, 487–489
   consumer involvement in, 217–219
   Consumer's Medical Resource (CMR),
      16, 139, 217–218, 220
   by consumers versus physicians, 708
   for disabled individuals, 397
   efficiency of, 448–449
   for elderly, 394–395
   Medical Decision Support (MDS),
      511–512
   shared, 534
   support for, 90, 447–448, 677
   threats to optimal, 454–455
   Web-based, 220–222
Deductibles, 102, 282
Deferred compensation plans. *See*
   Cafeteria plans; 401(k) plans
Definable diagnoses, 596
Defined benefit (DB) funds, 5, 8–9, 11,
   17, 33–37, 74–75, 210
Defined contributions (DC) plans, 4,
   17–18, 210, 768
   administrative implications of, 273
   choices offered in, 28–29
   features offered to employees of, 19
   managed, 779–780
   moving to, 215–216
   section 401(k) plans, 285
   tax law on
      administrative implications of, 273
      application of, 270–271
      implementation of, 271–273
      other relevant rulings, 273–275
      summary of, 275–277
Definity Health, 94, 134, 156, 768
Delayed care, 740–741
Delivery systems
   improvements in, 677–678, 819
   integrated, 637–638
   just–in–time delivery systems,
      678–679
   learning integrated delivery systems
      (LIDS), 701, 702
   Shouldice Hospital, 627–632

Demand
    for choices, 753–755
    of consumers, 414–415
    education and, 723
    information and, 754
    market side of, 769
    reduction of, for medical services,
        523–525
    for risk adjustments by consumers, 316
Deming, W. Edwards, 469, 557
Democratized investing, 6–7
Demographics
    European, 340
    Internet users, 430
    pressures of, to health care financing,
        351–352
    of uninsured consumers, 731, 736,
        741, 742–743, 790
Denial of coverage, 86, 520, 722
Department of Biomedical Informatics
    (Vanderbilt), 676–677
Design and construction of hospitals,
    657–658
Designer drugs, 143–145. See also
Pharmaceuticals industry
Design of coverage/plans
    benefits, 90
    design practices, 566
    initiatives, government (U.S.),
        147–149
    insurance coverage, 744–746
        benefits of ideal insurance, 236–239
        casualty insurance model, 232–233
        covered services, 233
        ideal plans, 226–234
        medical savings accounts (MSAs),
            230–231
        terms of exit, 233–234
        third-party payment, 231–232
        traditional models, obsolescence of,
            224–226
    redesigned benefit options, 220
    of risk adjustment, 256–257
    tax credits, 757–758
Destiny Health, 85, 93–94
Diabetes, 603, 605
    care enhancement and, 645–648,
        645–649
    comorbidities with, 105–106
    costs of, 119–120, 371
    Diabetes Center (Massachusetts
        General Hospital), 120

Diabetes Control and Complications
    Trial, 119–121
    KPSC Diabetes Care Management
        Program, 663
    loss of work due to, 555
    market for care of, 444
    standards of care measures, 646–647
Diabetes Control and Complications Trial
    (DCCT), 645–648
Diagnoses
    early, through genome research, 713
    ICD–9 coding, 247, 673–674
    imprecise nature of, 717
    late, 708
    pricing setting by, 591–592
    technologies based on, 315
    tracking by diagnosis–related
        categories, 470–471
Diagnosis related groups (DRGs), 244,
    246, 250, 324, 574
Diagnostics, 705, 722–723
Different-prices-for-different-needs
    formula, 72, 80, 81, 82
Diffusion, barriers to
    of AmeriChoice plan, 785–786
    CareCounsel, 499–500
    genomics-based medicine, 722–723
    Healthtrac, 529–530
    information, 425–426
    Kaiser, 666
    Washington State Health Care
        Authority (HCA), 305–306
Dimensions of quality of care, 445–446
Direct-to-consumer (DTC) advertising, 705
Disappearance of Health Insurance story,
    159–160
Discharges from hospitals, 741
Disclosure of information, 799–802,
    821–823
Discovery Health plan, 231, 331, 332,
    335–336
Discretionary spending accounts, 281–282
Discrimination risks, 722
Disease management. See also Chronic
    diseases
    acute care, 205–206, 503–505, 567
    as approach to chronic illness, 561–568
    asthma, 621–625
    Bentley approach to catastrophic care,
        596–597
    care enhancement program from,
        645–649

Disease Management Program: Asthma
(DMP:Asthma), 621–625
Disease Management Purchasing
Consortium, 593
Dissatisfaction. *See under* Satisfaction of
consumers
Diversification, geographical, 658–659
DNA, 710–711, 719, 723
Doctors
accessibility of, 431–432
awareness of consumer-driven market
of, 696–698
black lists of, 461
changing behavior of, 553–557
checking background of, 140–141
connectivity via Internet of,
433–434
dissatisfaction of, 323
genetic profiling/early diagnosis
by, 713
performance ratings of, 471
physician leadership, 641
problems of health insurance system
for, 43–44
reports of uncompensated care by, 739
resistance of, 539
shift from independence to team
member for, 636–637
skill sets of, 534
views on consumer purchasing of,
386–387
Doies, David, 43
Dr. Quality, 218–219
DRG creep, 324
DRGs (diagnosis related groups), 244,
246, 250, 324, 574
drkoop.com, 437
Drugs. *See also* Pharmaceuticals industry
current use of, 717
delivery of the right, 716–725
designer, 143–145
Food and Drug Administration (FDA),
578, 580
generic/branded drugs, 346–347
government controls on prescribing
(European), 347
personalized, 716
third-party payers, 397–398
Viagra, 331–332
Dual–income families, 285
Duke University, 46, 108–109
Dutch patients. *See* Netherlands

E
Early–stage health care firms, 92, 93–94
Early–stage policies, 83–89
East Bay Perinatal Medical Associates,
638–639
East coast matchmakers, 136–141
eBenX, 83
e-biomed, 607
EBRI (Employee Benefit Research Institute), 178–179
ECFC (Employers Council on flexible
compensation), 287
e-commerce, 434–435
Economic issues
creation of economic markets, 392
detrimental events in economic environment, 658–659
early twentieth century, 551
economic theory, 475
effects of consumerism on economy,
11–12
frozen charitable assets, 826–827
hardships for uninsured consumers,
739–740
inflation effects on health care,
767–768
U.S. economy, 731
U.S. spending on health care, 403
EDGAR system, 163–164
Education
about quality of care, 422
advances in, 701
CareCounsel's service, 493–495
demand and, 723
government support for, 669
for patients with chronic conditions,
564–565
support for, 825
of uninsured consumers, 736
Effectiveness of new technologies, 578
Efficacy
of AmeriChoice plan, 785
effects of consumer-driven health care
on, 404–405
evidence of, 424
explanations for, 101
Federal Employees Health Benefits
Program (FEHB), 293
of new technologies, 578
of Shouldice Hospital approach, 631
Washington State Health Care
Authority (HCA), 300–301, 304–305

Efficiency, 404–405, 448–449, 754–755, 801

Efficient Health Care Consumer Response Consortium, 434

e-health companies, 713–714

E-health decision support service, 221–222

Eight–hundred–pound gorilla image, 118–121

80/20 rule (Pareto principle), 265

Elderly. *See also* Medicare
    care in Europe of, 341
    long-term care, 396–397
    plans choices for, 394–395
    procedure choices for, 395–396
    provider choices for, 395
    RAND senior health programs, 530
    third-party payers/prescription drugs, 397–398

Electronic medical records (EMRs), 645–646, 701

Eli Lilly, 444

Elitist perspective of health care systems, 58

Ellwood, Paul, 205–206

Emotional issues, 447–448, 777

Employee Benefit Research Institute (EBRI), 178–179

Employee Retirement Income Security Act, 43

Employees. *See* Enrollees/employees

Employers
    benefits of CareCounsel for, 498–499
    coverage offered by, 40–41
    employer–driven model of health care, 790
    financial contributions by, 76–77
    focuses of new, 383
    funding by, for high-cost employees, 592–593
    guidelines for, 196
    large, 84, 314–315, 391, 655–656, 818
    long-term success of consumer-driven model for, 391–393
    meeting needs of, 318–319
    options for, 265
    payment of premiums by, 754
    premium contributions by, 824
    private sector, 40
    provision of health insurance by, 42–43
    reluctance of, 383–386
    restrictions placed by, 372
    retention of employees by, 284–285
    roles of, 17–19, 214–215, 236
    self–funding of health care costs by, 77–78, 90
    small, 22–23, 41, 227, 733, 752
    strategies for encouraging consumerism, 215–220
    of uninsured consumers, 734–735
    willingness to offer insurance by, 160

Employers Council on flexible compensation (ECFC), 287

Employment-based health care coverage, 539–540

Employment status, 733–734, 737–738

Empowerment
    of consumers, 86, 203–204, 408, 432, 708–715
    of patients, 431–432, 552–553, 556–557
    of PCPs, 86

EMRs (electronic medical records), 645–646, 701

Endangered health of uninsured consumers, 739–742

End Results Idea (Codman), 608

End-stage renal disease (ERSD), 663–664

Enrollees/employees
    adjusting payments according to needs of, 77
    approaches to plan offerings for, 265
    confidence of, in employers' choices, 178–179
    Employee Benefit Research Institute (EBRI), 178–179
    Employee Retirement Income Security Act, 43
    equal subsidies for plans, providing, 76–77
    expected monthly costs per, 300
    Federal Employees Health Benefits Program (FEHB), 94
    high-cost, employer funded health care for, 592–593
    incentives for enrolling sicker, 309–316
    incentives for making good choices, 75–76
    insurance benefits for, 22
    interest of, in consumer-driven approach, 387
    Internal Revenue Code ruling, 272–273
    meeting needs of, 318–319

restrictions on investing for, 22
roles of, in defined contributions
    plans, 18
strategies for encouraging
    consumerism in, 215–220
tax burdens of, 733
voucher systems, 266–267, 275–276
Enrollment, mandatory, 792
Enthoven, Alain, 95
Entrepreneurs in health insurance,
    130–136
Entry terms (to insurance plans),
    226–227
ERSD (end-stage renal disease), 663–664
Ethical issues, 141, 722–723
Ethnicity/race of uninsured consumers,
    735
Europe
    cause of problems in health care in,
        352–354
    consumers' perceptions of health care,
        706
    differences in systems, 343–351
    government interference in, 345–346
    managed care systems in, 322–323
    mediocrity in, 346–347
    one-class systems, 87
    private sector, 347–351
    reforms, 351–352
    solidarity costs of, 338–343
Evidence-based medicine, 469–472, 675,
    678–679
Evolution of consumer-driven health
    care, 307, 384–385
Examples. See Case studies/examples
Exemptions for insurance coverage, 41
Expectations
    customer-defined, 416
    for future performance, 417
    for hospital care, 443–444
    misplaced, 306
    patient, 443–444
Expenses/expenditures. See also Cost
    effectiveness; Costs; Financial issues
    discretionary/nondiscretionary, 331–332
    health care in United States, 660, 821
    by Hospital Corporation of American
        (HCA), 657–658
    managing, 327–328
    out-of-pocket medical expenses, 31–32
    shifting burden of, away from
        consumers, 406

of U.S. health care system, 404
    by U.S./European governments, 342
Experimental treatments, 599
Experiments. See Research/studies/
    surveys
Eye surgeries, 219–220

F
FACCT (Foundation for Accountability),
    419–427, 603, 608
Failures, 96, 107, 635. See also Problems
FASB (Financial Accounting Standards
    Board), 802, 817
FDA (Food and Drug Administration),
    578, 580
Federal Employees Health Benefits
    Program (FEHB)
    criticisms of, 294–296
    description of, 292
    efficacy of, 293
    evidence of need, 291
    mentioned, 94, 134–135, 372,
        476–477, 488, 759, 799
    other approaches to, 293
    recommendations for, 296
    societal impact of, 294
Fee-for-service model, 224, 225–226,
    253, 376
Fee schedules, changes in, 312
FEHB. See Federal Employees Health
    Benefits Program (FEHB)
Fidelity Investments, 18–19, 20, 21
Financial Accounting Standards Board
    (FASB), 802, 817
Financial issues. See also Costs;
    Expenses/expenditures; Funding issues;
    Income; Prices/pricing
    availability of capital, 657–658
    bankruptcies, 369
    budgets, health care systems based
        on, 327–328
    consumer-driven financial products,
        136
    debt, 341–343, 753, 819
    Financial Accounting Standards Board
        (FASB), 149, 706
    health care budgets, 539
    impact of consumerism on U.S.
        financial system, 7–10
    inflation effects on health care,
        767–768
    Kaiser revenues, 661

Financial issues *(continued)*
　management of new financial realities, 700
　production of services, 112
　spending, impact of deductibles on, 102
Five D's of consumers' wants, 524
Flat-fee arrangements, 613–614
Flemish Bloc (VB), 343
Flexible spending accounts (FSAs), 148, 279–280, 286–288. *See also* Medical savings accounts (MSAs)
Flexner Report, 550–552
FlexScape program (BC of California), 160
Florida, 186
Focused factories, 235, 263, 374, 636
　affordability of, 118
　for AIDS, 79–80
　capacity of facilities, 114–115
　centers of excellence and, 235–236
　for chronic diseases/chronically ill, 590–593
　creation of, 103
　direction of, 637–638
　goals of, 112–113
　implementation of, 638–641
　marketing strategies of, 235–236
　for poor/sick, 112–118
　support for, 105–110
　turf warfare in, 116–118
Focuses of care
　chronic diseases, 562–564
　consumer-focused products, 318–321
　by employers, 383
　focused health care delivery model, 627–632
　quality-focused competition, 425
　relational coordination for, 687–688
　on sick people, 80
　site-focused care, 582
　study on, 688–690
Focus groups, 423
Food and Drug Administration (FDA), 578, 580
Forbes, Steve, 771–772
Foundation for Accountability (FACCT), 419–427, 603, 608
401(k) plans, 8–9, 10–11, 155, 273, 282, 285, 779. *See also* Pension funds
FPOE (Freedom Party), 343
Fragmentation of care, 57, 79–80, 106–107
Framing effects of outcomes, 455

France, 325, 326
Freedom Party (FPOE), 343
Free-rider taxes, 760
Freestanding companies, 657
"Free" systems of health care, 339–341
FSAs (flexible spending accounts), 148, 279–280, 286–288. *See also* Medical savings accounts (MSAs)
Full-choice model of benefits, 286
Functional genomics, 710
Funding issues
　charitable grants, 826
　differences in funding employee accounts, 280–286, 327
　employer funding of FSAs, 280
　European, 344–347
　fund evaluations, 6–7
　private sector funding (Europe), 347
　raising taxes, 39
　self-funding by employers, 77–78, 90
Future of health care
　chronic disease management, 207–208
　congestive heart failure case study, 211–212
　consumers' needs, 635
　effects on efficiency/effectiveness, 404–405
　emerging systems, 373–375
　emerging technologies, 208–209
　focused factories, 641–642
　forces shaping new consumers, 405–407
　HCA's intentions for, 304–305
　implications for, 415
　information utopia in, 418
　integrated delivery systems, 637–638
　on the Internet, 428–429, 435–437
　marketing of Best Doctors services, 464–465
　MSAs, 336
　needs of, to be addressed, 715
　pharmaceutical manufacturers, 442
　potential scenarios, 407–409
　rethinking the system, 205–209
　right care approach, 204–205, 210
　role of information in, 440–442

G
GAAP (generally accepted accounting principles), 184
Gatekeeper concept, 50
Gates, Bill, 164

GeneChip system, 720
Generally accepted accounting principles (GAAP), 184
Genes, 724
Genetic maps, 724
Genetic profiles, individual, 708–715
Genetics, 724
Genomes, 724
Genomics, 710–711, 717, 718, 719–720, 724
Genset, 720
George, William W. (Bill), 130–131, 141
Georgia, 827
Germany, 323, 328, 344, 352
Gifford, John, 184
Global Health Care Alliance, Inc., 617–618
Globalization effects on uninsured consumers, 738
Global pricing, 614
Glucose testing. *See* Diabetes
Goals
    focused factories, 112–113
    of management of quality of care, 451
    of pharmaceutical companies, 719–721
    for products/large targets, 524–525
    of regulation of health care, 775
    shared, 686
Golden Rule of Central Florida Health Care Coalition, 469
Gore, Al, 58
Gorilla image, 118–121
Government. *See also* Legal issues/legislation; Political issues
    actions of, 556, 764–765, 821
    coverage for federal employees, 236
    designing initiatives, 147–149
    determining best policy, 818
    financial agencies, 294
    functions of, 827
    funding differences, 327
    guidelines for, 196
    international, 346–347, 351, 364
    as over*seer*s of change, 196
    on privacy, 590–591
    regulatory issues, 263, 464
    roles of, 145–149, 181–186, 380–381, 388–389, 765–766, 820–827
    spending by, 342
    uncentralization/decentralization of, 146–147
    universal health care naysayers, 179–181

Grady Health System, 106
Greater Cleveland Hospital Association, 250
Greenspan, Alan, 165
Group plans
    care systems, 310
    costs to employers of, 732–733
    economies of group buying, 236
    group health insurers, 177–179
    Health Insurance Plan (New York), 377
    high-cost, 87–89
    Kaiser Permanente Plan (California), 184, 377
    problems with purchasing group plans, 265–266
Guidelines
    care guideline for physicians, 549–550
    clinical, 596
    for consumer-driven health care, 196–197
    National Asthma Clinical Practice Guidelines, 665
    physician misunderstandings of, 554

H
Hamilton, Brutus, 111
Harvard Community Health Plan, 46–47
Haunted House story, 154–156
HCA. *See* Hospital Corporation of American (HCA); Washington State Health Care Authority (HCA) under Washington State
HCA Health Care Indemnity (captive insurance), 657
HCFA (Health Care Financing Administration), 614–615
Healing and the Mind (television series), 517
Health accounts, 220, 223
Health Action Council, 250
Health Affairs, 48
HealthAllies, 138, 769
Healthaxis.com, 135
Health-based premium payments, 299–302
Health Benefits Fund, 292
Healthcare Assistance Program, 492–498
Health Care Authority. *See* Washington State Health Care Authority (HCA)
healthcarebuy.com example, 221–222

Health Care Financing Administration (HCFA), 614–615. *See also* Centers for Medicare and Medicaid Services (CMS); U.S. Centers for Medical and Medicare Services
Health care SEC model, 797–804, 811–814
Health care systems
  based on budgets, 327–328
  Buyers Health Care Action Group (BHCAG), 310–312
  California Association of Hospitals and Health Systems, 249
  California Public Employees Retirement System (CalPERS), 767–768
  changes for patients in, 713–714
  choices of, by variable, 481–482, 483
  comparisons of, 311, 354–355
  differences in, 343–351
  dissatisfaction of consumers with, 510–511
  elitist perspective of, 58
  emotional issues of, 777
  European
    Belgium, 36
    births of, 732
    differences in systems, 343–351
    "free" systems of, 339–340, 340–341
    managed care systems in, 322–323
    one-class systems, 87
    Switzerland, 350
    United Kingdom, 323
  expenses of, 404
  future of, 205–209, 373–375, 415, 637–638
  Grady Health System, 106
  impact of Internet on, 511
  implementation of, 456, 457
    for chronic disease management, 567–568
    evidence-based, 678–679
    Personal Care Model, 786
  market-driven, 568
  Medical Manager System, 617
  Minneapolis/St. Paul area, 478
  Partners Healthcare System, 47
  Personalized Healthcare System (PHS), 89
  power principles for, 416–417
  problems of, 43–44, 351, 352–354, 363
  productivity of, 404–405
  Public Employees Retirement System (PERS) study, 526–527
  remedies for curing, 75–77
  self-managed, 349, 525–526
  sickness fund systems, 345
  single-payer health care systems, 343, 345
  social insurance-based, 343–344
  Twin Cities Metro Area, 311
  for uninsured consumers, 732–733
  universal
    access issues, 180–181
    achieving, in America, 742–746
    British, 180
    naysayers, 179–181
    uninsured consumers and, 789–791
    in United States, 761
  views of U.S., by Europeans, 338
  Vivius Personalized Healthcare System (PHS), 89, 134
Healthgrades.com, 556
Health insurance model, 319
Health Insurance Plan (New York), 377
Health Internet Ethics (Hi-Ethics), 141
Health Maintenance Organization (HMO) Act of 1973, 765–766, 770
Health maintenance organizations. *See* HMOs
Health management accounts, 609
Health of Seniors survey, 530
Health Partners Regional Affiliated, 88
Health Plan Employer Data and Information Set (HEDIS), 166
Health plans. *See also* Health care systems; Insurance coverage
  average contributions to, 332
  BHCAG, 93–94
  catalogues, 90
  choice of, for elderly, 394–395
  comprehensive medical plans, 292
  Health Plan Employer Data and Information Set (HEDIS), 166
  helping consumers to choose, 487–489
  provision of, by employers, 818
  resistance of, 387
Health Quality Choice Program (Cleveland). *See* Cleveland Health Quality Choice Program (CHQC)
Health reimbursement arrangements (HRAs), 276–277, 280–281
Health Savings Accounts (HSAs), 282, 283
Health Savings Security Accounts (HSSAs), 282, 283

Health Security Act, 743
Health security model, 318, 319
HealthSync system, 133–134
Healthtrac, Inc., 523–528
Healthwise approach
  areas of care in, 532–533
  challenges to mainstream replication
    of, 539–540
  cost/quality outcomes, 537–539
  Healthwise Handbooks, 536
  Healthwise Knowledgebase, 535
  mission/message of, 533–536
  new generation of health care through,
    540
Heart. *See* Cardiac care
Heart Hospital of Milwaukee, 114–115
HEDIS (Health Plan Employer Data and
  Information Set), 166
Henikoff, Leo, 79–80
Hernia repair, 627–632
HER 2 protein, 723
Herschman, Ray, 130, 131–134, 141
Hershey Foods case study, 248
Herzlinger, Regina "Regi," 262–269
Hewitt Associates, 491, 492
Hi-Ethics (Health Internet Ethics), 141
High-cost conditions, 216–217
High-deductible plans, 282
Highmark Blue Cross Blue Shield, 519
High-risk enrollees, 146
High-throughput factories, 704
Hill-Burton Act, 826
Hill Physicians Medical Group,
  636, 638
HIV/AIDS, 79–80, 595, 597, 664–665
HMOs
  appropriateness of model, 224–226
  experiments with, in Switzerland,
    349–350
  Kaiser, 184
  organization of, 372
  original concept of, 205–206
  Pareto principle (80/20 rule) for
    premiums, 265
  stability of, 46–47
Home care services, 598, 652
Honeywell, 213–218
Horizon Expert Orders, 677
Horizontal integration of care, 263,
  651–653. *See also* Integration of care
Hospital Corporation of American (HCA),
  653–660

Hospitals
  academic, 670, 699–702
  admissions for uninsured consumers,
    740
  adoption of new techniques by, 575
  American Hospital Association (AHA),
    115, 652
  California Association of Hospitals and
    Health Systems, 249
  California Hospital Outcomes Project
    case study, 248–250
  deaths of uninsured consumers in, 741
  design and construction of, 657–658
  Diabetes Center (Massachusetts
    General Hospital), 120
  focus of care/relational coordination
    in, 683–692
  Great Cleveland Hospital Association,
    250
  Heart Hospital of Milwaukee, 114–115
  Hospital Corporation of American
    (HCA), 653–660, 657–658
  hospitals belonging to systems, 653
  length of stay issues, 180, 672, 673,
    675, 685
  mergers, 47, 704
  multipurpose versus focused factory,
    113
  National Jewish Medical and Research
    Center, 619–625
  patient expectations for, 443–444
  ratings of, 113–114
  risk adjustment issues of, 244–245
  services/discharges of uninsured
    consumers, 741
  Shouldice Hospital, 627–632
  St. Luke's Episcopal Hospital
    (Houston), 614–615
  training of staff, 213
  Vanderbilt Medical Center, 669–679
  views on consumer purchasing
    of, 386
Hospital Survey and Construction Act,
  826
Hospital systems, definition of, 652
HR. *See* Human Resources (HR)
HRAs (health reimbursement arrange-
  ments), 276–277, 280–281
HSAs (Health Savings Accounts), 282, 283
HSSAs (Health Savings Security
  Accounts), 282, 283
Humana, 107

Human genomes, 710. *See also* individual genetic profiles
Human Resources (HR), 488
  control of insurance options by, 132–133
  corporate benefits staff, 491–492
  employee benefits, 655–656
  HR mavens, 176–177
Hyde, Stephen, 262–269

I
IBM, 440
ICD-9 coding, 247, 673–674
Ideal health insurance plans, 226–234
Illinois, 792–793
Illness burdens, variations in, 313
Immunization/vaccinations, 229
Implementation of systems, 456, 457, 567–568, 678–679, 786
Incentives
  for consumer cost-consciousness, 268
  incentive-based wellness programs, 85–86
  for innovations by providers, 46, 80–83
  of insurance pools, 234
  for insurers/providers, 77
  for judicial use of MSAs, 378
  for medical management, 508
  of old insurance systems, 87–88
  for overconsumption, 345
  for patients in fee-for-service model, 225
  for *see*king the sick, 309–316
  for shopping wisely, 75
  tax, 790–791
Income. *See also* Financial issues
  dual-income families, 285
  Employee Retirement Income Security Act, 17, 43
  family, 733
  income tax laws (2002), 18
  and likelihood of coverage, 751
  tax credits for low-income consumers, 756
  of uninsured consumers, 734, 737
Index funds, 5, 7
Indicators of quality of care, 243
Individual-based coverage system, 744–746
Individual genetic profiles, 708–715
Individual insurance market, 178
Individual mandates for tax credits, 760

Infantile consumerism, 779
Inflation effects on health care, 767–768
Information. *See also* Data/databases; Internet
  about quality, 467–474
  access to evidence-based, 535
  approaches to meeting need for, 424–426
  availability of, 169–170
  block-out of, 455
  CareCounsel's service, 493–495
  for care providers, 676–677
  catastrophic care, 598–599
  for choosing health care options, 12
  combining information technology and evidence-based medicine, 469–472
  on comparative physician quality, 461–462
  and consumer demand, 754
  on consumer satisfaction, 480
  consumers with adequate/inadequate, 408
  converting of, into diagnostics, 718
  disclosure of, 799–802
  ease of access, 429
  for employees, 196
  evidence of need for, 422–423
  Foundation for Accountability (FACCT), 420–427
  free-flowing, 238–239
  government agency for disseminating, 149
  guidebooks, 94
  Health Plan Employer Data and Information Set (HEDIS), 166
  importance of having, 325–326
  Internet as source of, 208
  as key to change, 468–469
  lack of, 419
  Lung Facts, 621
  meeting needs for, 424–425
  need for consumer-accessible, 816–817
  networks, 760
  obtaining from patients, 247–248
  patient information systems, 566–567
  on performance, 760
  present/future roles of, 440–442
  providing relevant, 76
  relationships between providers/ patients and, 447–448

revolutionary insurance systems, 129–130
role of, 410–418
sharing of, 609, 713
sources, 163–170
systems, 659
technologies, 374–375
WIZ Order, 671
Information age medicine, 557–558
Information society, 413–414
Information technology (IT), 659
Information therapy, 535–536
Informed choice model, 324–326
Initiatives, FACCT, 420–422
Innovations, 388
    creation of new, 103
    early innovators, 89–92
    effects of, 98
    examples of, 374
    integrated information records, 104–105
    lack of, 804
    personalized medicine, 109–110
    pharmaceutical/medical, 352–353
    by providers, 46, 80–83, 89
    rising market of innovators, 768–770
    services for the poor, 135–136
    in South Africa, 135–136
    technological, 573–574
Institute of Medicine (IOM), 552, 606
Insurance coverage
    choices of, 29
    choosing different, 83–85
    costs of premiums, 47
    covered services, 233
    demand for, 753–755
    denial of, 722
    designing, for information age
        benefits of ideal insurance, 236–239
        casualty insurance model, 232–233
        covered services, 233
        ideal plans, 226–234
        medical savings accounts (MSAs), 230–231
        terms of exit, 233–234
        third-party payment, 231–232
        traditional models, obsolescence of, 224–226
    different (See Different-prices-for-different-needs formula)
    disappearance of, 159–160
    for discretionary procedures, 219–220

employer-based, 42–43
employment-based, 539–540
exemptions for, 41
Medicaid, 40
offered by employers, 40–41, 752
for sick people, 33–37
system of, in America, 732–733
upgrading of, by employees, 291
Insurance industry, versus other businesses, 132
Insurers
    as engines of change, 196
    guidelines for, 196
    non-HMO, 157
    pressure from, 555
    refusal to pay by, 35
    registration of, 803–804
    resistance of, 387
    roles of, 381
    stability of HMOs, 46–47
    transaction price information for, 803
Integrated information records, 103, 104–105
Integrated Personal Medical Fund (PMF), 85
Integration of care, 79–80
    diabetes care enhancement, 645–648
    for HIV/AIDS, 664–665
    horizontal, 263, 651–660
    vertical, 107, 172–173, 652, 657
Interconsultation service, 460
Intermediaries, 135, 406
International issues
    Access Health Group (AH) client relationships, 508
    barriers to international consumer-driven health care, 365
    Belgium, 36
    births of health care systems, 732
    comparisons of health care systems, 343–351, 354–355
    health care funding, 346–347
    international views of consumer-driven health care, 363–364, 365–366
    Netherlands, 351
    roles of governments, 364
Internet
    common uses of, 754
    computer–assisted medical care, 378
    consumer use of, 414–415, 704–706, 708
    current state of health care on, 432–435

Internet *(continued)*
    direct-to-consumer (DTC) advertising
        on, 705
    for distribution of standards of care,
        678–679
    e-biomed, 607
    as enabler, 220–222
    future use of, 440, 701
    government role in medical
        information on, 380–381
    growth of, 429–430
    health care environment of, 430
    Healthwise Knowledgebase, 535
    Healthwise links, 537
    impact of, on U.S. health care system, 511
    increased use of, 464
    influences on health care offerings via,
        437
    information sharing via, 609
    as information source, 208
    information sources on, 139–141
    LUNG LINE, 620–621
    Medical Manager System, 617
    medtropolis.com, 657
    news media on, 555–556
    overview of use of, 428–429
    quality of information on, 706
    reasons for using, 820
    sharing of information via, 713–714
    surfing for information on, 557
    trends in patient empowerment and,
        431–432
    Web links from CareCounsel, 494
Interventions, 388–389, 777
Investing in Health (World Development
    Report/World Bank), 363
Investments, employee, 4
Investors, 18–19, 368–369
Involuntary versus voluntary uninsured
    consumers, 736–737
IOM (Institute of Medicine), 552, 606
IRS. *See under* Tax issues
IT (information technology), 659

J
J. D. Power and Associates, 410–418, 822
Jackson Hole conferences, 96, 758
Japan, 411–412
JCAHO (Joint Commission on
    Accreditation of Healthcare
    Organizations), 648–649, 654–655, 685

JDRF (Juvenile Diabetes Research
    Foundation), 603
Joint Commission on Accreditation of
    Healthcare Organizations (JCAHO),
    648–649, 654–655, 685
Jupiter Media Metrix, 429–430
Just-in-time delivery systems, 678–679
Just-say-no health insurance, 49–50, 59
Juvenile Diabetes Research Foundation
    (JDRF), 603

K
Kaiser Family Foundation/Harvard
    University Public Opinion Update
    survey, 491
Kaiser Permanente Plan, 184, 377
Kaiser Permanente Southern California
    (KPSC), 661–667
Kendall, David, 145–149
Kennedy, John F., 410
Kidney disease, 663–664
Koch, Michael, 675

L
Laparascopic surgery, 629
Lasik surgery, 219–220
Leadership, 578–579, 641
Leapfrog Group, 177, 424–425
Learning integrated delivery systems
    (LIDS), 701, 702
Learning strategies for new technologies,
    576–578
Legal issues/legislation. *See also* Tax
    issues
    anti-managed care legislation, 369
    Assembly Bill 524 (California), 249
    Balanced Budget Act (1997), 248, 251,
        253, 422–423, 792
    births of international health care
        systems, 732
    cases
        Adkins v. United States, 273–274
        Cernik v. Commissioner, 275
        Laverty v. Commissioner, 274–275
        United States v. Wells Fargo Bank,
            274
    childbirth length of stay laws, 180
    community rating laws, 267, 757
    Employee Retirement Income Security
        Act, 17, 43
    fighting physician-sponsored laws, 554

Health Insurance Portability and
    Accountability Act, 293
Health Maintenance Organization and
    Resources Development Act of 1973
    (Public Law 93–222), 294
Health Maintenance Organization
    (HMO) Act of 1973, 765–766, 770
Hill-Burton Act, 826
Hospital Survey and Construction Act,
    826
judgments for inadequate/
    inappropriate medical care, 464
laws with mandated benefits, 767
liability of employers, 42–43
medical savings accounts (MSAs),
    279–280, 288–289
Medicare Catastrophic Coverage Act,
    799
patient rights to know surgical
    procedures, 552–553
Patients' Bill of Rights, 770
Racketeer Influenced and Corrupt
    Organizations Act (RICO), 43
regulatory processes, 90
Switzerland Insurance Law, 349
tax laws, 270–273
use-it-or-lose-it provisions of
    FSAs/MSAs, 289, 771
Length of stay issues, 180, 672, 673, 675,
    685, 741
letstalk.com, 417
Levin, Mark, 143–145
Lewin Group, 15
Lichtenstein Hernia Institute, 628
LIDS (learning integrated delivery
    systems), 701, 702
Life expectancy, 563, 742
LifeLine (Honeywell), 217–218
Lifestyle Advantage, 519
Lifestyle changes for cardiac care, 516–521
Limited Access story, 162–163
Limits of managed care, 322–323
Linde, Ken, 85, 91
Living wills, 210
Long-term care, 34, 396–397
Long-term commitments to insurance
    plans, 234
Loyalty programs (South Africa), 335–336
Lumenos, 768
Lung cancer, 244–245
LUNG LINE, 620–621

M
Managed care, 46
    alternatives to, 322–328
    business challenges of, 659–660
    companies, 377
    compared to U.S. securities market,
        802–804
    complaints about, 798–799
    to consumer-driven care from, 214–215
    European systems, 322–323
    gatekeeper concept, 50
    improvements to, 314
    managed care model, 319
    versus managed cost, 557
Managed Care Consult Line, 621
Managed competition, 95–96
Managed defined contribution plans,
    779–780
Management of diseases. See Disease
    management
Management of new technologies,
    576–579
Mandated health coverage, 266, 760, 767
Mandatory participation, 267–268
Manseuto, Joe, 6
Marginal consumers, 12
Markets/marketing issues
    achieving desirable characteristics for,
        803–804
    competitive markets, 13–14
    creation of economic markets, 392
    diabetes care markets, 444
    direct-to-consumer (DTC) advertising,
        705
    drug therapy, 721
    focused factories, marketing strategies
        of, 235–236
    free markets, consumers' needs and,
        818–819
    health care versus other markets,
        164–16166
    ideal health insurance plans, 234–236
    implementation of consumer-driven,
        456
    individual versus group markets,
        177–178
    information market size, 423–424
    market context of benefits, 492
    Market Driven Health Care
        (Herzlinger), 107
    market-driven systems, 568

Markets/marketing issues *(continued)*
  marketing of Best Doctors services,
    462–463, 464–465
  market mapping, 476
  market mechanisms, 12–14, 345–346
  market-oriented health care, 147–148
  market sizes, 423–424
  nonprofit markets, 135
  pharmaceuticals, 712–713
  plastic surgery market, 819
  regulatory issues of, 777
  rising market of innovators, 768–770
  securities market example, 800–801
  size of, in targeting consumers, 783
  small-group market, 227
  South African MSA market, 336
  stratification of market, 160
  transfer pricing, 171–174
  uninsured markets, 752
Markowitz, Harry, 6–7
Massachusetts Health Quality Partnership
  (MHQP), 247, 425
Matching doctors to patients. *See* Best
  Doctors
Matisonn, Shaun, 85
Mayo clinic, 235
MDS (Medical Decision Support), 511–512
Measures. *See also* Buyers Health Care
  Action Group (BHCAG); Ratings
  Central Florida Health Care Coalition's,
    469–470
  FACCT's, 420–421
  investment performance, 6–7, 185
  measuring tools, 169
  of performance, 800
MedCath Corporation, 112, 113–116
MEDecision, 473
Media coverage, 555–556, 582–583, 816
Medicaid, 369, 756
  asthma patients, 623
  eligibility criteria for, 40
  expenditure growths of, 40
  increasing rates for, 792
  non-acceptance of, by doctors, 791
  price setting by, 824
Medical care system. *See* Health care
  systems
Medical Decision Support (MDS), 511–512
Medical events, uninsured, 31
Medical management, potential impact
  of, 507–509

Medical Manager System, 617
Medical plans. *See* Health plans
Medical records, 245, 246–247,
  645–648
Medical savings accounts (MSAs). *See
  also* Flexible spending accounts (FSAs)
  Archer medical savings accounts
    (MSAs), 279, 281–282
  creation of, 767
  HRAs, 282–283
  mentioned, 230–231, 237, 288–289,
    374, 377, 768, 770–771, 795, 818
  mixing/matching accounts, 280–281
  in South Africa, 330–336
  spending account contributions, 267
Medical underwriting, 234, 236
Medicare, 111, 369, 756
  adjustment of capititated payments
    case study, 252–256
  capitated health plan enrollment and,
    253
  coronary care expenses, 519–521
  denial of coverage/access, 520
  FEHB as model for reform in, 476
  Medicare Catastrophic Coverage Act,
    799
  Medicare + Choice, 252–253
  Participating Heart Bypass Demonstra-
    tion Project, 614–615
  payment for alternative medicine
    interventions, 521
  price setting by, 823–824
  publishing of data by, 423
  rate per beneficiary, 49–50
  reasons for risk adjustment in, 256
  risk adjustment methods of, 246
  screening tests for beneficiaries, 608
  2003 reforms, 282
Medications. *See* Drugs; Pharmaceuticals
  industry
Medicine/medical practice
  Academy of Medicine, 250
  alternative medicine programs,
    520–521
  condition-based, 709–710
  ethic of, 795
  evidence-based, 469–472, 675,
    678–679
  genomics-based, 722–723
  information age, 557–558
  mental, 630–631

personalized, 103, 109–110, 111–112, 143–145, 709, 716
population-based, 106, 108
predictive, 717
preventive, 710, 711, 712–713
statistical, 709
symptom-based, 709–710
MedisGroups, 247, 248
MEDSTAT Group, 527
Medtronic, 131, 206
medtropolis.com, 657
Mentally handicapped care, Social Pedagogic Services (SPDs) (Netherlands), 326
Mental medicine, 630–631
Menus for choice/enrollment, 759
Mergers, hospital, 47
Merrill Lynch, 80, 86, 94
MHQP (Massachusetts Health Quality Partnership), 247, 425
Millennium Pharmaceuticals, 109, 144, 720–721
Minimally invasive cardiac surgery, 572–576
Minimum, standard, required data set (MSRDS), 822–823
Minimum pricing/benefits, 823–824
Minnesota, 183, 476
Mixing/matching of FSAs/HRAs, 280–281
Models
    acute-care models, 567
    appropriateness of HMO model, 224–226
    for assessing relative risk among health plans, 299–300
    capitated pricing model, 600
    case management model, 671–675
    casualty insurance model, 232–233
    catastrophic care model, 595–601
    collaborative management model, 561–562, 568
    comparisons of, 319
    consumer-choice model, 794–795
    consumer-driven model, 382–383, 385–387, 391–393
    cost-plus indemnity model, 824
    employer-driven model of health care, 790
    FACCT model of communication, 421
    fee-for-service model, 224, 225–226, 253, 376
    FEHB as model for reform in Medicare, 476
    focused health care delivery model, 627–632
    401(k) plans as model, 10–11
    full-choice model of benefits, 286
    health care SEC model, 797–804, 811–814
    health security model, 318–321, 319
    informed choice model, 324–326
    managed care model, 319
    managed defined contribution plans, 779–780
    measures of model performance, 256
    obsolescence of traditional, 224–226
    "one size fits all" model, 288
    Personal Care Model (PCM), 146, 781–788
    population care management (KPSC) model, 662–667
Moral issues, 229
Morningstar rating system, 6–7, 163–164
Mortality rates. See Deaths/mortality rates
MSAs. See Medical Savings Accounts (MSAs)
MSRDS (minimum, standard, required data set), 822–823
Multicenter Lifestyle Demonstration Project, 517–519
Multipurpose hospitals, 113
Multiyear insurance policies, 32
Mutations, 724
Mutual fund companies, 20
MyHealthBank, 94

N
Naifeh, Steven, 136–137, 141, 457
National Asthma Clinical Practice Guidelines, 665
National Committee for Quality Assurance (NCQA), 305, 424–425, 551, 685
National health care systems, Belgium, 36
National Health Service (Britain), 354
National Heart, Lung, and Blood Institute, 517
National Institutes of Health (NIH), 517, 606
National Jewish Medical and Research Center, 619, 620–625
National Medical Care Expenditure Survey, 733

National Quality Forum, 456
National Quality Scholars Program (Vanderbilt), 677–678
NCQA (National Committee for Quality Assurance), 305, 424–425, 551, 685
Needs of consumers. *See also* Consumers/consumerism
  changing, 421
  with chronic conditions, 564–565
  different-prices-for-different-needs formula, 72
  evidence of, 291, 299, 302–303, 422–423
  in free markets, 818–819
  Healthwise consumers', 533
  meeting information needs, 424–425
  reduction of, 523–525
Needs statements, 782–783
Net. *See* Internet
Netherlands, 87, 325, 326, 351
Networks
  advance selection, 90
  base, 222
  CardioVascular Care Providers (CVCP), 613–618
  information, 760
  in–network versus out-of–network care, 479
  provider, 477, 598
  social, 686
  time of need, 90
New Jersey, 183
New York, 168, 182–183, 243–244, 247, 582, 800
NIH (National Institutes of Health), 517, 606
Nixon administration, 765
Nonprofit markets, 135
North Dakota, 178
Norwood, Charles, 42
Nucleotides, 724
Nurse care managers, 645
Nurses, 581–582

O

Objective data, 76
Obstacles. *See* Barriers/obstacles
Obstetrics, 444
Occupational communities, 686–687
OECD (Organization for Economic cooperation and Development), 341

Office of Personnel Management (OPM), 292
Ohio, 169, 183
Old Mutual of South Africa, 136
O'Leary, Dennis, 184
One-class systems (Europe), 87
One-price-for-all pricing, 72, 81, 82, 94–95
Online information. *See* Internet
Opinion leaders, 579
OPM (U.S. Office of Personnel Management), 292
Opponents of consumer-driven health care, 163–175
Optate, 219
Optimistic bias, 455
Orders, writing of, 676–677
Organization for Economic cooperation and Development (OECD), 341
Organizations (March and Simon), 686
Organization Study Committee (Association of Academic Health Centers), 700
Ornish, Dean, 111
Outcomes, 167
  achieving satisfactory, 449
  from American Healthways programs, 646–647
  in chronic disease management, 207–208
  clinical, 216–219
  clinical pathways system for improving, 672
  doctor/patient relationships and, 494–495
  drug therapy, 721
  efficiency, 690
  framing effects of, 455
  Healthwise approach, 537–539
  ICU, 251
  improving, 113
  indicators of, 243
  measures of, by interest groups, 169, 593
  pressure for data on, 325
  publishing of health, 817
  quality of care and, 449–450
  standardization for, 596
  Swiss, 350
Outlook for programs, 625
Out-of-pocket medical expenses, 31–32, 75

Outpatient care, 254, 473, 596, 597–598, 629
Oxford Health Plans, 582, 799

P

Paediatric Asthma Caregivers Quality of Life Questionnaire, 622–623
PAHO (Pan American Health Organization), 363, 366
Pan American Health Organization (PAHO), 363, 366
Pareto principle (80/20 rule), 265
Parkinson's disease, 527
Park Nicolette, 88–89
Partners Healthcare System, 47
Partners Health Initiative, 538
Partnerships, of start-up consumer-driven firms, 90
Path to a cure framework, 604–605
Pathways, clinical, 672, 676
Pathworx, 672
Patients. *See also* Consumers/consumerism
   as buyers of health care, 235
   changes in health care system for, 713–714
   confused/misinformed, 685
   connectivity via Internet of, 434
   dissatisfaction of, 323
   eligibility of, for new technologies, 578
   empowerment of, 431–432, 552–553, 556–557
   expectations of, 443–444
   ignorance of medical issues of, 556
   myocardial infarction, 664
   participation of, in care, 566
   patient-as-partner role, 534
   patient-as-provider role, 536–537
   patient-centered insurance, 236, 237
   patient-derived data, 245, 247–248
   patient information systems, 566–567
   patient power, 376
   quality of care and outcomes, 449–450
   relationships with providers of, 447–448
   resistance of, 539
   right to decide of, 376–379
   safety of, 116
   satisfaction ratings of, 169, 446–447
   trend toward informed, 409
Patients' Bill of Rights, 770
Pauly tax credit, 758. *See also* Tax issues

Payers, 441
   discretion for services of, 377
   options for, in France, 326
   preventive medicine focus for, 711
   single-payer systems (Europe), 343, 345, 351
   third-party, 377, 397–398, 721
Payments
   based on medical condition, 269
   by insurers, 555
   new mechanisms for, 464
   to providers, 87–89
   risk–adjusted, 314
PCM (Personal Care Model), 146, 781–788
PCPs (primary care providers/physicians), 30, 86, 208, 332, 637, 784
Peak Health, 78
Peer-based assessment of quality of care, 459–460
Peer review organizations (PROs), 556
Pennsylvania, 166, 168, 183
Pension funds, 9, 17, 19–21
Performance
   athletic, 111–112
   disclosure of, 182, 760
   improvement through adoption of new technologies, 580
   information disclosure on, 800
   investment, measuring, 185
   monitoring of, 416
   physician, 471
   ratings on providers, 168
   recording rules for data on, 456
   standards versus control of, 776
   tomorrow's standards of, 417
Per-member per-month (PMPM) basis for treatment, 600
Persistence, in *seeking* quality, 470–471
Personal care accounts, 387, 768
Personal care managers, 784
Personal Care Model (PCM), 146, 781–788
Personal health care accounts (PHAs), 90
Personalized Healthcare System (PHS), 89
Personalized medicine/medical technologies, 103, 109–110, 111–112, 143–145, 709, 716
Persons with AIDS (PWAs), 556
Perspectives
   academic health center's, 699–702
   consumer, 370

Perspectives *(continued)*
  on health management, 369
  of investors, 368–369
PERS (Public Employees Retirement
  System) study, 526–527
Pharmaceuticals industry, 109–110
  consumer-driven, 143–145
  copays, increasing, 431
  cost increases, 110
  criticisms of, 117–118
  drug manufacturers, 442
  Eli Lilly, 444
  generic/branded drugs, 346–347
  genome research in, 710
  goals of pharmaceutical companies,
    719–721
  innovations in, 352–353
  marketing issues, 712–713
  mergers, 721
  Millennium Pharmaceuticals, 109, 144,
    720–721
  price controls, 345
Pharmacogenomics, 724
PHAs (personal health care accounts), 90
PHS (Personalized Healthcare System), 89
Physician Line, 621
Physician practice management (PPM)
  groups, 652
Physicians. *See* Doctors
Pine, Michael, 251
Pinnacle Choice, 769
PIP-DCGs (principal in-patient diagnostic
  cost groups) method, 254
Plans. *See* Health plans
PlanScape PPO program, 320
Plastic surgery market, 819
PMF (Integrated Personal Medical
  Fund), 85
PMPM (per-member per-month) basis
  for treatment, 600
PMRI. *See* Preventive Medicine Research
  Institute (PMRI)
Point-of-service (POS) option, 231
Policies
  administrative
    access to health care (European), 354
    Agency for Health Care Policy and
      Research (AHCPR), 488, 553–557
    bed bank (Georgia), 827
    for consumer choice, 263
    determining best, 818

development of, 770
    health benefits policy by IRS, 755
    health insurance portability, 824
    health policy theories, 78–79
    mistakes of politicians, 353–354
    options for setting, 826–827
    policy analysis of health care, 743
    pricing for government–funded
      health care, 594
    Progressive Policy Institute (PPI),
      179, 606
    tax policy reforms, 755–757
    for uninsured consumers, 780
  insurance plan
    early-stage, 83–89
    multiyear insurance, 32
    terms of, 75, 89, 226–227, 227–228,
      233–234
Political issues
  of consumer-driven health care
    current problems of, 766–768
    for elderly, 397–398
    favoring change to consumer-driven
      market, 698
    government roles in, 764–765,
      770–771
    rising markets of innovators in,
      768–770
    summary of, 771–772
  government expenditures on health
    care, 342–343
  Health Security Act, 743
  mistakes in policy–making, 353–354
  parties' views on market–oriented
    health care, 147–148
  politicians' use of health care
    controversies, 774–775
  of tax credits, 761
  of universal health care coverage,
    743–744
Poor/nearly poor people
  access issues for, 791–793
  eligibility issues for, 790–791
  focused factories for, 112–118
  innovative services for, 135–136
  insurance for, 38–41
Population-based medicine, 106, 108.
  See also Demographics
Population care management, 505–506,
  662–665, 666
Population management, 644–645

Populations, underserved, 685
Population-specific results of case management, 675
PopulationWorx software, 645–646
Portability of health insurance, 293, 824
Portability of pension plans, 18
Poverty, 825
Power, J. D., III, 410–418
Power issues, 177, 436–437
Power principles for health care industry, 416–417
PPI (Progressive Policy Institute), 179, 606
PPM (physician practice management) groups, 652
Practice improvement, 607–608, 712–713
Preconceptions about consumer-driven health care, 153–154
Predictive medicine, 717
Pregnancy care, 639
Premiums
    contributions by employers, 754, 824
    costs/price of, 49–50, 320, 722
    health-based payments, 299–302
    Pareto principle (80/20 rule) for, 265
    payment of, 302–305
    price of, 47, 49–50
    reductions in, 50
Prepaid health care, 769–770
Prescription coverage, 331–332, 397–398
Presentation formats, FACCT's, 421
Prevention regimens, 32, 205–206, 710
Preventive Medicine Research Institute (PMRI), 516–519
Prices/pricing. *See also* Costs; Financial issues
    abandonment of minimum pricing, 823–824
    bundled services, 46
    for chronically ill, 591–592
    determining of, for providers, 77
    different-prices-for-different-needs formula, 72, 80, 81, 82
    distortion of, 76
    dropping insurance due to rising premiums, 320
    of health insurance, 77–83
    HealthSync example, 133–134
    issue of, to consumers, 388
    one-price-for-all pricing, 72, 81, 82
    package pricing (Texas Heart Institute), 612–618

policies for government-funded health care, 594
    of premiums, 722
    price controls, 369
    price-cutting, 47
    pricing power, 128
    raising prices, 128
    reforms in pricing, 80
    risk-adjusted, 80–83, 94–95
    shifting price burdens, 824
    structures for catastrophic care, 599–600
    of tests ordered, 676
    transfer pricing, 171–174
    uniform, 79
Primary Care Outcomes Research Institute, 494
Primary care providers/physicians (PCPs), 30, 86, 208, 332, 637, 784
Principal in-patient diagnostic cost groups (PIP-DCGs) method, 254
Privacy, 175–176, 590–591, 823
Private sector, 95, 170–171, 347–351, 802, 804, 821
Privatization without capitalization, 351–352
Problems
    adverse selection concept, 591, 752
    of breakfast insurance metaphor, 67–68
    of capitalization, 352–354
    chronic, 388
    of consumer-directed health arrangements, 397
    of consumer-driven concept, 385–387
    of defined benefit (DB) funds, 74–75
    discrimination/denial of health coverage, 722
    in European health care systems, 351, 352–354
    of existing international systems, 363
    fragmentation, 106
    free-rider problem, 370
    of FSAs, 287–288
    of health insurance system for doctors, 43–44
    lack of choices, 60–61
    of lack of disease management, 44–45
    of managed care approach, 636
    with purchasing group plans, 265–266
    risk allocations, 395
    of Swiss health care system, 350

Procedures, medical, 219–220, 395–396, 471

Product categories, of Access Health Group (AH), 503–507

Productivity, 206. *See also* Innovations
of athletes, 111–112
and costs, implications of, 382
explanations for, 102–104
improvements in, 323–324
increases in, 328
rewards for, 109
of U.S. health care system, 404–405

Profits, "skimming," 115–116

Prognostic, 708–709

Prognostic disease management, 708–709

Progressive Corporation, 95

Progressive Policy Institute (PPI), 179, 606

PROPATH Parkinson's disease trial, 527

PROs (peer review organizations), 556

Protocols, cancer treatment, 640

Provider networks, 477

Providers
calculations of illness burdens by, 313
cardiovascular care, 613–614
of care for uninsured consumers, 738–739
changes in orientation of, 371
choice of, 395
competition among, 214–215
concerns of, 167–168
connectivity of, 436
determining prices for, 77
distribution of care among, 566
as engines of change, 196
full-service, 115–116
grading, 167–168
guidelines for, 196
implications of new technologies for, 581–582
information on, for consumers, 803
intellectual capacity of, 166
international systems of, 732
Kaiser Permanente Plan (California), 184, 377, 661–667
low-performance, 800
methods of payment by, 75
payments to, 87–89
preventive medicine focus for, 712–713
pricing by, 14
provider organizations, 75–76
relationships with patients of, 447–448
roles of, 381, 441–442, 550–552, 553–557, 670–671
for uninsured consumers, 738–739

Provider support coordinators, 645

Publications, trade, 91

Public Employees Retirement System (PERS) study, 526–527

Public health support, 824–825

Public interest, focused factories and, 113–116

Purchasers, differences among, in risk adjustment mechanisms, 301

Purchasing, 219–220, 364, 656

PWAs (persons with AIDS), 556

Q

Quackwatch.com, 140–141

Quality assurance, 653–654, 654–655

Quality measures, 422

Quality of care. *See also* Satisfaction of consumers
advancing agenda for, 472
aspects of service quality, 482
assessing, 420
Atlas system, 469–470
case examples, 512–515
consumer-driven definition of, 450–451
controversies over recommendations of, 437
definition/dimensions of, 444–450
FACCT's quality measures, 420–421, 422
factors needed for, 510
Healthwise approach, 538–539
indicators of, 243
lack of best care, 607–608
National Committee for Quality Assurance (NCQA), 424–425, 551
outpatient, 473
patient-assessed, 688
peer-based assessment of, 459–460
provider understanding of, 671
raising, through consumer-driven health care, 105–111
reductions in, 339–340
search for, 467–469
stars in, 443–451
strategies for improving, 119
study on, 454
variations in, 549–550

Quality of life, 622–624, 716
Questionnaires, 525–526, 622–623, 688–689

R

Race/ethnicity, of uninsured consumers, 735
Rack rates, 138
Radical innovations, 573
RAND Corporation, preventive care, 530, 552
Ratings. *See also* Measures
    by Buyers Health Care Action Group (BHCAG), 479
    Morningstar rating system, 6–7, 163–164
    patient satisfaction, 169, 424–425
    provider performance, 168
    user ratings information, 76
Rationing of health care, 129
Reagan administration, 817
Records. *See* Medical records
Redesigned benefit options, 220
Reductions in quality of care, 339–340
Referrals/referral services
    asthma management, 622
    Best Doctors, 136–137, 459–460
    CareCounsel, 496
    empowerment of PCPs for, 86
    HealthAllies, 137–138
    health care information services, 139–141
    leakage of referrals by PCPs, 30
Reforms
    European health care, 351–352
    Medicare, 282, 476
    policy analysis of health care, 743
    pricing, 80
    reasons for, 751–753
    in regulation of health care, 776
    regulatory, 817–818
    tax policy, 755–757
Refundable tax credits, 374
Regional power of health care services, 436–437
Registration of insurers, 803–804
Regulation of health care, 801. *See also*
    Government; Legal issues/legislation
    for consumer choice, 263
        effects of, on consumer's choices, 706
        laws with mandated benefits, 767

oversight programs for, 817
    problems of, 798
    proposed, 464, 811–812
    role of, 774–778
    South African MSA market, 336
Reimbursement systems, 117, 312, 378, 539, 615, 669. *See also* Flexible spending accounts (FSAs)
Relational coordination theory, 686–687, 690
Relationships
    among genetic factors, tracking, 710
    provider/patient, 447–448
    between providers and consumers, 584–585
    relational coordination, 686–687
Remedies for curing health insurance system, 75–77
Renal disease, KPSC Renal Care Management Program, 663–664
Renewal of insurance, terms of, 227–228
Report cards for quality of care, 450, 477, 479, 583
Research/studies/surveys
    Access Health Group (AH) programs, 504, 505, 506–507
    accountable health research, 606–607
    AmeriChoice strategies, 146
    Bank of America study, 527
    British health care experiences, 180–181
    charges of ordered tests, 676
    choices of health coverage, 29
    chronic condition care, 564–565
    computer use by doctors, 139–140
    consumer health care e-commerce, 434
    costs of diabetes treatment, 119–120
    declined coverage, reasons for, 753
    deductibles and spending, 102
    Diabetes Control and Complications Trial (DCCT), 120, 645–648
    doctor/patient relationships, 494–495
    doctors' volume of patients, 44
    elderly people with diabetes, care for, 105–106
    employees' confidence in employers' choices, 178–179
    Fidelity Investments study of DC plans, 18–19
    focus of care, 688–690
    Health of Seniors survey, 530

Research/studies/surveys *(continued)*
    health plan information, 167
    Healthtrac self–management program,
        526–528
    HMO medical directors, 565
    home visitation, 798
    hospitals belonging to systems, 653
    on human genomes, 710–711
    impact of consumer-based competi-
        tion, 59
    impact of health care market evolu-
        tion, 700–701
    importance of research to health,
        602–603
    Internet use/users, 429–430
    Kaiser Family Foundation/Harvard
        University Public Opinion Update
        survey, 491–492
    lifestyle changes for cardiac care,
        516–521
    MEDSTAT Group, 528
    misunderstandings of surgical guide-
        lines, 554
    Multicenter Lifestyle Demonstration
        Project, 517–519
    National Medical Care Expenditure
        Survey, 733
    on new technologies, 571
    obtaining health care by uninsured
        consumers, 739–740
    outcomes/mortality rates, 168–169
    performance disclosures, 182
    pharmaceuticals cost increases, 110
    physician accessibility, 431–432
    physician performance, 471
    posting of, on Internet (e-biomed), 607
    preventive care, 552
    productivity of U.S. health care
        system, 404–405
    PROPATH Parkinson's disease trial,
        527
    Public Employees Retirement System
        (PERS) study, 526–527
    quality of care, 454
    rates of cesarean sections, 186
    ratings of California hospitals, 113–114
    reduction of need/demand for medical
        services, 523–525
    social science predictions, 454–457
    success of cardiovascular surgeries,
        613–614

    technology adoption, 579–580
    telephone survey by Choice Plus,
        480–484
    2000 Health Confidence Survey,
        178–179
    uninsured consumers, 740–741, 742, 751
    use of Internet for health information, 16
    value attachment to quality compar-
        isons, 455–456
Resistance issues, 387, 388, 398, 539,
    624–625
Resources, 76–77, 496, 537–538, 784
Restrictions on medical care/information,
    817
Retirement Medical Benefit Accounts
    (RMBAs), 282
Retirement plans/planning, 17–18, 17–23,
    43, 216. *See also* Defined contributions
    (DC) plans; 401(k) plans
Revolutions/revolutionaries in health
    care, 142–143
    about, 128–129
    Best Doctors, 136–137
    Clancy, Dean, 148
    consumer revolution, automotive
        industry, 411–412
    consumer revolutions, health care,
        412–415
    entrepreneurs in insurance, 130–136
    HealthAllies, 137–138
    health care information services,
        139–141
    innovative services for the poor,
        135–136
    revolutionary mosaic, 129–130
    role of government in, 145–149
    strategies, 129
    technology revolutions, 141–145
Right care approach, 204–205, 210, 549
Rights of consumers, 346, 376–379,
    410–411
Risk adjustments, 170–175, 183, 185
    by Buyers Health Care Action Group
        (BHCAG), 315–316
    California Hospital Outcomes Project
        case study, 248–250
    Cleveland Health Quality Choice Pro-
        gram (CHQC) case study, 250–252
    criticisms of, 256–257
    demand for by consumers, 316
    in designing a tax credit, 757–758

determining risks, 243–246
Medicare case study, 252–256
need for data, 245–248
payments, 299–302
private sector in European health care, 347–351
reasons for, 256
risk-adjusted prices, 80–83, 94–95, 195
Switzerland system, 349
Risk corridors, 600
Risk factors
allocation of risk, 395
assessing risk profiles, 327
beta (risk measurement), 6–7
of capitated pricing model, 600
categories of risk, 95
to early adopters of consumer-driven model, 383
genetic variations as, 708–709
health risk assessments, 783–784
for insurers, 265
of investments, 6
potential, 242–243
reducing, 227–228
risk-stratified pricing, 591
of small employers, 735
targeting at-risk populations, 217
transference of risk to employees, 223
unsupported, 250
Risk-reward equation, 657
RMBAs (Retirement Medical Benefit Accounts), 282
Roadmapping, science, 606–607
Robert Wood Johnson Foundation, 480
Roles
consumers, 196
of economy as a whole, 382
employers', 195–196
of genes in disease initiation, 719
government, 145–149, 181–186, 196, 380–381, 388–389, 820–827
of information, 410–418, 440–442
medical technologies, 382
of organizational learning in adopting new technologies, 580
Ryan, George, 792–793

S
Safety, 116, 575–576
Safety nets, for uninsured consumers, 97–98, 754–755, 790

Salick, Bernard, 235
Satellite treatment centers, 598
Satisfaction of consumers, 57–58. *See also* Consumers/consumerism
assessment of care by patients, 688–689
with Best Doctors, 462
collection of information on, 479
dissatisfaction, 323, 369, 510–511
European, 322–323
with FEHB, 293
NCQA Member Satisfaction Survey, 305
patient ratings of, 169, 446–447
studies on, 473–474
ways of accomplishing, 447–448
Savings accounts, 156, 279–283. *See also* Medical savings accounts (MSAs)
Scare stories
Class Warfare story, 161–162
Disappearance of Health Insurance story, 159–160
Haunted House story, 154–156
Limited Access story, 162–163
Screw the Sick story, 157–159
Wrong Time and Wrong Place story, 156
SCHIP (State Children's Health Insurance Program), 759, 792
Science roadmapping, 606–607
Screw the Sick story, 157–159
Scruggs, Richard "Dickie," 43
SEC, health care, 797–804
Securities and Exchange Commission (SEC), 169, 184, 706, 801, 812–813, 817. *See also* Health care SEC model
Security, health security model, 318–321
Selective chaos, 36
Self-care, 58, 524, 534, 536–537
Self-directed care, 381, 382–383
Self-employed persons, uninsured, 37–38, 790
Self-funded health care costs, 77, 90, 283, 393
Self-insurance, 228–230, 230–231
Self-managed health care systems, 349, 525–526
Self-policing for quality, 472
Seniors. *See* Elderly
Sense-making theory, 686

Services. *See also* Referrals/referral
    services
    bundled, 46, 80
    CareCounsel's, 493–495
    competition among, 474
    consumer-driven versus managed
        competition, 95–96
    Consumer's Medical Resource (CMR),
        511–512
    corporate support, 660
    covered, 233
    e-health decision support, 221–222
    fee-for-service model, 224, 225–226,
        253, 376
    full-service providers, 115–116
    health care information, 139–141
    Healthtrac, Inc.'s products, 525–526
    home care, 598
    hospital, 741
    innovative, 135–136
    Interconsultation, 460
    Kaiser's, 661
    National Health Service (Britain), 354
    new coronary care, 656
    payers' discretion for, 377
    point-of-service (POS) option, 231
    production of, 112
    product line of Access Health Group
        (AH), 503–507
    quality of, 482
    referral, 463–464
    regional, 436–437
    research and development of new, 657
    restriction of, 567
    retirement planning, 21–23
    shared, 654–655
    Social Pedagogic Services (SPDs)
        (Netherlands), 326
    supportive, 791–792
    U.S. Centers for Medical and Medicare
        Services, 520
    value of traditional, 697
Sheltered savings accounts, 156
Shouldice Hospital, 627–632
Sickness fund systems (Europe), 345
Sick people
    coverage for, 33–37, 80
    focused factories for, 112–118
    ignoring the obvious for, 118–121
    reimbursement levels for, 591
    Screw the Sick story, 157–159

Silent revolution in health care, 128–130
Silent World of Doctor and Patient, The
    (Katz), 552–553
Single nucleotide polymorphisms (SNPs),
    710, 711, 720, 725
Single-payer health care systems
    (Europe), 343, 345
Site-focused care, 582
Skilled nursing facilities (SNFs), 652
"Skimming" profits, 115–116
Slavitt, Andy, 137–138, 141
Smith, Gregory White, 136–137, 141, 457
SNFs (skilled nursing facilities), 652
SNPs (single nucleotide polymorphisms),
    710, 711, 720, 725
Social capital theorists, 686
Social insurance-based health care system
    (Europe), 343–344
Social networks, 686
Social science research, 454–457
Societal impacts
    of care enhancement program,
        647–648
    Federal Employees Health Benefits
        Program (FEHB), 294
    quality-focused competition, 425
    of Shouldice Hospital approach,
        631–632
    Washington State Health Care
        Authority (HCA), 307
Socrates dialogues, 262–269
Solidarity, costs of European, 338–343
Solucient, 113, 821–822
Solutions
    administrative services only (ASO)
        funding, 592–593
    for fragmentation problem, 106
    impediments to, 818
    innovative, 388
    Internet-based, 220–222
    relying on consumers for, 417
South Africa, 93–94, 135–136, 231,
    330–336, 335–336
Specialized care
    for catastrophic illness, 596–597
    by insurers in insurance, 236–237
    Shouldice Hospital, 627–632
    site-focused care, 582
Specialized functions, non-medical,
    654–655
Specialty provider networks, 598

Spending, 225, 333. *See also* Expenses/
    expenditures
Sperling, Kenneth, 60
St. Croix Valley Healthcare, 88
St. Luke's Episcopal Hospital (Houston),
    614–615
Stakeholders, 306
Standardization of products, 364
Standardized data, 821–823
Standards of care measures, 643,
    646–647, 678–679
Star quality, 443–451
Start-up health care ventures, 90, 91
State Children's Health Insurance
    Program (SCHIP), 759, 792
State grants for tax credits, 758–759
State programs, risk–adjusting capitated
    payments, 255
Statistical medicine, 709
Statistics
    Blue Cross Blue Shield program costs,
        141–142
    costs of chronic conditions, 562–563
    insurance offered by small
        employers, 41
    job-based insurance coverage, 738
    measures of model performance, 256
    Medicaid coverage, 40
    percentage of uninsured consumers,
        38–39
    price of premiums, 49–50
    reasons for no insurance, 750–751
    three disease states, 718
    uninsured who work, 41
Status quo naysayers, 175–179
Strategies
    competitive provider, 219
    designing risk adjustment, 256–257
    FACCT, 427
    improving quality of care, 119
    increasing learning potential in new
        technology adoption, 577
    revolutionary, 129
    tax credits, 749–750 (*See also under*
        Tax issues)
    turning employees into consumers,
        215–220
Stress effects of health danger, 455
Studies. *See* Research/studies/surveys
Subimo, 218–219, 220
Subsidies for plans, 76–77, 348–349, 760

Success factors for consumer-driven
    plans, 91, 391–393
Supplemental insurance, 462
Suppliers of pension funds, 19–21
Support, 447–448, 713–714, 824–825
Surgeries
    access to cardiac surgery for women,
        517
    coronary artery bypass graft (CABG)
        surgery, 244, 247
    hernia repair, 627–632
    hysterectomies, 640–641
    inappropriate, 551, 556
    Lasik, 219–220
    minimally invasive cardiac surgery,
        572–576
    misunderstandings of surgical guide-
        lines, 554
    open heart surgery, 142–143
    patient rights to know surgical proce-
        dures, 552–553
    plastic surgery market, 819
    prostatectomies, 675
    success of cardiovascular, 613–614
Surveys. *See* Research/studies/surveys
Switzerland, 89, 327–328, 348–350
Symptom-based medicine, 709–710
System of coverage in America, 732–733.
    See also Health care systems

T
T. Rowe Price, 20
"Take Care of Yourself," 524, 525
Tax issues. *See also* Legal issues/
    legislation
    adverse consequences to changing
        health plans, 388
    cafeteria (flexible benefit) plans, 286
    credits/personal care accounts, 387
    defined contributions (DC) plans
        administrative implications of, 273
        application of, 270–271
        implementation of, 271–273
        other relevant rulings, 273–275
        summary of, 275–277
    federal tax laws, 238, 262
    free-rider tax, 760
    health care exclusion, 766
    HRAs, 282–283
    incentives for universal health care,
        790–791

Tax issues *(continued)*
   income tax laws (2002), 18
   IRS
      eligible medical expenses (section
        213), 287
      health benefits policy by, 755
      insurance rulings by, 732–733
      1943 tax ruling, 766
      section 125, 271–272, 285, 286
   Medicaid/Medicare, 820–821
   medical savings accounts (MSAs), 231,
      279, 281–283, 288–289
   mixing/matching accounts, 280–281
   pretax contributions, 18, 84–85
   raising, as funding option, 39
   sheltered savings accounts, 156
   state-level, 238–239
   tax credits, 794–795
      additional measures for, 759–760
      background of plan, 749–750
      designing, 757–758
      policy reforms, 755–757
      refundable, 374
      state grants, 758–759
      success of, 761
Teaching hospitals, 669–679, 699–702,
   738
Technical complexity of plans, 306
Technocratic naysayers, 185
   government-controlled, universal
      health care naysayers, 179–181
   information sources, 163–170
   risk adjustment, 170–175
   status quo naysayers, 175–179
Technologies
   adoption of new, 576–579
   for chronic disease management, 208
   data gathering, 324–325
   diabetes management, 120–121
   differences in costs through, 315
   effects of new, 701
   emerging, 208–209, 714–715
   genomic, 710–711
   impact of new, 570–571
   implications of new, 580–584
   IT (information technology), 659
   medical technology manufacturers, 441
   minimally invasive cardiac surgery,
      572–576
   role of medical, 382
   spread of innovative, 579–580

Technology revolutions, 141–145
Telephone counseling, 494
Terms of policies, 75
   entry into insurance plan, 226–227
   exiting plans, 233–234
   renewal of plan, 227–228
   Swiss health insurance system, 89
Tertiary care facilities, 597–598, 599
Testing for HIV, 665
Texas Heart Institute, 142–143,
   612–618
Thawing of charitable assets, 826–827
Theories, 78–79, 686–687
Therapeutics, 717, 722–723
Third-party administrators (TPAs), 77–78,
   83, 86, 228–230, 393
Third-party payers, 377, 397–398, 721
Third Wave, The (Toffler), 413–414
Thought worlds, 686
Time of need networks, 90
Tools, 433, 535, 654–655
Total health care management, 644
Trade publications, 91
Training, 213, 567, 576–579. *See also*
   Education
Transfer pricing, rise and fall of, 171–174
Transition to consumer-driven health
   care, 371–372
Treasury Department, 282–283
Treatment, 119–120, 395–396
   cancer, 597–598, 600, 640
   costs, 371, 596
   experimental, 599
   per-member per-month (PMPM) basis
      for, 600
   satellite treatment centers, 598
   undertreated populations, 106
Trends
   401(k) plans, 285
   health benefits, 285
   job-based insurance coverage, 738
   in patient empowerment, 431–432
   reversal of current, 377
   role of information, 410–418
   suppliers' reactions to, 409
Trials. *See* Research/studies/surveys
Triangle of consumer-driven health care,
   365–366
Trust issues, 468–469, 477, 510
Turf warfare, 116–118
Twin Cities Metro Area, 311, 800

U

UM (utilization management), 506–507, 671–672

Uncompensated care, 739

Underserved populations, 685, 783

Understanding Variation: The Key to Managing Chaos (Wheeler), 557

Undertreated populations, 106

Unemployed consumers, tax credits for, 756

Uninsured consumers, 34–35, 699–700. *See also* Consumers/consumerism; Patients; Tax credits under tax issues
  care by academic medical centers of, 738
  consumer-choice model for, 794–795
  defined contribution plans for, 780
  demographics of, 736
  employer size, 734–735
  employment status of, 733–734
  endangered health of, 739–742
  health care providers for, 738–739
  income of, 734
  percentage of, 38–39
  race/ethnicity of, 735
  reasons for growing numbers of, 737–738
  reducing number of, 775–776
  safety nets for, 97–98
  self-employed, 37–38
  system of coverage in America, 732–733
  and universal health coverage, 789–791
  voluntary versus involuntary, 736–737

Uninsured medical events, 31

Union Carbide, 86–87, 94

Union issues, Internal Revenue Code ruling, 272–273

United Health Group, 781

United Kingdom, 323, 328, 345, 354

United States
  economic issues, 403, 731
  expenditures on health care in, 404, 660, 821
  financial system of, 7–10
  need for consumer-driven health care system in, 816–819
  PCPs in South Africa compared to, 332
  rights (consumers'), 410–411
  statistics on illness in, 523

Universal health care systems
  access issues of, 180–181
  achieving, in America, 742–746
  British, 180
  naysayers, 179–181
  uninsured consumers and, 789–791
  in United States, 761

URAC (American Accreditation Health Care Commission), 141

Urological disorders, 675

U.S. Centers for Medical and Medicare Services, 520

U.S. Chamber of Commerce, 21

U.S. Department of Commerce, 430

U.S. Healthcare, 158

U.S. Office of Personnel Management (OPM), 292

U.S. Securities and Exchange Commission (SEC). *See* Securities and Exchange Commission (SEC)

U.S. Treasury Department, 276

Used car example, 477–478

Use-it-or-lose-it aspect of FSAs, 287–288, 771

User ratings information, 76

Uterine disease, 640–641

Utilization management (UM), 506–507, 671–672

V

Vaccinations. *See* Immunization/vaccinations

Vanderbilt Medical Center, 669–679

Vanguard Group, 5–6, 20, 155

Venture capital firms, 91

Vertical integration of care, 107, 172–173, 652, 657. *See also* Horizontal integration of care; Integration of care

Viagra, 331–332

Visions of consumer-driven health care, 385–387

Vivius Personalized Healthcare System (PHS), 89, 134

Voluntary versus involuntary uninsured consumers, 736–737

Voucher systems, 266–267, 275–276, 398, 780

W

Wages, definition of, 272–273

Waiting times, 37

Washington state, 186
    payment of plan premiums, 302–305
    Washington State Health Care
        Authority (HCA)
        barriers to diffusion of, 305–306
        changes in consumer reporting of,
            304
        consumer assessment of health
            plans, 302–305
        health-based premium payments,
            299–302
        overviews of approaches of,
            298–299, 303–304
        societal impacts, 307
Watson Wyatt Worldwide, 8–9
Web. *See* Internet
WellMed, 219
Wellness/loyalty programs, 335–336, 436
Wellness programs, 85–86, 206
WellPoint plan, 84–85, 93–94, 318, 319–320
Welters, Tony, 145–149

Western health care, 508
White Paper on plan risk management, 79
WHO (World Health Organization), 363,
    366
WIZ Order system, 671, 675–677
Women
    access to cardiac surgery for, 517
    benign uterine disease, 640–641
    cancer of reproductive tract, 639–640
    feminist movement, 444, 556
    focused factories for women's health,
        638–639
Working uninsured, 41, 790–791
Workplace Pulse Survey, 287
World Health Organization (WHO), 363,
    366
Writing of orders, 676–677
Wrong Time and Wrong Place story, 156

X
Xerox, 155